Advances in Synthetic Healthcare Data:

Opportunities, Challenges, and Emerging Trends

Munir Ahmad
https://orcid.org/0000-0003-4836-6151
Survey of Pakistan, Pakistan

IGI Global
Scientific Publishing
Publishing Tomorrow's Research Today

Vice President of Editorial	Melissa Wagner
Director of Acquisitions	Mikaela Felty
Director of Book Development	Jocelynn Hessler
Production Manager	Mike Brehm
Cover Design	Jose Rosado

Published in the United States of America by
IGI Global Scientific Publishing
701 East Chocolate Avenue
Hershey, PA, 17033, USA
Tel: 717-533-8845 | Fax: 717-533-7115
Website: https://www.igi-global.com E-mail: cust@igi-global.com

Library of Congress Cataloging-in-Publication Data

LCCN: 2025036239 (CIP Data Pending)
ISBN13: 9798337356419
Isbn13Softcover: 9798337356426
EISBN13: 9798337356433

British Cataloguing in Publication Data
A Cataloguing in Publication record for this book is available from the British Library.

Table of Contents

Detailed Table of Contents

Barno Matchanova, Urgench State Pedagogical Institute, Uzbekistan
Nilufar Niyazova, Mamun University, Uzbekistan
Latofat Salayeva, Urgench State University, Uzbekistan
Munir Ahmad, Survey of Pakistan, Pakistan
Muzaffar Shojonov, Urgench State University, Uzbekistan

Synthetic genomic and omics datasets, encompassing genomics, transcriptomics, proteomics, and metabolomics, enable researchers to replicate the complex biological variability of real-world data while safeguarding sensitive patient information. Leveraging advanced generative models such as Generative Adversarial Networks (GANs), Variational Autoencoders (VAEs), and diffusion-based frameworks, scientists can now create realistic artificial datasets suitable for algorithm training, model validation, and cross-institutional collaboration. This chapter explores the principles, methodologies, and applications of synthetic genomic and omic data, emphasizing their transformative role in personalized medicine, drug discovery, and clinical trial simulation. It also discusses ethical, technical, and regulatory challenges, proposing future research directions toward multi-omics integration, privacy-preserving architectures, and global data-sharing frameworks.

Shaikat Das Joy, American International University-Bangladesh, Bangladesh
Noboranjan Dey, American International University-Bangladesh, Bangladesh
Md. Reazul Islam, University at Albany, State University of New York, USA
Mirza Asif Mahmud, American International University-Bangladesh, Bangladesh
Mahfujur Rahman, American International University-Bangladesh, Bangladesh
Kazi Tanvir, American International University-Bangladesh, Bangladesh
Dipta Gomes, American International University-Bangladesh, Bangladesh

Synthetic healthcare data offers a transformative solution to the privacy and accessibility constraints of real patient data. This chapter comprehensively examines its generation, from traditional statistical methods to advanced AI like GANs, VAEs, and Transformers. It explores critical applications in clinical trial simulation, medical imaging, and AI training. The analysis extends beyond technology to address pivotal barriers: ethical concerns of bias, evolving GDPR/HIPAA regulations, validation challenges, and interoperability with systems like HL7 FHIR. It concludes that responsible adoption hinges on merging technical rigor with ethical governance and cross-disciplinary collaboration to build trustworthy, innovative digital health ecosystems.

This chapter digs into the methods for creating synthetic health records using generative artificial intelligence (AI) approaches, stressing its critical role in improving healthcare research while protecting patient privacy. Synthetic health data are intentionally manufactured datasets that closely resemble real-world electronic health records but do not include actual patient information, allowing for safe data exchange and analysis. The chapter examines popular generative AI techniques such as generative adversarial networks and variational autoencoders, demonstrating how these models capture complicated statistical characteristics and correlations in healthcare data. It examines the use of synthetic EHRs in medical AI research, clinical simulations, and software testing. Furthermore, the chapter discusses data quality issues, ethical concerns, and balancing privacy and usefulness. Overall, generative AI is a transformational tool for overcoming data accessibility hurdles and encouraging innovation in health informatics.

Diabetic retinopathy (DR) is a serious eye condition linked to diabetes, resulting from high blood sugar levels. It can cause varying degrees of vision impairment, potentially leading to blindness. Early symptoms include blurred vision, changes in color vision, and dark spots. Detecting DR early is crucial to preventing vision loss, as it typically appears as small red spots on the retina from hemorrhages or

Synthetic data is rapidly emerging as a transformative enabler of artificial intelligence in healthcare, addressing long-standing challenges of privacy, accessibility, and data scarcity. By generating realistic yet non-identifiable datasets, it supports innovation in clinical research, diagnostics, precision medicine, and public health planning. Emerging trends, including hybrid real-synthetic models, federated learning, and cross-border collaborations, highlight its growing role in building scalable and equitable AI systems. To maximize impact, policymakers must establish clear regulations. Institutions should integrate synthetic data into their digital health strategies, and developers must ensure transparency and fairness. As adoption expands, synthetic data remains a cornerstone of ethical and sustainable AI-driven healthcare services.

Multiple sclerosis, Parkinson's disease, and Alzheimer's disease are difficult to manage because there are no accurate treatments available and they worsen over time. It is very important to identify these illnesses early and observe their progression over time. Traditional methods for diagnosing these diseases usually rely on the subjective evaluation of medical professionals and different symptoms that emerge later. Recently, AI, particularly machine learning (ML) and deep learning (DL), are developing into a powerful tool for to treat these illnesses. This paper looks at how AI can be used to study different types of brain scans, such as MRI, PET, and EEG. By combining these types of data, AI can help doctors make more accurate diagnoses of brain-related diseases. This chapter highlights how important it is to keep working on testing, improving, and using these technologies in the right way so they can have the best possible impact in real medical practice.

The role of machine learning is no longer limited to the field of computation. Machine learning has a huge potential in every possible field. The field of medicine is not an exception. Machine learning can be used to predict if a person is affected by COVID-19 or not as well as predict the number of cases of COVID-19 on a given day. The existing solutions give the result based on a particular machine learning model and other statistical models. This has many disadvantages, as the single machine learning model chosen, say for example logistic regression, to predict if a person is affected by the disease or not and to predict the number of cases may or may not give accurate results. This is where the importance of our solution comes in. Here the proposed solution is a hybrid model, which is the combination of machine learning models such as Naive Bayesian, logistic regression, random forest, etc. The results demonstrate that hybrid ML models can provide reliable and scalable tools for aiding clinical decision-making and public health policy.

Diabetic Retinopathy (DR) is a diabetes complication that affects the eyes and damaged blood vessels in the retina which can lead to vision loss and even blindness. Machine learning algorithms for DR detection have some limitations, such as lagging in feature extraction and selection. Data are taken from the Diabetic retinopathy detection dataset, which is available at www.kaggle.com for training and evaluate the model. Deep Learning methods, such as Diabetic Retinopathy Network 13 (DRNet13), a CNN-based architecture model performed exceptionally well, attaining the best result. But not concentrate on retinal images that have mild DR-related abnormalities may be less resilient to minor alterations in the appearance of the lesion or differences in image quality. In proposed technique combining the novel DRNet13 architecture with an attention mechanism to enhance diagnostic performance. Proposed technique outperform the existing methods,

S. Srinivasan, Department of Humanities and Social Sciences, Graphic Era University, Dehradun, India
R. Vallipriya, Department of Biochemistry & Biotechnology, Tamil Nadu Teacher Education University, Bharathidasan University, Trichy, India

In India, most tuberculosis (TB) patients initially seek treatment in the private sector before transitioning to the public sector. This study analyzes four years of state-wise, district-wise, and TU-wise TB notification data from Tamil Nadu, particularly Trichy District, using the Ni-kshay portal. The data reveals an improved trend in TB notifications from both sectors. TB is a notifiable disease, and the study emphasizes establishing a robust surveillance system to ensure treatment adherence in private facilities. Despite improvements, collecting TB notifications from the private sector remains challenging, highlighting the need to accelerate and expand notification efforts. Increasing active case identification at the state level is essential to improve TB notification and ensure adherence to standard treatment practices. Data management in digital reporting—particularly within the private sector—faces challenges due to EHR and Ni-kshay system upgrades and associated complications.

M. Kamaladevi, SASTRA University, India
V. Venkataraman, SASTRA University, India
S. Meganathan, SASTRA University, India
P. Umamaheswari, SASTRA University, India

Diabetes is a chronic medical condition characterized by elevated blood sugar levels, resulting from insufficient insulin production or ineffective use of insulin by the body. Predicting diabetes at early stage save human life. To improve the prediction, feature weighting algorithm and Hyperparameters tuned Boosting algorithm are used. In proposed work dataset are taken from Kaggle link (https://www.kaggle.com) and it is imbalanced in nature. To balanced data SMOTE algorithm is applied. Select the more relevant feature through feature weighting method and tune the hyperparameter like learning rate, number of estimators, and tree depth, influencing the ensemble's performance of Boosting algorithms like a AdaBoost, Gradient Boosting (GBM), XGBoost, LightGBM and CatBoost provides higher accuracy when compare with state of art machine learning algorithm. Among these methods hyperparameter tuned CatBoost algorithm shows 81% accuracy, ROC_AUC score is 0.84, Recall score of 0.8 which will be higher than the general boosting algorithm.

A. Sumathi, Department of CSE, SRC, SASTRA University, India
P. Umamaheswari, SASTRA University, India
M. Kamaladevi, SASTRA University, India

Gestational Diabetes Mellitus (GDM) is a form of diabetes that arises during pregnancy in women with no prior history of the condition. It is caused by the body's inability to produce sufficient insulin to meet the increased metabolic demands of pregnancy. If left undetected or poorly managed, GDM can lead to serious health complications, including high maternal blood glucose, increased risk of cesarean delivery, neonatal hypoglycemia, and long-term susceptibility to obesity and type 2 diabetes for both mother and child. Early and accurate prediction of GDM is therefore essential for timely intervention and improved maternal-fetal outcomes. A pipeline-based predictive model is proposed, integrating Principal Component Analysis (PCA) for dimensionality reduction with a Random Forest classifier for robust prediction. The use of synthetic healthcare data enables the development and testing of the model in a controlled environment, enhancing reproducibility and scalability and its integration into clinical decision support systems for personalized prenatal care.

Rajeswari Jayaraman, Sri Sivasubramaniya Nadar College of Engineering, India
J. Raja, Adhiparasakthi Engineering College, India
N. Ramya, Sri Sairam Engineering College, India

A major challenge in medical data analytics is identifying critical regions for segmentation and efficient feature extraction. Discontinuous regions of interest lead to uncertainty in results. This is addressed by applying Contrast-CNN for pixel-level fine shaping, which incorporates Contrast Limited Adaptive Histogram Equalization (CLAHE) in each critical region. CLAHE enhances image texture and resolves discontinuity. Once regions are identified, transfer learning is used to emphasize and extract features from affected lung images. A lung mask shape model is trained using various transformations—scaling, rotation, and lateral shifts—on normal and tuberculosis images. A Fusion-based CNN architecture is proposed to extract features for classification, combining VGG19's pixel-wise comparison strengths with ResidualNet's learning ability. The final predictions are processed through a fully connected layer to classify images as either normal or tuberculosis. This model offers a state-of-the-art solution for TB-affected lung image classification.

Gestational Diabetes is one of the major growing metabolic syndromes that affects pregnant mothers and their growing Infants worldwide. Traditional monitoring methods often require regular visits and keeping manual records up-to-date, and they have some short-term fluctuations, reduce timely intervention, and place an extra burden on patients for accurate logging and recall. Sustainable environment monitoring systems leverage wearable biosensors, continuous glucose monitors, cloud-based electronic health records, and AI-driven analytics to provide constant, real-time, and personalized monitoring. The sustainable monitoring system provides continuous, real-time tracking of health care data in GDM, also helps in providing personalized care, promotes early identification of risks, and reduces manual effort by improving patient engagement and outcomes. This Chapter explores how advanced technology with monitoring systems can be Integrated into maternal systems can be Integrated into maternal routine care.

Steganography, the practice of hiding information within non-secret data, appears to be a promising method for safeguarding sensitive medical information buried in diagnostic images. Steganographic techniques can be used in medical imaging to hide patient metadata, diagnostic notes, and digital watermarks in image files such as DICOM, X-ray, MRI, and CT scans. This allows for secure and seamless transmission across healthcare networks. A combination of encryption and steganography is proposed for secure transmission. First, the message is scrambled using Alpha Numeric Scrambling (ANS) Sequence technique and then encrypted. Then the encrypted text is embedded in an image cover medium using the Two-bit LSB technique and transferred to the receiver. The performance of the proposed algorithm is evaluated in terms of entropy, peak signal to noise ratio and mean square error.

When damaged kidneys are unable to filter blood effectively, waste and fluid buildup result. This is known as renal disease. It can be acute or chronic and is frequently associated with excessive blood pressure and diabetes. Because CT scans are more accurate than ultrasound, they are crucial for detecting anomalies such tumors, stones, cysts, and structural alterations. In order to create a strong diagnostic framework, this research will use deep learning and image processing techniques to identify key signs and a generative AI model to recommend treatments.

Preface

INTRODUCTION

It is my great pleasure to introduce *Advances in Synthetic Healthcare Data: Opportunities, Challenges, and Emerging Trends*. This edited volume brings together leading voices across disciplines to examine one of the most dynamic and consequential developments in modern healthcare: the emergence of high-fidelity synthetic data as a catalyst for innovation, collaboration, and responsible AI deployment.

The chapters collected here explore the opportunities and tensions inherent in a field defined by rapid technological progress and complex societal needs. As we confront persistent challenges around accessing, sharing, and safeguarding real-world healthcare data, synthetic data has emerged as a compelling alternative—one that preserves the statistical richness of clinical information while mitigating privacy risks and regulatory burdens. Yet its adoption raises new questions about validity, bias, governance, and trustworthiness. This book seeks to navigate these intersecting issues with clarity, critical perspective, and practical insight.

Drawing from the rich discussions and contributions of our authors, this volume offers a comprehensive survey of state-of-the-art synthetic data generation techniques, with a particular focus on AI-enabled models that now define the cutting edge of the field. Readers will find balanced examinations of current applications, from clinical research and digital health to population studies and public policy, alongside thoughtful analyses of ethical considerations and emerging regulatory frameworks. Throughout, the chapters highlight both the promise and the limitations of synthetic data, emphasizing the importance of rigorous evaluation, transparent methodologies, and interdisciplinary collaboration.

Our aim in assembling this book has been to provide a foundational resource for those seeking to understand how synthetic healthcare data can help address critical challenges—ensuring privacy, enhancing reproducibility, and expanding equitable access to high-quality datasets. By capturing best practices, open questions, and illustrative success stories, we hope to support the development of trustworthy data infrastructures that will shape the next generation of AI tools, clinical trials, and collaborative research networks.

This volume is intentionally crafted for a broad audience. Researchers and students in data science, biomedical informatics, artificial intelligence, and public health will find essential guidance as they explore new avenues for data-driven discovery. Clinicians, hospital IT professionals, and medical researchers will gain practical insights into integrating synthetic data into clinical and operational settings. Policymakers and regulators will encounter timely discussions on ethics, privacy, and governance. Innovators in digital health and emerging startups will discover technical and strategic perspectives critical to responsible product development.

I extend my sincere gratitude to the contributors, reviewers, and collaborators whose expertise and dedication made this book possible. It is my hope that this volume not only informs but inspires—encouraging readers to engage deeply with the opportunities and responsibilities that accompany synthetic healthcare data, and to help shape a future where data-driven innovation advances health for all.

ORGANIZATION OF THE BOOK

Chapter 1 introduces a deep learning–based system designed to advance early lung cancer diagnosis and personalized treatment planning. By integrating Convolutional Neural Networks with generative AI, the authors demonstrate how modern imaging analytics can elevate diagnostic accuracy and support more informed clinical decision-making. Their work highlights an urgent global health challenge and presents an AI-driven framework poised to enhance survival outcomes through earlier, more precise detection.

Chapter 2 explores the rapidly expanding domain of synthetic genomic and multi-omics data, emphasizing its critical role in precision medicine and biomedical discovery. Leveraging advanced generative models—including GANs, VAEs, and diffusion architectures—the chapter illustrates how synthetic omics datasets can replicate complex biological variability while preserving privacy. The authors thoughtfully examine methodological advances, research applications, and the ethical and regulatory pathways needed to support global-scale data sharing and multi-omics integration.

Chapter 3 offers a comprehensive examination of synthetic healthcare data generation, validation, and integration, presenting it as a foundational enabler for ethical and scalable digital health innovation. The chapter spans traditional statistical techniques to state-of-the-art generative AI, illustrating synthetic data's benefits across clinical simulation, imaging, and AI model development. Importantly, the authors contextualize these technologies within the realities of privacy regulations, interoperability standards, and the need for trustworthy governance frameworks.

Chapter 4 provides a focused analysis of generative AI methodologies for producing synthetic electronic health records, detailing how models such as GANs and VAEs capture the high-dimensional complexity of clinical data. The chapter underscores synthetic EHRs as essential resources for AI research, system testing, and clinical simulation, while also interrogating questions of data quality, ethical use, and the balance between realism and privacy. The authors position generative AI as a transformative lever for accelerating safe and responsible health informatics innovation.

Chapter 5 addresses the growing burden of diabetic retinopathy, presenting a deep learning–based approach for early detection through retinal imaging. The authors demonstrate how CNNs can efficiently extract features indicative of retinal damage without extensive annotation, enabling timely intervention and improved screening accuracy. Their contribution highlights the continuing power of computer vision methods to augment clinical workflows in chronic disease management.

Chapter 6 synthesizes emerging advances in AI-driven synthetic health data generation, comparing diverse generative frameworks—from GANs and VAEs to diffusion models and transformers. Through a rigorous assessment of fidelity, utility, and privacy, the chapter reveals both the strengths and limitations of each paradigm and outlines promising research directions in multimodal patient representation. The authors make a compelling case for synthetic data as a cornerstone of future-ready healthcare AI.

Chapter 7 examines synthetic data as a transformative catalyst for modern health services, particularly in enabling ethical, scalable AI solutions. The chapter situates synthetic datasets within broader trends, such as federated learning and hybrid real-synthetic modeling, underscoring their importance for global health equity. The authors also articulate the policy, institutional, and technical commitments required to ensure transparency, fairness, and effective adoption across healthcare ecosystems.

Chapter 8 explores the promise of AI-driven early diagnosis and risk prediction for neurodegenerative diseases, where traditional assessment methods often fail to detect early symptoms. By integrating machine learning and deep learning across multimodal imaging—MRI, PET, and EEG—the authors present a pathway for improving diagnostic accuracy and disease monitoring. The chapter underscores the value of continued research, validation, and integration to bring these emerging tools meaningfully into clinical practice.

Chapter 9 presents a novel stacking-based machine learning framework for COVID-19 prediction, illustrating the advantages of hybrid models over single-model approaches. By combining algorithms such as Naive Bayes, logistic regression, and random forests, the authors provide a more robust diagnostic and forecasting tool suited to real-world public health demands. Their findings emphasize the importance of model diversification for improving reliability in pandemic response.

Chapter 10 advances the field of diabetic retinopathy detection with a novel fusion of DRNet13 and attention mechanisms, resulting in improved resilience to subtle abnormalities and variations in image quality. The chapter demonstrates how targeted architectural enhancements can address longstanding limitations in feature extraction and early-stage lesion identification, offering a pathway toward more accurate and sensitive DR screening systems.

Chapter 11 provides a detailed evaluation of tuberculosis surveillance in India, focusing on the integration of EHR systems with the national Ni-kshay platform. Drawing on multi-year datasets from Tamil Nadu, the authors highlight improvements in disease notification while identifying persistent gaps in private-sector reporting and digital system adoption. The chapter reinforces the need for stronger surveillance, streamlined reporting workflows, and robust cross-sector coordination in TB control.

Chapter 12 explores enhanced diabetes prediction through feature weighting and hyperparameter-tuned boosting algorithms. By balancing an imbalanced dataset using SMOTE and systematically optimizing key model parameters, the authors demonstrate significant performance gains—particularly with CatBoost. Their work illustrates how methodological rigor in feature selection and model tuning can yield more accurate and clinically actionable predictive tools.

Chapter 13 introduces a pipeline-based prediction model for gestational diabetes mellitus using synthetic healthcare data, integrating PCA-based dimensionality reduction with Random Forest classification. The authors illustrate how synthetic data facilitates safe experimentation, reproducibility, and scalability, highlighting the model's potential role in clinical decision support for personalized prenatal care and early intervention.

Chapter 14 presents a streamlined fusion-driven CNN architecture for tuberculosis segmentation and classification, addressing challenges posed by discontinuous regions of interest in chest imaging. By incorporating CLAHE-enhanced preprocessing, transfer learning, and a hybrid CNN model combining VGG19 and ResidualNet, the authors offer an advanced solution for improving TB detection accuracy and robustness.

Chapter 15 examines sustainable, technology-enabled monitoring systems for high-risk pregnancies affected by gestational diabetes. By leveraging wearable biosensors, continuous glucose monitoring, cloud-based EHRs, and AI analytics, the chapter outlines a vision for real-time, patient-centered care that reduces burdens on expectant mothers while enhancing safety, early risk identification, and overall maternal health outcomes.

Chapter 16 explores secure medical data transmission through a combined Alpha-Numeric Scrambling (ANS) and steganography framework. The authors demonstrate how embedding encrypted patient information within medical images can strengthen confidentiality in digital health networks, evaluating their approach across entropy, PSNR, and MSE metrics. This chapter highlights the expanding role of advanced cryptographic techniques in safeguarding healthcare data.

Chapter 17 concludes the volume with an AI-based system for detecting and planning treatment for kidney disease using CT imaging. By integrating deep learning for diagnostic analysis with generative AI for treatment recommendation, the authors present a comprehensive framework for improving renal disease management. Their contribution exemplifies the convergence of imaging analytics and AI-driven clinical decision support.

CONCLUSION

As we bring this volume to a close, it is clear that the field of synthetic healthcare data—and the broader ecosystem of AI-driven innovation in medicine—is undergoing a profound and defining transformation. The chapters collected here illustrate not only the remarkable technical progress made across imaging, genomics, clinical prediction, and secure data exchange, but also the urgency with which we must approach the ethical, regulatory, and human dimensions of this work. Throughout the volume, our contributors underscore a consistent message: synthetic data and intelligent systems are not merely computational tools, but foundational elements of a future in which healthcare is more equitable, more precise, and more responsive to the needs of patients and practitioners alike.

Taken together, these contributions illuminate a landscape rich with possibility. They demonstrate how synthetic datasets can accelerate discovery, enhance clinical decision-making, and unlock the potential of AI in settings constrained by privacy, data scarcity, or fragmented infrastructure. They also reinforce that responsible innovation demands thoughtful validation, transparency, interdisciplinary collaboration, and robust governance frameworks that safeguard trust while enabling progress. As editor, I am inspired by the ways in which each chapter pushes the boundaries of what is possible, while remaining grounded in the realities and responsibilities of healthcare practice.

It is my hope that this volume serves not only as a reference, but as a catalyst—encouraging researchers, clinicians, technologists, and policymakers to engage with these emerging tools in intentional and imaginative ways. The future of healthcare will be shaped by our ability to harness synthetic data and AI with rigor, empathy, and foresight. May the insights shared here guide that journey and inspire the next generation of innovations that will advance health and well-being for communities around the world.

Chapter 1
Design and Development of a Deep Learning-Based System for Lung Cancer Diagnosis and Automated Treatment Suggestion

Varsha Vyankatesh Manglaram
Walchand Institute of Technology, Solapur, India

L. M. R. J. Lobo
https://orcid.org/0000-0002-8572-2082
Walchand Institute of Technology, Solapur, India

Vijay Athavale
https://orcid.org/0000-0002-6812-5198
Walchand Institute of Technology, Solapur, India

Shubham Vyavahare
https://orcid.org/0009-0009-4451-6635
Walchand Institute of Technology, Solapur, India

Rajani Yemul
https://orcid.org/0009-0000-3712-5518
Walchand Institute of Technology, Solapur, India

DOI: 10.4018/979-8-3373-5641-9.ch001

ABSTRACT

Lung cancer is a worldwide healthcare issue and is responsible for almost one in five cancer deaths. Early identification and personalized treatment are key to improving survival rates, but traditional diagnosing is often slow, very fallible, and not easily scalable. Lung cancer occurs when there is unrestrained growth of cancerous cells within the lung, and eventually results in death. Lung cancer symptoms include, but are not limited to, chest pain, shortness of breath, a persistent cough, and unexplained weight loss. The proposed system utilizes deep learning models, utilizing Convolutional Neural Networks (CNN's) which allows for a robust mechanism to classify CT scan images as normal, benign, or malignant. Following a diagnosis, a Transformer-based Generative AI module suggests appropriate treatments, such as chemotherapy or immunotherapy, depending on the patient's health. This study outlines an intelligent diagnostic system that uses generative artificial intelligence (AI) and convolutional neural networks (CNNs) to detect lung cancer and prescribe a customized course of treatment. With the use of medical imaging technologies and Generative AI predictive modeling, the system is intended to help healthcare providers make data driven choices that may result in better patient outcomes and lower death rates.

1. INTRODUCTION

Lung cancer is a disease that starts in the lungs, which are part of the respiratory system and allow us to breathe. The disease state starts when lung cells grow uncontrollably to form the tumor in the lung and potentially start to spread (called metastasis) to other parts of the body. Normally lung cells grow in a regulated way as the body needs them, for example replacing damaged cells in the lungs.

Lung cancer remains one of the most lethal cancers globally, and lung cancer is most commonly diagnosed at an advanced stage where the options for treatment are limited. Although new imaging techniques (such as CT scans and biopsies) are more accurate, standard diagnostic tests are frequently too expensive, take too long, and are often subject to human interpretation. This is an area where the development of intelligent, automated, and scalable diagnostic systems is timely to help clinicians with their timely, accurate decisions.

Recent developments in deep learning - in particular convolutional neural networks (CNNs) for image classification, and U-Net for medical image segmentation provide a significant opportunity to improve the accuracy of cancer detection. At the same time, the rise of generative artificial intelligence (AI) can provide a method to customize not only early detection, but ultimately treatment recommendations based on unique patient characteristics. Coupling these technologies could support moving dispensable the time between early detection and personalized treatment planning, which could have the potential to increase survival rates and lower the global burden of lung cancer as a whole.

The goal of this research is to design an AI-based diagnostic and treatment recommendation service that can classify lung CT scans into normal, benign or malignant with a high level of accuracy while also utilizing generative AI to provide recommendations for treatment modalities including, chemotherapy, immunotherapy and surgeries. By bringing together diagnostic imaging and generative decision support into a single system, the proposed platform seeks to simplify clinical workflows and provide data-driven, patient-centered care.

This research will address the following research questions:

1. How accurately can deep learning models (CNN and U-Net) detect and classify lung cancer from CT scan images in comparison to currently existing methods of diagnosis?
2. Can using generative AI help to improve the personalized treatment recommendations developed after diagnosis?
3. What would be the possibilities of setting up this system online to support healthcare professionals and patients with real-time decision making?

The answers to these questions will contribute to discourse in the emerging area of AI-assisted healthcare and demonstrate the ways in which intelligent systems can support decision making for early detection of lung cancer and the planning of treatment.

Over the past two decades, cancer research has progressed remarkably, especially in our understanding of the complex biology that allows tumorigenesis to occur. In 2022, Hanahan provided depth and dimension to his original "Hallmarks of Cancer" by incorporating several newer hallmarks such as polymorphic microbiomes and senescent cells. This more decisive definition of tumorigenesis provided a better understanding of how tumours develop and progress. Understanding these proposed Hallmark advances may guide future therapeutic approaches and research initiatives (Hanahan, 2022).

Birajdar and Lobo (2023) explore how deep learning can significantly enhance cancer research by enabling more accurate prediction and analysis of medical data. They emphasize that "intelligent systems based on deep learning models provide a powerful tool for early detection and treatment planning"

Deepa et al. (2024) developed Fossil_Net, a convolutional neural network-based model that improved predictive and classification functions to predict and classify lung cancer from CT scans. Their solution demonstrates efficacy that improves diagnostic performance based upon reference approaches. Their study supports the importance of using deep learning to more accurately detect cancers, potentially removing human interpretation from the process and quickening clinical decision-making process.

Shinde and Lobo (2019) present a secured prediction system for human diseases by applying a genetic algorithm approach within data mining techniques. In recent years, there have been many advances in cancer research resulting in better techniques and instruments for diagnosis and treatment. Nevertheless, lung cancer remains a health threat worldwide because of high incidence and mortality. The issue with lung cancer is that it begins in the lungs, and without diagnosis or treatment as soon as possible, it will metastasize to multiple areas of the body very rapidly. Smoking may be a factor involved, but possible causes include toxin exposure, pollution, and genetics.

Lobo and Markandeya (2023) present the case for an expert system that uses machine learning prediction algorithms to improve the accuracy and efficiency of medical diagnosis and consultancy. They state that sophisticated systems can assist health professionals by providing reliable decision support, and ultimately provide better care to patients.

Lung cancer remains one of the most difficult stages to detect because the earliest symptoms are so mild and the appearance of tumours can vary extensively. Sai et al. (2024) proposed a multi-model method as shown in Figure 1 for detecting lung cancer using machine learning techniques in that their approach uses multiple models together to improve the diagnostic accuracy. Their approach improves diagnosis accuracy and efficiency through combining sophisticated data preparation, classification algorithms, and image analysis. This approach represents a significant step forward in applying artificial intelligence to important health-related problems.

Figure 1. Lung Cancer Prediction model

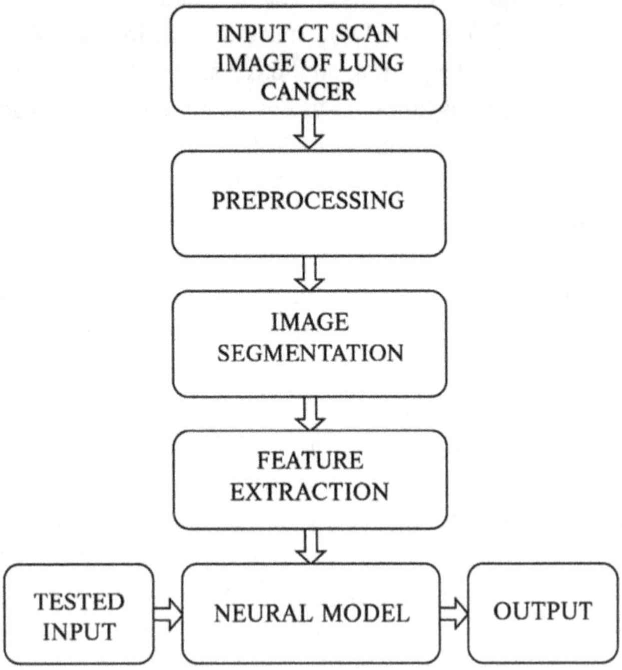

There is an urgency for lung cancer detection, as early detection of lung cancer has increased probability of successful treatment and enhanced prognosis for survival. Generally, existing lung cancer diagnostics, including imaging scans and biopsy approaches, are labor-intensive, and time-consuming, as well as potentially resulting in human error. As a result, artificial intelligence and machine learning techniques have repeatedly and increasingly been explored and implemented within the health care domain. Deep learning algorithms, particularly convolutional neural networks, have shown great potential for digressing or processing medical images and detecting cancerous nodules with high levels of accuracy. Early detection of lung cancer in a pragmatic manner substantially decreases the opportunity for favorable outcomes and surviving lung cancer.

2. RELATED WORK

Nageswaran et al. (2022) utilized machine learning classification and image processing techniques to help diagnose and predict lung cancer with increased accuracy and efficiency in the clinical diagnostics setting. Ahmed et al. (2019) experienced the same increase in performance classifying lung cancer using supervised learning and data mining techniques on a multidimensional dataset.

Tisha and Ani in (2024), stressed how machine learning can allow for the early detection of lung cancer by leveraging predictive models to enhance diagnostic accuracy and decrease diagnosis times. A systematic review on how machine learning has evolved in lung surgery was given by Taha et al., (2022) who suggested the importance of incorporating technology into surgical decision-making and outcome predictions is growing.

The work of Narain Ponraj et al. (2018), which focused on using LBP and LOOP-based textural feature extraction methodologies, demonstrated how these approaches could benefit the performance of image-based lung cancer detection in the classification of CT lung images.

Ardila et al. (2019) produced an end-to-end lung cancer screening system using low-dose chest CT scans and 3D deep learning, allowing them to match the performance of expert radiologists.

Wang et al. (2020) proposed a deep learning alternative to improve diagnosis of nodules in CT lung scans that outperformed standard detection algorithms. The authors illustrated the potential of AI to improve radiologist identification of lung cancer in early stages while also reducing false positives. Zhang et al. (2019) examined the potential for hybrid PET/CT imaging to improve detection of lung cancer by merging functional and anatomical imaging with regards to lung cancer detection. Their study showed that utilizing the bimodality of imaging resulted in improved lesion definition and localization, which ultimately leads to improved clinical decision-making. Liu et al. (2022) created a deep learning-based detection system to perform detection of lung cancer in chest X-rays, which performed with excellent accuracy in malignancy detection patterns. Their approach also allows for scalable and cost-effective start of screening, especially in resource-limited healthcare settings.

Heckel et al. (2024) detail the state of the art of deep learning approaches to improve and accelerate MRI reconstruction in this scoping review. They consider end-to-end neural networks, self-supervised learning, and other approaches to producing better images in shorter scan times. The authors also starkly point out issues such as distribution shift and generalizability to other imaging modalities or other MRI imaging set-ups. This work encourages the inclusion of artificial intelligence into clinical workflows in radiology to produce better and faster diagnosis.

Using PET-based radiomics and machine learning, Hyun et al. (2019) predicted lung cancer histological subtypes via a non-invasive approach to tumor classification, advancing the field of radiomic traits to understanding how to tailor tumor-specific treatment strategies. Bibikova & Fan (2023) researched the possibilities of circulating tumor DNA liquid biopsy as an alternative to more invasive techniques for early detection of lung cancer. Their research indicates that liquid biopsy may have practical clinical potential for earlier detection and monitoring of lung cancer with limited dependence on imaging-based approaches.

To support medical professionals in classifying lung cancer more effectively, Chitale et al. (2023) developed and implemented ensemble approaches based convolutional neural networks (CNNs). The study illustrated how the application of many machine learning approaches could improve classification accuracy and support decision-making informatics for clinical practice.

To determine the best performing models for predicting the progression of the disease, Puri et al. (2025) performed a comparison analysis including several regressor techniques for the detection of lung cancer. Their findings indicate that regression-based machine learning techniques can improve the predictive outcome performance and increase diagnostic accuracy.

In an extensive review of machine learning approaches to classify lung diseases from chest X-ray images, Imam Basha and Jana (2025) evaluated the advantages and disadvantages of different models including support vector machines, convolutional neural networks, and ensemble models. The authors emphasized that image-based diagnostics will become more pertinent in pulmonary clinical care with the increasing familiarity with non-invasive and scalable options. The authors highlighted that deep learning and explainable artificial intelligence create greater accuracy and deeper understanding of automated image classification systems - which in turn, facilitates clinical decisions and early disease diagnosis.

A hybrid approach incorporating deep learning and classical machine learning methods was proposed by Sonal et al. (2025) for the evaluation and classification of lung cancer. With improved accuracy, this method illustrates the strengths of hybrid models of AI methods in medical image processing.

To aid and improve the assessment of lung cancer, Liu et al. (2025) introduced a brand-new multivariate time series classification framework called SIR-3DCNN. This framework provides an important snapshot of the feasibility of 3D convolutional neural networks for the complex analysis of medical data by harnessing spatiotemporal features to improve diagnostic accuracy.

Muna et al. (2025) presented an artificial intelligence approach for cancer analysis that incorporated safe data processing and innovative computational methods with emphasis on early detection and prognosis. Their methodology chimed in the importance of integrating artificial intelligence and security for credible medical judgement in intelligent health systems.

Altuhaifa et al. (2023) conducted a comprehensive review of machine learning techniques in terms of predicting lung cancer survival based on clinical information. Their review highlights the significance of using patient specific data to increase the accuracy of prognostic variables and help with patient-centered treatment planning.

Wulczyn et al. (2021) demonstrated the ability of AI to provide both strong predictive performance and transparency in the clinical decision-making process by developing an interpretable deep learning model for prediction of survival in colorectal cancer. In their study, they offered an informative basis for building trust in AI-enabled prognostic tools for numerous types of cancer.

Field et al. (2024) developed a federated learning model for survival prediction of non-small cell lung cancer based on actual clinical data from multiple institutions. Their study evaluated the ability of the model to contribute to the decision-making process about radiation therapy, in addition to considering how this research is applicable to decentralized and privacy-preserving health systems.

Wani et al., (2023) made a major contribution to medically relevant interpretable deep learning systems through DeepXplainer, which is a lung cancer detection system that uses explainable artificial intelligence (XAI) techniques. Their developed framework for AI detection showcases a potential for clinicians to gain insights into the AI model's predictions for improved transparency and trustworthiness in its usability as a diagnostic tool.

A machine learning-based explainable application, called XML GBM Lung, was presented by Rikta et al. (2023) that strives to embed the package with interpretability while still optimizing accuracy in lung cancer prediction. Their study actually highlights how important explainable models are for acceptance and diagnostic confidence in clinical practice.

Li et al. (2022) provided a comprehensive overview of machine learning uses in lung cancer, including application examples for diagnosis, treatment, and prognosis. Their work shows the different ways AI can be integrated into clinical practices and assist in personalized medicine in the course of lung cancer treatment.

To obtain an understanding of positives and negatives of the models, Urs and Babu (2024) indicated a performance analysis of machine learning algorithms for classifying different types of lung cancer. Their results improve algorithm choice when developing an accurate subtype classification in clinical practice.

Abdullah and Jaddi (2020) evidenced the power of bio-inspired computing to solve complex real-world problems through a dual-inspired kidney algorithm to predict cancer and predict water quality. Their approach led to competitive accuracy particularly in the medical diagnostic task of cancer diagnosis.

Yu et al. (2020) created a hybrid model which predicted lung cancer from CT images through an adjustable heuristic hierarchical mathematical model, supplemented with deep learning models. They demonstrated improved feature extraction and classification performance, illustrating the advantage of hybridizing deep neural networks and mathematical models in medical imaging.

Topol (2019) highlights the intersection of human and artificial intelligence to improve diagnostic accuracy, personalize treatments, and improve clinical efficiency. Topol foresees AI as an adjunct to health care professionals rather than a replacement. In addition, the article emphasizes the need for ethical and regulatory frameworks to drive the use of AI in healthcare.

Gong et al. (2024) explored a segmentation based on deep learning with a CT radiomics ensemble learning model to improve prediction of brain metastasis in patients with non-small cell lung cancer (NSCLC). The authors showed the importance of adding radiomics features to a deep learning model improved prediction performance. This combining approach could support more accurate and timely clinical decision-making for treatment.

Babar et al. (2024) proposed a federated active learning system with transfer learning to enhance lung diagnosis at the edge, enabling intelligence to optimize, and privacy to be maintained, at the remote site of healthcare. By training models collaboratively, their system can facilitate what others cannot with sharing data whilst reaching a diagnostic accuracy comparable to other methods.

Jindal et al. (2023) established a federated learning-based CNN model for diagnosing multiple lung diseases, demonstrating the model's ability to train it on decentralized datasets while preserving patient privacy. In so doing, their approach achieves high confidence diagnoses on sensitive data without centralization thus stretching the boundaries for collaborative AI in healthcare.

Kumar et al. (2018) were able to classify lung cancer with high accuracy using deep learning methods that took advantage of complex feature representations yielded from imaging data. Their work demonstrates that deep learning can be used early and effectively to improve automated cancer classification.

Tjoa and Guan (2021) provided a thorough assessment of explainable artificial intelligence (XAI) in the medical space, identifying how important it is for artificial intelligence systems to have interpretability especially in high-stakes applications like health care in which transparency and trust are key components of the patient clinician relationship.

Gupta et al. (2021) undertook the development of a conversational chatbot which employed natural language processing (NLP) techniques to support cancer diagnostic processes and patient support more broadly, showcasing how NLP allows for patient cantered, user-friendly and interactive health and wellbeing delivery. Their solution provides an example of how AI-based communication tools can increasingly enhance initial symptom evaluation and patient engagement.

Esteva et al. (2019) provided an overall review of deep learning applications in health care. The authors emphasized the technology's ability to change diagnoses, medical imaging and predictive analytics. The review demonstrates how deep learning models have greater advantages over the traditional methods' scalability and accuracy, which would aid when used for AI-assisted clinical decisions. Sairam and Egala (2024) provided a comprehensive review on deep-learning based methods for analyzing medical images. Their report shows the evidence that convolutional neural networks (CNNs), and other architectures have consistently improved the accuracy and speed of diagnostic imaging, as well as some current limitations and future directions for research in that area. This further supports the case for the potentially transformative role of AI in healthcare diagnostics.

Gao et al. (2025), conducted a systematic review on the current use of deep learning techniques for the detection and segmentation of pulmonary nodules on medical imaging studies. The authors outline the current state of deep learning methods relevant to pulmonary nodule detection, with respect to convolutional neural networks (CNNs) and their role in improving lung cancer diagnostic accuracy and early diagnosis, standards are given concerning the regime of current work, as the proliferation of automated services and future technology may distinguish between similar procedures; while the authors recommend fully automated systems could benefit radiologists by always having access to consistent and objective image interpretation reports. The authors also outline present limitations, such as the variability in imaging data and that larger datasets and more available images with annotations in the future is needed; and a few directions for future work as well, highlighting a growing position of the role of AI, as an adjunct to aid successful clinical decisions and measure patient outcomes in thoracic imaging.

Huang, Chung, and Xu (2025) created a deep learning model of object detection for the early detection of lung cancer. The focus of this study was to identify regions of suspiciousness in medical imaging, with high levels of precision and efficiency. Their findings contribute to the understanding of how advanced AI methods can improve accuracy and provide earlier detection of medical abnormalities; ultimately allowing for intervention at a much earlier stage than ever before. The findings are also a positive milestone for the increased use of deep learning models in clinical diagnostic literature.

Wulaningsih et al. (2024) did a systematic review and meta-analysis to evaluate deep learning models designed to predict the risk of malignancy in CT detected pulmonary nodules. They found that the performance of these models had good accuracy in differentiating benign from malignant nodules, and that the models might help in early detection of cancer. However, the authors identified that additional verification in a variety of clinical settings is warranted to allow generalizability.

3. METHODOLOGY

The proposed system is designed to diagnose lung cancer by integrating patient CT scan images, and subsequently suggesting personalized treatment using Generative AI in Figure 2. The overall architecture includes three core components:

data preprocessing, disease classification using machine learning models (ANN and CNN), and treatment recommendation through a generative language model.

A. Data Collection and Pre-processing

The system makes use of a hybrid dataset including structured data and unstructured data i.e. CT scan images. The image data will go through preprocessing techniques that include, converting to grayscale, denoising, resizing and increasing contrast, to allow the CNN model to better extract features.

B. Diagnosis Using Machine Learning Models

For the classification task, the system employs two deep learning models:

- **Artificial Neural Network (ANN)**: Used to analyze structured symptom data to anticipate lung cancer diagnosis likelihood.
- **Convolutional Neural Network (CNN)**: Used on CT scan images, detects cancerous regions in the images and classifies them into normal, benign, or malignant.

Both models use supervised learning methods to train the data, and then the outputs of both models are combined to improve diagnostic accuracy. Performance can be evaluated in a number of ways, including accuracy, precision, recall, and F1-score.

C. Treatment Suggestion Using Generative AI

Upon diagnosis, the Generative AI model is then leveraged to create personalized treatment plans. The model uses diagnosis results, type of cancer, and patient-specific information to recommend the type of therapy for the cancer. Examples of possible therapies are surgery, chemotherapy, targeted therapies, or immunotherapy therapies. The Generative AI model has the ability to generate text-based output driven by current medical guidelines and research knowledge in a dynamic manner.

D. System Deployment and User Interface

The entire solution has been created as a web-based application for care practitioners and patients. The interface allows users to enter their symptoms, upload CT scans and display the diagnosis and the treatment. The application also incorporates a chatbot to answer questions about symptoms, diagnosis or therapy. The system has also been designed to support dynamic datasets, which allows future functionalities to add new symptoms or diseases.

Figure 2. Lung Cancer Prediction and Treatment Suggestion Process

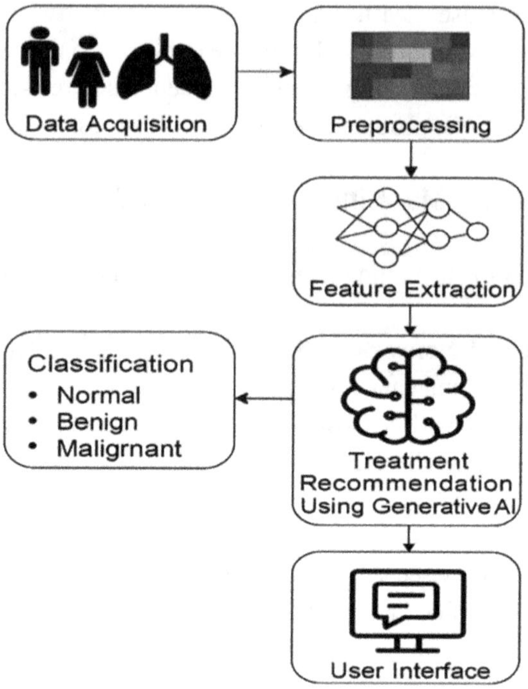

The proposed system is divided into two models: Model 1 — Lung Cancer Diagnosis from CT Scan Images, and Model 2 — Text Generation using a Generative AI Model.

The diagram Model Figure 3 illustrates a two-way deep learning pipeline for lung cancer diagnosis from CT scan images, integrating segmentation and classification processes. Here's a detailed explanation of how the two stages work together:

Figure 3. Lung Cancer Diagnosis from CT Scan Images

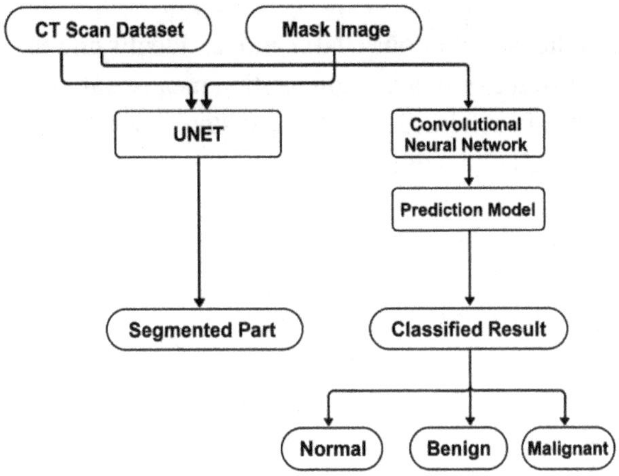

CT Scan Dataset & Mask Image:

- **CT Scan Dataset**: These are the actual medical images obtained from CT (Computed Tomography) scans of patients' lungs. They provide detailed cross-sectional views of the lung tissues.
- **Mask Image**: These are manually or automatically created binary images used to highlight the regions of interest within the CT scans—such as suspected tumors or nodules. The masks serve as ground truth labels for training the segmentation model.

UNET:

- UNET is a specialized deep learning model intended for image segmentation problems. As the structure of UNET is U-shaped, it is an appropriate image analysis model for biomedical images, as it captures global and local features of the image. In this system, UNET takes as input both the CT scan images and the mask images, learns the pattern of abnormalities, and produces an output that isolates or "segments" the relevant region (for example, a tumor or lung nodule) of interest. This step is necessary to ensure that subsequent analyses of the CT scan are only on the features that are potentially abnormal.

Segmented Part:

- This image is the output of our UNET model, identifying the region of interest (e.g. lung lesion or tumor). Segmentation means that we are only using the important parts of each image for the next steps, increasing the accuracy and efficiency of the classification.

Convolutional Neural Network (CNN):

- A CNN is a popular deep neural network to leverage for image recognition tasks. The CNN will take the segmented portion (the area of interest from the lungs) as input and will swim through numerous convolutional layers. The convolutional layers will have the purpose of autonomously extracting and learning important features such as shape, texture, and intensity patterns that reveal conditions of lung tissue that are either normal or abnormal.

Prediction Model:

- The **prediction model** is built using the CNN and is trained to classify the segmented regions based on the features learned.This model uses a labeled dataset (with known outcomes: normal, benign, malignant) to learn the distinctions between different lung conditions. Once trained, it can accurately predict the condition of unseen CT scan segments.

Classified Result:

The **final output** of the system is a classification label that identifies the nature of the detected region.

There are three possible diagnostic outcomes:

- **Normal**: No suspicious or abnormal tissue is found. The lung appears healthy in the CT scan.
- **Benign**: The system detects a benign (non-cancerous; non-malignant) tumor. Most benign tumors do not spread to other parts of the body and in most cases would not need to be treated immediately.
- **Malignant**: The system detects a malignant (cancerous) tumor. Malignant tumors are dangerous because they are able to grow quickly and spread (metastasis) to other parts of the body. Early detection is the key to successful treatment.

Figure 4. Text Generation using a Generative AI Model.

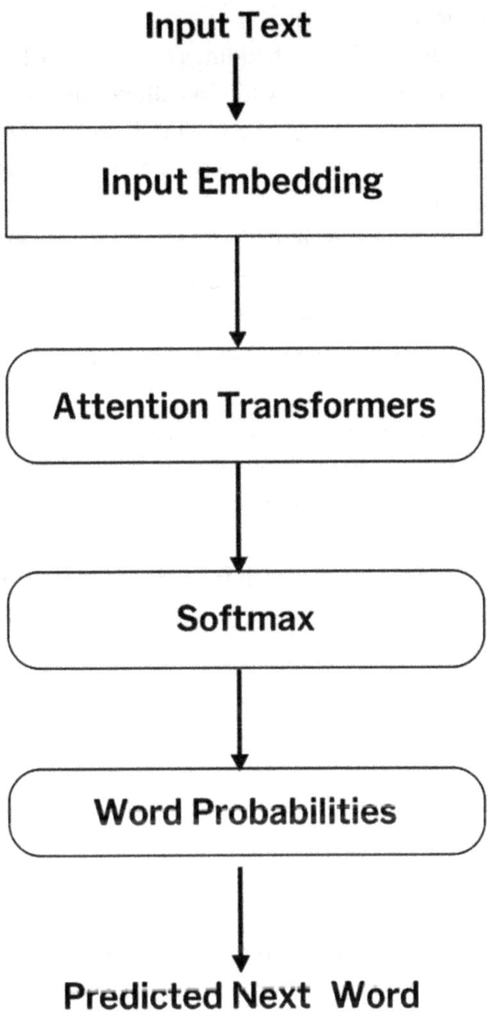

The Above Figure 4 shows model no.2 of Generative AI here after the prediction of disease this model Suggest Appropriate treatments. Generative AI refers to a subset of artificial intelligence that focuses on creating new content based on learned patterns from existing data. This can include generating text, images, audio, video. Text generation in generative AI involves creating human-like written content based on input prompts.

Input Text: This model follows a similar procedure with the sequence of input text. It could be a partial sentence or phrase which will be used as contextual information to predict the next word.

Attention Transformers: The embeddings are sent to a Transformer model, or more specifically an attention model. Attention allows the model to pay attention to different parts of the input sequence to create a prediction. Attention is beneficial as it allows the model to determine how words (and context) are related to each other, even if the words are far apart.

SoftMax Layer: The output from the attention transformer is passed through a Softmax function which converts the output, raw scores (logits), into a probability distribution over words. This is helpful because it allows the model to define the probability linked to each possible next word, and then rank those words in terms of likelihood.

Word Probabilities: After the Softmax function is applied to the output of the attention transformer, the model outputs now return a set of probabilities for every word in the vocabulary. This probability represents how likely each word is to be the next word in the sequence, given the contextual information.

Predicted Next Word: The word with the highest probability is selected as the predicted next word. The model could continue being this process iteratively to create entire sentences or paragraphs, and that is simply what inferences for many text generation tasks such as chatbots.

3.1. Algorithm

The projected model, which makes use of big data sets and a deep learning algorithm to build its output, is for the estimation Lung Cancer and provides the classification in its output.

U-Net is an advanced deep learning model that is frequently used for image segmentation tasks in medical contexts, with lung cancer detection being an example. In this case, U-Net enables practitioners of all degrees of experience to quickly and accurately detect and localize lung regions and possible cancerous nodule from the input CT scan image. This process involves the U-Net architecture, which utilizes an encoder-decoder structure. The encoder learns and extracts important features, and the decoder reconstructs the segmented areas of interest in the input image while also guaranteeing that information in the spatial domain is preserved, based on the skip connections used in the model. This architectural model enables the generation of accurate segmented masks, which are essential for distinguishing lung regions in the image from other irrelevant background regions.

Convolutional Neural Networks (CNNs) are a special type of deep learning model for processing visual, or image data. In detecting lung cancer, CNNs classify CT scan images. However, unlike standard algorithms that require hand-crafted features, CNNs learn patterns in the data itself, which separate normal tissue, benign nodules, and malignant tumors. The architecture of a CNN consists of multiple layers, including convolutional layers which apply filters to identify patterns such as edges or textures, pooling layers which reduce the spatial topology, and fully connected layers which provide the classification output. Consequently, a CNN can learn complex features of a medical image, where standard algorithms need to hand-craft features. Using segmented lung regions from a pre-trained model (e.g., a U-Net), the CNN focuses on only a small piece of the whole lung volume and should decrease the mis-classification of normal lung regions into cancerous regions, providing better accuracy of the detection of cancerous conditions. CNNs are powerful tools to detect complex features, and once a model has been trained on a diverse dataset, they can efficiently detect subtle changes in medical images.In this approach, individual CT scan slices or cropped regions of interest (ROIs) containing Lung are used as input to the CNN. The model is trained to classify each image or region into one of three categories: normal, Bening and malignant. The training data must consist of labeled images for each class, with expert annotations to ensure accuracy.

The Intersection over Union (IoU) metric can be used to evaluate the accuracy of segmenting the lung cancer region from CT images. IoU is commonly used and accepted performances metrics for image segmentation tasks in general, and for medical imaging tasks in particular. It considers how much the predicted segmentation mask (the one created by the model that you trained) overlaps with the ground truth annotation (provided either by human experts or yourself).

A higher IoU score will allow for better identification of the cancer region indicated by the model (the predicted mask) will be closer to the real cancerous region in the lung regions of the CT images. As a result, it will indicate if the segmentation model (for example UNet) is doing a better job segmenting out the anticipated regions that were previously identified as "abnormal" or otherwise "affected/contaminated".

Definition of IoU

IoU is calculated using the formula:

$$\text{IoU} = \frac{\text{Area of Overlap (Intersection)}}{\text{Area of Union}}$$

Where:

- Intersection is the number of pixels common to both the predicted mask and the ground truth mask.

- Union is the total number of pixels present in either the predicted or ground truth masks (combined area).

To compute IoU:

- The segmentation masks must first be converted into binary arrays, where:
    - o **0** represents background pixels (normal lung tissue),
    - o **1** represents the region of interest (suspected cancerous area).

IoU is important for model training and evaluation to ensure the segmentation model (UNet) finds the borders of tumors or nodules in the lung, as tumor size, shape, and location can be different with each patient. In addition, data augmentation techniques are often applied to train a model, including rotation, scaling, and flipping, that will improve the robustness and generalization of the model. This will provide the UNet model with varying patterns to learn from and will help prevent overfitting.

The UNet model will automatically segment lung tumors from CT scans after it has been trained to predict very high IoU values, aiding radiologists and physicians to detect early-stage lung cancer, plan treatment, and track disease progression.

3.1.1. Segmentation

The deep learning model U-Net can uncover cancerous nodules in CT scans while also segmenting lung areas. To create accuracy masks, U-Net uses an encoder-decoder structure with skip connections to distinguish lung tissues as a foreground from the background. U-net performance is evaluated using IoU whereby a higher score means better segmentation which in turn assists in diagnosis.

Segmentation is the process of selecting and highlighting specific areas in an image such as the lungs or cancerous nodules in a CT scan. In order to differentiate lung tissue from the background which ultimately helps identify cancer utilizing models, such as U-Net, segmentation allows machine learning to concentrate only on critical areas and provides the most accurate representation for each segment to improve diagnosis.

Convolutional neural networks (CNNs) are used for classification of CT scan images as benign or malignant or normal. They are able to find patterns in lung cancer or automatically learn features from images. CNN improves accuracy when segmented images are used as it can only focus on lung regions when the U-Net architecture is used for segmentation. The accuracy, precision, recall, and F1-score are measured after the model is trained with labeled data. Transfer learning and data augmentation are two methods to improve performance. CNNs can also be used for quick direct classification when there is no need to segment and identify structures within the images.

3.1.2. Classification

Classification is one of the vital steps of automated identification of lung cancer with CT scans. It consists of placing images into one of three categories: benign (non-cancerous nodules), malignant (cancerous lesions), or normal (healthy lungs). This uses Convolutional Neural Networks (CNNs), deep learning models designed to ingest and analyze visual data.

CNNs consist of several layers that learn to extract features from medical images such as edges, textures and shapes. The model learned to identify the features that separate the three groups because it was trained on a set of annotated CT scans. Once training is complete, the CNN is able to classify new unannotated CT scans. The measure of performance uses metrics such as accuracy, precision, recall, and F1-score. Since the classification stage is a critical part of early cancer detection and treatment selection.

4. EXPERIMENTAL SETUP

4.1 Software Requirements:

- o **VS Code (Development):** VS Code is lightweight yet powerful for development, especially when working with machine learning and deep learning libraries like TensorFlow.
- o **TensorFlow:** TensorFlow is primarily used for deep learning and machine learning problems, such as classification, perception, understanding, discovery, prediction, and creation.
- o **Python 3.10:** It brings performance improvements and new syntax features like pattern matching, which can help with cleaner and more efficient code.

4.2 Hardware Requirements:

- o **Processor i3/i5:** Processor i3/i5 is used for best performance. The i3/i5 is a powerful machine suitable for developing machine learning models.
- o **RAM 16GB and above:** With 16 GB of RAM, there would be enough memory to run a few lightweight programs simultaneously. It allows opening multiple browser tabs and handling various operations efficiently.

- **GPU 8GB VRAM Graphics Card with CUDA Support:** An 8GB VRAM GPU with CUDA support will allow for efficient parallel computing, making deep learning tasks like training classification models much faster. With your analytical approach, you might find it helpful to optimize batch sizes and leverage mixed precision training to further enhance performance.

5. RESULTS AND DISCUSSIONS

To coordinate with the system's utilities, the system is created in Python utilizing generic code The data set required is downloaded from Kaggle.

The accuracy is a ratio based on predicted output and actual output for a system which is labeled as.

$$A = \frac{Nc}{Nt}$$

Where A is Accuracy, Nc is Number of correctly identified data points and Nt is Total number of data points

For e.g. If there are 97 classified data points properly classified and 100 data points consider for the experimentation

accuracy = 97 / 100 = 0.97 or 97%

The F1-Score is particularly useful in image processing tasks, as it provides a balance between precision and recall. In object detection, for example, a high precision score is important to avoid false positives.

The traditional F1-Score is designed as follows:

$$\text{F1} - \text{Score} = 2 \times \frac{\text{Precision} * \text{Recall}}{\text{Precision} + \text{Recall}}$$

It can first define the accurate positives (TP), wrong positives (FP), and wrong negatives (FN) as follows in order to simplify the equation:

$$\text{Precision} = \frac{\text{TP}}{\text{TP} + \text{FP}}$$

$$\text{Recall} = \frac{\text{TP}}{\text{TP} + \text{FN}}$$

Calculated Precision is as follows:

Precision = Accurate Positives / (Accurate Positives + Wrong Positives) ... (a)

Precision = 542 / (542 + 8).
Precision = 0.985455
It can analyze the Recall as follows:

Recall = Accurate Positives / (Accurate Positives + Wrong Negatives) ... (b)

Recall = 542 / (542 + 19).
Recall = 0.966132.
Finally, it can analyze the F1- Score as follows:

F1-Score = ((Two * Precision * Recall) / (Precision + Recall)) ... (c)

F1-Score = ((2 * 0.985455* 0.966132) / (0.985455+ 0.966132)).
F1-Score = (2 * 0.952079) / 1.951587.
F1-Score = 1.904158/ 1.951587.
F1-Score = 0.975698.

Table 1 indicates the parameters like precision, recall, and F-score for different classification of Lung Cancer Shows Evaluation chart representing Precision, Recall and F1 Score for the Lung Cancer as normal benign and Malignant.in Figure 5.

Table 1. Class-Specific Evaluation Metrics (Source: author)

Classification of Lung Cancer	Precision	Recall	F1-Score
Malignant	0.985455	0.966132	0.975698
Normal	0.971223	0.973558	0.972389
Benign	0.876923	0.95	0.912

Figure 5. Classification Performance Evaluation Metrics.

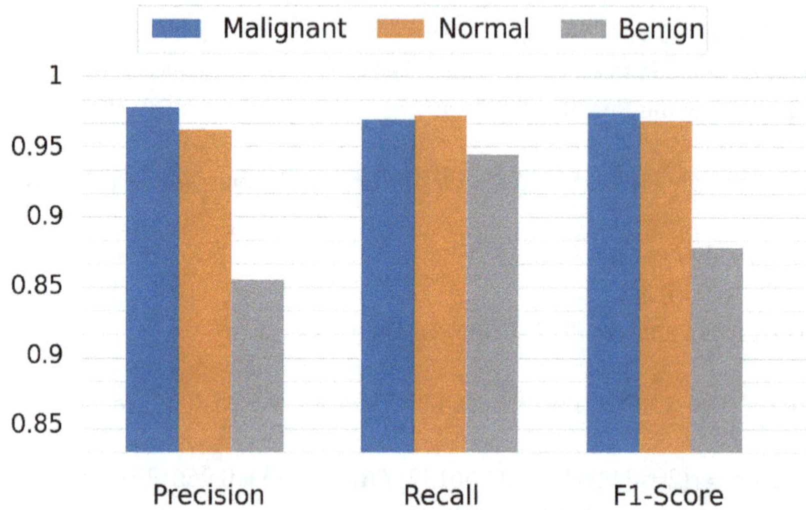

Figure 6. Confusion Matrix for Lung Cancer

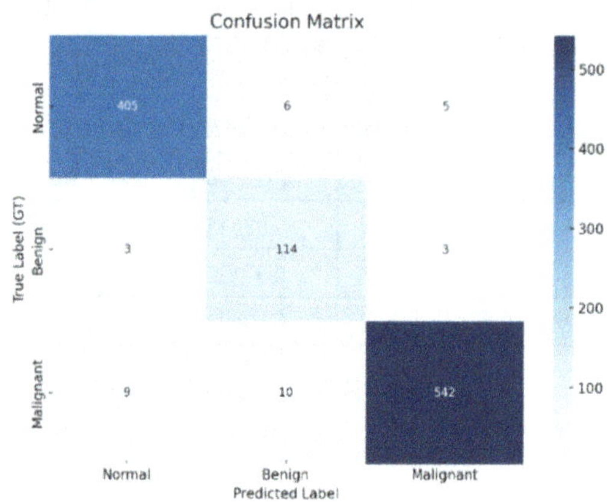

Here is the graphical representation of the confusion matrix based on your data. It shows the model's performance in classifying lung CT images into Normal, Benign, and Malignant categories.

The confusion matrix shown above Figure 6 illustrates the classification performance of the proposed lung cancer detection system across three categories: Normal, Benign, and Malignant. Out of 416 actual normal cases, the model correctly identified 405 as normal, while 6 were misclassified as benign and 5 as malignant. For the benign class, 114 out of 120 were correctly predicted, with 3 incorrectly labeled as normal and 3 as malignant. In the malignant category, the model achieved high accuracy by correctly classifying 542 out of 561 cases, with 9 misclassified as normal and 10 as benign. The high values along the diagonal of the matrix indicate strong performance, particularly in detecting malignant cases. This matrix highlights the model's effectiveness in distinguishing between different types of lung conditions based on CT scan images, which is critical for timely and treatment recommendations.

The Table 2 below displays some of the findings from the literature review produced by various writers.

Table 2. Results for Accuracy Obtained Utilizing Different Machine Learning Techniques.

Format of Input Data	Processing Technique	Feature's extraction	Accuracy
Scanned Images of Lung Cancer	Normalization and augmentation	Normal, Benign, Malignant	97%

Compared with other systems, the CNN-based architecture has a reported accuracy of 97% which surpasses the 95% accuracy that Kumar et al. (2018) reported for lung cancer classification using deep learning. The increase in accuracy indicates that the combination of segmentation using U-Net and CNN-based classification improves diagnostic accuracy.

Table 3. Comparisons of Existing Systems with Standard Literature.

Model of Machine Learning Using CNN Algorithm			
Name of model	**Author Reference**	**Accuracy Achieved by other authors**	**Accuracy Achieved**
CNN	Kumar et al. (2018)	95%	97%

In order to assess the efficacy of the proposed system, the performance was compared against previously published machine learning and deep learning methods in the literature. Kumar et al. (2018) presented CNNs to classify lung cancer with an accuracy of 95% accuracy while Ardila et al. (2019) demonstrated good accuracy with a 3D deep learning model input with low-dose CT images. Similarly, Radhika et al. (2019) compared machine learning methods and while moderate accuracy increases were demonstrated, their methods were outperformed by deep learning methods. In this case the proposed CNN with U-Net segmentation performed better with an accuracy of 97%, precision of 98.5% and f1 score of 0.97. It is noteworthy that the proposed method integrated segmentation to extract the lung regions with the classification capabilities of a CNN to detect nodules minimizing noise and providing finer diagnostics. In summary, this comparison demonstrates that the proposed system provides a new level of accuracy for AI-supported lung cancer detection and analysis.

The main simulation parameters utilized in the CNN-based lung cancer detection framework are presented in Table 4. The table contains a summary of the dataset split strategy, the configuration of convolutional layers, optimizer settings, and training regimen, which dictates the learning behavior and performance of the model.

Table 4. Simulation variables.

Specifications	**Amounts**
CNN Variables	
Training data variation	70%, 20%, 10%,
Max epochs	2000
Number of filters in convolution 2d layer	16
Solver name	Adam learning rate 3×10^{-4}
Minibatch size	8

Table 5, Table 6, demonstrate Dataset details, summary of CNN of each data for the developed model. Normal means the lungs are healthy with no signs of cancer, Benign refers to a non-cancerous growth that is usually harmless, Malignant indicates cancer that can spread and needs immediate treatment.

Table 5. Dataset details.

Dataset 1	
Total image count	**1097**
Number of classes	3 (Normal, Benign, Malignant)
Size of the image	512 x 512
Normal image count	416
Benign image count	120
Malignant image count	561

Table 6. CNN Summary.

Layer	**Details**
Input Layer	512x512x3
2D Convolution	3x3x3 with stride 1x1
Activation Function	ReLu
Fully Connected Layer	128x3
Activation Function	SoftMax
Loss	Categorial Cross entropy

Figure 7. Examples of lung CT scans (top) and corresponding segmented images (bottom) for (i)Normal, (ii) Benign, and (iii) Malignant lung cases.

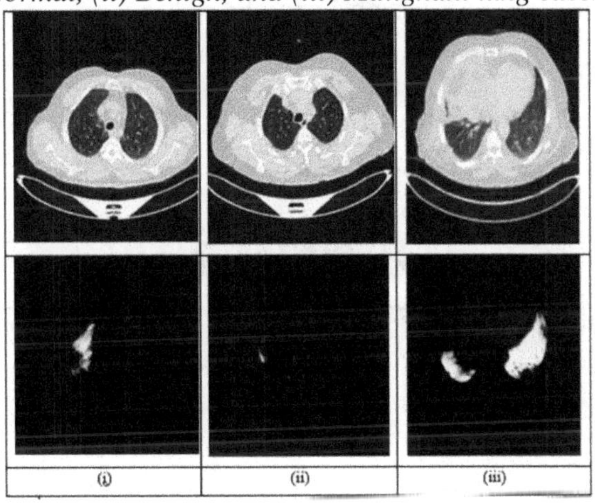

Figure 7 shows representative examples of lung CT scan images and their segmented outputs for three distinct diagnostic categories of lung tumors: (i) Normal, (ii) Benign, and (iii) Malignant. The first row contains raw axial CT slices of the thorax, and the second row shows the respective segmented images from a deep learning-based segmentation model (such as U-Net).

For the Normal case (i) which returns a CT scan with clear lung fields and no indications of abnormal growth, the segmented image highlights very few regions, demonstrating there are no nodules or suspicious tissue.

For the Benign case (ii), the scan shows the presence of nodular structures which do not present as cancerous and posse

ss imperfect localized density changes (increase/decrease), and the segmented output identifies these regions as isolated regions to avoid ambiguity against malignant features.

In contrast, for Malignant case (iii) we can identify dense, irregular parenchyma masses characteristic of cancerous lesions. The segmentation clarifies these regions resulting in better automated classification and treatment planning.

This visual comparison accentuates segmentation exhibiting ways in which improve the clinician's diagnostic process by automatically identifying suspicious areas to allow the clinician to distinguish between normal, benign, or malignant cases.

Figure 8. Choose image From Dataset

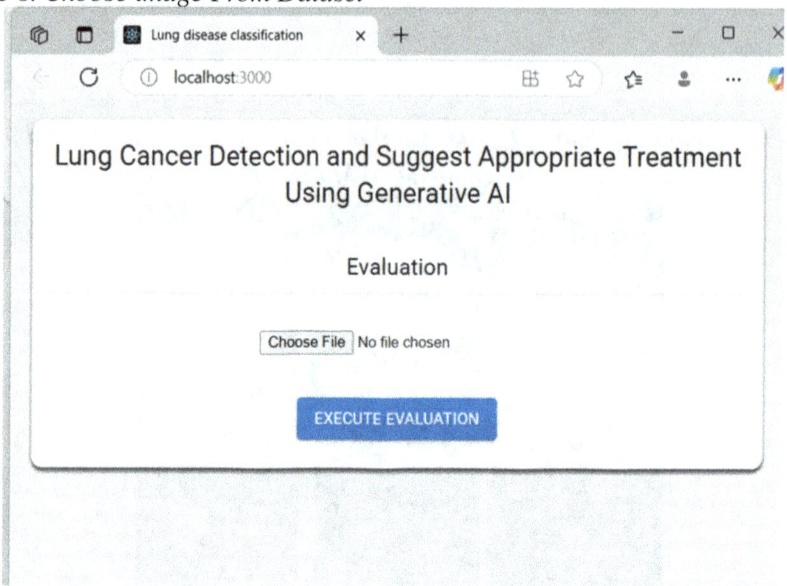

In the Figure 8 the system provides a user-friendly web interface for lung cancer detection and treatment suggestion. Users can upload lung CT scan images through a file input section and click the "EXECUTE EVALUATION" button to initiate the diagnosis.

Figure 9. After Selection of input Image

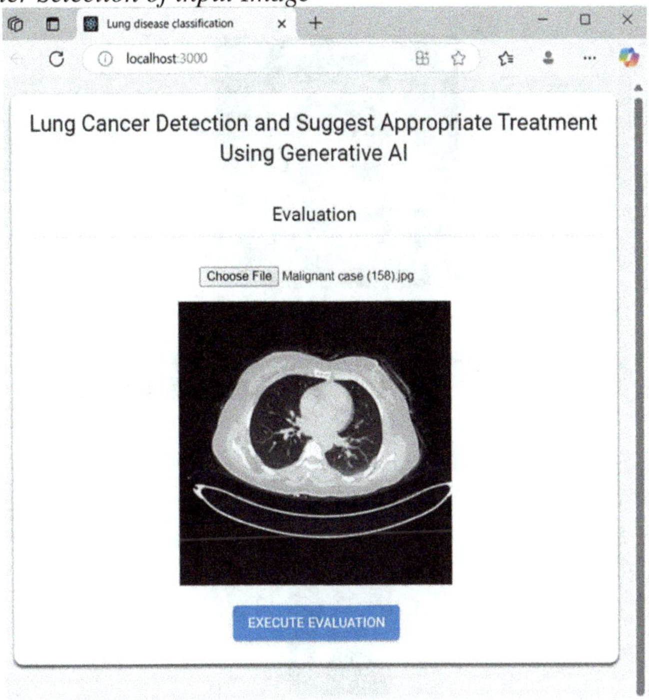

In the Figure 9 this screen shows how a user can upload a lung scan image for cancer detection. Once an image is selected, it is displayed on the screen. By clicking the "EXECUTE EVALUATION" button, the system analyzes the scan using AI to detect lung cancer and suggest appropriate treatment.

Figure 10. Lung Cancer classification and Segmentation

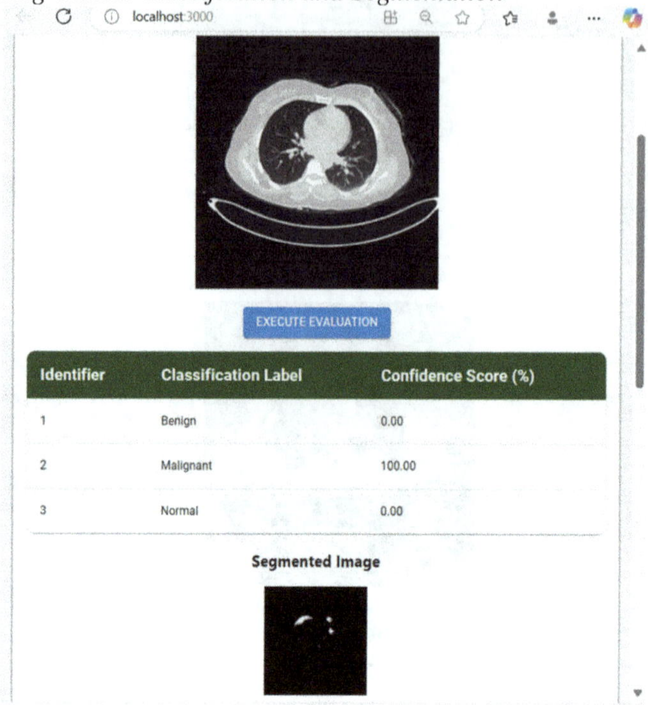

After uploading the lung scan and clicking the "EXECUTE EVALUATION" button, the system displays the result. It shows in the Figure 10 classification labels (Benign, Malignant, Normal) along with their confidence scores. In this case, the system has detected the image as Malignant with 100% confidence. A segmented image is also shown below, highlighting the affected area in the scan.

Figure 11. Treatment Recommendation

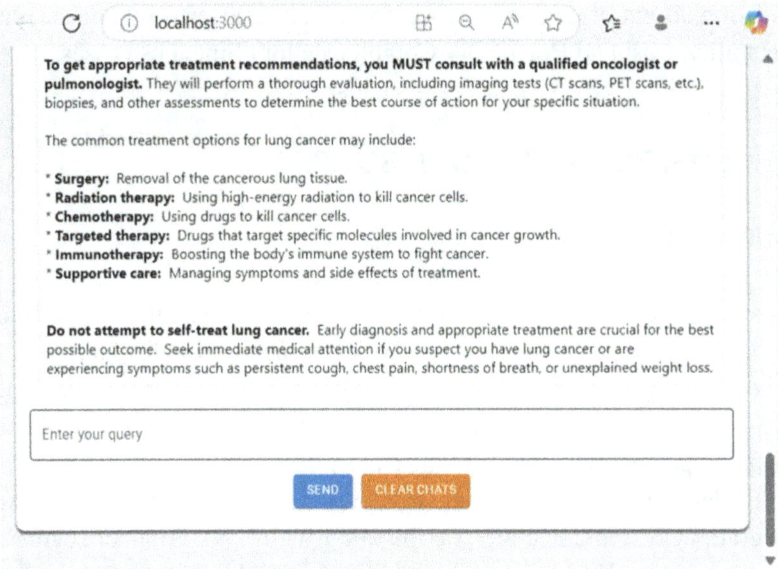

In the Figure 11 the system advises users to consult a qualified doctor (oncologist or lung specialist) for proper treatment. Doctors may use tests like CT scans or biopsies to decide the best treatment. Some common treatment options for lung cancer include:

- **Surgery:** Removing the cancer from the lungs.
- **Radiation therapy:** Using strong energy rays to destroy cancer cells.
- **Chemotherapy:** Using medicine to kill cancer cells.
- **Targeted therapy:** Special drugs that attack cancer cells directly.
- **Immunotherapy:** Helping the body's immune system fight cancer.
- **Supportive care:** Reducing pain and side effects of other treatments.

The system also warns not to treat lung cancer on your own. It says early diagnosis and proper medical care are very important. If someone has symptoms like constant cough, chest pain, or trouble breathing, they should see a doctor immediately.

Research Limitations

The proposed system has limitations. The system works with publicly available databases, (i.e. LIDC-IDRI and Kaggle) meaning its generalizability may be limited, and results are dependent on the quality of CT images and dedication to proper annotation. The system performs at high computing rates, the system processes only CT images, the system was formulated to provide a generalized treatment recommendation absent of unique patient information. Concerns remain surrounding interpretability, trust and Regulatory Compliance for clinical use cases.

6. CONCLUSION AND FUTURE SCOPE

6.1. Conclusion

This study offers an AI-based framework that uses generative algorithms and CT scan image to diagnose lung cancer and recommend suitable treatment alternatives. The system uses a CNN classifier to classify the images into normal, benign, or malignant and a UNET model to precisely segment lung areas from CT scans.

Enhancing patient outcomes for lung cancer necessitates early and accurate detection. To detect lung abnormalities, we developed an AI system in this research that integrates CNN architecture classification with UNET model segmentation of CT scan images. With outstanding precision, recall, and overall accuracy, the system easily differentiates between benign, malignant, and normal cases. The technology closes the gap between screening and clinical decision-making by applying generative AI to provide personalized therapy suggestions as a function of the diagnostic outcome along with detection. Experimental results with segmentation and classification accuracy in excess of 97% demonstrated the robustness of the proposed system and indicated the promise of the system as a reliable diagnostic aid tool in medical imaging.

6.2. Future Scope

In the future, the system could also integrate other medical data; for example, PET scans, health records, etc., which would increase the accuracy of the system. It will improve as it becomes smaller and faster for mobile devices and use in rural health care. Better AI models and explainable AI will also make the system more robust as well as provide more value for physicians to use.

AI DISCLOSURE

This book chapter, " *Design and Development of a Deep Learning Based System for Lung Cancer Diagnosis and Automated Treatment Suggestion* " was primarily authored by [Varsha Manglaram, Dr. L.M.R.J. Lobo, Dr. Vijay Anant Athavale, Mr. Shubham Vyavahare, Mrs. Rajani Yemul.] with intellectual contributions, analysis, and writing done by the authors. Artificial Intelligence (AI)-based tools, including but not limited to ChatGPT and other text-processing software, were used to assist in specific aspects of the writing process. Portions of this paper were developed with the assistance of artificial intelligence tools. Canva was used for creating diagrams, and Grammarly was utilized for language refinement and summarization support. However, the conceptualization, analysis, interpretation of results, and conclusions presented in this paper are solely the work of the authors. The AI tools were used only to support the writing and presentation process, and all final content has been thoroughly reviewed and approved by the authors.

ACKNOWLEDGMENT

The authors acknowledge the Department of Information Technology, Walchand Institute of Technology, Solapur, India for provision of support and resources for, the project. Special appreciation to L.M.R.J. Lobo by assisting with quality guidance and feedbacks throughout the research. The research made use of the lung CT scan images taken from the LIDC-IDRI dataset, which is publicly available through The Cancer Imaging Archive (TCIA) and other datasets available from Kaggle, to train and test the models. The authors also used open-source tool like TensorFlow to train the models and evaluate the system. The authors thank their peers and co-researchers for their valuable suggestions and technical support for the different component of this work.

REFERENCES

Ahmed, S. R. A., Barazanchi, I. A., Mhana, A., & Abdulshaheed, H. R. (2019). Lung cancer classification using data mining and supervised learning algorithms on multi-dimensional data set. [PEN]. *Periodicals of Engineering and Natural Sciences*, *7*(2), 438. DOI: 10.21533/pen.v7i2.483

Altuhaifa, F. A., Win, K. T., & Su, G. (2023). Predicting lung cancer survival based on clinical data using machine learning: A review. *Computers in Biology and Medicine*, *165*, 107338. Advance online publication. DOI: 10.1016/j.compbiomed.2023.107338 PMID: 37625260

Ardila, D., Kiraly, A. P., Bharadwaj, S., Choi, B., Reicher, J. J., Peng, L., & Corrado, G. S. (2019). End-to-end lung cancer screening with three-dimensional deep learning on low-dose chest computed tomography. *Nature Medicine*, *25*(6), 954–961. https://pubmed.ncbi.nlm.nih.gov/31110349/. DOI: 10.1038/s41591-019-0447-x PMID: 31110349

Babar, F. F., Jamil, F., Alsboui, T., Babar, F. F., Ahmad, S., & Alkanhel, R. I. (2024, May). Federated active learning with transfer learning: Empowering edge int Gaoelligence for enhanced lung cancer diagnosis. In *Proceedings of the 20th International Wireless Communications and Mobile Computing Conference (IWCMC)* (pp. 1333–1338). IEEE. https://doi.org/DOI: 10.1109/IWCMC61514.2024.10592390

Bibikova, M., & Fan, J. (2023). Liquid biopsy for early detection of lung cancer. *Chinese Medical Journal Pulmonary and Critical Care Medicine*, *1*(4), 200–206. DOI: 10.1016/j.pccm.2023.08.005 PMID: 39171286

Birajdar, P. S., & Lobo, L. M. R. J. (2023). Advancing cancer research: Intelligent prediction and analysis system based on deep learning. [JETIR]. *Journal of Emerging Technologies and Innovative Research, 10*(8). https://www.jetir.org/indexx?v=10&i=8&j=August%202023

Chitale, R., Shah, B., Bhalgat, S., Pandey, A., & Jakhete, S. A. (2023, August). Utilization of CNN and ensemble methods to support medical practitioners in categorizing lung cancer: A research paper. In *Proceedings of the 7th International Conference on Computing, Communication, Control and Automation (ICCUBEA)* (pp. 1–5). IEEE. https://doi.org/DOI: 10.1109/ICCUBEA58933.2023.10392016

. Deepa, V., & M. C., F. (2024). Fossil_Net: Lung cancer prediction and classification from CT images using convolutional neural networks. In 2024 2nd International Conference on Computing and Data Analytics (ICCDA) (pp. 1–5). IEEE. https://doi.org/DOI: 10.1109/ICCDA64887.2024.10867395

Esteva, A., Robicquet, A., Ramsundar, B., Kuleshov, V., DePristo, M., Chou, K., Cui, C., Corrado, G., Thrun, S., & Dean, J. (2019). A guide to deep learning in healthcare. *Nature Medicine, 25*(1), 24–29. DOI: 10.1038/s41591-018-0316-z PMID: 30617335

Field, M., Vinod, S., Delaney, G. P., Aherne, N., Bailey, M., Carolan, M., Dekker, A., Greenham, S., Hau, E., Lehmann, J., Ludbrook, J., Miller, A., Rezo, A., Selvaraj, J., Sykes, J., Thwaites, D., & Holloway, L. (2024). Federated learning survival model and potential radiotherapy decision support impact assessment for non–small cell lung cancer using real-world data. *Clinical Oncology, 36*(7), e197–e208. DOI: 10.1016/j.clon.2024.03.008 PMID: 38631978

Gao, C., Wu, L., Wu, W., Huang, Y., Wang, X., Sun, Z., Xu, M., & Gao, C. (2025). Deep learning in pulmonary nodule detection and segmentation: A systematic review. *European Radiology, 35*(1), 255–266. DOI: 10.1007/s00330-024-10907-0 PMID: 38985185

Gong, J., Wang, T., Wang, Z., Chu, X., Hu, T., Li, M., Peng, W., Feng, F., Tong, T., & Gu, Y. (2024). Enhancing brain metastasis prediction in non-small cell lung cancer: A deep learning-based segmentation and CT radiomics-based ensemble learning model. *Cancer Imaging; the Official Publication of the International Cancer Imaging Society, 24*(1), 1. Advance online publication. DOI: 10.1186/s40644-023-00623-1 PMID: 38167564

Gupta, P., Kumar, D., Malviya, M., & Choudhury, T. (2021). Cancer chatbot: An NLP-based conversational system for cancer diagnosis and support. *IEEE Access : Practical Innovations, Open Solutions, 9*, 145857–145869.

Hanahan, D. (2022). Hallmarks of cancer: New dimensions. *Cancer Discovery, 12*(1), 31–46. DOI: 10.1158/2159-8290.CD-21-1059 PMID: 35022204

Heckel, R., Jacob, M., Chaudhari, A., Perlman, O., & Shimron, E. (2024). Deep learning for accelerated and robust MRI reconstruction: A review. Magnetic Resonance Materials in Physics. *Biology and Medicine (Aligarh), 37*(3), 335–368. DOI: 10.1007/s10334-024-01173-8 PMID: 39042206

Hyun, S. H., Ahn, M. S., Koh, Y. W., & Lee, S. J. (2019). A machine-learning approach using PET-based radiomics to predict the histological subtypes of lung cancer. *Clinical Nuclear Medicine, 44*(12), 956–960. DOI: 10.1097/RLU.0000000000002810 PMID: 31689276

Imam Basha, S. K., & Jana, S. (2025). Review: Machine learning-based lung diseases classification by using chest X-ray image. In *Proceedings of the 2025 International Conference on Visual Analytics and Data Visualization (ICVADV)* (pp. 1241–1245). IEEE. https://doi.org/DOI: 10.1109/ICVADV63329.2025.10961453

Jindal, V., Kukreja, V., Singh, D. P., Vats, S., & Mehta, S. (2023, October). Pushing diagnostic frontiers: Federated learning CNN for diverse lung disease. In *Proceedings of the 2023 4th IEEE Global Conference for Advancement in Technology (GCAT)* (pp. 1–6). IEEE. https://doi.org/DOI: 10.1109/GCAT59970.2023.10353284

Kumar, R.. (2018). Lung cancer classification using deep learning. *Procedia Computer Science, 132*, 1228–1236. DOI: 10.1016/j.procs.2018.05.118

Li, Y., Wu, X., Yang, P., Jiang, G., & Luo, Y. (2022). Machine learning for lung cancer diagnosis, treatment, and prognosis. *Genomics, Proteomics & Bioinformatics, 20*(5), 850–866. DOI: 10.1016/j.gpb.2022.11.003 PMID: 36462630

Liu, H., Zhang, Y., Wang, X., Chen, J., & Li, Q. (2022). Deep learning-based detection of lung cancer in chest X-rays. *Biomedical Signal Processing and Control, 76*, 103977. DOI: 10.1016/j.bspc.2022.103977

Liu, R., Wang, S., Tian, F., & Yi, L. (2025). SIR-3DCNN: A framework of multivariate time series classification for lung cancer detection. *IEEE Transactions on Instrumentation and Measurement, 74*, 1–13. Advance online publication. DOI: 10.1109/TIM.2025.3563000

Lobo, L. M. R. J., & Markandeya, D. L. (2023). Expert system for medical diagnosis and consultancy using prediction algorithms of machine learning. In Algorithms for intelligent systems (pp. 381–391). https://doi.org/DOI: 10.1007/978-981-99-1435-7_33

Muna, A., Amjad, A., Abdulhafeez, J., & Ishaque, M. (2025). AI-powered cancer analysis: A secure and innovative approach to early diagnosis and prognosis. In *Proceedings of the 2025 2nd International Conference on Advanced Innovations in Smart Cities (ICAISC)* (pp. 1–8). IEEE. https://doi.org/DOI: 10.1109/ICAISC64594.2025.10959580

. Nageswaran, S., Arunkumar, G., Bisht, A. K., Mewada, S., Kumar, J. N. V. R. S., Jawarneh, M., & Asenso, E. (2022). Lung cancer classification and prediction using machine learning and image processing. BioMed Research International, 2022, Article 1755460. https://doi.org/ (Retracted in BioMed Research International, 2024, Article 9851527. https://doi.org/)DOI: 10.1155/2022/1755460

NarainPonraj. D., Christy, E., A, G., S, G., & Sharu, M. (2018). Analysis of LBP and LOOP based textural feature extraction for the classification of CT lung images. In 2018 4th International Conference on Devices, Circuits and Systems (ICDCS). IEEE. https://doi.org/DOI: 10.1109/ICDCSyst.2018.8605138

Puri, C., Sharma, M., & Reddy, K. T. V. (2025). Lung cancer detection: A comparative approach using regressor methods. In *Proceedings of the 2025 4th International Conference on Sentiment Analysis and Deep Learning (ICSADL)* (pp. 722–726). IEEE. https://doi.org/DOI: 10.1109/ICSADL65848.2025.10933212

Radhika, P. R., Nair, R., & Gangadharan, V. (2019). A comparative study of lung cancer detection using machine learning algorithms. In *2019 Fifth International Conference on Electrical Energy Systems (ICEES)* (pp. 1–4). IEEE. https://doi.org/ DOI: 10.1109/ICECCT.2019.8869001

Rikta, S. T., Uddin, K. M. M., Biswas, N., Mostafiz, R., Sharmin, F., & Dey, S. K. (2023). XML-GBM lung: An explainable machine learning-based application for the diagnosis of lung cancer. *Journal of Pathology Informatics*, *14*, 100307. Advance online publication. DOI: 10.1016/j.jpi.2023.100307 PMID: 37025326

. Sai, O. B. S., Vighnesh, D., Varshitha, N. N., Nandhini, P., & J. S., I. T. (2024). A multifaceted approach to lung cancer diagnosis using machine learning techniques. In 2024 4th International Conference on Sustainable Expert Systems (ICSES) (pp. 658–663). IEEE. https://doi.org/DOI: 10.1109/ICSES63445.2024.10763190

Sairam, M. V. S., & Egala, R. (2024). A review on medical image analysis using deep learning. *Engineering Proceedings*, *66*(1), 7. DOI: 10.3390/engproc2024066007

Shinde, S. G., & Lobo, L. M. R. J. (2019). A secured prediction system for human diseases using a genetic algorithm approach to data mining. *International Journal of Emerging Technologies and Innovative Research*, *6*(1), 266–274. https://www.jetir.org/papers/JETIRW006059.pdf

Sonal, D., Pattanaik, S., Nayak, K., Vyas, R. R., Sharma, T., & Kohli, A. (2025). An approach for detecting and classification of lung cancer using deep learning and machine learning. In *Proceedings of the 2025 IEEE 14th International Conference on Communication Systems and Network Technologies (CSNT)* (pp. 53–58). IEEE. https://doi.org/DOI: 10.1109/CSNT64827.2025.10968546

Taha, A., Flury, D. V., Enodien, B., Taha-Mehlitz, S., & Schmid, R. A. (2022). The development of machine learning in lung surgery: A narrative review. *Frontiers in Surgery*, *9*, 914903. DOI: 10.3389/fsurg.2022.914903 PMID: 36171812

Tisha, S. N., & Ani, S. A. (2024). Predictive Insights: Empowering early detection of lung cancer using machine learning excellence. 2017 IEEE Region 10 Symposium (TENSYMP), 1–6. https://doi.org/DOI: 10.1109/TENSYMP61132.2024.10752136

Tjoa, E., & Guan, C. (2021). A survey on explainable artificial intelligence (XAI): Toward medical XAI. *IEEE Transactions on Neural Networks and Learning Systems*, *32*(11), 4793–4813. DOI: 10.1109/TNNLS.2020.3027314 PMID: 33079674

Topol, E. J. (2019). High-performance medicine: The convergence of human and artificial intelligence. *Nature Medicine*, *25*(1), 44–56. DOI: 10.1038/s41591-018-0300-7 PMID: 30617339

Urs, M. P. R., & Babu, G. N. K. S. (2024). Performance analysis and classification of lung cancer types using machine learning. *2024 International Conference on Knowledge Engineering and Communication Systems (ICKECS)*, 1–5. https://doi.org/DOI: 10.1109/ICKECS61492.2024.10617015

Wang, X., Li, Y., Zhang, H., Chen, J., & Liu, Q. (2020). Enhanced nodule detection in lung CT scans using deep learning. *AI*, *1*(1), 24–38. DOI: 10.3390/ai1010003

Wani, N. A., Kumar, R., & Bedi, J. (2023). DeepXplainer: An interpretable deep learning based approach for lung cancer detection using explainable artificial intelligence. *Computer Methods and Programs in Biomedicine*, *243*, 107879. Advance online publication. DOI: 10.1016/j.cmpb.2023.107879 PMID: 37897989

Wulczyn, E., Steiner, D. F., Moran, M., Tan, F., Flament-Auvigne, I., Brown, T., & Chen, P. H. C. (2021). Interpretable survival prediction for colorectal cancer using deep learning. *NPJ Digital Medicine*, *4*(1), 1–26. DOI: 10.1038/s41746-021-00427-2 PMID: 33875798

Yu, H., Zhou, Z., & Wang, Q. (2020). Deep learning assisted predict of lung cancer on computed tomography images using the adaptive hierarchical heuristic mathematical model. *IEEE Access : Practical Innovations, Open Solutions*, *8*, 86400–86410. DOI: 10.1109/ACCESS.2020.2992645

Zhang, Y., Li, H., Chen, X., Wang, J., & Liu, Q. (2019). Hybrid PET/CT imaging for enhanced lung cancer diagnosis. *IEEE Transactions on Biomedical Engineering*, *66*(10), 2905–2913. DOI: 10.1053/j.semnuclmed.2009.03.003

Chapter 2
Synthetic Genomic and Omics Data Applications in Precision Medicine and Biomedical Research

Barno Matchanova
Urgench State Pedagogical Institute, Uzbekistan

Nilufar Niyazova
Mamun University, Uzbekistan

Latofat Salayeva
Urgench State University, Uzbekistan

Munir Ahmad
https://orcid.org/0000-0003-4836-6151
Survey of Pakistan, Pakistan

Muzaffar Shojonov
https://orcid.org/0009-0000-2061-2555
Urgench State University, Uzbekistan

ABSTRACT

Synthetic genomic and omics datasets, encompassing genomics, transcriptomics, proteomics, and metabolomics, enable researchers to replicate the complex biological variability of real-world data while safeguarding sensitive patient information. Leveraging advanced generative models such as Generative Adversarial Networks (GANs), Variational Autoencoders (VAEs), and diffusion-based frameworks, scientists can now create realistic artificial datasets suitable for algorithm training,

DOI: 10.4018/979-8-3373-5641-9.ch002

model validation, and cross-institutional collaboration. This chapter explores the principles, methodologies, and applications of synthetic genomic and omic data, emphasizing their transformative role in personalized medicine, drug discovery, and clinical trial simulation. It also discusses ethical, technical, and regulatory challenges, proposing future research directions toward multi-omics integration, privacy-preserving architectures, and global data-sharing frameworks.

INTRODUCTION

The convergence of synthetic data generation and omics sciences, encompassing genomics, transcriptomics, proteomics, and metabolomics has opened new frontiers in precision medicine and biomedical research. Omics datasets capture the complexity of biological systems at multiple molecular layers, offering unprecedented insights into human health, disease mechanisms, and therapeutic responses. However, these datasets are often large, high-dimensional, and sensitive due to their biological and personal nature. Such attributes create substantial challenges in data accessibility, reproducibility, and privacy preservation, hindering the collaborative potential of biomedical research.

Traditional biomedical data sharing is constrained by ethical, legal, and technical limitations that restrict access to patient-level omic data. As a result, researchers frequently encounter obstacles related to small sample sizes, data imbalance, and underrepresentation of rare conditions. Moreover, strict privacy regulations such as GDPR and HIPAA impose further restrictions on data exchange across institutions. Synthetic data generation has emerged as a promising solution to these barriers by creating artificial datasets that retain the statistical and biological characteristics of real data without exposing sensitive information. This capability addresses a critical need for data democratization and reproducibility in precision medicine.

The integration of synthetic data into omics research holds transformative potential. It enables scalable training and validation of machine learning models even when real datasets are scarce or protected. Synthetic genomic and omic data can augment rare disease cohorts, simulate hypothetical clinical trial scenarios, and support federated learning environments that eliminate the need for direct data sharing. By facilitating secure, realistic, and reusable biomedical datasets, synthetic data contributes to accelerating discoveries, enhancing model generalizability, and reducing biases in precision healthcare.

The primary objectives of this chapter are to explain the theoretical foundations and methodologies of synthetic data generation within omic sciences, examine how synthetic omic data supports research reproducibility, data privacy, and equitable access, illustrate real-world applications in precision medicine such as disease modeling, biomarker discovery, and clinical decision support, and discuss the ethical, technical, and regulatory challenges associated with synthetic biomedical data. The chapter is structured to provide a logical progression from foundational concepts to advanced applications. Section 2 introduces the principles of omics sciences and their role in precision medicine, while Section 3 explores the main methodologies of synthetic data generation, including generative adversarial networks (GANs), variational autoencoders (VAEs), and diffusion models. Section 4 presents case studies and applications of synthetic omic data in biomedical research and healthcare innovation. Section 5 addresses ethical, regulatory, and data governance considerations related to synthetic biomedical datasets, and finally, Section 6 concludes with key insights, emerging trends, and future research directions.

LITERATURE REVIEW

Evolution of Synthetic Data in Biomedical Research

The notion of synthetic data originates from mid-20th-century statistical simulation techniques aimed at understanding complex systems, but its formal incorporation into biomedical research accelerated with the rise of generative modelling methods — notably Variational Autoencoders (VAEs), Generative Adversarial Networks (GANs), and more recently diffusion-based generative frameworks. Initially, synthetic data work in biomedical domains focused primarily on patient-level records and imaging modalities (for example in electronic health records and radiology) to circumvent issues of privacy, data sharing and sample scarcity. For instance, Brett Beaulieu-Jones and colleagues demonstrated that generative deep neural networks could simulate synthetic participants in a clinical trial while preserving privacy constraints (Beaulieu-Jones et al., 2019; Rajotte et al., 2022).

As omics technologies matured and deep learning techniques became more proficient at modelling high-dimensional nonlinear dependencies, synthetic data generation gradually expanded into molecular biology. The capacity to mimic complex, structured omic datasets opened new vistas for reproducibility, data sharing and augmentation in biomedical research.

Synthetic Genomic Data

Synthetic genomic data generation represents a rapidly evolving intersection of genomics, data science, and privacy-preserving machine learning. Its central goal is to reproduce genome-scale characteristics—such as allele frequency spectra, linkage disequilibrium (LD) patterns, haplotype blocks, and population stratification—without revealing real individuals' genotypes. Unlike traditional simulation frameworks (e.g., coalescent models or forward genetic simulators like SLiM or msprime) that rely on predefined population parameters, modern deep generative models learn these complex patterns directly from empirical data, allowing them to emulate the underlying statistical distributions of genetic variation at scale (Adrion et al., 2020).

A landmark contribution by Yelmen et al., (2021) demonstrated that Generative Adversarial Networks (GANs) and Restricted Boltzmann Machines (RBMs) can generate artificial genomes closely resembling real human population structure and allele frequency distributions. Their study used phased haplotype data from the 1000 Genomes Project and trained models to reproduce genome-wide variant matrices. The synthetic genomes preserved essential genomic diversity, enabling downstream applications such as ancestry inference and principal component analysis (PCA), while mitigating re-identification risks. Importantly, Yelmen and colleagues showed that the synthetic genomes exhibited realistic pairwise genetic distances and population-specific clustering patterns, indicating that generative models can faithfully reproduce both within- and between-population variance, a critical requirement for population genetics and evolutionary inference.

Subsequent studies have refined these approaches. (Groß & Wunder, 2023) developed a privacy-preserving VAE architecture capable of producing synthetic genotypes under differential privacy constraints, maintaining statistical similarity to real data while bounding the risk of individual-level leakage. Similarly, (Kenneweg et al., 2024) used diffusion-based generative models to iteratively learn to denoise synthetic genotype matrices from random noise, achieving higher fidelity and diversity than GAN-based methods. Diffusion models have been particularly effective in capturing long-range genomic correlations, something GANs often fail to represent due to mode collapse or limited receptive field size. These architectures are now being adapted for large-scale whole-genome synthesis, offering near-realistic genotype distributions that can be used to benchmark polygenic risk score (PRS) models, genome-wide association studies (GWAS) pipelines, and population stratification correction algorithms.

Building on this, (Oprisanu et al., 2022) evaluated various synthetic genomic data generation methods, comparing their ability to preserve data utility (e.g., allele distributions, PCA-based ancestry clustering) and privacy (e.g., resistance to membership inference attacks). Their findings highlighted a persistent utility–privacy trade-off, where models achieving high fidelity often risk privacy leakage, while highly private models may underperform in preserving genomic structure. A more recent advancement is the RESHAPE framework proposed by (Cavinato et al., 2024), which synthesizes haplotype reference panels by simulating descendants of known genomes. This method disrupts genome–phenome links and allows safe data sharing across institutions while maintaining essential population-level genetic variation. RESHAPE marks a significant step toward privacy-preserving yet realistic synthetic genomes applicable in genome-wide association studies (GWAS) and fine-mapping analyses.

Despite these advances, key challenges remain. The balance between privacy and utility is a persistent tension: overly constrained models may produce biologically implausible genomes, while overfit models may inadvertently leak information about real individuals. Evaluating the realism, utility, and privacy leakage of synthetic genomes thus requires robust benchmarking—often combining statistical similarity metrics (e.g., allele frequency divergence, LD decay curves) with adversarial privacy tests (e.g., membership inference attacks). Furthermore, ensuring that synthetic genomes capture rare variants, structural variations, and epigenomic annotations remains a major research frontier, particularly as the field moves toward multi-omic synthetic data integration.

Synthetic Omics Data

Omics datasets, including transcriptomics, proteomics, metabolomics and multi-omic integrations, capture dynamic molecular processes and complex interplays across different biological layers. Generating synthetic omics data generally involves neural network architectures (e.g., conditional VAEs, GANs, diffusion models) that learn multi-omic dependencies, expression distributions, and experimental noise characteristics. For example, Marouf et al. (2020) developed a conditional single-cell GAN (cscGAN) to generate synthetic single-cell RNA-seq data, capturing non-linear gene-gene dependencies and enabling data augmentation of rare cell-types, ultimately improving downstream tasks like marker-gene detection and classifier robustness (Marouf et al., 2020)

In proteomics, simulation efforts often focus on instrument and acquisition realism (peak shapes, retention time, fragmentation spectra). Tools that simulate LC–MS/MS experiments (e.g., Synthedia) and peptidomics pipelines provide in-silico data useful for method development, benchmarking of search engines, and testing of downstream statistical workflows. These simulators use mechanistic models, statistical noise models, or hybrid ML-driven components to mirror real proteomics output. The proteomics community has also emphasized repositories and standardized formats (e.g., iProX) that support sharing both real and simulated proteomics data for reproducibility (Leeming et al., 2023).

Moreover, simulation frameworks continue to evolve: Shakola et al. (2022) proposed a general benchmarking framework for synthetic RNA-seq data generators, underscoring the growing methodological maturity of synthetic omic data approaches (Shakola et al., 2022). Metabolomics simulation has likewise emphasized realistic mass-spectrometry signal generation and downstream chemometric properties. Virtual mass-spectrometer frameworks and simulated LC-MS datasets allow evaluation of pre-processing, peak picking and annotation strategies; such tools are especially helpful when experimental acquisition is costly or when method comparisons require controlled, repeatable datasets (Wandy et al., 2023). Across multi-omic and integrated settings, recent efforts use conditional, multi-modal VAEs/GANs and joint latent representations to model cross-modal dependencies (for example, linking genotype → transcriptome → proteome relationships). However, the field still lacks widely accepted benchmarks for multi-omic synthetic data fidelity, making comparative evaluation an active area of research (Neely et al., 2023).

Synthetic Data in Precision Medicine

In the domain of precision medicine, where interventions are increasingly tailored to individual molecular profiles, the role of synthetic genomic and omic data is especially compelling. Synthetic datasets can be used to augment rare disease cohorts, simulate clinical trial scenarios, balance imbalanced classes, and support federated learning frameworks where raw data cannot be transferred. Importantly, synthetic data can enable cross-institutional collaborations under data-sharing constraints, facilitating model training, validation and testing in a privacy-preserving manner. The alignment with regulatory frameworks such as General Data Protection Regulation (GDPR) (Francesca, 2019) and Health Insurance Portability and Accountability Act (HIPAA) amplifies the utility and relevance of synthetic biomedical data in modern healthcare research (Lutkevich, 2019; Said et al., 2024). Case studies and reviews show that synthetic datasets can yield downstream model performance comparable to models trained on real data when generation preserves relevant signal (e.g., disease vs control discriminants) and when evaluators use rigorous fidelity metrics. The emergence of diffusion models for genotype synthesis and improvements in multi-modal conditional generation have widened the toolset available to precision medicine researchers (Yelmen et al., 2021).

In the era of precision medicine, where treatments, diagnostics, and preventive interventions are increasingly tailored to the molecular, genetic, and environmental profiles of individual patients, synthetic genomic and omic data are emerging as powerful enablers of innovation and scalability. These artificial datasets, designed to emulate the statistical and biological properties of real patient data, address critical challenges of data scarcity, privacy, and representativeness that have long constrained precision medicine research.

Synthetic datasets can augment underrepresented cohorts (e.g., rare diseases, pediatric cases, or minority populations) by expanding sample sizes without requiring additional patient recruitment. They also simulate clinical trial scenarios and help balance class distributions in imbalanced biomedical datasets, conditions frequently encountered when modeling disease progression or treatment response (Figueira & Vaz, 2022; Murtaza et al., 2023). In genomic prediction and drug response modeling, synthetic data serve as an effective tool for data augmentation, enhancing model robustness while reducing overfitting to limited or biased datasets (van Breugel et al., 2024).

A major application area lies in federated and privacy-preserving learning frameworks, where real data cannot be transferred across institutional or national boundaries. Synthetic data enables cross-institutional collaboration by allowing the sharing of realistic, yet de-identified, data surrogates. For instance, researchers can jointly train predictive models or validate algorithms across distributed hospital networks without exposing protected health information (Kiran et al., 2025; Little et al., 2023). This capability directly supports compliance with regulatory frameworks such as the General Data Protection Regulation (GDPR) in the European Union and the Health Insurance Portability and Accountability Act (HIPAA) in the United States, which impose strict constraints on identifiable data handling and transfer (Price & Cohen, 2019; Voigt & Von dem Bussche, 2017).

Empirical studies show that models trained on high-fidelity synthetic biomedical datasets can achieve comparable downstream performance to those trained on real data, provided the synthetic generation process preserves clinically relevant signals such as disease–control discriminants or molecular biomarkers (Goncalves et al., 2020; Walonoski et al., 2018). Recent advancements in diffusion-based models and multi-modal generative architectures further enhance the biological plausibility of synthetic data by integrating genomic, transcriptomic, and clinical information in a coherent latent space (Luo et al., 2025). These hybrid approaches enable simulation of patient trajectories and molecular profiles under various treatment conditions, offering unprecedented opportunities for in silico experimentation and decision support in personalized healthcare.

Ethical and Regulatory Considerations

Although synthetic data offers substantial promise, it also raises important ethical, technical, and regulatory questions. Firstly, poorly generated synthetic datasets may still leak individual-level information if generative models over-fit or mirror real data too closely. Ensuring a **balance between utility and privacy** is therefore critical. Studies on synthetic electronic health records found that while some methods preserved statistical properties well, others (notably some GAN-based models) failed to generate high-utility data or adequately protect privacy (Goncalves et al., 2020).

Synthetic data reduce many re-identification vectors but are not automatically risk-free. Membership-inference and model-extraction attacks demonstrate that synthetic datasets can leak information if generative models overfit or if evaluation of privacy risk is incomplete. Empirical studies of membership inference against synthetic health data recommend adversarial testing and quantitative privacy metrics (e.g., membership inference risk, empirical nearest-neighbor metrics) as part of any release pipeline. Researchers have proposed attacker models as evaluation metrics to quantify practical privacy risk; the literature shows a trade-off between privacy (lower leakage) and utility (higher fidelity), and highlights the need for standardized privacy-utility reporting in biomedical synthetic data work. Regulatory perspectives increasingly treat well-validated synthetic datasets as potential enablers for secondary research use if accompanied by transparent governance and privacy risk assessments (e.g., adherence to GDPR/HIPAA principles where applicable) (Zhang et al., 2022).

Table 1 shows some of the methods described in the literature review section as a summary table.

Table 1: Representative methods and key studies

Method / Class	Data type/scope	Key contribution/finding	Citation
GANs (including conditional GANs)	Single-cell RNA-seq	cscGAN generates realistic single-cell profiles, augments rare cell types, and improves downstream tasks.	(Marouf et al., 2020)
GANs / RBMs for genomes	Human genotype/ population structure	Artificial genomes reproduce allele frequencies, LD, and population structure with low measured privacy leakage.	(Yelmen et al., 2021)
VAE / hybrid VAE-GAN	Tabular, multi-omic	Comparative analyses show tradeoffs: VAEs are often easier to train but may underfit fine structure; GANs capture sharp distributions but risk mode collapse.	(Kiran & Kumar, 2023)
Proteomics simulators (mechanistic/statistical)	LC-MS/MS proteomics (DIA)	Simulates DIA LC-MS runs for method benchmarking; supports evaluation of acquisition and analysis pipelines.	(Leeming et al., 2023)
Metabolomics simulators / virtual MS	Untargeted metabolomics LC-MS	In-silico comparison of acquisition methods using virtual mass spectrometer frameworks.	(Wandy et al., 2023)
Privacy evaluation/ attacks	Synthetic health data	Membership inference attacks against synthetic health data illustrate concrete privacy risks and suggest testing frameworks.	(Zhang et al., 2022)
Reviews/method surveys	Health / clinical data	Comprehensive review of synthetic methods across healthcare modalities; discusses evaluation metrics and open challenges.	(Pezoulas et al., 2024)

METHODOLOGICAL FRAMEWORK

Overview

The methodological foundation for synthetic genomic and omic data generation integrates computational biology, machine learning, and data privacy principles to balance realism with confidentiality. The process begins with data representation and preprocessing, a critical step where complex, high-dimensional biological information—such as genomic sequences, transcriptomic profiles, proteomic spectra, and metabolomic signatures—is encoded into computationally tractable forms. This often involves normalization, dimensionality reduction, feature encoding, and transformation into numerical matrices or latent embeddings that preserve biological relationships. For example, genomic variants may be represented as one-hot encoded sequences, while transcriptomic data may require log normalization and batch correction to eliminate experimental bias. Proper preprocessing ensures that generative models capture genuine biological signals rather than noise or confounders, setting a foundation for accurate and interpretable synthetic data generation (Goncalves et al., 2020).

The second stage, model training and generation, leverages generative modeling paradigms such as Variational Autoencoders (VAEs), Generative Adversarial Networks (GANs), and the more recent diffusion models to learn the underlying distributions of biological data. VAEs encode complex omic data into low-dimensional latent spaces, facilitating the reconstruction of biologically plausible samples that retain population-level diversity. GANs, consisting of a generator and discriminator in an adversarial setup, have been widely used to generate synthetic gene expression and genotype data, producing outputs nearly indistinguishable from real datasets. More recently, diffusion models have demonstrated superior stability and fidelity, enabling the capture of fine-grained molecular variations and complex dependencies in multi-omic systems. These models can also be conditioned on metadata—such as disease labels, demographic traits, or environmental exposures, allowing researchers to simulate realistic subpopulations for precision medicine applications (van Breugel et al., 2024).

The final stage, evaluation and validation, ensures that generated datasets achieve a balance between biological fidelity and privacy preservation. Evaluation typically involves multiple layers: (i) fidelity metrics, such as distributional similarity (e.g., KL divergence, Wasserstein distance), correlation structure preservation, and predictive equivalence; (ii) biological relevance tests, where synthetic samples are assessed for their ability to replicate known biological associations, gene–pathway coherence, or disease markers; and (iii) privacy assessments, including membership inference attacks and re-identification risk analysis to verify that individual-level information is not leaked. Some frameworks further integrate explainability and auditability layers to document data provenance and model behavior, supporting regulatory compliance and ethical oversight. Collectively, these stages establish a robust, reproducible pipeline for generating biologically meaningful, privacy-preserving synthetic datasets that can be safely shared and analyzed across genomic, transcriptomic, proteomic, and metabolomic research domains.

Data Representation and Preprocessing

High-throughput omic data—ranging from genomic sequences to proteomic spectra—require systematic encoding and preprocessing to make them suitable for generative modeling. The way these biological signals are represented directly affects how well generative models can learn and reproduce underlying biological variability, dependencies, and multi-scale interactions. Each omic layer presents unique challenges: genomic data are discrete and sequence-based, transcriptomic data are continuous and highly variable, and proteomic or metabolomic data often contain sparse, instrument-dependent noise. Consequently, preprocessing pipelines must be tailored to the biological and computational characteristics of each data type to ensure fidelity, interpretability, and cross-study generalization (Athieniti & Spyrou, 2023; Baião et al., 2025; Marouf et al., 2020; Yelmen et al., 2021).

Genomic Variants

Genomic data, such as Single Nucleotide Polymorphisms (SNPs), structural variants, and haplotypes, are foundational for synthetic data generation in population genomics and precision medicine. SNP data are typically converted into genotype matrices where each allele (e.g., AA, AG, GG) is encoded numerically or using one-hot representations to maintain categorical distinctions. More sophisticated representations, such as haplotype blocks or phased sequences, allow models to capture linkage disequilibrium (LD), recombination patterns, and population-specific variant correlations, which are crucial for realistic genomic synthesis. Additionally, embedding-based approaches have been introduced to represent genomic loci in continuous latent spaces, enabling models like diffusion-based generators to learn long-range dependencies across chromosomes. These representations are often supplemented with metadata such as ancestry or phenotype labels to condition the generation process for disease-specific simulations (Yelmen et al., 2021).

Transcriptomic Data

For transcriptomic data derived from RNA-sequencing (RNA-seq), preprocessing focuses on transforming raw count data into biologically meaningful, normalized matrices. Common normalization schemes include Transcripts Per Million (TPM), Fragments Per Kilobase of transcript per Million mapped reads (FPKM), and Counts Per Million (CPM), which standardize expression levels across samples and genes. To address experimental variability and batch effects that can obscure biological signals, methods such as ComBat, Harmony, and Seurat's integration pipelines are employed to harmonize datasets from different laboratories or platforms. Logarithmic transformation is often applied to stabilize variance and bring expression distributions closer to normality. These preprocessing steps ensure that the generative model learns transcript-level co-expression structures, pathway dynamics, and disease–control discriminants rather than technical noise or batch-specific artifacts (Marouf et al., 2020).

Proteomic and Metabolomic Data

Proteomic and metabolomic data—frequently derived from mass spectrometry (MS) or nuclear magnetic resonance (NMR) spectroscopy—pose distinct preprocessing challenges due to signal sparsity, dynamic range, and measurement variability. Typically, spectra are converted into feature abundance matrices or intensity vectors, where each column corresponds to a molecular feature or ion peak and each row represents a sample. Peak alignment, baseline correction, and normalization (e.g., total ion count or probabilistic quotient normalization) are applied to mitigate technical variability. Missing value imputation and outlier detection are also essential, as mass spectrometry data often contain dropouts or machine-specific artifacts. Once cleaned and standardized, these representations enable generative models to reconstruct or simulate biologically coherent molecular profiles that capture physiological or pathological variations (Athieniti & Spyrou, 2023; Baião et al., 2025).

Dimensionality Reduction and Latent Encoding

Before training generative models, high-dimensional omic datasets undergo dimensionality reduction to uncover intrinsic biological structure and improve computational efficiency. Classical methods, such as Principal Component Analysis (PCA) and Independent Component Analysis (ICA), extract dominant variance components, while non-linear techniques, like t-SNE and Uniform Manifold Approximation and Projection (UMAP), preserve both local and global relationships in complex expression landscapes. More recently, autoencoder-based embeddings and contrastive learning frameworks have been adopted to learn dense, biologically meaningful latent representations that retain important co-expression and interaction patterns. This step is pivotal for ensuring that generative models focus on informative biological signals rather than redundant or noisy features, ultimately leading to the synthesis of high-fidelity, biologically realistic data (Moon et al., 2019).

Generative Modeling Approaches

The generation of synthetic genomic and omic data relies on a range of deep generative modeling paradigms designed to capture complex, high-dimensional biological dependencies while ensuring privacy preservation. Each modeling family—Generative Adversarial Networks (GANs), Variational Autoencoders (VAEs), diffusion models, transformer-based architectures, and hybrid or federated frameworks—offers distinct strengths in terms of distributional learning, interpretability, and scalability. Together, these methods constitute the methodological core of modern synthetic biology pipelines, enabling simulation of genotype-phenotype relationships, rare disease data augmentation, and privacy-conscious data sharing in precision medicine contexts (Goncalves et al., 2020; van Breugel et al., 2024).

Generative Adversarial Networks (GANs)

GANs have become one of the most influential paradigms for synthetic omic data generation due to their capacity to approximate complex, non-linear biological distributions without explicit likelihood modeling. A GAN comprises two neural networks—a generator that produces synthetic samples and a discriminator that distinguishes real from fake data—trained in an adversarial process that pushes the generator toward realistic outputs. Variants such as conditional GANs (cGANs) allow conditioning on metadata like tissue type, disease status, or patient demographics, thereby enabling context-specific synthesis. In genomics, GANs have successfully reproduced population allele frequency spectra and linkage disequilibrium patterns, while in transcriptomics, models such as scGAN and cscGAN have generated realistic single-cell RNA-seq data that preserve cell-type clustering and gene co-expression networks (Marouf et al., 2020). Despite their success, GANs require careful tuning to prevent mode collapse and ensure that generated samples reflect the full biological diversity of the training data (Goodfellow et al., 2014).

Variational Autoencoders (VAEs)

VAEs provide a probabilistic framework for learning latent representations of omic data, mapping complex biological profiles into a lower-dimensional manifold from which synthetic samples can be generated. Unlike GANs, VAEs explicitly model the data distribution through an encoder–decoder architecture that learns both reconstruction fidelity and latent regularization via the Kullback–Leibler divergence term. This structure makes VAEs particularly suited for capturing continuous biological variability, such as gene expression gradients or molecular pathway transitions. Conditional variants (CVAEs) allow the generation of disease- or tissue-specific profiles, making them valuable tools for simulating hypothetical biological conditions and exploring potential interventions. VAEs have been widely applied to single-cell transcriptomics and metabolomics, where their smooth latent spaces facilitate biological interpretation and trajectory inference. Recent developments, including β-VAEs and disentangled VAEs, further enhance interpretability by isolating independent sources of biological variation, enabling controlled synthetic generation (Kingma & Welling, 2014; Lopez et al., 2018; Way & Greene, 2018).

Diffusion and Transformer Models

Diffusion models represent an emerging class of generative frameworks that iteratively learn to reverse a noise diffusion process to reconstruct realistic data samples. Their mathematical stability and capacity for high-fidelity generation have recently extended from image domains to genomic and omic datasets. Diffusion-based models for genotype synthesis have shown promise in replicating full genotype matrices while preserving allele correlations and haplotype integrity, outperforming GANs and VAEs in sample diversity and quality (Ho et al., 2020; Jumper et al., 2021). Parallelly, transformer-based architectures, originally developed for natural language processing, have been adapted to sequence modeling in genomics, capturing long-range dependencies and regulatory motifs across DNA and RNA sequences. These models leverage attention mechanisms to understand hierarchical biological context, such as enhancer–promoter interactions or pathway-level dependencies. When integrated, diffusion and transformer approaches provide a powerful toolkit for modeling genome-scale complexity and temporal dynamics in multi-omic data (Rao et al., 2021).

Hybrid and Federated Frameworks

To address data privacy, institutional boundaries, and model generalizability, hybrid and federated frameworks have gained traction in synthetic omics. Hybrid architectures combine complementary generative mechanisms—such as VAE-GAN hybrids that balance distributional fidelity and realism—to enhance biological accuracy. In federated learning, model parameters are trained collaboratively across decentralized datasets hosted by different institutions without exchanging sensitive data, ensuring compliance with data protection regulations like GDPR and HIPAA. Synthetic data can serve as intermediaries in federated systems, enabling local models to share statistical insights rather than raw samples. This integration is particularly valuable in precision medicine, where multi-institutional collaboration is necessary to achieve robust model generalization across diverse patient populations. By combining generative modeling with privacy-preserving computation (e.g., differential privacy or secure aggregation), hybrid and federated frameworks pave the way toward scalable, ethical, and equitable biomedical AI systems (Guan et al., 2024).

Evaluation Metrics

Evaluating synthetic genomic and omic data requires a multi-dimensional framework that balances statistical fidelity, biological plausibility, and privacy protection—each of which determines the practical usability and ethical safety of synthetic datasets in biomedical research. The evaluation process not only measures the similarity between real and synthetic data distributions but also ensures that generated datasets preserve essential biological signals while minimizing the risk of re-identification or information leakage. As synthetic data become increasingly integrated into biomedical pipelines, transparent, quantitative, and standardized evaluation metrics are critical for benchmarking their reliability and trustworthiness.

Statistical Fidelity

Statistical fidelity metrics assess how well synthetic data replicate the statistical properties of real datasets. These include univariate and multivariate distributional similarity measures, such as Jensen–Shannon Divergence (JSD), Kullback–Leibler Divergence (KLD), Earth Mover's Distance (EMD), and Kolmogorov–Smirnov (KS) tests that compare feature-wise or joint probability distributions. For high-dimensional omic data, Principal Component Analysis (PCA) or Uniform Manifold Approximation and Projection (UMAP) embeddings are used to visualize global structure and ensure that real and synthetic samples overlap in latent space (Marouf et al., 2020). In genomic contexts, metrics such as allele frequency spectra, linkage disequilibrium (LD) decay curves, and haplotype block concordance are particularly informative for evaluating whether synthetic genotypes preserve population-level structure and correlations (Yelmen et al., 2021). Furthermore, correlation matrices or Mutual Information (MI) estimates across features can quantify the extent to which dependencies among genes, proteins, or metabolites are retained. High statistical fidelity implies that the generative model effectively captures the underlying data manifold without overfitting or memorizing individual records.

Biological Plausibility

Beyond statistical similarity, synthetic omic data must retain biologically meaningful relationships and dynamics that are relevant to the underlying system being modeled. Biological plausibility evaluates whether generated data maintain gene–gene, protein–protein, or metabolite–metabolite interaction networks consistent with known biological knowledge. For example, synthetic transcriptomic data should reproduce co-expression modules observed in real samples, while proteomic data should reflect pathway-level abundance correlations. Network-based analyses, such as graph similarity indices, module preservation statistics, and enrichment consistency tests (e.g., via Gene Ontology or KEGG pathways), are used to verify that generated datasets uphold biological interpretability (Lopez et al., 2018). In single-cell applications, cluster integrity and marker gene conservation are assessed using Adjusted Rand Index (ARI), Silhouette Scores, and Differential Expression Concordance. These biological validation steps ensure that synthetic datasets are not only statistically realistic but also mechanistically coherent—an essential criterion for downstream analyses like biomarker discovery and drug response modeling.

Privacy Risk Assessment

Since one of the core motivations for generating synthetic biomedical data is privacy preservation, it is essential to rigorously quantify and mitigate re-identification risks. Privacy evaluation involves determining whether synthetic data unintentionally expose information traceable to individuals in the training set. Standard methods include membership inference attacks (MIA), where adversaries attempt to infer if a particular sample was part of the original dataset, and attribute inference attacks, which test whether sensitive features can be reconstructed. Tools such as distance-based record linkage (e.g., Euclidean or Hamming distance thresholds) and nearest-neighbor overlap ratios can estimate how closely synthetic samples resemble real individuals (Yoon et al., 2020). Differential privacy frameworks further formalize privacy guarantees by bounding the information leakage during model training using parameters (ε, δ), with smaller ε indicating stronger privacy protection. In biomedical contexts, achieving a balance between data utility and privacy—where synthetic datasets remain analytically valuable yet untraceable—is the gold standard.

Utility and Downstream Task Evaluation

A final layer of evaluation involves measuring the practical utility of synthetic data in real analytical workflows. This is achieved by substituting synthetic data for real data in predictive or inferential pipelines and comparing performance metrics such as accuracy, AUROC, F1-score, and precision-recall across models. For instance, classifiers trained on synthetic transcriptomic data should yield comparable predictive accuracy for disease vs. control classification tasks as those trained on real data, indicating that relevant biological signal has been preserved (Gonçalves et al., 2020). Similarly, in genomics, synthetic genotype matrices can be tested in Genome-Wide Association Study (GWAS) pipelines to assess whether significant loci identified in real data are recoverable from synthetic samples (Chakraborty et al., 2023). High concordance between real and synthetic analytical outcomes signals strong functional equivalence—a key determinant for adoption in precision medicine research and federated learning environments.

Validation in Biomedical Pipelines

Validation represents the crucial translational phase where synthetic omic data are evaluated within real-world biomedical pipelines to ensure their practical utility, biological relevance, and compliance with ethical and regulatory standards. Unlike quantitative evaluation metrics, validation within biomedical contexts emphasizes end-to-end usability—how well synthetic datasets integrate into genomic association studies, predictive modeling workflows, and precision medicine applications. One major validation pathway involves incorporating synthetic data into Genome-Wide Association Studies (GWAS) or fine-mapping analyses, comparing downstream results with those derived from real data. High concordance in allele frequency distributions, linkage disequilibrium structures, and identified risk loci supports biological plausibility and indicates minimal distortion of genomic patterns (Chakraborty et al., 2023).

In predictive modeling tasks, such as disease classification, drug response prediction, or biomarker discovery, synthetic datasets are used to augment limited real-world training cohorts. Performance consistency between models trained on synthetic and real data—measured through accuracy, AUROC, or precision-recall curves—demonstrates transferability and generalization capacity (Chen et al., 2021). Cross-domain validation, where synthetic transcriptomic or proteomic data are integrated with orthogonal datasets (e.g., imaging or clinical metadata), tests interoperability and the preservation of multi-omic correlations. Furthermore, federated validation frameworks allow benchmarking synthetic data across institutions without centralizing sensitive datasets, reinforcing privacy-preserving collaborative research (Rieke et al., 2020).

Validation also extends to ethical and regulatory compliance, particularly under frameworks such as the General Data Protection Regulation (GDPR) and the Health Insurance Portability and Accountability Act (HIPAA), where synthetic datasets must demonstrate sufficient privacy guarantees. Biological experts further assess interpretability by verifying whether gene regulatory networks, protein–protein interaction patterns, or metabolomic clusters generated from synthetic data correspond to known biological mechanisms. Ultimately, validation within biomedical pipelines ensures that synthetic omic data are not only statistically consistent but also biologically informative, ethically compliant, and ready for deployment in clinical and translational research settings (Yelmen et al., 2021; Goncalves et al., 2020).

DISCUSSION

Applications in Precision Medicine

Synthetic genomic and omic data have emerged as transformative tools in precision medicine, offering scalable and ethically compliant solutions for data-driven healthcare. In disease risk prediction, synthetic single-nucleotide polymorphism (SNP) datasets help address the chronic underrepresentation of non-European populations in genomic studies, thereby improving model robustness and fairness across diverse ancestries (Chakraborty et al., 2023). By expanding training cohorts with synthetic genomes that preserve allele frequency distributions and linkage disequilibrium patterns, predictive algorithms achieve better calibration for rare or population-specific variants. In drug discovery, synthetic transcriptomic profiles simulate cellular responses to candidate compounds, enabling early estimation of drug efficacy and toxicity before in vitro or in vivo validation (Zhavoronkov et al., 2019). Such simulated responses support mechanism-of-action exploration and reduce laboratory costs associated with early-phase screening. Furthermore, in clinical trial simulation, synthetic patient cohorts replicate heterogeneous clinical and omic profiles, facilitating virtual trial design optimization, power analysis, and recruitment feasibility assessments (Walsh et al., 2022). These applications demonstrate how synthetic data expand the translational reach of computational biology in precision medicine pipelines.

Enhancing Data Diversity and Balance

A key advantage of synthetic data generation lies in its ability to address data imbalance and diversity limitations in biomedical datasets. Rare diseases, minority genomic subpopulations, and underrepresented tissue types often suffer from limited sample availability, leading to biased or underperforming predictive models. Generative frameworks such as GANs and diffusion models mitigate this issue by producing biologically plausible synthetic samples that expand minority classes while preserving authentic data distributions (Benaim et al., 2023). Augmented datasets have shown improved model generalization across heterogeneous populations and reduced overfitting to dominant phenotypic clusters. Moreover, cross-omics data synthesis—where transcriptomic data are generated conditionally on genomic or proteomic features—enhances biological coherence and ensures that inter-layer variability reflects realistic physiological patterns. This capacity to create balanced, representative datasets is essential for equitable precision medicine, where population-level inclusivity and model fairness are critical scientific and ethical imperatives.

Privacy-Preserving Data Sharing

Privacy remains a major constraint in genomic research due to the high re-identifiability of individual sequences. Synthetic omics data offer a promising solution by enabling data sharing without exposing sensitive personal information. By generating datasets that maintain global statistical properties while removing individual-level identifiers, institutions can share genomic and clinical information across borders in compliance with GDPR, HIPAA, and other privacy frameworks (Bogdanovic et al., 2024). Integration of differential privacy mechanisms—such as noise injection in latent spaces or parameter-level regularization—further strengthens anonymity while preserving analytical utility (Abay et al., 2018). These privacy-preserving synthetic datasets support global biomedical collaboration, allowing researchers to jointly develop predictive models, validate biomarkers, and replicate studies without violating patient confidentiality. This paradigm fosters open innovation and accelerates translational research, especially in international consortia and multi-institutional projects where direct data sharing is otherwise restricted.

Challenges and Limitations

Despite substantial progress, synthetic omic data generation faces notable scientific and operational challenges. Ensuring biological realism in high-dimensional, multi-layered data remains difficult, as generative models may oversimplify non-linear dependencies or introduce artificial correlations. Maintaining multi-omics coherence—for example, ensuring that synthetic transcriptomic or proteomic layers are biologically consistent with underlying genomic variations—requires advanced conditional modeling and integrative architectures (Xu et al., 2023). Synthetic artifacts such as implausible gene expression patterns or unrealistic variant frequencies can distort downstream analyses, highlighting the need for rigorous validation pipelines. Moreover, standardization gaps persist: there is no universally accepted benchmark or quality metric for evaluating synthetic biological datasets across studies or platforms. This hinders reproducibility and cross-comparability, limiting clinical translation.

Addressing these limitations calls for concerted efforts toward community-driven standards, harmonized evaluation protocols, and transparent model reporting.

Integrative Potential with AI-Driven Medicine

The future of synthetic omic data lies in its integration with AI-driven biomedical systems. As large language models (LLMs) and multi-modal transformers increasingly incorporate biological and clinical data, synthetic omic datasets will serve as indispensable training resources, ensuring diversity, scalability, and compliance in AI model development (He et al., 2024). For instance, digital twin systems—virtual representations of individual patients—can leverage synthetic genomic and transcriptomic data to simulate disease trajectories and personalize treatment recommendations. In diagnostic applications, AI models trained on hybrid real-synthetic datasets demonstrate enhanced interpretability and resilience to data scarcity. Synthetic data also facilitates continuous model updating without exposing protected health information, supporting adaptive learning in clinical environments. This synergy between synthetic biology and artificial intelligence is poised to redefine precision medicine, enabling ethically responsible, data-rich innovation in diagnostics, therapeutics, and personalized care.

CONCLUSION AND FUTURE DIRECTIONS

Synthetic genomic and omic data represent a transformative evolution in the landscape of precision medicine, systems biology, and biomedical data science. Through the application of advanced generative models—such as GANs, VAEs, and diffusion architectures—researchers can now produce high-fidelity biological datasets that capture the complex distributions and dependencies inherent in real omic profiles. These synthetic datasets enable the development and validation of predictive algorithms in scenarios where access to authentic data is restricted by privacy, ethical, or logistical constraints. By creating realistic, scalable, and representative datasets, synthetic biology bridges critical data gaps, supporting equitable participation in genomic research and enhancing the reproducibility of biomedical findings across diverse populations.

Beyond accessibility, synthetic omic data underpin a new paradigm of responsible data innovation, balancing discovery potential with the imperative of privacy preservation. The capacity to share and analyze synthetic data without compromising individual identity safeguards fosters an environment of open collaboration across institutions, nations, and disciplines. Integrating differential privacy, federated learning, and secure generative frameworks ensures that synthetic datasets maintain statistical and biological fidelity while remaining resistant to re-identification or adversarial exploitation. This paradigm shift empowers the scientific community to move from data scarcity and silos toward an ecosystem of ethically governed, computationally enriched knowledge exchange.

Looking ahead, future research directions emphasize the integration of multi-omics and longitudinal data generation frameworks. Synthetic modeling that simultaneously captures genomic, transcriptomic, proteomic, and metabolomic layers will enable more holistic simulations of cellular systems and disease mechanisms. Similarly, the capacity to model temporal dynamics—representing disease progression, treatment response, or environmental influence over time—will significantly enhance clinical and translational applications. The incorporation of biologically informed priors into generative architectures, such as embedding pathway maps, regulatory networks, or spatial transcriptomic context, will produce models that are not only statistically accurate but also mechanistically interpretable. These advances will transform synthetic data generation from a purely statistical task into a truly biological modeling endeavor.

However, realizing the full potential of synthetic omic data requires a parallel evolution in regulatory, ethical, and methodological frameworks. Establishing international standards for data validation, benchmarking, and interpretability is essential for ensuring cross-study comparability and scientific integrity. Ethical guidelines must delineate acceptable use cases, governance structures, and oversight mechanisms for synthetic biomedical data—particularly as these datasets become more realistic and potentially re-identifiable. Collaborative initiatives involving academia, industry, and regulatory agencies will be vital to ensure that synthetic data ecosystems align with public trust and societal benefit.

REFERENCES

Adrion, J. R., Cole, C. B., Dukler, N., Galloway, J. G., Gladstein, A. L., Gower, G., Kyriazis, C. C., Ragsdale, A. P., Tsambos, G., Baumdicker, F., Carlson, J., Cartwright, R. A., Durvasula, A., Gronau, I., Kim, B. Y., McKenzie, P., Messer, P. W., Noskova, E., Del Vecchyo, D. O., & Kern, A. D. (2020). A community-maintained standard library of population genetic models. *eLife*, *9*, e54967. Advance online publication. DOI: 10.7554/eLife.54967 PMID: 32573438

Athieniti, E., & Spyrou, G. M. (2023). A guide to multi-omics data collection and integration for translational medicine. In *Computational and Structural Biotechnology Journal* (Vol. 21). DOI: 10.1016/j.csbj.2022.11.050

Baião, A. R., Cai, Z., Poulos, R. C., Robinson, P. J., Reddel, R. R., Zhong, Q., Vinga, S., & Gonçalves, E. (2025). A technical review of multi-omics data integration methods: From classical statistical to deep generative approaches. *Briefings in Bioinformatics*, *26*(4), bbaf355. Advance online publication. DOI: 10.1093/bib/bbaf355 PMID: 40748323

Beaulieu-Jones, B. K., Wu, Z. S., Williams, C., Lee, R., Bhavnani, S. P., Byrd, J. B., & Greene, C. S. (2019). Privacy-preserving generative deep neural networks support clinical data sharing. *Circulation: Cardiovascular Quality and Outcomes*, *12*(7), e005122. Advance online publication. DOI: 10.1161/CIRCOUTCOMES.118.005122 PMID: 31284738

Cavinato, T., Rubinacci, S., Malaspinas, A. S., & Delaneau, O. (2024). A resampling-based approach to share reference panels. *Nature Computational Science*, *4*(5), 360–366. DOI: 10.1038/s43588-024-00630-7 PMID: 38745108

Figueira, A., & Vaz, B. (2022). Survey on Synthetic Data Generation, Evaluation Methods and GANs. *Mathematics 2022, Vol. 10, Page 2733*, *10*(15), 2733. DOI: 10.3390/math10152733

Francesca, T. (2019). *Comparing privacy laws: GDPR v. CCPA*. https://futurium.ec.europa.eu/en/european-ai-alliance/open-library/comparing-privacy-laws-gdpr-v-ccpa

Goncalves, A., Ray, P., Soper, B., Stevens, J., Coyle, L., & Sales, A. P. (2020). Generation and evaluation of synthetic patient data. *BMC Medical Research Methodology*, *20*(1), 108. Advance online publication. DOI: 10.1186/s12874-020-00977-1 PMID: 32381039

Goodfellow, I. J., Pouget-Abadie, J., Mirza, M., Xu, B., Warde-Farley, D., Ozair, S., Courville, A., & Bengio, Y. (2014). Generative Adversarial Nets. *Advances in Neural Information Processing Systems, 27.* https://www.github.com/goodfeli/adversarial

Groß, B., & Wunder, G. (2023). Differentially private synthetic data generation via lipschitz-regularised variational autoencoders. *2023 IEEE Smart World Congress (SWC)*, 1–8.

Guan, H., Yap, P. T., Bozoki, A., & Liu, M. (2024). Federated learning for medical image analysis: A survey. In *Pattern Recognition* (Vol. 151). DOI: 10.1016/j.patcog.2024.110424

Ho, J., Jain, A., & Abbeel, P. (2020). Denoising diffusion probabilistic models. *Advances in Neural Information Processing Systems, 2020-December.*

Jumper, J., Evans, R., Pritzel, A., Green, T., Figurnov, M., Ronneberger, O., Tunyasuvunakool, K., Bates, R., Žídek, A., Potapenko, A., Bridgland, A., Meyer, C., Kohl, S. A. A., Ballard, A. J., Cowie, A., Romera-Paredes, B., Nikolov, S., Jain, R., Adler, J., & Hassabis, D. (2021). Highly accurate protein structure prediction with AlphaFold. *Nature*, *596*(7873), 583–589. Advance online publication. DOI: 10.1038/s41586-021-03819-2 PMID: 34265844

Kenneweg, P., Dandinasivara, R., Luo, X., Hammer, B., & Schönhuth, A. (2024). Generating Synthetic Genotypes using Diffusion Models. *ArXiv Preprint ArXiv:2412.03278.*

Kingma, D. P., & Welling, M. (2014). Auto-encoding variational bayes. *2nd International Conference on Learning Representations, ICLR 2014 - Conference Track Proceedings*. DOI: 10.61603/ceas.v2i1.33

Kiran, A., & Kumar, S. S. (2023). A Comparative Analysis of GAN and VAE based Synthetic Data Generators for High Dimensional, Imbalanced Tabular data. *2023 2nd International Conference for Innovation in Technology, INOCON 2023*. DOI: 10.1109/INOCON57975.2023.10101315

Kiran, A., Rubini, P., & Kumar, S. S. (2025). Comprehensive Review of Privacy, Utility, and Fairness Offered by Synthetic Data. *IEEE Access : Practical Innovations, Open Solutions*, *13*, 15795–15811. DOI: 10.1109/ACCESS.2025.3532128

Leeming, M. G., Ang, C. S., Nie, S., Varshney, S., & Williamson, N. A. (2023). Simulation of mass spectrometry-based proteomics data with Synthedia. *Bioinformatics Advances*, *3*(1), vbac096. Advance online publication. DOI: 10.1093/bioadv/vbac096 PMID: 36698761

Little, C., Elliot, M., & Allmendinger, R. (2023). Federated learning for generating synthetic data: A scoping review. *International Journal of Population Data Science, 8*(1), 2158. DOI: 10.23889/ijpds.v8i1.2158 PMID: 38414544

Lopez, R., Regier, J., Cole, M. B., Jordan, M. I., & Yosef, N. (2018). Deep generative modeling for single-cell transcriptomics. *Nature Methods, 15*(12), 1053–1058. Advance online publication. DOI: 10.1038/s41592-018-0229-2 PMID: 30504886

Luo, J., Yang, L., Liu, Y., Hu, C., Wang, G., Yang, Y., Yang, T.-L., & Zhou, X. (2025). Review of diffusion models and its applications in biomedical informatics. *BMC Medical Informatics and Decision Making 2025 25:1, 25*(1), 1–21. DOI: 10.1186/s12911-025-03210-5

Lutkevich, B. (2019). What is HIPAA (Health Insurance Portability and Accountability Act)? In *WhatIs.com.*

Marouf, M., Machart, P., Bansal, V., Kilian, C., Magruder, D. S., Krebs, C. F., & Bonn, S. (2020). Realistic in silico generation and augmentation of single-cell RNA-seq data using generative adversarial networks. *Nature Communications, 11*(1), 166. Advance online publication. DOI: 10.1038/s41467-019-14018-z PMID: 31919373

Moon, K. R., van Dijk, D., Wang, Z., Gigante, S., Burkhardt, D. B., Chen, W. S., Yim, K., van den Elzen, A., Hirn, M. J., Coifman, R. R., Ivanova, N. B., Wolf, G., & Krishnaswamy, S. (2019). Visualizing structure and transitions in high-dimensional biological data. *Nature Biotechnology, 37*(12), 1482–1492. Advance online publication. DOI: 10.1038/s41587-019-0336-3 PMID: 31796933

Murtaza, H., Ahmed, M., Khan, N. F., Murtaza, G., Zafar, S., & Bano, A. (2023). Synthetic data generation: State of the art in health care domain. In *Computer Science Review* (Vol. 48). DOI: 10.1016/j.cosrev.2023.100546

Neely, B. A., Dorfer, V., Martens, L., Bludau, I., Bouwmeester, R., Degroeve, S., Deutsch, E. W., Gessulat, S., Käll, L., Palczynski, P., Payne, S. H., Rehfeldt, T. G., Schmidt, T., Schwämmle, V., Uszkoreit, J., Vizcaíno, J. A., Wilhelm, M., & Palmblad, M. (2023). Toward an Integrated Machine Learning Model of a Proteomics Experiment. In *Journal of Proteome Research* (Vol. 22, Issue 3). DOI: 10.1021/acs.jproteome.2c00711

Oprisanu, B., Ganev, G., & De Cristofaro, E. (2022). On Utility and Privacy in Synthetic Genomic Data. *29th Annual Network and Distributed System Security Symposium, NDSS 2022*. DOI: 10.14722/ndss.2022.24092

Pezoulas, V. C., Zaridis, D. I., Mylona, E., Androutsos, C., Apostolidis, K., Tachos, N. S., & Fotiadis, D. I. (2024). Synthetic data generation methods in healthcare: A review on open-source tools and methods. *Computational and Structural Biotechnology Journal, 23,* 2892–2910. DOI: 10.1016/j.csbj.2024.07.005 PMID: 39108677

Price, W. N., & Cohen, I. G. (2019). Privacy in the age of medical big data. In *Nature Medicine* (Vol. 25, Issue 1). DOI: 10.1038/s41591-018-0272-7

Rajotte, J. F., Bergen, R., Buckeridge, D. L., El Emam, K., Ng, R., & Strome, E. (2022). Synthetic data as an enabler for machine learning applications in medicine. In *iScience* (Vol. 25, Issue 11). DOI: 10.1016/j.isci.2022.105331

Rao, R., Liu, J., Verkuil, R., Meier, J., Canny, J. F., Abbeel, P., Sercu, T., & Rives, A. (2021). MSA Transformer. *BioRxiv*, 2021.02.12.430858. DOI: 10.1101/2021.02.12.430858

Said, A., Yahyaoui, A., & Abdellatif, T. (2024). HIPAA and GDPR Compliance in IoT Healthcare Systems. *Communications in Computer and Information Science, 2071 CCIS*, 198–209. DOI: 10.1007/978-3-031-55729-3_16

Shakola, F., Palejev, D., & Ivanov, I. (2022). A Framework for Comparison and Assessment of Synthetic RNA-Seq Data. *Genes*, *13*(12), 2362. Advance online publication. DOI: 10.3390/genes13122362 PMID: 36553629

van Breugel, B., Liu, T., Oglic, D., & van der Schaar, M. (2024). Synthetic data in biomedicine via generative artificial intelligence. *Nature Reviews Bioengineering*, *2*(12), 991–1004. DOI: 10.1038/s44222-024-00245-7

Voigt, P., & Von dem Bussche, A. (2017). The EU General Data Protection Regulation (GDPR): A Practical Guide. In *The EU General Data Protection Regulation (GDPR): a Practical Guide*. DOI: 10.1007/978-3-319-57959-7

Walonoski, J., Kramer, M., Nichols, J., Quina, A., Moesel, C., Hall, D., Duffett, C., Dube, K., Gallagher, T., & McLachlan, S. (2018). Synthea: An approach, method, and software mechanism for generating synthetic patients and the synthetic electronic health care record. *Journal of the American Medical Informatics Association : JAMIA*, *25*(3), 230–238. Advance online publication. DOI: 10.1093/jamia/ocx079 PMID: 29025144

Wandy, J., McBride, R., Rogers, S., Terzis, N., Weidt, S., van der Hooft, J. J. J., Bryson, K., Daly, R., & Davies, V. (2023). Simulated-to-real benchmarking of acquisition methods in untargeted metabolomics. *Frontiers in Molecular Biosciences*, *10*, 1130781. Advance online publication. DOI: 10.3389/fmolb.2023.1130781 PMID: 36959982

Way, G. P., & Greene, C. S. (2018). Extracting a biologically relevant latent space from cancer transcriptomes with variational autoencoders. *Pacific Symposium on Biocomputing*, *0*(212669), 80–91. Advance online publication. DOI: 10.1142/9789813235533_0008 PMID: 29218871

Yelmen, B., Decelle, A., Ongaro, L., Marnetto, D., Tallec, C., Montinaro, F., Furtlehner, C., Pagani, L., & Jay, F. (2021). Creating artificial human genomes using generative neural networks. *PLOS Genetics*, *17*(2), e1009303. Advance online publication. DOI: 10.1371/journal.pgen.1009303 PMID: 33539374

Zhang, Z., Yan, C., & Malin, B. A. (2022). Membership inference attacks against synthetic health data. *Journal of Biomedical Informatics*, *125*, 103977. Advance online publication. DOI: 10.1016/j.jbi.2021.103977 PMID: 34920126

Chapter 3
Synthetic Healthcare Data in Generation, Validation, and Integration for Ethical and Scalable Health Innovation

Shaikat Das Joy
https://orcid.org/0009-0001-1657-3140
American International University-Bangladesh, Bangladesh

Noboranjan Dey
https://orcid.org/0009-0007-1991-9198
American International University-Bangladesh, Bangladesh

Md. Reazul Islam
University at Albany, State University of New York, USA

Mirza Asif Mahmud
https://orcid.org/0009-0006-6947-4003
American International University-Bangladesh, Bangladesh

Mahfujur Rahman
https://orcid.org/0000-0002-3245-8767
American International University-Bangladesh, Bangladesh

Kazi Tanvir
https://orcid.org/0009-0001-0612-6101
American International University-Bangladesh, Bangladesh

Dipta Gomes
https://orcid.org/0000-0003-3019-6051
American International University-Bangladesh, Bangladesh

ABSTRACT

Synthetic healthcare data offers a transformative solution to the privacy and accessibility constraints of real patient data. This chapter comprehensively examines its

DOI: 10.4018/979-8-3373-5641-9.ch003

generation, from traditional statistical methods to advanced AI like GANs, VAEs, and Transformers. It explores critical applications in clinical trial simulation, medical imaging, and AI training. The analysis extends beyond technology to address pivotal barriers: ethical concerns of bias, evolving GDPR/HIPAA regulations, validation challenges, and interoperability with systems like HL7 FHIR. It concludes that responsible adoption hinges on merging technical rigor with ethical governance and cross-disciplinary collaboration to build trustworthy, innovative digital health ecosystems.

1. INTRODUCTION

The increasing dependence on data-driven decision-making in healthcare, from clinical research to Artificial Intelligence (AI)-enhanced diagnostics and public health initiatives, has elevated the demand for comprehensive, high-quality health data. However, the ethical, legal, and logistical issues that come with collecting and sharing real patient data are major concerns and pose fundamental research challenges. Privacy concerns, strict regulations (*GDPR*, 2016), requirements for patient consent, and institutional data silos often hinder researchers, physicians, and developers from accessing essential data necessary for innovation (Gonzales et al., 2023). Synthetic healthcare data has emerged as a promising alternative approach that preserves the statistical characteristics of real data while reducing the risks associated with personally identifiable information (Bhanot et al., 2021).

This chapter begins by reviewing the most recent methods for generating synthetic healthcare data, including both AI-driven and conventional approaches. Following the exploration of traditional methods such as statistical modeling, multiple imputation, agent-based modeling, and probabilistic simulations, the discussion transitions to innovative AI-powered techniques transforming synthetic data generation. The performance of Transformer-based models, Variational Autoencoders (VAEs), and Generative Adversarial Networks (GANs) in replicating medical time-series data, clinical narratives, and Electronic Health Records (EHRs) is compared in detail (Lu et al., 2025a; Xu et al., 2019). The chapter then shifts to a thorough comparison of these methods with an emphasis on practical applications. Examples include data augmentation for machine learning models in pathology and radiology, synthetic cohorts to simulate clinical trials, and synthetic data for rare disease research where real datasets are limited. To illustrate the practical value, these examples demonstrate advantages like facilitating safe cross-institutional research collaborations, reducing data imbalance, and accelerating the development of AI models (Xu et al., 2019). To organize the narrative, the chapter next outlines critical barriers and considerations that are listed below:

- **Ethical Challenges:** Discusses informed consent, data provenance, and the potential misuse of synthetic data for manipulative or biased AI development. It also explores ethical questions around representational fairness, especially for underrepresented populations in source data (Seeram & Kanade, 2024).
- **Regulatory and Governance Issues:** Investigates current and emerging regulatory frameworks, including the role of synthetic data in FDA approvals, European Data Strategy guidelines, and WHO-led initiatives for ethical health data sharing (*GDPR*, 2016).
- **Validation and Trust:** Explore frameworks for data quality assessment, such as privacy-utility trade-offs, fidelity metrics, and similarity evaluations using downstream AI model performance. Emphasis is placed on the need for transparent benchmarking and reproducibility (Bhanot et al., 2021).
- **Integration into Real-World Systems:** Reviews interoperability challenges with existing health information systems, including HL7 FHIR and DICOM standards. Real-world examples include the use of synthetic patient records for training clinical decision support systems (CDSS), federated learning environments for AI training, and national synthetic health datasets for epidemiological simulations (Knevel & Liao, 2023).
- **Public and Professional Perception:** Finally, the chapter reflects on the societal dimensions of synthetic data. Public trust, clinician acceptance, and transparency in data labeling (i.e., clearly distinguishing synthetic vs. real data) are critical to ethical deployment. The chapter examines survey studies and user feedback from healthcare professionals, highlighting perceived risks and expectations related to the use of synthetic data in clinical environments (Gonzales et al., 2023).

Throughout the chapter, emphasis is placed on comparative insights—not just among technical methods but across geographic, institutional, and regulatory contexts to highlight the breadth of perspectives. To further clarify, the use of synthetic data in startup environments is compared to that in government health agencies and academic hospitals, offering a multi-stakeholder perspective as the analysis moves from technical to organizational considerations.

1.1. Major Contributions

- Compare the advantages and disadvantages of contemporary AI-driven synthetic data generation methods with more conventional statistical methods.
- Offers practical case analysis for applications in public health, diagnostics, and clinical research.

- Provide insights into changing legal frameworks by critically examining ethical, regulatory, and governance issues.
- Examine interoperability tactics and validation frameworks for incorporating synthetic data into healthcare IT ecosystems.
- Examine professional and public perceptions, emphasizing issues of transparency and trust.

1.2. Chapter Organization

To guide the reader through the content, the chapter begins with motivations and challenges in data generation in Section 1, proceeds to traditional methods such as statistical modeling and rule-based simulations in Section 2, and then advances to AI-driven techniques, including GANs, VAEs, Transformers, and Large Language Models, in Section 3. Building on these methods, the narrative then explores real-world applications, including clinical trials, medical imaging, and AI/ML training, in Section 4. The chapter next transitions to ethical and privacy concerns in Section 5, regulatory and governance frameworks, including GDPR and HIPAA compliance in Section 6, and validation and trust frameworks for data quality and privacy assurance in Section 7. Section 8 further addresses interoperability and integration challenges in healthcare IT systems and standards such as HL7 FHIR and DICOM, while Section 9 covers professional and public perceptions emphasizing transparency and trust. The conclusion synthesizes insights and outlines future directions, focusing on technical, ethical, and regulatory alignment for responsible adoption of synthetic data in healthcare innovation.

2. FOUNDATIONS OF SYNTHETIC DATA IN HEALTHCARE

The promise of data-driven innovation has risen with the growing digitalization of healthcare, but high-quality patient data remains insufficient for research in a private preserving, representative way. To address these challenges, synthetic healthcare data has become a compelling solution to these problems (Giuffrè & Shung, 2023) and is thus positioned to boost research, privacy protection, and fair AI development in modern healthcare. In modern healthcare, synthetic data is becoming a backbone for queries and innovation.

Synthetic data is a critical technology in health care systems because of a high privacy protection related framework on personal health information (PHI) as HIPAA regulation in United State and GDRP regulations Community case study 1 about COVID-19 case by (Pasculli et al., 2025). With the recent and evolving regulatory frameworks regarding the use of Artificial Intelligence (AI) in both drug and medical device development, the distinction between data derived from authentic and artificial sources, and the use of process-driven and/or data-driven algorithmic processes, is emerging as a critical consideration in clinical research and regulatory discourse. A critical literature review that reveals evidence of the current ambivalence in using the term "synthetic" (and related terms) to refer to "true/observed" data in the context of clinical trials and AI-generated data (or "artificial" data). This paper, stemming from a critical evaluation of perspectives from the scientific literature and recent regulatory initiatives, seeks to elucidate this distinction by exploring their respective utilities, regulatory stances, and emerging needs, as well as the potential of both data types to advance medical science and therapeutic development. Synthetic data fills that gap by enabling data sharing without raising concerns about patient privacy.

2.1. Definition and Types of Synthetic Data

Synthetic Healthcare Data is information that closely resembles real-world health data in terms of distributional and structural characteristics but does not in any way reveal the details of any particular individual or breach any private health information (Yan et al., 2022). Such data can include information as benign as patients' demographic details, medical and social histories, diagnoses, laboratory values, and medication administration records, or as complex as clinical episode narratives. Unlike real anonymized data, which is derived from real patients, synthetic data is generated entirely by models trained on real data or by rule-based systems, so you cannot trace it back to the actual individuals.

2.1.1. Types of Synthetic Healthcare Data

2.1.1.1. Fully synthetic data

Data in this category is created exclusively using models trained on real patient data, with no real patient records included. These are especially well-suited when reducing re-identification risk is a core focus. Fully synthetic data is typically used in regulatory testing, algorithm benchmarking and is highly relevant for data sharing across borders (McDuff et al., 2023).

2.1.1.2. Synthetic Data

In such datasets, only the sensitive fields (e.g., diagnosis and Zip code) are generated; other columns of the database remain as is. This approach gives better fidelity; however, if not carefully evaluated can be risky for indirect re-identification (Bhanot et al., 2021).

2.1.1.3. Hybrid Data

It is a mixture of real and synthetic records used to enrich datasets. The approach is especially useful for underrepresented diseases and rare events with little or no real data (Prasanna Das et al., 2022). Hybrid-data is also used to solve class imbalance in machine learning (ML) tasks.

There are several criteria that high-quality synthetic data must meet to remain useful, secure, and ethically sound as presented in Table 1.

2.2. Comparison with Traditional Anonymization Techniques

Conventional approaches, such as anonymization, redaction, or pseudonymization, suppress direct identifiers but are inevitably susceptible to linkage attacks that exploit quasi-identifiers in auxiliary datasets (Mikel Hernandez et al., 2022). Conversely, synthetic data is completely new records that do not belong to anyone. It offers better privacy if the synthetic model is strong. Meanwhile, not all synthetic data is GDPR- or HIPAA-compliant. It is possible that synthetic data, even if only allowing indirect identification, can still be defined as personal data under regulatory frameworks. As such, synthetic datasets should be assessed biometrically using privacy risk assessment frameworks.

Old techniques are easier and simpler to implement, but they still will not cut it in the current privacy threat model. Linkage attacks on major data or in combination with auxiliary information can accurately re-identify individuals in de-identified datasets (Jadon & Kumar, 2023). Comparison between the Synthetic and Traditional approaches is provided in Table 2.

Table 1. Essential Features of Synthetic Healthcare Data

Feature	Explanation
Statistical Fidelity	Retains Distributions, Correlations and Clinical Sensibility (e.g. Disease-Age Relation) Correlation analysis, the distributional similarity tests, utility metrics are tools to measure this (Lu et al., 2025)
Privacy Preservation	Does not require memorization of real records as in differential privacy or PATE-GAN (Gonzales et al., 2023)
Fairness and Bias Control	Guarantees fair participation in all populations, especially of the most at-risk individuals (Rujas et al., 2025).
Completeness and Scalability	Enables the creation of large, diverse, and geographically representative datasets, even for rare diseases.
Provenance and Documentation	Open disclosure of how the data was generated, how these parameters are computed, and what exactly this type of data is used for (Yan et al., 2022).

2.3. Regulatory and Ethical Pressures to Adopt

2.3.1. GDPR (EU)

GDPR permits getting away from the compliance obligations when data is truly anonymized. The non-identifiability of synthetic data, even when combined with auxiliary data, is an example (Pasculli et al., 2025).

2.3.2. HIPAA (USA)

The synthetic data that do not have PHI, is out of the scope of HIPAA. This permits multiset data collection for research involving multiple centers (Giuffrè & Shung, 2023).

2.3.3. Ethical Considerations:

- Fuller access to data facilitates the development of AI that can be have more inclusive deployments by breaking through institutional data silos (Gonzales et al., 2023).
- Reduces patient burden by cutting back on redundant data collection.
- Allows for more balanced AI as it has constructs of minority by using synthetic mine examples and facilitating demographic parity (Prasanna Das et al., 2022).
- Strengthens research equity by leveling the playing field for low-resource settings in accessing datasets.

In general, to prevent misuse of synthetic data, we need a proper governance model in place. Model card disclosures, such as waivers, validation protocols, and audit mechanisms for consent, should be fully aligned with Responsible AI guidelines and data stewardship principles. Furthermore, globally standardized guidelines are required to validate and certify synthetic datasets for clinical purposes, as discussed in the research (Yan et al., 2022).

Table 2. Synthetic Data vs Traditional Data

Attribute	Traditional Anonymization	Synthetic Data
Risk of Re-identification	High, particularly when linking assaults are present.	Low (if correctly generated)
Utility for ML	Often diminished because of disguising	High: maintains key patterns
Guarantees of Privacy	Weak (based on heuristics)	Robust (statistical and model-based)
Exemption from Regulation	Hardly allowed	With validation, exempt
Adaptability in Sharing	Limited because of problems with compliance	High (fit for release to the public)

3. TECHNIQUES FOR GENERATING SYNTHETIC HEALTHCARE DATA

The process of generating synthetic healthcare data spans a wide range, from simple statistical simulations to advanced AI-based generative models. The better approach would also differ across use cases, depending on the type of healthcare dataset, the level of privacy guarantees required, and the intended application (Lu et al., 2025).

3.1. Paradigms of Synthetic Data Generation

There are two main paradigms guiding the current trend for synthetic data generation:

1. Traditional Statistical Methods
2. Simulation-Based Approaches

3.1.1. Traditional Statistical Methods

One of the earliest and most widely used methods for generating synthetic healthcare data is statistical modeling and imputation. These are called parameter resampling methods, which consist of fitting statistical distributions to the observed data and generating new samples based on the estimated parameters. The method outputs synthetic data that preserves the statistical properties of the original dataset while protecting individual-level information. A common example is simulating continuous healthcare variables, such as lab test results or vital signs, with multivariate normal distributions. Synthetic records are generated using a Gaussian copula to preserve the correlations among variables. One type of imputation is regression-based missing data techniques, and methods such as multiple imputation by chained equations (MICE) are widely used to fill in gaps or create full synthetic datasets from incomplete inputs observed for non-response members (Giuffrè & Shung, 2023).

Statistical modeling approaches are best applied to low-dimensional, structured data like electronic health records (EHR), and one of the most popular solutions, especially in the R language, is the synthpop package, which generates synthetic microdata that both preserves data utility and privacy. Other tools, such as Amelia and Python-based libraries like the Synthetic Data Vault (SDV) and scikit-learn, can support different forms of imputation and the creation of synthetic data. These techniques are valued for their transparency and interpretability, which are important for compliance with industry regulations and for reproducibility in science. Furthermore, these methods depend heavily on proper model selection and parameter specification, which often lead to bias (Lu et al., 2025).

3.1.2. Simulation-Based Approaches

A fundamental perspective on synthetic data generation in the healthcare sector is rule-based simulation, which uses expert-defined logic, clinical guidelines, and probabilistic decision trees to geographically represent holistic patient pathways (Dahmen & Cook, 2019).

Synthetic data generation of patient experiences from birth to death, including embedded diseases, interventions, medications, and outcomes. The ability to generate full longitudinal patient histories allows it to shine in the evaluation of healthcare IT systems, as a tool for training machine learning models and for building decision-support tools. Synthesized data is realistic and can be interpreted by domain experts, as the rules themselves are based on real clinical practices. Although it has its own strengths, rule-based systems are by no means perfect. They required a large amount of domain knowledge to set them up and maintain them, but they did not adapt well to new or unexpected data patterns. Additionally, the hardcoded rules limit the variation in generated data, which in turn influences the model's generalizability. Therefore, rule-based approaches are frequently integrated with more versatile data-driven tools to humanize synthetic datasets (Jadon & Kumar, 2023).

3.2. Generative AI Methods Using Deep Learning

3.2.1. Generative Adversarial Networks (GANs)

GANs introduce a disruptive change in the way synthetic data is currently generated by training neural networks to learn intricate patterns of real datasets (Goodfellow et al., 2016). From a general point of view, in 2014 GANs consist of two networks that compete: the generator, which attempts to generate synthetic samples that are close to real data, and the discriminator, which has been trained on both original and fake data. This process continues until the discriminator can no longer differentiate between real and generated data (Basri, 2024).

Over the years, GANs have been modified and applied to both structured and unstructured data in the healthcare domain. Models such as MedGAN are designed to generate discrete EHR data, and CTGAN improves over GAN on imbalanced and categorical tabular datasets. PATE-GAN is Privacy-Aware based on the Private Teacher Ensembles (PATE) framework and provides differential privacy guarantees, which are essential for complying with data protection regulations such as GDPR and HIPAA (Rujas et al., 2025).

Recent advancements like HealthGAN and SyncGAN are the advent of more advanced architecture that allow mechanistic analysis on multi-modal data (e.g., time-series and imaging modalities). Allowing the provision of more sophisticated manufacture of synthetic datasets reflecting clinical phenomenon. Despite the powerful capabilities of GANs, they are struggling with problems such as training instability and mode collapse (i.e., the generator only produces a limited set of data), overfitting real patient data, due to which there is a risk that privacy will be leaked (Figueira & Vaz, 2022).

Researchers use a variety of techniques to overcome these difficulties - e.g. differential privacy (McDuff et al., 2023), regularization, ensemble learning and so on. Add noise during training, clip the gradients during training too and use federated learning are further tools that can be applied while protecting sensitive confidential data, but keeping it in a useful shape.

3.2.2. Variational Autoencoders (VAEs)

Another great generative modeling approach, but this time based on probabilistic encoding and decoding. Variational Autoencoder (VAEs) learn to encode data into a summary statistic or latent space, then decode this representation with the decoder part and thus learn about the underlying distribution of your data. They are well-suited for generating continuous and high-dimensional data, like here physiological signals or imaging data.

VAEs offer more stable training dynamics compared to GANs and are less likely to collapse, making them the better alternative when it comes to modeling synthetic healthcare data. VAEs have been used in the clinical imaging domain too to generate synthetic MRI and CT scans that conform anatomical fidelity without exposing patient privacy (Rujas et al., 2025a). In fact, VAEs have been employed by researchers to generate synthetic bio signals from different modalities - such as electrocardiograms (ECGs), heart rate variability, and glucose monitoring data.

The latent space in VAEs provides a smooth and continuous profile of different patient states, transitioning from one disease state (type 1) to another (type 2), making it especially suitable for synthesizing patient trajectories or hypothetical profiles. Moreover, VAEs could be integrated with domain-specific priors or labels to yield conditional VAEs [CVAEs] improving their utility in the healthcare scenarios (Mohd Aman et al., 2021).

3.2.3. Transformers and Large Language Models (LLMs)

Transformer-based architectures have recently been introduced and have revolutionized the modeling of sequential healthcare data due to the advances that they bring into NLP. Recently, transformers were later widely adopted in EHR and time-series due to the flexible handling of irregular time, the remarkable success of it in resolving long-range dependencies (Nazera et al., 2025). These models firstly focus on adapting the transformer architecture to patient health records framing codes and visits as sequences of words and sentences (Knevel & Liao, 2023). The extensive simulation studies indicate that through fine-tuning the self-supervised implementation of these models, we can in fact generate completely synthetic sequences conforming to the probabilistic constraints specified by real EHR data. In addition, transformers can traverse the interactions between medications, diagnoses and lab results over time which further increases synthetic longitudinal dataset quality.

Large Language Models (LLMs), such as GPT-3 and GPT-4, are being adapted for healthcare. Internally, they can create artificial clinical stories, simulate discharge notes and mimic that all-important patient-doctor conversation. These capabilities can be useful when training clinical NLP models or enriching few-shot datasets for low-prevalence conditions. Still, LLMs are not perfect - they tend to hallucinate, significantly trivialize, and diverge from factual narratives and therefore can become dangerous for clinical applications. The resulting models may produce reasonable but incorrect medical content and will thus require rigorous validation (Figueira & Vaz, 2022).

However, LLMs and transformers are at the top of the current state-of-the art techniques for generating synthetic data. Structured and unstructured data can never be both seamlessly integrated, combined with their ability of holistic healthcare model does not only provide new research and education opportunities for evaluating system tests.

The choice of the technique for synthetic data generation varies depending on the type of data, as well as its purpose and constraint on privacy. Over the years traditional methods such as market research and surveying have been used but the human-scale interpretability and simplicity also mean scalability cannot be achieved; AI-driven methods have become popular; some claim they are futuristic thinking - scalable no doubt in terms of collecting data at scale which results realistic testing. Striking a balance between these two factors, a hybrid approach that utilizes domain knowledge with the power of generative modeling may offer the best resolution.

3.3. Hybrid Techniques

Early work integrating VAEs and GANs into hybrid frameworks such as the VAE-GAN or combining LLM with structured clinical data has since been established as an important strategy to improve the fidelity, generalization, and diversity of synthetic healthcare data. Such hybrid architecture strikes a balance, as much generative power as possible, with the right amount of control, for addressing both data realism and privacy preservation. For example, VAE-GAN architecture draws upon the reliability and ordered latent space properties of VAEs along with the high-fidelity output capacity of GANs to have some steam in advancing complex modality generation - imaging and bio signals for instance. Likewise, combining LLMs with typical structured tabular data creates rich, contextual patient records but also retains clinical cohesion. Hybrid models have demonstrated the ability to enhance quality (Dahmen & Cook, 2019), interpretability, and compliance with privacy mandates. Synthetic Data Techniques by modality has been presented in Table 3.

Table 3. Synthetic Data Techniques by Modality

Modality	Preferred Technique	Rationale
Tabular EHR	CTGAN (Xu et al., 2019), MedGAN (Choi et al., 2017), PATE-GAN (Knevel & Liao, 2023; Susser et al., 2024).	Still captures categorical and numerical dependencies with privacy protection
Clinical Text	GPT-based LLMs (Brown et al., 2020; Jayun Hyun et al., 2021)	Produces summary and note with natural context of language.
Time-series/ Biosignals	Transformers (Chandra et al., 2024), SyncGAN (Pasculli et al., 2025)	Ensure temporal dependencies and signal continuity are preserved.
Multi-modal Records	HealthGAN (Mackay, 2025), LLM + Structured Input (Aldausari et al., 2023)	Includes data types for full-patient level simulations

3.4. Tools and Platforms

The effective, concrete utilization of synthetic health care data in clinical, academic, and commercial applications is being driven by several tools and platforms. Here is a comparison of several main platforms in use illustrated in Table 4.

Table 4. Tools and their Use Case

Tool	Description	Use Case
Synthea	Patient simulator based on rules	Epidemiological research and simulated medical records
MDClone	On-profit platform for artificial intelligence	Reusing data from research and hospitals
Gretel.ai	Synthetic data production pipeline from start to finish	Protecting privacy in machine learning and training datasets
HealthGAN	Framework for EHR synthesis based on GANs	Multimodal data production
SynSys	ML for Behavior and Time-Series Data	Smart healthcare simulations (Dahmen & Cook, 2019)

Although the technology driving synthetic healthcare data has advanced significantly, there are several critical challenges ahead before this frontier is responsibly and scalable realized.

Validation is one of the biggest hurdles. Yet to date, there are no widely accepted benchmarks or gold standards for measuring the expertise of synthetic data. This in turn results in variance in evaluation and credibility on all platforms for any kind of data consumption. Future work could develop community-led benchmarking frameworks and openly-accessible evaluation datasets (Yan et al., 2022b).

Another serious dilemma that lies is the bias and fairness of synthetic data. The use of synthetic data has the risk of reproducing or even magnifying the social and systemic biases contained in the original datasets. And even the synthetic data sets used in lieu of real patient data could make these biases worse without design strategies that ensure fair representation, like conditional GANs or bias-controlled loss functions. Alternatives include Bt-GAN, proposed to attenuate bias by learning from biased feedback in a way that is ostensibly fair and instance-agnostic, where demographic and outcome balancing is enforced during generation while training (Lu et al., 2025).

Explainability and transparency are the biggest issues as well. Unlike posterior seeded generator chains, deep generative models often exhibit as opaque black box procedures preventing interpretation of outputs or understanding of data generation process. Without this visible approach, HCP adoption by health institutes and subsequent regulatory approval can be limited. The practices like model cards, synthetic data audits and provenance tracking are also increasing momentum in order to encourage accountability and et traceability (Lu et al., 2025).

Another future direction would be towards the integration of synthetic data with other secure technologies. It hath been a far better literature is not suitable always for making a model robust or clinical decision. If used in conjunction with federated learning, secure multi-party computation (SMPC), or homomorphic encryption, a combination of these can enable more complete privacy-preserving pipelines. This also can enable real-time updates and distributed collaborations while ensuring data governance policies are enforced (James et al., 2021). Globally, regulatory bodies are in the process of refining their definitions of anonymized or de-identified data so synthetic data generators must be increasingly adaptive to comply. For legal defensibility, public trust (Yan et al., 2022), aligning synthetic data practices with frameworks (GDPR, HIPAA and likely yet-to-be passed AI-specific legislation) is necessary.

4. APPLICATION DOMAINS IN HEALTHCARE

Synthetic data in healthcare is increasingly viewed as a foundational element of digital health innovation, addressing the tension between data paucity and the ethical mandates of patient privacy. Based on synthetic but realistic and privacy-preserving patient profiles, clinical courses, and medical images, such processed synthetic data can provide an alternative, scalable as well and privacy-respectful data source to real data. Its use cases include the clinical research funnel, medical imaging, and AI/ML training, where it supports trial simulation, recruitment optimization, diagnostics training, algorithm validation, and privacy-preserving model development. These applications collectively demonstrate the transformative impact and challenges of synthetic data in validation, generalization, and regulatory trust.

4.1. Clinical Research

4.1.1. Trial Simulation

Now, trials are the relief upon stanchion of medical innovation, but they also suffer due to extensive timelines, expense, and lagging recruitment. Using synthetic data, in-silico trial simulations can be performed so that investigators can design studies, assess the feasibility of endpoints, and provide an estimation for statistical power calculations without the expense of real-world trial enrollment. The patient trajectories, the response to medications, and the distribution of outcomes can be replicated by generative models like GANs and VAEs. (Chandra et al., 2024) serve as evidence that ClinicalGAN can not only imitate longitudinal patient monitoring signals but also help the researchers to predict dropout rates and to evaluate drug effect observability in multi-center clinical trials. Through replicating rare adverse effects and variance amongst responders, these artificial trials decrease the likelihood of underpowered or confounded research. And, of the same importance, synthetic trial environments facilitate the examination of regulatory strategies. Organizations such as the FDA are showing an increasing willingness to consider synthetic controls if the generated cohorts are biased to truth against the real-world comparators. In addition, synthetic trial simulations act not only as methodological instruments, but as a route to regulation innovation.

4.1.2. Recruitment Optimization

Recruitment continues to be a bottleneck in clinical trials, sometimes leading to early termination of a trial due to time or cost issues. By simulating data, researchers can provide predictions of the feasibility of recruitment and effective inclusion/exclusion criteria.

(Kumar et al., 2024) developed synthetically generated recruitment cohorts based on population demographics to help sponsors predict if underrepresented groups can be included within planned timescales. The report observed that the synthetic cohorts corrected the demographic imbalances that are frequently observed in oncology studies, thus making them more applicable across a larger patient population.

In rare diseases, where patient numbers are extremely limited, the upside could be even larger. (Mishra & Venkatesh, 2024) highlighted that the use of synthetic trial datasets can supplement small patient cohorts, generating pseudo-controls to complement genuine cases. This relieves the torment of vulnerable patients yet allows for stringent statistical analysis. The optimization of recruiting cohorts with synthetic data, therefore, serves a double purpose to speed up the trial initiation and enhance clinical representation equity.

4.2. Medical Imaging

4.2.1. Synthetic Scans for Diagnostic Training

Medical images suffer from these three issues seriously, like medical data privacy and labeling cost, and data imbalance. Training radiologists or pathologists usually involves enormous pools of labeled images, but access is restricted due to confidentiality. Synthetic imaging overcomes this by creating privacy-preserving yet diagnostically valid images.

(Hanna et al., 2025) identified synthetic pathology slides as one of the frontiers in digital pathology education. Their review highlighted the potential of synthetic histopathology data to be scalable for infrequent diseases and as a means by which trainees can experience diagnostically important, yet infrequent patterns without violating patient confidentiality. Likewise, generative models have been used in radiology to generate CT/MRI images that maintain important tissue textures and anonymize specific features.

Moreover, these datasets facilitate uniform training by setting the same example to learners across the institutions, which minimizes diagnostic variation.

4.2.2. Algorithm Testing and Validation

Artificial Intelligence in imaging efforts need a big, varied, and uniform dataset to benchmark algorithms. Synthetic imaging repositories could be designed to mimic edge cases, which are underrepresented in clinical archives (e.g., a typical tumor morphology or rare pediatric cases).

(Wang et al., 2024) proposed a multimodal deep learning approach to psychiatric imaging by incorporating synthetic scans with other clinical modalities to enhance the diagnostic prediction. This synthetic multimodal dataset was well generalized to real cohorts, proving the power of synthetic data for improving cross-domain learning.

Synthetic imagery also facilitates stress testing of algorithms under controlled conditions. For instance, an algorithm for diagnosis can be evaluated on thousands of simulated rare abnormalities to evaluate its sensitivity and specificity over the range of clinical cases. This method suffers less from the scarcity and bias of real test sets.

4.3. AI/ML Model Training

4.3.1. Augmentation and Generalization

In healthcare applications, AI systems often suffer from a shortage of data, data imbalance, and biased data. A related challenge is that some data may be underrepresented relative to others, be it patient demographics, disease types, disease variants, or types of imaging modalities (when the data is for use in machine learning applications).

Synthetic data improves generalization by diversifying the training space. For instance, diabetic retinopathy datasets can be augmented with synthetic retinal scans to aid a model in diagnosing early diseases well across populations. Several studies in the clinical space (Chandra et al., 2024; Hanna et al., 2025) emphasize that GAN-based augmentation can help balance datasets, reduce overfitting, and improve robustness when models are tested across diverse clinical sites.

4.3.2. Privacy-Preserving Learning

Medical data privacy is a long-standing problem in AI training, in that even when the data is de-identified, it is possible to suffer from dataset re-identification through linkage attacks. One promising solution is synthetic data-recording, where synthetically generated patient records (statistically valid ones) are produced, and there are no direct patient identifiers.

(Hanna et al., 2025) emphasized that synthetic datasets are increasingly becoming the gold standard for privacy-preserving ML in pathology and genomics. Meanwhile, (Chandra et al., 2024) demonstrated that adversarial models can generate data that is statistically identical to real clinical signals while also being devoid of any pattern that can be used to identify the ground truth, and thus they can be used to anonymize data while preserving predictive value.

This potentially privacy-preserving feature is essential for cross-institutional cooperation. Hospitals can share synthetic data without breaking HIPAA or GDPR, facilitating worldwide AI progress without legal or ethical roadblocks.

5. CHALLENGES AND CONSIDERATIONS OF USING SYNTHETIC DATA

In these fields, generated healthcare data exhibits four common advantages:

a) Scalability: that is, allow for quick scaling up on training, validation, and training datasets.
b) Equity: to guarantee inclusion of rare diseases and of minority populations.
c) Confidentiality: Protecting patient privacy pursuant to regulations.
d) Emphasis on innovation: catalyzing the development of new research designs and algorithmic advances.

Yet challenges persist. There is an urgent need for validation frameworks that ensure synthetic data represent real-world distributions, but do not reinforce biases. The threat of distributional shift when synthetic and real data become disconnected remains a technical and ethical issue. Furthermore, regulatory approval is still developing; although synthetic controls are being well received, no universal regulatory guidelines have been implemented for validating protocols. Table 5 summarizes domains of application and main contributions of recent works related to clinical research and medical imaging. It identifies trial simulation, recruitment optimization, and algorithm testing as potential research applications, and the cost-savings, reduction in time to initiate trials, and increased robustness of algorithms as strengths of these applications.

Table 5. Application Domains and Impact of Recent Studies in Healthcare.

Studies	Domain	Application	Key Benefits
(Chandra et al., 2024)	Clinical Research in Trial Simulation	In-silico trial design, outcome prediction, and regulatory testing	Reduces costs and underpowered studies; anticipates design flaws
(Kumar et al., 2024; Mishra & Venkatesh, 2024)	Clinical Research in Recruitment Optimization	Forecasting recruitment feasibility, balancing demographics, and rare disease support	Accelerates trial initiation; improves representation equity
(Hanna et al., 2025)	Medical Imaging in Synthetic Scans	Synthetic pathology slides, radiology scans for training, and rare case exposure	Scalable training datasets; protects patient privacy
(Wang et al., 2024)	Medical Imaging in Algorithm Testing	Benchmarking algorithms, generating rare anomalies, and reproducible validation	Stress-test algorithms under controlled conditions; enhances robustness

6. CASE STUDY AND USE CASES

The integration of synthetic data into clinical and research settings has emerged as a transformative approach to address the challenges associated with real-world medical data. Synthetic data, generated through advanced computational models, replicates the statistical properties of real patient data without compromising privacy. This capability is particularly valuable in scenarios where access to real data is limited due to privacy concerns, regulatory constraints, or data scarcity.

6.1. Real-world implementation of synthetic data in a clinical or research setting

Synthetic data plays a significant role in the design and simulation of clinical trials. By creating virtual patient groups, researchers can simulate different trial scenarios and optimize key parameters such as sample size, treatment protocols, and outcome measures. This approach helps identify potential issues and refine trial protocols before actual implementation, which improves efficiency and reduces costs. The development of TrialSynth, a Variational Autoencoder (VAE) model, has shown how synthetic clinical trial data can be used to simulate complex patient trajectories and responses to treatments (Gao et al., 2024). Artificial Intelligence (AI) and Machine Learning (ML) models require large, diverse datasets for training and validation. Synthetic data serves as a valuable resource in this context by offering abundant examples that mirror real-world data distributions. This is especially important in medical imaging and electronic health records (EHRs), where annotated data is often scarce. Studies have shown that synthetic datasets can effectively train AI models for tasks such as disease classification and predictive analytics, which helps improve model robustness and generalizability (Giuffrè & Shung, 2023). Real-world medical datasets often suffer from class imbalances and biases, which can lead to skewed model predictions and compromised fairness. Synthetic data generation techniques, such as Bias-transforming Generative Adversarial Networks (Bt-GAN), have been developed to address these issues. Bt-GAN incorporates fairness constraints during data generation to make sure synthetic datasets represent diverse patient populations and reduce bias in downstream predictive models (Ramachandranpillai et al., 2024). Rare diseases and adverse events are often underrepresented in clinical datasets, which makes research and model development challenging. Synthetic data allows researchers to create comprehensive datasets that include rare conditions, which helps study these infrequent but critical health issues. By simulating a wide range of clinical scenarios, synthetic data helps develop models that can identify and predict rare events, improving patient safety and care outcomes.

6.1.1. Ethical and Regulatory Considerations

While synthetic data offers numerous advantages, its adoption in clinical and research settings requires careful consideration of ethical and regulatory aspects. It is crucial to avoid the inadvertent re-identification of individuals. Implementing robust anonymization techniques and following privacy-preserving frameworks like Differential Privacy is essential to maintain patient confidentiality. Regulatory bodies must establish clear guidelines for the use of synthetic data in clinical research to ensure consistency, transparency, and accountability. This includes defining standards for data quality, validation processes, and the ethical use of synthetic datasets in research and clinical applications (Giuffrè & Shung, 2023). The implementation of synthetic data in clinical and research settings represents a significant advancement in medical research methodologies. Synthetic data provides a way to generate realistic, privacy-preserving datasets. It helps address critical challenges like data scarcity, privacy concerns, and model bias. As technology evolves, the integration of synthetic data is set to improve the efficiency and inclusiveness of clinical research. This will lead to better patient outcomes and advancements in medical science.

6.2. Challenges faced, lessons learned, outcomes achieved.

6.2.1. GANerAid - Realistic Synthetic Patient Data for Clinical Trials

One of the major challenges in using Generative Adversarial Networks (GANs) for generating synthetic patient data is ensuring the data accurately reflects the diversity and complexity of real-world patient populations. Early implementations of GANs for clinical trials struggled to capture the full heterogeneity of patient populations, particularly in terms of disease progression, treatment responses, and demographic diversity (Akiya et al., 2024).

The lesson learned from these challenges was the importance of incorporating domain-specific clinical knowledge into the design of the GAN models. By adjusting the architecture and introducing feedback from medical experts, it became possible to generate synthetic data that better mirrored the variety and complexity seen in real clinical trials. The outcome achieved was the creation of a refined GANerAid model that generated synthetic datasets that closely matched real-world clinical trial populations. This allowed for more precise trial designs and optimized recruitment strategies, ultimately reducing the time and costs associated with clinical trials (Akiya et al., 2024).

6.2.2. Bt-GAN - Mitigating Bias in Synthetic Health Data

A significant challenge in the use of synthetic data for healthcare is the potential amplification of biases present in real-world data. Bt-GAN has been designed to address this issue by incorporating fairness constraints during data generation. However, initial attempts showed that without fairness constraints, synthetic datasets tended to over-represent certain demographic groups, leading to biased predictive models when applied to healthcare scenarios (Ramachandranpillai et al., 2024).

Fairness needs to be incorporated into the data generation process from the beginning. Advanced bias-mitigation techniques, such as score-based weighted sampling, were implemented to ensure that the synthetic data accurately represented diverse patient populations. As a result, Bt-GAN improved the fairness of predictive models by generating more balanced and representative synthetic datasets. This not only reduced bias in healthcare predictions but also helped establish trust in the use of synthetic data for healthcare applications (Ramachandranpillai et al., 2024).

6.2.3. Large Language Models (LLMs) for Generating Clinical Text Data

Generating realistic synthetic clinical text data, particularly for electronic health records (EHRs), is challenging due to the complexity and domain-specific nature of medical language. Early versions of large language models (LLMs) struggled with generating coherent and accurate clinical text, which could compromise the utility of synthetic data in training machine learning models. Without fine-tuning on healthcare-specific data, LLMs produced text that was often unrealistic or incoherent (Barr et al., 2025).

Fine-tuning LLMs with specialized healthcare data are critical for generating high-quality clinical text. After this fine-tuning, the models were able to produce realistic clinical narratives, including doctor's notes, diagnostic descriptions, and patient histories. This allowed the generation of high-quality synthetic EHR data that can be used for training AI models without compromising patient privacy. The creation of more accurate and reliable synthetic clinical data has significant potential for training predictive models, clinical decision support systems, and other healthcare applications (Barr et al., 2025). A comparison of Synthetic data Generation Techniques has been provided in Table 6.

Table 6. Comparison of Synthetic Data Generation Techniques. Challenges, Lessons, and Outcomes`

Case Study	Challenge	Lesson Learned	Outcome Achieved
GANerAid (Akiya et al., 2024)	Ensuring diversity in synthetic data	Incorporating clinical expertise into model design	Improved trial simulation accuracy and recruitment strategies
Bt-GAN (Ramachandranpillai et al., 2024)	Addressing bias in synthetic data	Integrating fairness constraints into data generation	Reduced bias in predictive models, promoting equitable healthcare
LLMs for Clinical Text (Barr et al., 2025)	Generating realistic clinical narratives	Fine-tuning models on healthcare-specific data	Enabled generation of high-quality synthetic EHR data for AI training

7. INTEGRATION INTO REAL-WORLD SYSTEMS

7.1. Interoperability with EHRs and Health Information Exchanges

Integrating synthetic healthcare data into real-world health systems necessitates achieving seamless interoperability with Electronic Health Records (EHRs) and Health Information Exchanges (HIEs). EHRs are integral to modern healthcare, storing a vast array of structured and unstructured patient data across various clinical workflows. For synthetic data to contribute meaningfully to healthcare innovations such as model training, decision support system validation, and population health analysis it must align with the standards, formats, and governance structures that define clinical systems and healthcare information exchange networks.

7.2. Standards and Data Models

To enable interoperability, synthetic datasets must comply with established healthcare data standards such as HL7 v2, HL7 Clinical Document Architecture (CDA), and the increasingly adopted Fast Healthcare Interoperability Resources (FHIR) standard. FHIR, due to its modular design, RESTful API compatibility, and resource-based representation, has emerged as the standard of choice for health data exchange in modern clinical environments (Tabari et al., 2024). It simplifies the integration of synthetic data into healthcare systems by aligning synthetic records with standardized clinical entities such as patients, encounters, and clinical observations. Mapping synthetic datasets to FHIR resources ensures data portability and reduces the need for extensive reformatting when transferring data between disparate systems.

In addition to adopting standards for data structure, interoperability also requires using controlled terminologies such as SNOMED CT, LOINC, and ICD-10 for clinical (Pezoulas et al., 2024). These standards guarantee that synthetic diagnoses, lab results, and treatment plans are semantically compatible with the healthcare system's existing vocabulary, thereby enhancing the understanding of synthetic data within clinical contexts. The integration of synthetic data with these frameworks ensures that it mirrors the richness and complexity of real patient data while remaining accessible for health professionals and computational models alike.

7.3. Integration with Health Information Exchanges

Health Information Exchanges (HIEs) are essential for enabling the secure sharing of patient data across institutions, which is critical for improving care coordination, reducing duplicative tests, and fostering population health insights (Rosenthal et al.,

2024). Synthetic data plays a pivotal role in assessing the scalability and performance of HIEs by allowing simulations of large volumes of health data to ensure that the systems can oversee diverse datasets across multiple organizational settings. These synthetic datasets provide a safe environment for exploring advanced health use cases such as predictive modeling, cohort discovery for clinical trials, and emergency management scenario simulations, without compromising real patient confidentiality.

Synthetic data integration within HIEs also allows assessing the performance of data-sharing protocols and ensures that health data flows smoothly between systems under real-world conditions. This interaction between synthetic data and HIEs facilitates system optimization and helps evaluate how well different platforms oversee the interoperability challenges that are prevalent in healthcare IT ecosystems.

7.4. Technical and Organizational Challenges

Despite the considerable potential, achieving interoperability with EHRs and HIEs is fraught with technical and organizational challenges. Many EHR systems are still siloed, using proprietary APIs and rigid data formats that complicate seamless data exchange (G. Lee et al., 2024). This lack of standardization necessitates that synthetic data generators produce FHIR-compliant bundles that also include metadata for data provenance, versioning, and transformations, ensuring traceability within integrated systems.

Moreover, healthcare organizations often face significant resource constraints when it comes to integrating and validating synthetic datasets with their existing infrastructure. These constraints are particularly pronounced in smaller or resource-limited institutions that prioritize clinical operations over IT integration efforts. As a result, collaboration between synthetic data vendors, health IT specialists, and healthcare providers is essential to overcoming these integration hurdles (Trowman et al., 2024).

7.5. Ethical and Governance Considerations

Interoperability efforts must be carefully governed to ensure that synthetic data is used ethically within health systems. Although synthetic data is de-identified, it remains critical to establish robust governance frameworks that regulate its integration with EHRs and HIEs. Key aspects of these frameworks include defining protocols for data validation, ensuring data security and privacy, and outlining the roles of external vendors in deploying synthetic data within real-world environments. Furthermore, there must be safeguards to prevent the accidental re-identification of patients, particularly when synthetic datasets are used for clinical trials or other high-stakes applications.

Governance frameworks should also address the use of synthetic data in live systems, ensuring that data integrity and quality are maintained throughout the lifecycle of its integration. Ethical concerns regarding the transparency and accountability of AI-driven decision support systems, particularly those trained on synthetic data, must be acknowledged and mitigated through clear oversight and regulatory compliance.

8. OPPORTUNITIES IN REAL WORLD SYSTEMS AND CURRENT APPROACHES

8.1. Opportunities for Scalable Health Innovation

When executed with careful consideration of the technical, organizational, and ethical challenges, the interoperability of synthetic healthcare data with EHRs and HIEs unlocks significant opportunities for scalable health innovation. Synthetic data can serve as a testing ground for new clinical decision support tools, offering a risk-free environment to evaluate their performance before they are deployed on real patient data (Susser et al., 2024). These tools can be used to enhance predictive analytics, support clinical trial recruitment, and optimize care delivery across diverse health systems.

Moreover, synthetic datasets embedded within HIEs can support large-scale public health initiatives, such as simulating the spread of infectious diseases or modeling the impact of health interventions. By enabling safe, scalable testing, synthetic data accelerates the development and deployment of health innovations that improve patient outcomes, reduce healthcare costs, and enhance system efficiencies, all while protecting patient privacy and promoting trust in health data exchanges.

8.2. Use of Synthetic Data in Federated Learning and Collaborative Research

Federated learning (FL) has emerged as a promising paradigm for training machine learning models across decentralized devices or data sources while preserving data privacy. The integration of synthetic healthcare data in federated learning offers a unique opportunity to enhance collaborative research and model development without the need for sharing sensitive patient information. This approach enables the creation of robust, privacy-preserving models that can benefit from diverse datasets, such as those generated from different healthcare systems, institutions, or research networks. By leveraging synthetic data in FL, collaborative research can progress without compromising patient confidentiality, a critical concern in healthcare data sharing.

8.3. Federated Learning: A Privacy-Preserving Model

In traditional machine learning, data is centralized in one location for model training. However, in federated learning, the training process occurs directly on local devices or data sources, and only model updates are shared rather than raw data. This process allows healthcare institutions, hospitals, and research organizations to collaboratively train models without needing to exchange or centralize patient data, thus mitigating privacy concerns. The use of synthetic data in this context serves as an additional layer of privacy protection, as it reduces the reliance on real patient data and ensures that sensitive health information is never shared between participants.

Synthetic datasets can be used as "stand-ins" for real-world data in federated learning models, particularly when there is a lack of sufficient local data or when working with rare diseases or conditions. Synthetic data can effectively augment local datasets, ensuring that the federated learning model is trained on a more balanced and diverse dataset. Moreover, synthetic data can simulate edge cases or rare events, which are often underrepresented in real-world datasets but crucial for robust model performance in healthcare applications, such as disease prediction, risk assessment, or treatment recommendations.

8.4. Enhancing Collaborative Research Through Synthetic Data

Federated learning is increasingly used in collaborative research, where multiple research institutions or healthcare providers come together to train machine learning models on distributed data sources. Synthetic data can facilitate this collaboration by acting as a bridge between institutions with different capabilities or regulations for sharing data. For example, researchers from multiple institutions might not be able to share real patient data due to privacy laws (such as HIPAA in the U.S. or GDPR in Europe). In such cases, synthetic data can enable the sharing of model insights and research findings without violating privacy regulations.

Synthetic data also plays a crucial role in accelerating collaborative research by enabling the simulation of large datasets that would be challenging to collect otherwise. For instance, in multi-center clinical trials or studies involving multiple healthcare systems, it can be challenging to obtain large-scale datasets that are both diverse and representative of different patient populations. By generating synthetic data that mirrors these populations, researchers can conduct experiments or validate hypotheses across a broader range of scenarios than might otherwise be possible, even when real data is limited.

8.5. Addressing Data Imbalance and Bias

One of the primary challenges in healthcare machine learning is the inherent data imbalance, where some conditions or demographics are underrepresented in datasets. This imbalance can lead to biased models that perform poorly for certain patient groups or clinical scenarios. The introduction of synthetic data in federated learning can mitigate this issue by allowing the generation of diverse and balanced datasets that are tailored to the specific needs of the research or healthcare application.

For example, synthetic data can be generated to oversample underrepresented conditions or patient groups, improving the model's ability to make accurate predictions across all demographic and clinical categories. In federated learning, these synthetic datasets can be created locally at each institution or healthcare provider, enhancing the overall diversity and fairness of the collaborative model.

8.6. Technical Challenges in Federated Learning with Synthetic Data

Despite the advantages, integrating synthetic data into federated learning presents several technical challenges. One significant challenge is ensuring the quality and representativeness of synthetic data. The synthetic data generated for federated learning must closely mirror the real-world data that would be used in the model, both in terms of structure and underlying patterns. This requires advanced techniques in data generation, such as generative adversarial networks (GANs) or variational autoencoders (VAEs), to ensure that synthetic data is realistic and usable for model training.

Additionally, federated learning models require robust communication protocols to share model updates across distributed nodes. The incorporation of synthetic data can complicate this process, as the synthetic data must be treated as an extension of the real data to ensure that updates reflect genuine insights. Furthermore, privacy-preserving mechanisms, such as differential privacy, must be employed to ensure that even the synthetic data does not inadvertently reveal sensitive patient information through model updates.

8.7. Ethical and Regulatory Considerations

The use of synthetic data in federated learning and collaborative research must be guided by strong ethical and regulatory frameworks. While synthetic data is designed to mitigate privacy concerns, researchers must ensure that it does not introduce new ethical risks, such as the potential for synthetic data to be reverse-engineered or re-identified. Therefore, it is essential to establish clear guidelines for the generation, validation, and use of synthetic datasets in federated learning to prevent misuse and maintain trust among research participants and healthcare providers.

Governments and regulatory bodies are increasingly recognizing the potential of federated learning and synthetic data in healthcare. However, they must also develop standards and policies that govern their use. These regulations must balance the benefits of collaborative research and privacy-preserving data sharing with the need for patient protection, transparency, and accountability in healthcare systems.

The combination of federated learning and synthetic data has the potential to revolutionize healthcare research by enabling collaborative, privacy-preserving data sharing across institutions, while enhancing the quality of machine learning models. Moving forward, we expect to see further advancements in synthetic data generation techniques, more robust federated learning algorithms, and improved interoperability between synthetic data and clinical data sources. These advancements will unlock new opportunities for precision medicine, public health initiatives, and clinical decision-making, driving innovation in healthcare while maintaining strict privacy and security standards.

8.8. Deployment in Digital Health Applications and Decision Support Systems

The integration of synthetic healthcare data into digital health applications and decision support systems (DSS) has the potential to significantly enhance healthcare delivery. By simulating realistic patient data, synthetic data can be used for training, testing, and validating various models and tools, allowing healthcare organizations to deploy innovative technologies without compromising patient privacy or requiring access to real-world health records. This section explores how synthetic data can be deployed within digital health applications, including electronic health records (EHRs), telemedicine systems, and personalized health interventions, and within decision support systems to assist healthcare providers in clinical decision-making.

9. SYNTHETIC DATA IN DIGITAL HEALTH APPLICATIONS

Digital health applications are rapidly transforming healthcare by providing solutions that improve access, efficiency, and outcomes. These applications, which include EHR systems, telemedicine platforms, mobile health apps, and patient portals, rely heavily on data to provide personalized healthcare services. The use of synthetic healthcare data in these applications allows for testing and optimizing algorithms, user interfaces, and workflows before deploying them in real-world settings (Pezoulas et al., 2024).

Telemedicine platforms that enable remote consultations can be evaluated with synthetic data representing a variety of patient conditions, demographics, and comorbidities, ensuring that the algorithms perform effectively across different populations. Similarly, synthetic data can be used to simulate patient interactions in mobile health applications, such as symptom tracking apps or fitness monitoring tools, to assess their performance in predicting outcomes or guiding user behavior. By simulating patient data, developers and researchers can identify potential issues or biases in these applications without the ethical concerns associated with using real patient data.

In the context of EHRs, synthetic data allows for the training of predictive models that can forecast patient outcomes, suggest treatment plans, or identify potential drug interactions. These models can be integrated into EHR systems to provide real-time decision support for clinicians. The synthetic data ensures that these systems are robust, capable of handling diverse patient populations, and ready for deployment in clinical environments without risking exposure to sensitive patient information.

9.1. Synthetic Data in Decision Support Systems

Decision support systems are designed to assist healthcare providers in making informed clinical decisions by analyzing data and providing actionable insights. These systems can range from simple alert systems to complex, AI-powered tools that predict patient outcomes, suggest treatments, or identify patterns in patient data that might not be immediately apparent to healthcare professionals.

Synthetic healthcare data plays a critical role in the development, testing, and validation of these systems. Synthetic data can be used to simulate a wide range of scenarios that might be difficult or time-consuming to collect in real-world settings. For instance, when developing an AI-powered diagnostic tool for a rare disease, it is often challenging to find enough real-world data to train a model. Synthetic data generation techniques, such as generative adversarial networks (GANs), can create realistic datasets that simulate a broad array of disease manifestations, improving the model's ability to generalize across diverse patient populations (Rosenthal et al., 2024).

Furthermore, synthetic data can be used to evaluate the performance of decision support systems under various conditions, such as data sparsity, imbalanced datasets, or specific patient subgroups. For example, synthetic data can simulate low-resource environments or scenarios where only partial patient data is available, allowing decision support systems to be assessed for robustness and adaptability. This ensures that the final model can provide accurate and actionable recommendations even when working with incomplete or low-quality data.

9.2. Overcoming Data Limitations and Bias in Decision Support

One of the primary challenges in building reliable decision support systems is ensuring that they are trained on diverse and representative datasets. Healthcare data is often biased due to demographic imbalances, underrepresentation of certain conditions, or data privacy restrictions. Synthetic data helps overcome these limitations by enabling the creation of balanced datasets that include rare conditions, diverse populations, and edge cases. This diversity is essential for developing decision support systems that are equitable, robust, and able to manage the complexity of real-world clinical environments. For example, in predictive modeling for disease outbreaks, synthetic data can simulate the spread of a disease across different regions, demographics, and healthcare settings. This ensures that the decision support system can offer reliable predictions across a wide range of scenarios. Similarly, in personalized medicine applications, synthetic data can be used to create datasets that represent different genetic profiles, lifestyles, and environmental factors, allowing the system to tailor recommendations to individual patients.

9.3. Ethical Considerations and Data Privacy

The deployment of synthetic data in digital health applications and decision support systems is driven by the need to protect patient privacy while enabling innovation. Unlike real-world health data, synthetic data is generated in a way that does not contain identifiable patient information, thus reducing the risk of privacy breaches. However, it is crucial to ensure that the synthetic data used in health applications is realistic and does not inadvertently introduce biases or inaccuracies that could lead to flawed decision-making. For instance, when deploying a synthetic dataset for model training in a clinical decision support system, developers must ensure that the synthetic data maintains the same statistical properties as real patient data, such as correlations between variables and distributions of health outcomes. Failure to do so could lead to models that perform poorly in real-world settings. Additionally, ethical guidelines must be established to govern the generation, use, and sharing of synthetic data, ensuring that it is used responsibly and transparently across digital health applications.

9.4. Enhancing Collaboration in Health Innovation:

The use of synthetic data in digital health applications and decision support systems also promotes collaboration across healthcare providers, researchers, and technology developers. By using synthetic data, researchers can share models and insights without the need to exchange sensitive patient information, fostering collaborative innovation while maintaining patient confidentiality. Synthetic data can also facilitate the development of open-source tools and platforms for healthcare, enabling a wider range of organizations to contribute to and benefit from advancements in digital health technologies.

Moreover, the deployment of synthetic data within decision support systems allows for the continuous improvement and adaptation of these systems. As more synthetic data is generated and incorporated into the training of AI models, the systems can be fine-tuned to account for emerging health trends, new medical knowledge, and evolving patient needs. This ensures that healthcare decision support systems remain agile, adaptable, and capable of providing high-quality care in an ever-changing healthcare landscape.

9.5. Future Directions and Challenges

Looking ahead, the deployment of synthetic data in digital health applications and decision support systems will continue to evolve alongside advancements in AI, data science, and healthcare technology. Future research will focus on improving the realism and diversity of synthetic healthcare data, developing new algorithms for integrating synthetic data into decision-making processes, and addressing the ethical challenges related to the use of synthetic data.

The continued collaboration between healthcare providers, data scientists, and technology developers will be critical in ensuring that synthetic data can be effectively deployed to improve healthcare outcomes while safeguarding patient privacy and data security. A comprehensive representation of varied factors in deployment of Synthetic Data in Digital Health Applications has been presented in Table 7.

Table 7. Deployment of Synthetic Data in Digital Health Applications and Decision Support Systems.

Feature	Digital Health Applications	Decision Support Systems
Primary Purpose	Improve the functionality, testing, and validation of health applications (e.g., EHRs, telemedicine, mobile health apps).	Enhance clinical decision-making through predictive modeling, risk assessments, and treatment recommendations.
Synthetic Data Usage	Used to simulate patient data for testing interfaces, workflows, and application functionalities without real patient data.	Used for training machine learning models, ensuring balanced and diverse data for accurate predictions across varied scenarios.
Privacy and Security	Ensure privacy by generating data that does not contain real patient information, mitigating privacy risks.	Provides privacy-preserving model training without compromising sensitive health information.
Data Augmentation	Synthetic data enhances datasets, especially for rare conditions or diverse patient populations underrepresented in real data.	Synthetic data simulates rare conditions or demographic groups to ensure models are robust and generalized.
Scalability	can simulate large-scale datasets without the logistical and ethical issues of collecting real-world data.	Supports scalability in model training by providing diverse scenarios, enabling model testing across multiple conditions.
Bias Mitigation	Helps reduce bias by generating diverse datasets, particularly for underrepresented conditions or populations.	Ensures models are unbiased by balancing datasets to include all patient demographics, preventing skewed decision-making.
Regulatory Compliance	Meets data privacy regulations (e.g., HIPAA, GDPR) by using synthetic data instead of real patient data.	Ensures compliance with privacy laws by using synthetic data for model validation and decision support, avoiding direct data sharing.
Realism and Accuracy	Data must be realistic to ensure proper system performance and accurate simulations (e.g., using generative models like GANs).	Synthetic data must replicate clinical data distributions to ensure decision support models are accurate and dependable.
Use Cases	Testing of telemedicine systems, symptom tracking apps, predictive models in EHRs, mobile health apps, and clinical trials.	Diagnostic tools, risk prediction models, clinical decision-making, personalized treatment suggestions, and drug interactions.
Ethical Considerations	Minimizes ethical concerns by avoiding the use of real patient data in testing and validation stages.	Prevents ethical risks related to privacy breaches and ensures transparency in model development and deployment.

10. PRIVACY PRESERVING SYNTHETIC DATA IN HEALTHCARE

A promising answer to these enduring problems in biomedicine, like privacy restrictions and limited data access, is synthetic data, which are artificially created records that replicate the statistical characteristics of actual health data. By reproducing the characteristics and connections of source datasets, high utility synthetic datasets can facilitate "Analyses comparable to those obtained from real data" without disclosing actual subject information (Y. G. Lee et al., 2025; Zamzmi et al., 2025). Though they have significantly increased the realism of synthetic health data, recent developments in generative AI (GANs, VAEs, diffusion models, etc.) also raise questions regarding data fidelity, leakage, and fairness (Koetzier et al., 2024; Templin et al., 2024). To guarantee that synthetic datasets are valuable for tasks downstream without jeopardizing confidentiality, the field now places a strong emphasis on rigorous evaluation and provable privacy guarantees (such as differential privacy) (Santangelo et al., 2025; Wagner et al., 2024). Below, we examine the most popular privacy-preserving techniques for creating synthetic data (Table 8), important evaluation metrics (Table 9), and new guidelines and standards supporting the use of synthetic data in healthcare (Table 10).

10.1. Privacy-Preserving Generation Methods

A variety of methods produce synthetic healthcare data with different privacy guarantees. Table 7 summarizes representative approaches, their model types, (ε, δ)-DP assurances, core mechanisms, and distinctive features. Broadly, methods fall into:

a) **DP-enhanced generative models** (GANs, VAEs, diffusion) that incorporate noise or auditing for formal privacy.
b) **nNon-DP heuristic methods** (e.g., data obfuscation, resampling) that lack provable bounds but can still reduce risk.

Tian et al. use a denoising diffusion probabilistic model to synthesize realistic longitudinal EHR time series. By injecting noise into a mixed diffusion process, their model achieves empirically lower membership-reidentification risk than baselines, while preserving high fidelity (Tian et al., 2024). (Marino et al., 2025) employ DataSifter, a pipeline that generalizes and perturbs tabular data in multiple rounds (small/med/large obfuscation), yielding tunable privacy-utility tradeoffs. Purely generative methods like CTGAN (a conditional tabular GAN) use no formal DP: they capture complex data distributions but must rely on audit metrics (Marino et al., 2025). Simple oversampling such as SMOTE creates synthetic minority-class examples by interpolation; while effective for balancing classes, it offers no privacy guarantee beyond usual anonymization (Marchesi et al., 2025). Other DP-GAN variants (e.g. PATE-GAN) combine GANs with the PATE framework to achieve formal DP bounds, albeit often at a utility cost (Liu et al., 2025). In practice, healthcare datasets use a mix of these approaches depending on context (e.g., fully DP for regulatory submissions vs. heuristic synthetic augmentation for pilot studies).

Table 8. Privacy-Preserving Synthetic Data Generation Methods.

Method	Model Type	Privacy Guarantee	Mechanism	Key Features
Diffusion Model (EHR) (Tian et al., 2024)	Denoising diffusion	No formal DP (empirical)	Stochastic reverse diffusion	High-fidelity time-series, low membership risk
DataSifter (Marino et al., 2025)	Tabular perturbation	Adjustable (semi-DP)	Iterative variable generalization + noise	Tunable privacy-utility tradeoff, preserves key stats
CTGAN (Marino et al., 2025)	Generative Adversarial	No formal DP	Conditional GAN on copula transform	Captures complex joint distributions; baseline synthetic
SMOTE (Marchesi et al., 2025)	Oversampling (tabular)	None (anonymization only)	Synthetic minority interpolation	Balances class frequencies; improves representation
PATE-GAN (private GAN) (Liu et al., 2025)	Generative Adversarial	(ε, δ)-DP (via PATE)	Teacher-student ensemble with added noise	Formal DP auditing of GAN; higher privacy cost

10.2. Evaluating Synthetic Data Quality and Privacy

Ensuring synthetic data is both useful and safe requires rigorous evaluation. Current practice involves metrics of data fidelity (how well the synthetic distribution matches real data) and utility (performance on downstream tasks), balanced against privacy risk measures (Santangelo et al., 2025; Zamzmi et al., 2025). Key quantitative metrics include population-level statistics (e.g., feature distributions, correlation structure), predictive accuracy in machine-learning models, and similarity scores (e.g., Frechet Inception Distance for images). On the privacy side, one computes either DP epsilon or empirical tests (e.g. membership inference attack accuracy, re-identification risk) (Zamzmi et al., 2025). However, the field currently lacks standardized benchmarks. As Santangelo et al. note, "the lack of standardized evaluation metrics complicates selection of synthetic data models," and available metrics often fail to capture medical plausibility (Santangelo et al., 2025). Consequently, recent work emphasizes holistic assessment frameworks (Zamzmi et al., 2025), proposes an SMD Scorecard summarizing quality across seven criteria (fidelity, privacy, compliance, etc.) tailored to clinical use. Santangelo et al. introduce SynthRO, a user-friendly dashboard that computes diverse metrics and benchmarks candidate synthetic datasets, highlighting the importance of reproducible, transparent evaluation (Santangelo et al., 2025). Table 8 lists common quality and privacy metrics.

10.3. Applications for Equity and Global Collaboration

Synthetic data have unique roles in advancing health equity and enabling AI in low-resource contexts. By generating diverse patient records, synthetic approaches can bridge gaps in under-represented populations and mitigate biases inherent in real-world data (Marchesi et al., 2025; Ritoré et al., 2024). For instance, oversampling techniques like SMOTE or tailored GANs can amplify rare subgroups (e.g. minority ethnicities or uncommon conditions) to improve model fairness (Marchesi et al., 2025). Marchesi et al. demonstrate that using synthetic data led to more equitable performance for Black patients and women on sepsis prediction tasks (Marchesi et al., 2025). Similarly, "open" synthetic datasets can be shared across institutions or countries, democratizing AI research much like open-access data initiatives (Ritoré et al., 2024). In resource-limited settings or emerging consortia (e.g. rare disease networks), synthetic data offer a safe proxy for privacy-sensitive records, accelerating algorithm development and validation (Elvatun et al., 2025; Ritoré et al., 2024). (Elvatun et al., 2025) showed synthetic external control arms in oncology trials could replicate real-world results without exposing patient-level registry data, potentially speeding drug development while protecting privacy. Moreover, synthetic data facilitate international collaborations by allowing collaborative model training on aggregated synthetic proxies instead of raw data (Wagner et al., 2024). In education and training, digital twin simulations (virtual patients or care environments) rely on synthetic data to let clinicians safely practice interventions (Halpern et al., 2024; Kuriakose et al., 2024). These "living" models, informed by synthetic patient trajectories, promise personalized medicine and system-level optimization (e.g. hospital workflow), all while preserving individual anonymity (Halpern et al., 2024).

Table 9. Synthetic Data Evaluation Metrics.

Metric Type	Example Metric	Purpose	Insight
Statistical Fidelity (Santangelo et al., 2025)	Wasserstein distance; Kolmogorov-Smirnov statistic	Compare feature distributions	Detects shifts/mismatches in marginal distributions
Machine-Learning Utility (Marino et al., 2025)	Predictive model accuracy (AUROC, error) on synthetic vs real	Assess task performance	Indicates how well models trained/evaluated on synthetic data generalize
Fairness and Representation (Marchesi et al., 2025)	Class balance metrics (e.g., ratio of minority samples)	Evaluate demographic parity	Measures synthetic data's ability to correct underrepresentation

continued on following page

Table 9. Continued

Metric Type	Example Metric	Purpose	Insight
Differential Privacy (Liu et al., 2025)	ε (epsilon) value	Formal privacy guarantee	Quantifies privacy loss allowed during generation
Re-identification Risk (Zamzmi et al., 2025)	Membership inference AUC; Percentage of unique records	Empirical privacy check	Estimates chance an attacker matches synthetic entries to real subjects

10.4. Ethical, Legal and Regulatory Frameworks

As synthetic data grows, frameworks and standards emerge to guide best practices. The Hastings Center notes both "promise and peril" in synthetic health data: while detachment from real patients can protect privacy, ethical issues (bias, validity, accountability) persist (Susser et al., 2024; Wagner et al., 2024). There is broad consensus on the need for transparency and documentation: recent work introduces Synthetic Medical Data (SMD) Cards, standardized reports that accompany datasets to detail generation methods, limitations, and validation results (Wagner et al., 2024; Zamzmi et al., 2025). Tools like SynthRO implement such checklists automatically (Santangelo et al., 2025). On the policy side, guidelines from regulatory bodies are still nascent; some propose treating high-quality synthetic data as "non-human data" exempt from stringent privacy rules, provided they meet anonymization thresholds (Elvatun et al., 2025; Zamzmi et al., 2025). Internationally, coalitions (e.g. GA4GH, OECD) are exploring synthetic data recommendations, and professional organizations urge integrating Differential Privacy and reproducibility standards into all synthetic data pipelines (Liu et al., 2025; Zamzmi et al., 2025).

In summary, synthetic data hold enormous potential for enabling AI in healthcare while respecting patient privacy. Success depends on choosing suitable generation methods (Table 8), rigorously evaluating outputs (Table 9), and following emerging standards to ensure fairness, safety, and transparency (Table 10) (Liu et al., 2025; Zamzmi et al., 2025). As recent reviews emphasize, synthetic data are already used across diverse domains (from multi-omics and medical imaging to clinical trials and global health) (Pezoulas et al., 2024; Rujas et al., 2025a). Ongoing research and interdisciplinary collaboration will be needed to refine techniques, close privacy gaps, and fully realize the promise of synthetic data for healthcare innovation and equity.

CONCLUSION

This chapter has provided a comprehensive examination of synthetic healthcare data, spanning traditional statistical methods, simulation-based approaches, and state-of-the-art AI-driven techniques such as GANs, VAEs, Transformers, and Large Language Models. By comparing these approaches, the chapter highlighted their strengths and limitations in generating diverse, privacy-preserving datasets suitable for clinical research, diagnostics, and public health applications. Case studies and real-world implementations underscored how synthetic data can augment rare disease research, improve recruitment in clinical trials, balance datasets for AI/ML training, and enable cross-institutional collaboration while safeguarding patient confidentiality.

Beyond the technical dimensions, the chapter has addressed the critical ethical, regulatory, and governance considerations that shape the adoption of synthetic data in healthcare. It has also explored validation frameworks, interoperability challenges with clinical systems, and the perceptions of healthcare professionals and the public. Collectively, these discussions underscore that synthetic data is not only a technological innovation but also a socio-technical system requiring trust, transparency, and policy alignment.

In conclusion, synthetic healthcare holds immense promise as a catalyst for innovation, enabling privacy-preserving, scalable, and equitable research and clinical applications. Yet its transformative potential will only be fully realized when technical rigor, fairness guarantees, explainability, and regulatory clarity converge. By addressing these limitations through interdisciplinary collaboration, synthetic data can become a cornerstone of trustworthy, future-proof digital health systems.

Table 10. Standards and Frameworks for Synthetic Health Data.

Framework/Initiative	Type	Scope/Purpose	Key Features
SMD Scorecard (Zamzmi et al., 2025)	Reporting standard	Evaluates synthetic medical datasets on seven "Cs" (e.g., fidelity, privacy, compliance)	Provides a comprehensive quality report for any synthetic dataset
SynthRO Dashboard (Santangelo et al., 2025)	Evaluation toolkit	Open-source software for benchmarking synthetic tabular data	Automates multiple metrics, allows side-by-side model comparisons
FAIR Principles (extended) (Foraker et al., 2025)	Data standards	FAIR (findable, accessible, interoperable, reusable) applied to synthetic data	Emphasizes metadata, provenance, and documentation (proposed by community)

continued on following page

Table 10. Continued

Framework/Initiative	Type	Scope/Purpose	Key Features
OECD/WHO AI guidelines (Wagner et al., 2024)	Policy recommendation	Broad AI ethics guidelines (including data sharing, privacy)	Encourage safe AI use in health, implicitly covering synthetic data
Differential Privacy Benchmarks (Marino et al., 2025)	Technical standard	NIST-led challenge on DP synthetic data (general domain)	Provides baseline tasks and metrics to certify DP mechanisms

REFERENCES

Akiya, I., Ishihara, T., & Yamamoto, K. (2024). Comparison of Synthetic Data Generation Techniques for Control Group Survival Data in Oncology Clinical Trials: Simulation Study. *JMIR Medical Informatics*, *12*, e55118. DOI: 10.2196/55118 PMID: 38889082

Aldausari, N., Sowmya, A., Marcus, N., & Mohammadi, G. (2023). Video Generative Adversarial Networks: A Review. *ACM Computing Surveys*, *55*(2), 1–25. DOI: 10.1145/3487891

Barr, A. A., Quan, J., Guo, E., & Sezgin, E. (2025). Large language models generating synthetic clinical datasets: A feasibility and comparative analysis with real-world perioperative data. *Frontiers in Artificial Intelligence*, *8*, 1533508. Advance online publication. DOI: 10.3389/frai.2025.1533508 PMID: 39974356

Basri, M. A. (2024). *Evaluating the Usefulness of Synthetic Data in Healthcare: Applications in Predictive Modeling and Privacy Protection.*

Bhanot, K., Qi, M., Erickson, J. S., Guyon, I., & Bennett, K. P. (2021). The Problem of Fairness in Synthetic Healthcare Data. *Entropy (Basel, Switzerland)*, *23*(9), 1165. DOI: 10.3390/e23091165 PMID: 34573790

Brown, T., Mann, B., Ryder, N., Subbiah, M., Kaplan, J. D., Dhariwal, P., Neelakantan, A., Shyam, P., Sastry, G., Askell, A., Agarwal, S., Herbert-Voss, A., Krueger, G., Henighan, T., Child, R., Ramesh, A., Ziegler, D., Wu, J., Winter, C., . . . Amodei, D. (2020). Language Models are Few-Shot Learners. *Advances in Neural Information Processing Systems, 33*, 1877–1901. https://proceedings.neurips.cc/paper/2020/hash/1457c0d6bfcb4967418bfb8ac142f64a-Abstract.html

Chandra, S., Prakash, P. K. S., Samanta, S., & Chilukuri, S. (2024a). ClinicalGAN: Powering patient monitoring in clinical trials with patient digital twins. *Scientific Reports*, *14*(1), 12236. DOI: 10.1038/s41598-024-62567-1 PMID: 38806536

Choi, E., Biswal, S., Malin, B., Duke, J., Stewart, W. F., & Sun, J. (2017, November 6). Generating Multi-label Discrete Patient Records using Generative Adversarial Networks. *Proceedings of the 2nd Machine Learning for Healthcare Conference.* https://proceedings.mlr.press/v68/choi17a.html

Dahmen, J., & Cook, D. (2019a). SynSys: A Synthetic Data Generation System for Healthcare Applications. *Sensors (Basel)*, *19*(5), 1181. DOI: 10.3390/s19051181 PMID: 30857130

Elvatun, S., Knoors, D., Brant, S., Jonasson, C., & Nygård, J. F. (2025). Synthetic data as external control arms in scarce single-arm clinical trials. *PLOS Digital Health*, *4*(1), e0000581. DOI: 10.1371/journal.pdig.0000581 PMID: 39847598

Figueira, A., & Vaz, B. (2022). Survey on Synthetic Data Generation, Evaluation Methods and GANs. *Mathematics*, *10*(15), 2733. DOI: 10.3390/math10152733

Foraker, R., Morrow, J. D., Johnson, J. A., Wilcox, A. B., Forster, A. J., & Payne, P. R. O. (2025). Understanding synthetic data: Artificial datasets for real-world evidence. *BMJ Evidence-Based Medicine*, bmjebm-2024-113617. DOI: 10.1136/bmjebm-2024-113617

Giuffrè, M., & Shung, D. L. (2023a). Harnessing the power of synthetic data in healthcare: Innovation, application, and privacy. *NPJ Digital Medicine*, *6*(1), 186. Advance online publication. DOI: 10.1038/s41746-023-00927-3 PMID: 37813960

Gonzales, A., Guruswamy, G., & Smith, S. R. (2023). Synthetic data in health care: A narrative review. *PLOS Digital Health*, *2*(1), e0000082. DOI: 10.1371/journal.pdig.0000082 PMID: 36812604

Goodfellow, I., Bengio, Y., & Courville, A. (2016). *Deep learning*. The MIT Press.

Halpern, G. A., Nemet, M., Gowda, D. M., Kilickaya, O., & Lal, A. (2024). Advances and utility of digital twins in critical care and acute care medicine: A narrative review. *Journal of Yeungnam Medical Science*. Advance online publication. DOI: 10.12701/jyms.2024.01053 PMID: 39587767

Hanna, M. G., Pantanowitz, L., Dash, R., Harrison, J. H., Deebajah, M., Pantanowitz, J., & Rashidi, H. H. (2025a). Future of Artificial Intelligence—Machine Learning Trends in Pathology and Medicine. *Modern Pathology*, *38*(4), 100705. DOI: 10.1016/j.modpat.2025.100705 PMID: 39761872

Hernandez, M., & Hernandez, M. (2022). Incorporation of Synthetic Data Generation Techniques within a Controlled Data Processing Workflow in the Health and Wellbeing Domain. *Electronics (Basel)*, *11*(5), 812–812. DOI: 10.3390/electronics11050812

Hyun, J., Yongho Lee, Lee, Y., Ha Min Son, Son, H. M., Seo Hu Lee, Lee, S. H., Vinh Pham, Pham, V., Park, J. U., Ji Ung Park, Park, J. U., Tai-Myoung Chung, Chung, T. M., & Chung, T.-M. (2021). *Synthetic Data Generation System for AI-Based Diabetic Foot Diagnosis*. 2(5), 1–9. DOI: 10.1007/s42979-021-00667-9

Jadon, A., & Kumar, S. (2023, July 25). Leveraging Generative AI Models for Synthetic Data Generation in Healthcare: Balancing Research and Privacy. *2023 International Conference on Smart Applications, Communications and Networking (SmartNets)*. 2023 International Conference on Smart Applications, Communications and Networking (SmartNets), Istanbul, Turkiye. DOI: 10.1109/SmartNets58706.2023.10215825

James, S., Harbron, C., Branson, J., & Sundler, M. (2021). Synthetic data use: Exploring use cases to optimise data utility. *Discover Artificial Intelligence*, *1*(1), 15. Advance online publication. DOI: 10.1007/s44163-021-00016-y

Knevel, R., & Liao, K. P. (2023). From real-world electronic health record data to real-world results using artificial intelligence. *Annals of the Rheumatic Diseases*, *82*(3), 306–311. DOI: 10.1136/ard-2022-222626 PMID: 36150748

Koetzier, L. R., Wu, J., Mastrodicasa, D., Lutz, A., Chung, M., Koszek, W. A., Pratap, J., Chaudhari, A. S., Rajpurkar, P., Lungren, M. P., & Willemink, M. J. (2024). Generating Synthetic Data for Medical Imaging. *Radiology*, *312*(3), e232471. DOI: 10.1148/radiol.232471 PMID: 39254456

Kumar, C. U. O., Singh, I., & Suguna, M. (2024). Optimizing Patient Recruitment for Clinical Trials: A Hybrid Classification Model and Game-Theoretic Approach for Strategic Interaction. *IEEE Access : Practical Innovations, Open Solutions*, *12*, 10254–10280. DOI: 10.1109/ACCESS.2024.3351688

Kuriakose, S. M., Joseph, J. A. R., & Kollinal, R. (2024). The Rise of Digital Twins in Healthcare: A Mapping of the Research Landscape. *Cureus*. Advance online publication. DOI: 10.7759/cureus.65358 PMID: 39184791

Lee, G., Kweon, S., Bae, S., & Choi, E. (2024). Overview of the EHRSQL 2024 Shared Task on Reliable Text-to-SQL Modeling on Electronic Health Records. In Naumann, T., Ben Abacha, A., Bethard, S., Roberts, K., & Bitterman, D. (Eds), *Proceedings of the 6th Clinical Natural Language Processing Workshop* (pp. 644–654). Association for Computational Linguistics. DOI: 10.18653/v1/2024.clinicalnlp-1.62

Lee, Y. G., Kwak, M.-S., Kim, J. E., Kim, M. S., No, D. U., & Chai, H. Y. (2025). Synthetic data production for biomedical research. *Osong Public Health and Research Perspectives*, *16*(2), 94–99. DOI: 10.24171/j.phrp.2024.0335 PMID: 40262847

Liu, Y., Acharya, U. R., & Tan, J. H. (2025). Preserving privacy in healthcare: A systematic review of deep learning approaches for synthetic data generation. *Computer Methods and Programs in Biomedicine*, *260*, 108571. DOI: 10.1016/j.cmpb.2024.108571 PMID: 39742693

Lu, Y., Chen, L., Zhang, Y., Shen, M., Wang, H., Wang, X., van Rechem, C., Fu, T., & Wei, W. (2025a). *Machine Learning for Synthetic Data Generation: A Review* (No. arXiv:2302.04062). arXiv. https://doi.org//arXiv.2302.04062DOI: 10.48550

Mackay, P. (2025). *Compiling Complex Medical Reports using a Generic LLM: Exploring Hybrid Prompt Engineering Strategies for Language Improvement and Hallucination Mitigation* [Thesis, University of Lincoln]. DOI: 10.24385/lincoln.29596808.v1

Marchesi, R., Micheletti, N., I-Hsien Kuo, N., Barbieri, S., Jurman, G., & Osmani, V. (2025a). Generative AI mitigates representation bias and improves model fairness through synthetic health data. *PLoS Computational Biology*, *21*(5), e1013080. DOI: 10.1371/journal.pcbi.1013080 PMID: 40388536

Marino, S., Cassidy, R., Nanni, J., Wang, Y., Liu, Y., Tang, M., Yuan, Y., Chen, T., Sinha, A., Pandian, B., Dinov, I. D., & Burns, M. L. (2025). Medical data sharing and synthetic clinical data generation – maximizing biomedical resource utilization and minimizing participant re-identification risks. *NPJ Digital Medicine*, *8*(1), 526. DOI: 10.1038/s41746-025-01935-1 PMID: 40818998

McDuff, D., Curran, T., & Kadambi, A. (2023a). *Synthetic Data in Healthcare* (No. arXiv:2304.03243). arXiv. https://doi.org//arXiv.2304.03243DOI: 10.48550

Mishra, S., & Venkatesh, M. (2024). Rare disease clinical trials in the European Union: Navigating regulatory and clinical challenges. *Orphanet Journal of Rare Diseases*, *19*(1), 285. DOI: 10.1186/s13023-024-03146-5 PMID: 39085891

Mohd Aman, A. H., Hassan, W. H., Sameen, S., Attarbashi, Z. S., Alizadeh, M., & Latiff, L. A. (2021). IoMT amid COVID-19 pandemic: Application, architecture, technology, and security. *Journal of Network and Computer Applications*, *174*, 102886. DOI: 10.1016/j.jnca.2020.102886 PMID: 34173428

Nazera, F., Tanvir, K., & Kabir, Md. S., Hasan, Md. S., Hena, K. T., & Gomes, D. (2025). Hybrid Vision Transformer Naive Bayes Model for Mosquito Species Recognition with Virus Colony Search Optimization. *2025 International Conference on Quantum Photonics, Artificial Intelligence, and Networking (QPAIN)*, 1–6. DOI: 10.1109/QPAIN66474.2025.11171832

Pasculli, G., Virgolin, M., Myles, P., Vidovszky, A., Fisher, C., Biasin, E., Mourby, M., Pappalardo, F., D'Amico, S., Torchia, M., Chebykin, A., Carbone, V., Emili, L., & Roeshammar, D. (2025). Synthetic Data in Healthcare and Drug Development: Definitions, Regulatory Frameworks, Issues. *CPT: Pharmacometrics & Systems Pharmacology*, *14*(5), 840–852. DOI: 10.1002/psp4.70021 PMID: 40193292

Pezoulas, V. C., Zaridis, D. I., Mylona, E., Androutsos, C., Apostolidis, K., Tachos, N. S., & Fotiadis, D. I. (2024). Synthetic data generation methods in healthcare: A review on open-source tools and methods. *Computational and Structural Biotechnology Journal, 23*, 2892–2910. DOI: 10.1016/j.csbj.2024.07.005 PMID: 39108677

Prasanna Das, H., Tran, R., Singh, J., Yue, X., Tison, G., Sangiovanni-Vincentelli, A., & Spanos, C. J. (2022). Conditional Synthetic Data Generation for Robust Machine Learning Applications with Limited Pandemic Data. *Proceedings of the AAAI Conference on Artificial Intelligence, 36*(11), 11792–11800. DOI: 10.1609/aaai.v36i11.21435

Ramachandranpillai, R., Sikder, M. F., Bergström, D., & Heintz, F. (2024). Bt-GAN: Generating Fair Synthetic Healthdata via Bias-transforming Generative Adversarial Networks. *Journal of Artificial Intelligence Research, 79*, 1313–1341. DOI: 10.1613/jair.1.15317

Regulation—2016/679—EN - gdpr—EUR-Lex. (n.d.). Retrieved 6 September 2025, from https://eur-lex.europa.eu/eli/reg/2016/679/oj/eng

Ritoré, Á., Jiménez, C. M., González, J. L., Rejón-Parrilla, J. C., Hervás, P., Toro, E., Parra-Calderón, C. L., Celi, L. A., Túnez, I., & Armengol De La Hoz, M. Á. (2024). The role of Open Access Data in democratizing healthcare AI: A pathway to research enhancement, patient well-being and treatment equity in Andalusia, Spain. *PLOS Digital Health, 3*(9), e0000599. DOI: 10.1371/journal.pdig.0000599 PMID: 39283912

Rosenthal, S., Adler-Milstein, J., & Patel, V. (2024). Public Health Data Exchange Through Health Information Exchange Organizations: National Survey Study. *JMIR Public Health and Surveillance, 10*, e64969. DOI: 10.2196/64969 PMID: 39588746

Rujas, M., Martín Gómez Del Moral Herranz, R., Fico, G., & Merino-Barbancho, B. (2025a). Synthetic data generation in healthcare: A scoping review of reviews on domains, motivations, and future applications. *International Journal of Medical Informatics, 195*, 105763. DOI: 10.1016/j.ijmedinf.2024.105763 PMID: 39719743

Santangelo, G., Nicora, G., Bellazzi, R., & Dagliati, A. (2025a). How good is your synthetic data? SynthRO, a dashboard to evaluate and benchmark synthetic tabular data. *BMC Medical Informatics and Decision Making, 25*(1), 89. DOI: 10.1186/s12911-024-02731-9 PMID: 39966793

Seeram, E., & Kanade, V. (2024). Ethical and Regulatory Considerations. In E. Seeram & V. Kanade, *Artificial Intelligence in Medical Imaging Technology* (pp. 151–167). Springer Nature Switzerland. DOI: 10.1007/978-3-031-64049-0_9

Susser, D., Schiff, D. S., Gerke, S., Cabrera, L. Y., Cohen, I. G., Doerr, M., Harrod, J., Kostick-Quenet, K., McNealy, J., Meyer, M. N., Price, W. N.II, & Wagner, J. K. (2024). Synthetic Health Data: Real Ethical Promise and Peril. *The Hastings Center Report, 54*(5), 8–13. DOI: 10.1002/hast.4911 PMID: 39487776

Templin, T., Perez, M. W., Sylvia, S., Leek, J., & Sinnott-Armstrong, N. (2024). Addressing 6 challenges in generative AI for digital health: A scoping review. *PLOS Digital Health, 3*(5), e0000503. DOI: 10.1371/journal.pdig.0000503 PMID: 38781686

Tian, M., Chen, B., Guo, A., Jiang, S., & Zhang, A. R. (2024a). Reliable generation of privacy-preserving synthetic electronic health record time series via diffusion models. *Journal of the American Medical Informatics Association : JAMIA, 31*(11), 2529–2539. DOI: 10.1093/jamia/ocae229 PMID: 39222376

Trowman, R., Migliore, A., & Ollendorf, D. A. (2024). Designing collaborations involving health technology assessment: Discussions and recommendations from the 2024 health technology assessment international global policy forum. *International Journal of Technology Assessment in Health Care, 40*(1), e41. DOI: 10.1017/S0266462324000436 PMID: 39494818

Wagner, J. K., Cabrera, L. Y., Gerke, S., & Susser, D. (2024a). Synthetic data and ELSI-focused computational checklists—A survey of biomedical professionals' views. *PLOS Digital Health, 3*(11), e0000666. DOI: 10.1371/journal.pdig.0000666 PMID: 39565773

Wang, C., Tachimori, H., Yamaguchi, H., Sekiguchi, A., Li, Y., & Yamashita, Y. (2024). A multimodal deep learning approach for the prediction of cognitive decline and its effectiveness in clinical trials for Alzheimer's disease. *Translational Psychiatry, 14*(1), 105. DOI: 10.1038/s41398-024-02819-w PMID: 38383536

Xu, L., Skoularidou, M., Cuesta-Infante, A., & Veeramachaneni, K. (2019). *Modeling Tabular data using Conditional GAN* (No. arXiv:1907.00503). arXiv. https://doi.org//arXiv.1907.00503DOI: 10.48550

Yan, C., Yan, Y., Wan, Z., Zhang, Z., Omberg, L., Guinney, J., Mooney, S. D., & Malin, B. A. (2022a). A Multifaceted benchmarking of synthetic electronic health record generation models. *Nature Communications, 13*(1), 7609. Advance online publication. DOI: 10.1038/s41467-022-35295-1 PMID: 36494374

Zamzmi, G., Subbaswamy, A., Sizikova, E., Margerrison, E., Delfino, J. G., & Badano, A. (2025a). Scorecard for synthetic medical data evaluation. *Communications Engineering, 4*(1), 130. DOI: 10.1038/s44172-025-00450-1 PMID: 40691520

Chapter 4
Strategies for Generating Synthetic Health Records Using Generative Artificial Intelligence

Geetha Manoharan
https://orcid.org/0000-0002-8644-8871
SR University, India

Subhashini Durai
LEAD College of Management, India

ABSTRACT

This chapter digs into the methods for creating synthetic health records using generative artificial intelligence (AI) approaches, stressing its critical role in improving healthcare research while protecting patient privacy. Synthetic health data are intentionally manufactured datasets that closely resemble real-world electronic health records but do not include actual patient information, allowing for safe data exchange and analysis. The chapter examines popular generative AI techniques such as generative adversarial networks and variational autoencoders, demonstrating how these models capture complicated statistical characteristics and correlations in healthcare data. It examines the use of synthetic EHRs in medical AI research, clinical simulations, and software testing. Furthermore, the chapter discusses data quality issues, ethical concerns, and balancing privacy and usefulness. Overall, generative AI is a transformational tool for overcoming data accessibility hurdles and encouraging innovation in health informatics.

DOI: 10.4018/979-8-3373-5641-9.ch004

1 INTRODUCTION TO THE IMPERATIVE FOR SYNTHETIC DATA IN HEALTHCARE

The contemporary healthcare system is full of data. Electronic Health Records (EHRs), genomic information, images, and wearable data altogether create an unparalleled promise to speed up medical research, tailor therapy, and streamline healthcare delivery (Auffray et al., 2016). But all this data are largely in silos and out of reach. The sensitive character of patient information correctly brings it within the ambit of stringent privacy regulations such as the United States' Health Insurance Portability and Accountability Act (HIPAA) and Europe's General Data Protection Regulation (GDPR). Despite being crucial for protecting patients' rights, these regulations create significant obstacles to data exchange, which is crucial for conducting major medical research studies, developing machine learning models, and verifying software. The effects of this bottleneck in accessing data are far-reaching. Scientists for orphan diseases normally find it difficult to collect large enough datasets to be able to draw statistically significant conclusions. Implementers of predictive models with artificial intelligence on disease diagnostic or progression models have their efforts hampered by small and, in most cases, imbalanced datasets. In addition, actual health data in real-world settings is also plagued with biases—historical and systemic inequities in healthcare access and treatment—which, when employed in training AI models, perpetuate and even magnify these inequalities (Obermeyer et al., 2019).

1.1 Defining Synthetic Health Records

It is against this intricate backdrop that synthetic health records have cropped up as a game-changing substitute. A synthetic health record is a computationally created dataset that mirrors the properties, statistical features, and temporal dynamics of an average patient dataset but holds no real, identifiable patient data (Beaumont, 2021). It is not to create a one-to-one correspondence of actual patients but to construct a completely new population of "virtual" patients whose aggregate data will be statistically indistinguishable from the actual population.

Consider this metaphor: a good painter can be instructed by thousands of actual portraits to learn how to look at the rules of light, shadow, and human form. He or she can then produce an entirely new, realistic portrait of someone who never even existed. A generative AI model works the same way and is trained on a real patient database to learn the subtle multivariate relationships between diagnoses, medications, lab results, and demographics. It then applies what it has learned to fill in a new generation of realistic but completely artificial patients.

1.2 The Promise of Generative AI

Creating synthetic data of high quality is a complicated process. Medical data is considered difficult and complex because it exemplifies a data set that combines different types of information, including structured data, unstructured data, and temporal sequences (Rujas et al., 2025). Structured data includes lab results, billing codes are the unstructured data includes temporal sequences, which are patient journeys over time. Simple statistical methods mostly fail to represent all the detailed dependencies of the data. Generative Artificial Intelligence is one of the best solutions for this problem. Generative AI is a term used for the group of deep learning models that are totally different from discriminative ones, as they do not specialize in classification or prediction (e.g., identifying a tumor in an image). Instead, these models learn the underlying distribution of a given dataset and, therefore, can create new synthetic data samples (Goodfellow et al., 2014). The achievements of the models like Generative Adversarial Networks (GANs), Variational Autoencoders (VAEs), and lately Transformer-based architectures and Diffusion Models, in the ability to learn and imitate the complex data distributions, have been very impressive (Hasan et al., 2025). The synthetic health records with the level of detail and the wide range of applications that were never possible before can now be generated by using these sophisticated methods.

1.3 Chapter Overview

This new chapter gives the users very detailed instructions about the latest techniques to be implemented in different models of generative AI to create synthetic health records. The objective and structure of this chapter are to be a very detailed and yet a very accessible guide for medics, researchers, data scientists, and engineers.

The second section will introduce the big picture by describing the necessary concepts of the main generative AI models that are used in this domain.

Thirdly, specific mechanisms and procedures for adjusting these models to various data types would be the matter of Section 3. The paper also addresses the network structures of medical GANs (medGAN) and their offspring while discussing the general subfield of biomedical data.

Section 4 talks about the detailed and hands-on part of the process, starting from data preprocessing and feature engineering specific to EHRs, going through the process of model selection and finishing with training.

The next chapter, i.e., Section 5, will talk about the most vital issue of synthetic data generation, i.e., the problem of performance evaluation and validation. We plan to present a framework comprising three aspects—fidelity, utility, and privacy—on which the quality of data can be assessed.

In Section 6, the authors will focus on the complex ethical and regulatory issues, undoubtedly covering bias, fairness, transparency, and compliance.

Section 7 will talk about the numerous contemporary issues and openings for future investigations that could change the entire field in the coming times.

Overcoming these topics, the authors will demonstrate that generative AI is not just a technical tool but a crucial technological pioneer that can bring about the greatest benefits of medical data, thus opening new possibilities of a hybrid physician's mind that is free, collaborative, and safe for the privacy of the patient.

2 FOUNDATIONAL CONCEPTS IN GENERATIVE AI

To comprehend the strategies behind the generation of synthetic health records, one must first familiarize oneself with the core principles governing the generative models that support this process. These models are the engines that learn from real data to produce synthetic output. Although the field itself is vast and fast-moving, several key architectures form the basis of contemporary synthetic data generation: Generative Adversarial Networks (GANs), Variational Autoencoders (VAEs), and more recently, advanced paradigms such as Transformers and Diffusion Models.

2.1 Generative Adversarial Networks (GANs)

It is maybe the most influential generative architecture in the past decade: Generative Adversarial Network (GAN), proposed in 2014 by Ian Goodfellow and his friends. The core idea is brilliantly intuitive: it frames the learning process as a two-player game between a Generator and a Discriminator (Goodfellow et al., 2014).

The Generator (G): This neural network's job is to create synthetic data. It takes a random noise vector as input and attempts to transform it into a data sample (e.g., a synthetic patient record) that looks like it came from the real dataset. Think of the Generator as a forger trying to create counterfeit money.

The Discriminator (D): This network acts as the detective. It is a binary classifier that shows both real data samples from the training set and fake data samples from the Generator. Its goal is to correctly distinguish between the real and the fake.

The training process is a "zero-sum" game. The Generator constantly tries to produce more realistic fakes to fool the Discriminator. Simultaneously, the Discriminator gets better at spotting even the most subtle flaws in the Generator's creations. They are trained together in an adversarial loop. The Generator's success is the Discriminator's failure, and vice versa. These competitive dynamic pushes both networks to improve. Over many iterations, the Generator becomes so proficient that its output is virtually indistinguishable from the real data to the point where the Discriminator is no better than random chance (50% accuracy) at telling them apart. When this process reaches equilibrium, the Generator has been fully trained so that it becomes a master manipulator, able to generate continuous-consistent synthetic data.

The loss function for a standard GAN can be expressed as a minimax game:

```
GminDmax V(D, G)=Ex□pdata(x)[logD(x)] +Ez□pz(z)
[log(1-D(G(z)))]
```

Here, 14D(x) is the Discriminator's probability that real data 15x is real, and 16D(G(z)) is the Discriminator's probability that fake data generated from noise 17z is real.18 The Discriminator D tries to maximize this objective, while the Generator G tries to minimize it.

Relevance to Health Data: GANs are particularly powerful for generating realistic, high-dimensional data, but their training can be notoriously unstable. In healthcare, they have been adapted to handle the unique mix of discrete (e.g., diagnosis codes) and continuous (e.g., lab values) variables found in EHRs, leading to specialized variants like medGAN (Choi et al., 2017).

2.2 Variational Autoencoders (VAEs)

Introduced by Kingma and Welling (2013), the Variational Autoencoder (VAE) takes a different, more probabilistic approach to generation. VAEs are built on the concept of an autoencoder, which is a neural network designed to learn a compressed representation (encoding) of its input data. A simple autoencoder has two parts:

Encoder: Compresses the high-dimensional input data into a low-dimensional "latent space" representation.

Decoder: Reconstructs the original input data from this compressed latent representation.

While a standard autoencoder is good for compression, it is not generative. We cannot simply pick a random point in the latent space and expect the decoder to produce a realistic new sample. VAEs modify this architecture to be generative by making the latent space continuous and well-structured.

Instead of mapping an input to a single point in the latent space, the VAE encoder maps it to a probability distribution (typically a Gaussian distribution defined by a mean and a variance). This means that similar inputs will be encoded into nearby regions in the latent space. To generate a new data point, we can now sample a random point from this learned latent distribution and pass it to the decoder. Because the latent space is smooth and continuous, this decoded output will be a novel but plausible data sample.

The VAE is trained to optimize two objectives simultaneously, captured in its loss function:

1. **Reconstruction Loss:** This measures how well the decoder can reconstruct the original input from its latent representation. It ensures the model is learning to capture the important features of the data.
2. **Kullback-Leibler (KL) Divergence:** This is a regularization term. It forces the distribution learned by the encoder to be close to a standard normal distribution (mean of 0, variance of 1). This organizes the latent space, preventing the model from "cheating" by assigning each data point to a distinct, isolated region, and ensures that the entire latent space is populated with meaningful representations.

Relevance to Health Data: In general, VAEs are more stable than GANs and offer a structured latent space that can be utilized for tasks such as visualizing patient clusters or understanding disease progression. Despite their focus on reconstruction and regularization, their loss function may result in slightly sharper samples than GANs, even though they are considered more realistic.

2.3 Transformer-Based Models

Originally designed for natural language processing tasks like translation or text generation, Transformers have revolutionized AI with their revolutionary self-attention mechanism (Vaswani et al., 2017). The main innovation of the Transformer model is its capability of gauging the relevance of differing portions of an input sequence while processing it. This quality is very effective with sequential data, where the context for a given element depends on its relationship with other elements, regardless of distance. Within the context of health data, one could view a patient's electronic health record (EHR) as a varying sequence of events: visits, diagnoses, prescriptions, and lab tests. RNNs tend to struggle with long-term dependencies in such sequences (for example, from childhood diagnosis to adult-onset condition), but Transformers are the best at directly modeling any two events in a patient's history through self-attention and, thus, perfectly suited for representing complex temporal dynamics that arise in healthcare data.

Generally, when it comes to generative workflows, autoregressive Transformer models proceed by generating a sequence one element at a time, each new element being conditioned on all previously generated elements. Suppose, for instance, the model is generating a synthetic patient journey; in that case, it would generate a demographic profile first, then generate the first visit/diagnosis conditioned on that profile, then generate a subsequent lab test or prescription conditioned on the profile and first visit, and so on, gradually forming a realistic clinical narrative. Relevance to Health Data: Transformers are quickly becoming the state-of-the-art method for generating sequential health data because they can maintain long-range clinical and temporal coherence. Models like Gena-BERT (Li et al., 2020) have shown great promise in generating realistic sequences of medical codes.

2.4 Diffusion Models

More recently, and very successful are Denoising Diffusion Probabilistic Models (DDPMs), or Diffusion Models (Ho et al., 2020; Sohl-Dickstein et al., 2015). These are state-of-the-art in image generation and are now widely being used across other data modalities, such as tabular and medical data. The functioning of a diffusion model can be understood in two stages:

1. **Forward Process (Diffusion):** This is a deterministic process where you begin with an actual sample of data (e.g., patient record) and gradually increase a small amount of Gaussian noise at numerous time steps. At the conclusion of this process, the original sample of data has evolved into clean raw noise.
2. **Reverse Process (Denoising):** It is in this stage that knowledge acquisition takes place. The training a neural network performs is to undo the diffusion process. The network that is given a noisy sample as input and is made to figure out the small portion of noise that was added at a specific time step is the one that is being referred to. The denoising network can, through repeated use, starting from absolute noise, a clean and lifelike data sample, which is entirely new, can be slowly brought back by the model.

Diffusion models have their charm in this denoising modelling undertaken step by step. Instead of creating a complex structure of data in a single attempt as done in a GAN or VAE, the model learns a much simpler job of predicting and removing a minute amount of noise at every timestep. This adds to the stability of the training process and usually results in synthetic samples of better quality and higher diversity.

All the building blocks of health data imply: Diffusion models are significantly newer to the healthcare domain; however, they hold great promise. Their potential for generating tabular EHR data embodies excellent handling of complex distributions with high fidelity. Early studies have already been done, modeling synthetic patient records that are both realistic and privacy-preserving (Pinaya et al., 2022).

3 CORE STRATEGIES FOR SYNTHETIC EHR GENERATION

Generating synthetic Electronic Health Records (EHRs) is not a one-size-fits-all problem. The choice of generative model and strategy depends heavily on the nature of the data (static vs. sequential, discrete vs. continuous) and the intended use case for the synthetic data. This section explores the specific strategies for applying the foundational models discussed previously to the unique challenges of health data.

3.1 Generating Static, Tabular EHR Data

Many applications require a static snapshot of a patient cohort, represented as a table where rows are patients and columns are features (e.g., demographics, diagnoses, latest lab values). This tabular data is often a mix of continuous variables (age, blood pressure) and discrete or categorical variables (gender, ICD-10 diagnosis codes).

3.1.1 GANs for Tabular Data: medGAN, table-GAN, and CTGAN

Standard GANs were designed for continuous data like images and struggle with discrete variables. Applying them naively to tabular health data often fails because the gradient-based updates from the discriminator are not well-suited for the all-or-nothing nature of categorical features. To address this, several specialized GAN architectures have been developed.

medGAN (Medical Generative Adversarial Network): Proposed by Choi et al. (2017), medGAN was one of the first major attempts to apply GANs to realistic, high-dimensional EHR data. It incorporates autoencoders into the GAN framework to learn a more effective representation of the sparse, multi-label binary vectors common in medical coding (e.g., a patient having multiple diagnoses). It also uses batch normalization and shortcut connections to improve training stability and learn more meaningful representations from discrete medical codes.

CTGAN (Conditional Tabular GAN): CTGAN (Xu et al., 2019) was a major step forward for mixed-type tabular data. The model brings in two main features. Firstly, it has a conditional generator, where the model is conditioned on one of the discrete columns. This not only simplifies the complicated joint distribution learning problem but also makes it possible to solve these smaller conditional distribution problems independently. Secondly, it adopts a new mode-specific normalization method for non-Gaussian and multimodal continuous variables, which are typical in health data (for instance, the bimodal distribution of a lab value for healthy vs. diseased populations). The fact that CTGAN can precisely depict the complex interactions between mixed data types is what makes it a very strong and popular baseline for synthetic EHRs generation.

TVAE (Tabular VAE): While GANs are very popular, VAEs-based methods also exist. With CTGAN, the TVAE model employs a VAE to model tabular data. It uses an autoregressive neural network as a decoder for the sequential generation of columns, where the generation of each column is conditioned on the previously generated ones. This ensures that dependencies between variables are better captured.

3.2 Generating Sequential and Longitudinal Health Data

A patient's health is dynamic, often changing with time. Longitudinal data are central to studies on disease progression, treatment efficacy, and future outcome projections as they represent the patient's fate through a timeline of clinical events. Hence, the creation of plausible sequences requires models that can properly comprehend temporal dependencies.

3.2.1 Recurrent GANs (R-GANs) and TimeGAN

In a GAN, to be able to handle sequences, its generator and discriminator can be replaced with RNNs or recurrent neural networks, like LSTM (Long Short-Term Memory) or GRUs (Gated Recurrent Units).

Recurrent GANs (R-GANs): In such an architecture, RNNs will be both generator and discriminator. The generator takes an input sequence consisting of random vectors and returns an output sequence of synthetic clinical events, whereas the discriminator will consider a sequence from a disjunct union of both real and synthetic sequences and try to classify the entire sequence as real or fake. This makes the task for the generator not just to learn realistic individual events, but also plausible temporal transitions between the events (Esteban et al., 2017).

TimeGAN (Time-series Generative Adversarial Network): Yoon et al. (2019) presented TimeGAN, a refined architecture for the generation of realistic time series data. It integrates a module for unsupervised feature extraction (using an autoencoder) for learning the temporal representation at a lower-dimensional latent space, after which the adversarial learning will take place within this latent space, thereby improving both efficiency and stability of the training. A key contribution of TimeGAN is its incorporation of a “stepwise supervised loss”, which explicitly drives the generator to capture the stepwise conditional distributions in the data.45 This renders it very promising for medical time series where the next event might be highly conditioned upon the former.

3.2.2 Transformer-Based Sequential Generators

Transformers are very good in capturing long-range dependencies, which is one area where RNNs underperform. Hence, they stand state of the art in generating long and complex patient histories.

MEDICAL TRANSFORMERS (for example, Gena-BERT): Models based on BERT (Bidirectional Encoder Representations from Transformers) can also be used for generational purposes. For instance, one can train a model from real patient sequences with the task of predicting the "masked" clinical codes. After training, such a model would have a deep contextual understanding of clinical pathways to be capable of generating a new sequence that starts with a "begin-sequence" token and autoregressively samples the next most likely clinical code, feeding it back as input for the next step (Li et al., 2020). This can potentially produce very coherent and clinically plausible sequences of diagnoses, procedures, and medications.

SyntEHR: The hallmark example of such a model is SynthEHR, a Transformer architecture that leverages the GPT-2 design to learn patient trajectories from EHRs (Biswal et al., 2021). The patient journey is treated as a sequence of "tokens," where each token represents a medical concept (e.g., an ICD code). By training on a large corpus of real patient sequences, it learns the "grammar" of clinical care and can generate realistic, variable-length patient histories.

3.3 Advanced Strategies and Hybrid Models

Everyone is moving forward now toward hybrid architecture and toward complexity out of the single-model architecture that has been the standard in the past.

3.3.1 Diffusion Models for Tabular and Mixed Data

Diffusion models represent a new frontier for EHR generation. The stability of their training and the high quality of their output are very attractive. In the case of tabular data, the noise is usually added and removed on a feature-by-feature basis. There is a need for some special ways to mix continuous and discrete data types to handle them. For instance, Gaussian diffusion may be employed for the continuous columns, whilst a categorical counterpart (multinomial diffusion) is applicable for the discrete ones (Kotelnikov et al., 2023). These models have been able to demonstrate the proficiency of opening complex, multimodal distributions of health data more than those of GAN variants.

3.3.2 Privacy-Preserving Generative Models (DP-GAN, DP-VAE)

The creation of synthetic data was mainly influenced by the need to protect privacy. Though a generator trained on real data could one time record and yield back a rare, unique patient record theoretically a situation termed as "model inversion" or "membership inference" attacks. To assure privacy through formal, mathematical means, implementing Differential Privacy (DP) alongside generative models is an option. Differential Privacy is a highly dependable mathematical model that facilitates the estimation statistically similar output irrespective of any single individual's data been included in the input dataset (Dwork, 2008). For the case of generative models, this is accomplished by supplementing the noise in the gradients that are used for training. This approach, called Differentially Private Stochastic Gradient Descent (DP-SGD), is the method for training the models like DP-GAN and DP-VAE (Abadi et al., 2016).

A new synthetic dataset is presented now with a guarantee ((ϵ,δ)-differential privacy) that the probability of any individual being re-identified in the original training set is very low. There is however a basic trade-off: enhancing the privacy level (i.e., lowering the privacy budget ϵ) is most likely to lead to the sacrifice of data utility. Scientists can produce synthetic health records that range in their usability from software testing to novel clinical research by picking and customizing these approaches such as privacy-enhanced transformers for longitudinal data or specialized GANs for static tables.

4 PRACTICAL IMPLEMENTATION: A STEP-BY-STEP GUIDE

Generating high-quality synthetic health records is as much an engineering challenge as it is a data science problem. The process involves a series of critical steps, from wrangling raw, messy EHR data to carefully training and tuning a complex generative model. This section provides a practical, step-by-step guide to this implementation pipeline.

4.1 Step 1: Data Acquisition and Preprocessing

Real-world EHR data is rarely "AI-ready." It is often stored in complex relational databases (e.g., OMOP Common Data Model, FHIR) and is characterized by missing values, inconsistencies, and a wide variety of data types.

4.1.1 Defining the Cohort and Features

The first step is to define the target patient population (the cohort) and the relevant features. This requires close collaboration with clinical domain experts. For example, if the goal is to generate data for a study on type 2 diabetes, the cohort would be patients with a corresponding diagnosis code. Relevant features might include:

Demographics: Age, gender, race/ethnicity.

Diagnoses: ICD-9/10 codes for diabetes and common comorbidities (e.g., hypertension, hyperlipidemia).

Medications: NDC codes or generic names for relevant drugs (e.g., metformin, insulin).

Lab Results: Continuous values for tests like HbA1c, glucose, creatinine.

Procedures: CPT codes for relevant medical procedures.

4.1.2 Data Extraction and Structuring

Once defined, the data must be extracted from the source database and structured into a suitable format.

For Static/Tabular Data: The goal is to create a single flat table per patient. This often involves aggregation. For instance, for a patient with multiple HbA1c measurements, one might take the mean, median, or most recent value. Diagnoses and medications are often represented as multi-hot encoded binary vectors, where each column represents a specific code, and a '1' indicates its presence for that patient.

For Sequential/Longitudinal Data: The data must be structured as a sequence of time-stamped events for each patient. This involves creating a unified event table where each row is an event (e.g., 'DIAGNOSIS_ICD10_E11.9', 'MEDICATION_METFORMIN_500MG', 'LAB_HBA1C_7.5') with an associated patient ID and timestamp or visit number.

4.1.3 Handling Missing Data and Normalization

Missing data is ubiquitous in EHRs. A lab test might not have been ordered, or a diagnosis might not have been coded.

Imputation: Imputation is the act of filling in missing values by either simple methods such as mean, median, and mode or complicated ones such as k-nearest neighbors (KNN) or model-based imputation (e.g., MICE).

Explicit "Missing" Category: "Missing" as an explicit category: For certain categorical variables, "missing" can be construed as its own meaningful category.

Data also needs to be transformed for modeling.

Continuous Variables: These are typically scaled to a specific range, such as [0, 1] (Min-Max scaling) or standardized to have a mean of 0 and a standard deviation of 1 (Standard scaling). This is crucial for the stable training of deep neural networks.

Categorical Variables: These are converted into numerical format using one-hot encoding or entity embeddings.

4.2 Step 2: Model Selection

The choice of generative model is dictated by the data structure and the project's goals.

Use Case: Generating a static, cross-sectional patient table with mixed data types.

Good Choice: CTGAN or TVAE. These models are specifically designed to handle the mix of continuous and categorical variables and model their complex correlations effectively.

Alternative: Diffusion Models for tabular data are a powerful emerging option, potentially offering higher fidelity.

Use Case: Generating longitudinal patient journeys with sequences of medical codes.

Good Choice: Transformer-based models (e.g., GPT-style). They excel at capturing long-range dependencies and generating clinically coherent narratives.

Alternative: TimeGAN is a strong choice, particularly for multivariate time-series data that includes continuous values (e.g., sequences of vital signs).

Use Case: The synthetic data must come with a formal privacy guarantee.

Required Choice: A differentially private model like DP-GAN or a model trained with DP-SGD. The choice between them depends on the underlying data structure (tabular vs. sequential).

4.3 Step 3: Model Training and Hyperparameter Tuning

Training generative models is an iterative process of experimentation and refinement.

4.3.1 Training Configuration

Batch Size: The number of data samples processed in one iteration. This affects training speed and stability. GANs can be sensitive to batch size.

Learning Rate: Controls how much the model's weights are updated during training. A learning rate that is too high can cause unstable training, while one that is too low can result in a very slow or stalled learning process. Using a learning rate scheduler, which adjusts the rate during training, is common practice.

Optimizer: Algorithms like Adam or RMSprop are standard choices for training deep learning models.

Epochs: The number of times the entire training dataset is passed through the model. The right number of epochs is crucial to avoid underfitting (model hasn't learned enough) or overfitting (model has memorized the training data).

4.3.2 Dealing with Training Instabilities (Especially for GANs)

GAN training is notoriously challenging and can suffer from issues like:

Mode Collapse: The generator finds a few "safe" examples that can easily fool the discriminator and only produce those, leading to a lack of diversity in the synthetic data. For example, it might only generate male patients with diabetes, ignoring all other patient profiles. This can be mitigated by using techniques like minibatch discrimination or experimenting with different loss functions (e.g., Wasserstein loss).

Vanishing/Exploding Gradients: The discriminator becomes too good, too quickly, and its feedback to the generator becomes uninformative (vanishing gradients), or the training process becomes wildly unstable (exploding gradients). Techniques like gradient clipping, careful network initialization, and using normalization layers (e.g., batch norm, layer norm) can help.

4.3.3 Hyperparameter Tuning

The performance of a generative model is highly sensitive to its hyperparameters (e.g., number of layers, size of hidden units, learning rate). Finding the optimal combination is key.

Grid Search/Random Search: Systematically trying different combinations of hyperparameters.

Bayesian Optimization: A more intelligent search method that uses the results of past trials to choose the next set of hyperparameters to evaluate, making the search process more efficient.

4.4 Step 4: Synthetic Data Generation

Once the model is trained to a satisfactory level (as determined by monitoring its loss curves and preliminary evaluation metrics), it can be used to generate the synthetic dataset. This involves:

Sampling from the Latent Space: Feeding random noise vectors (for GANs/VAEs) or starting tokens (for Transformers) into the trained generator.

Generating the Data: The generator processes this input and outputs the synthetic data in its normalized/encoded format.

Post-processing/Inverse Transformation: The generated data must be transformed back into its original scale and format. This involves inverse scaling for continuous variables and decoding one-hot vectors back into their original categorical labels.

The result is a new, synthetic dataset, ready for the most important step: rigorous evaluation.

5 EVALUATION AND VALIDATION: THE TRIAD OF QUALITY

Generating a synthetic dataset is only half the battle. A synthetic dataset is useless—or even dangerous—if it is not a high-quality proxy for the real data. The evaluation process is therefore paramount and must be comprehensive. A robust validation framework assesses the synthetic data from three critical perspectives: Fidelity (resemblance to real data), Utility (usefulness for a specific task), and Privacy (protection of patient information). This triad ensures the synthetic data is both safe and effective.

5.1 Fidelity: Is Synthetic Data Realistic?

Fidelity, or "statistical similarity," measures how well synthetic data captures the statistical properties of the real data. The goal is to ensure the marginal distributions, correlations, and joint distributions are preserved.

5.1.1 Univariate and Bivariate Similarity

These are foundational checks to see if the basic statistics match up.

Marginal Distributions: Compare the distributions of individual features between the real and synthetic datasets. For continuous variables, this can be done visually using histograms or density plots and quantitatively using metrics like the

Kolmogorov-Smirnov (KS) test or Wasserstein distance. For categorical variables, compare the frequency counts or use a Chi-squared test.

Pairwise Correlations: Compare the correlation matrices (e.g., using Pearson correlation for continuous variables) of real and synthetic data. A visual comparison of heatmaps can be very insightful. The structural similarity of these matrices can be quantified.

5.1.2 Multivariate Similarity and Dimensionality Reduction

Real-world data lies on a complex, high-dimensional manifold. A good synthetic dataset should replicate this structure.

Principal Component Analysis (PCA): Perform PCA on both the real and synthetic datasets and compare the principal components. If the synthetic data is realistic, the top components should capture similar sources of variance.

t-SNE / UMAP Visualization: Use dimensionality reduction techniques like t-SNE or UMAP to project the high-dimensional real and synthetic data into a 2D or 3D space. Visually inspect whether the shape, density, and clustering of the synthetic data cloud resemble that of the real data. A good synthetic dataset will occupy the same "space" as the real data.

5.2 Utility: Is Synthetic Data Useful?

The ultimate test of a synthetic dataset is whether it can be used for the same downstream tasks as the real data and yield similar conclusions. This is often referred to as the "Train on Synthetic, Test on Real" (TSTR) paradigm.

5.2.1 Machine Learning Efficacy

Train a predictive model (e.g., a logistic regression model to predict hospital readmission, or a random forest for mortality prediction) on the real dataset. Evaluate its performance (e.g., AUROC, F1-score) on a held-out real test set. This establishes a performance benchmark. Train the same predictive model architecture on the synthetic dataset. Evaluate the model trained on synthetic data on the same real test set. The utility is measured by how close the performance of the model trained on synthetic data is to the benchmark model trained on real data. If the performance is very similar, the synthetic data has high utility for that specific machine learning task (Choi et al., 2017).

5.2.2 Clinical Study Replication

A more advanced utility test is to attempt to replicate the findings of a known clinical study or epidemiological analysis using only the synthetic data. For example, if a real dataset shows a known association between a certain medication and a reduced risk of a specific adverse event, the synthetic data should also demonstrate this association with a similar odds ratio or hazard ratio when analyzed with the same statistical methods (e.g., Cox proportional hazards model). Successfully replicating such findings provides strong evidence of the data's real-world utility.

5.3 Privacy: Is Patient Data Safe?

Even if synthetic data contains no 1-to-1 copies of real records, privacy can still be breached if the model memorizes sensitive information. Privacy evaluation aims to quantify this risk.

5.3.1 Distance to Closest Record (DCR)

This metric checks for direct data leakage. For each synthetic record, find the closest record in the real training dataset using a distance metric (e.g., Euclidean or Hamming distance). If many synthetic records are identical or nearly identical to real records, it indicates that the generator may have overfit and memorized parts of the training data. The distribution of these minimum distances for the synthetic data should be compared to the distribution of minimum distances between records within the real dataset itself.

5.3.2 Membership Inference Attacks

The second type of privacy audit is more advanced. The goal of a membership inference attack is to discern from the generative model whether a certain, specifically targeted patient's record was used in the construction of the original training dataset. The attacker then will build a classifier that takes the data record as input to give an output in the form of a probability further defined as "member" of the training set. This attack model is commonly trained on the behavior of the generative model in terms of both data it has seen and data it has not seen. If the attacker's classifier can predict membership with significantly better-than-chance (50%) accuracy, it indicates that the generative model has leaked information about its training data (Shokri et al., 2017). Therefore, the success of such attacks stands as a strong empirical measure for assessing the privacy risks in question.

5.3.3 Formal Privacy Guarantees

Off hand, privacy for models using differential privacy (e.g., DP-GAN) is not simply a matter of empirical evaluation but a mathematical guarantee. The privacy budget, referred to as epsilon (ϵ), sets a formal limit on the amount of new information a model can reveal about any single individual. Thus, the lower the value of ϵ, the stronger the privacy is. The most stringent kind of privacy acknowledgment is showing the (ϵ,δ) values that the model was trained on.

Through a thorough implementation of this threefold evaluation framework, the developers can obtain a comprehensive grasp of the quality of their synthetic data, thereby certifying that it is a realistic, usable, and safe substitute for the original patient data.

6 ETHICAL CONSIDERATIONS AND THE REGULATORY LANDSCAPE

Creating and utilizing synthetic health data, although technologically desirable, is not separate from the ethical and legal obligations that they hold. They are, indeed, moral and legal "citizens" in the viral network of the health care system, ethical responsibilities and legal regulations being part of that network. Without a cautious and careful way through this terrain, the results may be prejudiced, the trust of the public that there is compliance with the law may be weakened, and even laws enacted to ensure the safety of patients may be broken.

6.1 The Specter of Bias: Fairness and Equity

Perhaps the most significant ethical challenge is bias. Generative AI models learn from the data they are given. If the real-world health data used for training reflects existing societal biases and health disparities, the synthetic data will inevitably learn, replicate, and potentially amplify them.

Representation Bias: If a particular demographic group (e.g., a racial minority, a rural population) is underrepresented in the original dataset, the generative model will have less information to learn from for this group. Consequently, the synthetic data may poorly represent these individuals, leading to downstream AI models that are less accurate for them (Chen et al., 2023). For example, a synthetic dataset for a skin cancer detection model trained on data predominantly from light-skinned individuals will likely be less useful for validating algorithms on darker skin tones.

Historical Bias: Health data can reflect historical inequities. For instance, if a certain group has historically received a lower quality of care or has been systematically under-diagnosed for a condition, the model will learn these biased patterns as "ground truth." A synthetic dataset generated from this data might suggest that certain interventions are less effective for this group, not because they are biologically different, but because the historical data reflects a disparity in care.

Mitigation Strategies:

Bias Auditing of Source Data: Before training, the real dataset must be thoroughly audited for biases in representation and outcomes across different demographic subgroups.

Fairness-Aware Generative Models: Researchers are developing techniques to debias models during training. This can involve adding fairness constraints to the loss function, encouraging the model to generate data where outcomes are equitable across different protected groups (e.g., ensuring that the correlation between race and a negative health outcome in the synthetic data is weaker than in the biased real data).

Augmentation and Re-sampling: Techniques like oversampling underrepresented groups in the training data can help but must be done carefully to avoid simply creating unrealistic duplicates.

6.2 Accountability and Transparency

When synthetic data is used to develop or test a clinical tool, who is accountable if the tool fails or causes harm? The "black box" nature of some complex generative models can make it difficult to understand *why* they generated a particular type of data.

Traceability: It is essential to maintain clear documentation (datasheets for datasets) that details the source of the original data, the preprocessing steps taken, the specific generative model and hyperparameters used, and the results of the evaluation process (Gebru et al., 2021). This creates a transparent audit trail.

Interpretability: Research into making generative models more interpretable is ongoing. Understanding which features in the input data most influence the generated output can help diagnose and correct for biases or other undesirable model behaviors.

6.3 The Regulatory Framework: HIPAA and GDPR

Privacy regulations are the legal bedrock governing the use of health data. The application of these laws to synthetic data is a nuanced and evolving area.

HIPAA (Health Insurance Portability and Accountability Act): In the U.S., HIPAA's Privacy Rule protects "Individually Identifiable Health Information." Data is considered de-identified, and thus outside HIPAA's direct purview, if it meets one of two standards: (1) Safe Harbor, which involves removing 18 specific identifiers, or (2) Expert Determination, where a statistical expert certifies that the risk of re-identification is very small.

Synthetic data, by definition, contains no real patient information. Therefore, a properly generated and validated synthetic dataset is considered fully anonymized and would not be classified as Protected Health Information (PHI). This is its primary legal advantage. However, the *process* of generating synthetic data still requires access to the original, protected PHI, and this process must be conducted within a secure, HIPAA-compliant environment.

GDPR (General Data Protection Regulation): The EU's GDPR sets a high bar for data protection. It uses the concept of "personal data," which is broadly defined. While fully anonymous data falls outside the scope of GDPR, the process of "anonymization" itself is considered data processing. The regulation emphasizes that data should be considered anonymous only if the risk of re-identification is effectively zero.

This is where synthetic data with Differential Privacy (DP) guarantees becomes particularly valuable. DP provides a provable, mathematical argument against re-identification that aligns well with the rigorous standards of GDPR. Organizations using synthetic data in a GDPR context may find that using DP-enhanced models provides a stronger legal and ethical foundation for their claim of anonymization. In summary, the ethical use of synthetic health data requires a proactive approach. It demands a commitment to fairness, a rigorous process for bias detection and mitigation, and a clear understanding of how this novel technology fits within existing legal frameworks for patient privacy.

7 CURRENT CHALLENGES AND FUTURE DIRECTIONS

While generative AI has made remarkable strides in creating synthetic health records, the field is far from solved. Several key challenges remain, and the path forward is illuminated by exciting and innovative research directions that promise to create synthetic data of even greater quality, utility, and trustworthiness.

7.1 Current Challenges and Limitations

Capturing Extreme Rarity (The "Long Tail"): Generative models are trained to learn the primary modes of data distribution. They often struggle to adequately represent very rare events, diseases, or patient profiles—the "long tail" of the distribution. For a model trained on millions of records, a condition that appears only a dozen times might be treated as noise and be absent from the synthetic data. This is a critical limitation, as studying rare diseases is a key use case for synthetic data.

Complex Temporal Dependencies: While Transformers have improved the modeling of sequential data, capturing very long-term, complex, and irregular temporal patterns remains a challenge. For example, modeling the decades-long interplay between lifestyle factors, intermittent treatments, and the slow progression of a chronic disease requires a level of temporal understanding that pushes the limits of current architectures.

Handling Unstructured Data: The richest source of clinical information is often locked away in unstructured clinical notes, radiology reports, and discharge summaries. While generative language models can generate text, seamlessly integrating the generation of realistic, coherent clinical narratives with structured EHR data (diagnoses, labs) in a single, unified model is an active and complex area of research.

Scalability and Computational Cost: Training state-of-the-art generative models like large Transformers or Diffusion Models on massive, hospital-scale datasets requires immense computational resources (GPUs/TPUs) and significant engineering expertise, placing it out of reach for smaller research institutions or startups.

The Utility-Privacy Trade-off: As discussed, the application of differential privacy to ensure formal privacy guarantees often comes at a cost to data utility. Finding the "sweet spot" that provides meaningful privacy without degrading the data's usefulness to the point of being impractical is a persistent challenge. The optimal balance depends heavily on the specific use case and risk tolerance.

7.2 Future Directions and Emerging Trends

The future of synthetic health data generation is bright, with several research avenues poised to overcome current limitations.

Federated Learning for Synthetic Data Generation: A major bottleneck is the need to centralize sensitive patient data to train a generative model. Federated Learning (FL) offers a powerful alternative. In an FL setup, multiple institutions (e.g., hospitals) collaboratively train a single, shared generative model without ever moving their data from their local, secure servers. Each institution trains the model on its local data and shares only the model updates (gradients), not the data itself, with a central server that aggregates them. This allows for the creation of a generative model trained on a diverse, multi-institutional dataset, leading to more robust and generalizable synthetic data while inherently preserving privacy (Chang et al., 2020).

Causal Generative Models: Standard generative models are excellent at learning correlations but have no understanding of cause and effect. A synthetic dataset might correctly learn that yellow fingers are correlated with lung cancer, but it doesn't know that smoking is the common cause of both. Causal Generative Models, which incorporate principles of causal inference, aim to learn the underlying causal graph of the data. A synthetic dataset generated from such a model would not only be statistically realistic but could also be used for *silico* experiments, for example, simulating the effect of a new treatment by intervening on the causal graph, a task impossible with standard synthetic data.

Multimodal Data Generation: Patient health is inherently multimodal. The future lies in models that can jointly generate data across different modalities. Imagine a single generative model that can create a synthetic patient profile that includes not only their EHR data (diagnoses, medications) but also their corresponding synthetic chest X-ray images, genomic data, and wearable device signals.

Over time, as the boundaries of scientific inquiry continue to move, synthetic health data will still play a crucial role in the medical research and development sector, thereby cutting down the time required to deliver a healthcare system that is more equitable, efficient, and personalized.

8 DISCUSSION AND CONCLUSION

On the one hand, the healthcare sector is witnessing a deep-dive data transformation. On the other hand, there are equally far-reaching barriers to accessing real-world health data. Among them are privacy laws, issues of patient confidentiality, a scarcity of data for rare diseases, and data currently available, which exhibit biases that create huge obstacles for researchers, developers, and policymakers. Synthetic health records represent a potent solution to these barriers: these artificially generated data present a statistical picture and patterns of real patient data without any real individual information. The path traced through the terrain of synthetic health data generation symbolizes huge potential fuelled by the sophistication of generative artificial intelligence. We have progressed from a time when accessing data felt like climbing Mount Everest to the fact that we can now algorithmically generate high-fidelity proxies for real-world patient data that preserve privacy. This technological advancement has the potential to create equal opportunities for healthcare research, bring down the time taken for the creation of life-saving AI, and kick-start innovation, while firmly protecting one of the foundational rights of patient privacy (Bhuyan et al., 2025).

The different strategies covered in this chapter—from GANs' adversarial nature to VAEs' probabilistic quaintness, the sequential mastery by Transformers, and diffusion models' high-quality output—gave birth to a compelling toolkit. In contrast, it is a technical approach requiring structured and thoughtful careful preprocessing of the data. A principled model selection should be done cautiously, and even more so, a multi-tiered evaluation framework should be constructed on fidelity, utility, and privacy. A synthetic dataset is not worth much if it cannot undergo rigorous validation against those criteria. It also must be undertaken in the clear-eyed knowledge that we have ethical responsibilities. The specter of algorithmic bias is a very deep challenge that requires us to broaden our audits of our source data to develop fairness-aware models to ensure that synthetic data will close, not further widen, existing health disparities. It is not a stumbling block but a beaming visible signpost—the regulatory walls of HIPAA and GDPR—that ensures our innovations become based on trust and accountability.

The future is vibrant and full of possibilities. The combination of federated learning, causal inference, and large-scale multimodal models will, without a doubt, open up the next generation of synthetic data that will not only be richer and more robust but will also be more deeply intertwined with the process of medical discovery. We can harness the power of synthetic health records to reveal the untapped medical knowledge that lies hidden within our collective medical knowledge by properly adopting these technological breakthroughs, which will, in the end, lead to a healthier world for everyone.

REFERENCES

Abadi, M., Chu, A., Goodfellow, I., McMahan, H. B., Mironov, I., Talwar, K., & Zhang, L. (2016). Deep learning with differential privacy. *Proceedings of the 2016 ACM SIGSAC Conference on Computer and Communications Security*, 308–318. https://doi.org/DOI: 10.1145/2976749.2978318

Auffray, C., Balling, R., Barroso, I., Bencze, L., Benson, M., Bergeron, J., Bernal-Delgado, E., Blomberg, N., Bock, C., Conesa, A., Del Signore, S., Delogne, C., Devilee, P., Di Meglio, A., Eijkemans, M., Flicek, P., Graf, N., Grimm, V., Guchelaar, H.-J., & Zanetti, G. (2016). Making sense of big data in health research: Towards an EU action plan. *Genome Medicine*, *8*(1), 1–10. DOI: 10.1186/s13073-016-0323-y PMID: 26750923

Beaumont, J. (2021). *Synthetic data for the privacy-conscious Luddite*. Towards Data Science.

Bhuyan, S. S., Sateesh, V., Mukul, N., Galvankar, A., Mahmood, A., Nauman, M., Rai, A., Bordoloi, K., Basu, U., & Samuel, J. (2025). Generative artificial intelligence Use in healthcare: Opportunities for clinical excellence and administrative efficiency. *Journal of Medical Systems*, *49*(1), 10. DOI: 10.1007/s10916-024-02136-1 PMID: 39820845

Biswal, S., Singh, D., & Pentyala, S.. (2021). SynthEHR: A Transformer-based approach for generating synthetic electronic health records. *2021 IEEE International Conference on Bioinformatics and Biomedicine (BIBM)*, 2686-2693.

Chang, K., Shlezinger, N., & Eldar, Y. C. (2020). Federated learning for privacy-preserving medical data generation. *arXiv preprint arXiv:2009.07062*.

Chen, I., Johansson, F. D., & Sontag, D. (2023). Why is my model unfair? A systematic review of sources of unfairness in machine learning for healthcare. *Nature Medicine*, *29*(6), 1344–1354.

Choi, E., Biswal, S., Malin, B., Duke, J., Stewart, W. F., & Sun, J. (2017).[98] Generating multi-label discrete patient records using generative adversarial networks. *Machine Learning for Healthcare Conference*, 286–305. PMLR.

Dwork, C. (2008). Differential privacy: A survey of results. In *International Conference on Theory and Applications of Models of Computation* (pp. 1-19). Springer, Berlin, Heidelberg.

Esteban, C., Hyland, S. L., & Rätsch, G. (2017). Real-valued (medical) time series generation with recurrent conditional GANs. *arXiv preprint arXiv:1706.02633*.

Gebru, T., Morgenstern, J., Vecchione, B., Vaughan, J. W., Wallach, H., Daumé, H.III, & Crawford, K. (2021). Datasheets for datasets. *Communications of the ACM*, *64*(12), 86–92. DOI: 10.1145/3458723

Goodfellow, I., Pouget-Abadie, J., Mirza, M., Xu, B., Warde-Farley, D., Ozair, S., Courville, A., & Bengio, Y. (2014). Generative adversarial nets. *Advances in Neural Information Processing Systems*, •••, 27.

Hasan, S. S., Fury, M. S., Woo, J. J., Kunze, K. N., & Ramkumar, P. N. (2025). Ethical application of generative artificial intelligence in medicine. *Arthroscopy*, *41*(4), 874–885. DOI: 10.1016/j.arthro.2024.12.011 PMID: 39689842

Ho, J., Jain, A., & Abbeel, P. (2020). Denoising diffusion probabilistic models. *Advances in Neural Information Processing Systems*, *33*, 6840–6851.

Kingma, D. P., & Welling, M. (2013). Auto-encoding variational bayes. *arXiv preprint arXiv:1312.6114*.

Kotelnikov, A., Barannikov, S., Kiani, A., & Burnaev, E. (2023). TabDDPM: Modelling Tabular Data with Diffusion Models. *International Conference on Learning Representations*.

Li, Y., Rao, S., Solares, J. R. A., & Ramakrishnan, N. (2020). Gena-bert: A new method for generating electronic health records. *2020 IEEE International Conference on Healthcare Informatics (ICHI)*, 1-10.

Obermeyer, Z., Powers, B., Vogeli, C., & Mullainathan, S. (2019). Dissecting racial bias in an algorithm used to manage the health of populations. *Science*, *366*(6464), 447–453. DOI: 10.1126/science.aax2342 PMID: 31649194

Pinaya, W. H., Scarpiniti, M., Kikas, P., Tudosiu, P. D., Dighum, W., & Cardoso, M. J. (2022). Brain imaging generation with latent diffusion models. *arXiv preprint arXiv:2209.07162*. DOI: 10.1007/978-3-031-18576-2_12

Rujas, M., del Moral Herranz, R. M. G., Fico, G., & Merino-Barbancho, B. (2025). Synthetic data generation in healthcare: A scoping review of reviews on domains, motivations, and future applications. *International Journal of Medical Informatics*, *195*, 105763. DOI: 10.1016/j.ijmedinf.2024.105763 PMID: 39719743

Shokri, R., Stronati, M., Song, C., & Shmatikov, V. (2017). Membership inference attacks against machine learning models. *2017 IEEE Symposium on Security and Privacy (SP)*, 3–18. DOI: 10.1109/SP.2017.41

Sohl-Dickstein, J., Weiss, E., Maheswaranathan, N., & Ganguli, S. (2015). Deep unsupervised learning using nonequilibrium thermodynamics. *International Conference on Machine Learning*, 2256–2265. PMLR.

Vaswani, A., Shazeer, N., Parmar, N., Uszkoreit, J., Jones, L., Gomez, A. N., Kaiser, L., & Polosukhin, I. (2017). Attention is all you need. *Advances in Neural Information Processing Systems*, •••, 30.

Xu, L., Skoularidou, M., Cuesta-Infante, A., & Veeramachaneni, K. (2019). Modeling tabular data using conditional GAN. *Advances in Neural Information Processing Systems*, •••, 32.

Yoon, J., Jarrett, D., & van der Schaar, M. (2019). Time-series generative adversarial networks. *Advances in Neural Information Processing Systems*, •••, 32.

Chapter 5

Prediction and Primary Diagnosis of Diabetic Retinopathy From Retinal Images Using Deep Learning Algorithm

D. Rubidha Devi
https://orcid.org/0000-0001-9074-8984
SASTRA University, India

Priya Govindarajan
Amrita School of Computing, Amrita Vishwa Vidyapeetham, Mysuru, India

Vimala Devi P.
https://orcid.org/0000-0001-8422-6266
SASTRA University, India

M. Vanitha
https://orcid.org/0000-0002-5957-1970
SASTRA University, India

S. Parthasarathy
Mahatma Gandhi Medical College and Research Institute, India

ABSTRACT

Diabetic retinopathy (DR) is a serious eye condition linked to diabetes, resulting from high blood sugar levels. It can cause varying degrees of vision impairment, potentially leading to blindness. Early symptoms include blurred vision, changes

DOI: 10.4018/979-8-3373-5641-9.ch005

in color vision, and dark spots. Detecting DR early is crucial to preventing vision loss, as it typically appears as small red spots on the retina from hemorrhages or microaneurysms. This paper presents a method that utilizes Convolutional Neural Networks (CNN) to identify crucial features such as haemorrhages, exudates, bleeding, and microaneurysms, thereby enhancing the accuracy of diabetes-related predictions. The CNN approach enables the processing of real-time data, simplifying the extraction of key features from retinal images without necessitating extensive annotation or segmentation. This approach not only streamlines the detection and treatment process during the early stages but also provides a preliminary safeguard for patient health.

1. INTRODUCTION

Diabetes-related retinopathy (DR) affects over 422 million people worldwide, and it is estimated that one-third of these individuals will develop DR. According to the World Health Organization, by 2030, approximately 360 million people are predicted to be blinded by DR, which would account for 2.6% of global blindness. Early detection and treatment can significantly reduce the risk of blindness. Diabetes, caused by high blood glucose levels, leads to serious damage to blood vessels, which can result in various complications such as kidney problems, eye damage, bleeding gums, nerve damage, and heart issues (Yang et al., 2022) (Dutta et al., 2018). Changes in eating patterns help to spread diabetes over the world.

DR is caused by the rupture of eye capillaries induced by high blood glucose levels, which causes lesions in the retina and impairs vision. In the initial phases, the disease may develop silently, leading to significant vision loss or total blindness if not realized and treated (Diabetic Retinopathy Columbus I Diabetes Norfolk I Eye Physicians P.C., n.d.) swiftly . Exudates, which are apparent in retinal imaging, are important indications of the progression of DR. The presence and type of lesions on the retina, which include microaneurysms, haemorrhages, and exudates, indicate the severity of DR(Wu, 2013)(Usman Akram et al., 2014)(Alyoubi et al., 2020a). Retinal photographs and optical coherence tomography (OCT) are used in the diagnosis. Collaboration between retinal specialists, ophthalmologists, and endocrinologists is necessary. Early identification, which is critical for effective therapy, can be aided by computerized diagnostic approaches such as retinal screening. Floating spots, impaired vision, night blindness, and colour vision impairment are all common symptoms (Alyoubi et al., 2020a). DR is divided into two types, Non-proliferative (NPDR) and proliferative (PDR).

Convolutional Neural Network (CNN) (Mekala et al., 2021)(Lam et al., n.d.) algorithms have the potential to enhance the detection of diabetic retinopathy (DR) and offer an intermediate repair technique. Effective feature extraction requires data preprocessing, which includes converting input images to grayscale, removing noise, and applying median filtering. CNN algorithms are capable of categorizing and detecting retinopathy, resulting in significant time and cost savings compared to manual methods. The proposed approach aims to raise awareness of DR detection and emphasize the importance of accurate forecasts. As the prevalence of DR is projected to increase significantly by 2030, enhancing awareness and detection efforts is crucial. While many current research studies focus on accuracy, few incorporate a precautionary intermediate strategy. The method presented not only serves as a preventive measure for patients but also acts as a time-efficient solution for early diagnosis and treatment. This study highlights the importance of integrating artificial intelligence, particularly CNN algorithms, in DR detection to overcome the challenges associated with manual diagnosis, ultimately leading to improved patient outcomes. In conclusion, the suggested deep learning model based on CNN algorithms offers a promising solution for the detection and classification of DR. This automated approach can reliably diagnose and assess the severity of DR, transforming the existing diagnostic process by enabling timely treatments and potentially preventing vision loss in diabetic patients. Early studies of diabetic retinopathy primarily relied on conventional methods for feature discovery. However, recent advancements in machine and deep learning have shifted these strategies. Previously, DR detection involved manually extracting features from clinical photographs and feeding them into deep learning models for disease classification. Various researchers have proposed different techniques for predicting DR, reflecting the evolution of methodologies in this field.

Ting Luo et al. utilized biophysical techniques to measure the impact of non-proliferative diabetic retinopathy on retinal branching, comparing vascular branching in healthy and diabetic subjects (Luo et al., 2017a). Pedro Costa et al. introduced a novel approach based on multiple instance learning (MIL) frameworks for image annotation (Costa et al., 2018). Toufique Ahmed Soomro conducted a review of over eighty papers on retinal vessel detection, identifying the best 17 papers for retinal blood vessel segmentation (Soomro et al., 2019). Manoj Kumar Behera proposed an automated screening system using image processing to predict DR(Behera, 2020). Lifeng Qiao employed CNN algorithms for microaneurysm detection in clinical fundus images (Qiao et al., 2020). Samaneh Abbasi-Sureshjani used deep residual networks to identify diabetes from eye images, while Qaisar Abbas proposed an automatic severity level exposure of DR using processing steps on eye fundus photographs(Abbasi-Sureshjani et al., 2018)(Abbas et al., 2017a). Feng Li suggested a method for automated DR detection in retinal fundus photos through deep transfer learning(Li et al., 2019). Nguyen et al. used a multiple-layer feed-ahead network for DR severity classification (Nguyen et al., 1996). Zhang et al. employed SVM for categorizing non-lesion and lesion regions, and Soares et al. utilized two-dimensional Gabor wavelet images for feature extraction in vascular parts (Xiaohui & Chutatape, 2004)(Soares et al., 2006).

Various authors explored different approaches, including image pre-processing strategies proposed by Nayak et al. for lesion detection and DR severity assessment (Nayak et al., 2008). Barriga et al. developed a machine using PLS and amplitude and frequency modulation to find lesions in eye regions (Barriga et al., 2010). Priya et al. compared the effectiveness of PNN and SVM, with SVM found to be 97% more accurate (Priya & Aruna, 2012). Roychowdhury reduced feature count to classify diabetics in different models, and Srivastava utilized the Frangi filter method for obtaining characteristics from eye photos to train SVM (Roychowdhury et al., 2014) (Srivastava et al., 2015) . Santhakumar proposed a novel method of cutting images into rectangular shapes and inputting them into SVM for DR severity classification (Santhakumar et al., 2017). Pratt et al. extracted lesion features from augmentation methods, simplifying classification (Santoso & Nelloh, 2017). Abbas et al. introduced a deep visual feature (DVF) without processing steps, using gradient histogram region-wise and multiple layer networks for classification (Abbas et al., 2017b). Kanungo et al. compared the effects of hyperparameters on processed and trained images (Kanungo et al., 2017). Quellec et al. identified important pixels in retinal images using heat maps (Quellec et al., 2017). Zhao et al. combined bilinear network and interest mechanism for high accuracy (Abbas et al., 2017b). Orujov implemented the Mamdani (type-2) fuzzy rule for contour detection image processing (Orujov et al., 2020).

The selection of an appropriate algorithm for predicting diabetic retinopathy (DR) is influenced by a variety of factors, including the particular nature of the problem at hand as well as the unique properties and characteristics of the dataset being used. Diabetic retinopathy is a progressive eye disease caused by diabetes, and its early detection is crucial for preventing vision loss. While no universally applicable methodology can address all the complexities involved in predicting the onset and progression of retinopathy, convolutional neural networks (CNNs) have emerged as a popular choice, especially when working with large and diverse datasets. CNNs are designed to automatically detect intricate patterns and features in images, making them particularly well-suited for image classification tasks such as analyzing retinal scans. Numerous studies have been conducted to evaluate the effectiveness of various algorithms in the classification and detection of DR. Although researchers have explored different machine learning techniques, there is a growing consensus within the scientific community that CNNs provide superior performance in terms of accuracy and reliability for classifying diabetic retinopathy. Their ability to learn from vast amounts of imaging data allows for more precise and timely diagnoses, which is essential for patient outcomes in diabetes management

(Khan et al., 2021). In conclusion, the journey of predicting and classifying diabetic retinopathy (DR) has transformed dramatically, shifting from conventional techniques to cutting-edge deep learning methods. The choice of algorithm is intricately tied to the unique traits of the data at hand. While various algorithms have been explored in this evolving landscape, convolutional neural networks (CNNs) have emerged as a powerful choice, celebrated for their ability to enhance accuracy, particularly when navigating the complexities of large datasets. This evolution signifies a remarkable leap forward in the quest to understand and combat this sight-threatening condition.

2. METHODOLOGY

This study presents an innovative deep learning framework focused on the early detection and classification of Diabetic Retinopathy (DR) severity, utilizing detailed retinal images for analysis (Teo et al., 2021). The system is systematically organized into five essential modules, each playing a pivotal role in the overall process.

Noise Filtering: The process begins with the noise filtering module, where raw retinal images are meticulously preprocessed. This crucial step involves eliminating unwanted artifacts and disturbances that could obscure the subtle details within the images. By enhancing the image quality, this module lays the groundwork for accurate analytical outcomes.

Feature Extraction: Following the cleaning process, the feature extraction module employs sophisticated algorithms to identify and capture vital characteristics of the retina. This phase entails discovering intricate patterns, textures, and anomalies that are indicative of diabetic retinopathy, showcasing the delicate interplay of light and shadow that reflects the retina's underlying health.

Dataset Training: With essential features identified, the system transitions into the dataset training phase. Here, a diverse collection of retinal images, representing various manifestations of DR across its spectrum of severity, is utilized to train the model. This extensive dataset empowers the artificial intelligence to learn and adapt, refining its ability to recognize and differentiate between the nuances of Type-1 and Type-2 DR.

Dataset Testing: After the training phase, the model undergoes comprehensive testing with a separate set of retinal images. This evaluation phase is critical, challenging the model to apply its learned knowledge in real-world scenarios. By comparing its predictions against known outcomes, researchers can assess the model's accuracy and reliability, ensuring it can effectively navigate the complexities of various cases.

Disease Prediction: The final module culminates in the practical application of the system's capabilities. Using the insights gained during training, the Convolutional Neural Network (CNN) analyzes new retinal images to predict the presence and type of Diabetic Retinopathy. The model not only classifies the severity of the condition but also offers actionable precautionary recommendations for further management. The overarching goal of this advanced system is to enhance the accuracy of Diabetic Retinopathy prediction and diagnosis, a vital undertaking given the significant risk of vision loss or blindness associated with the condition. Accompanying this exploration is an architectural diagram in Figure 1, which visually represents the intricate processes involved in this cutting-edge approach

Figure 1. Architecture diagram of work

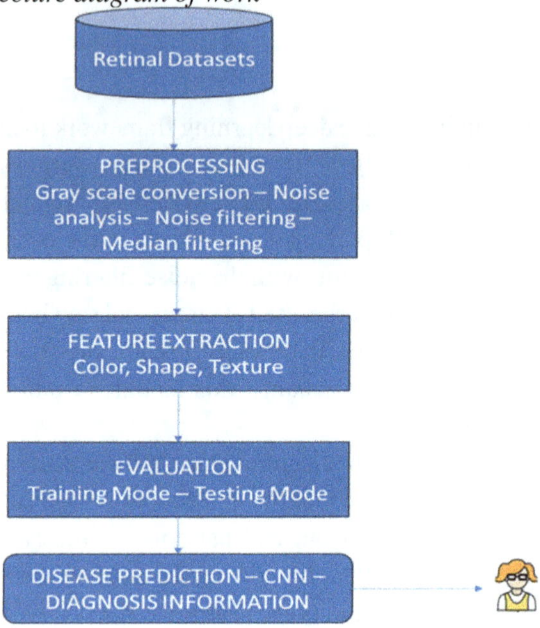

2.1. Dataset

The dataset was obtained from the Kaggle repository, and it contains various sources of noise in the tags and images. These noise issues may arise from factors such as out-of-focus shots, overexposure, or underexposure to light and environmental conditions. The primary objective is to eliminate these noises before proceeding with training. The quality of the images may affect the visual appearance of the left and right eyes. Figure 2 illustrates some samples from the dataset. This dataset consists of high-resolution eye images and is categorized into three classes, as shown in Figure 3.

Figure 2. Sample dataset

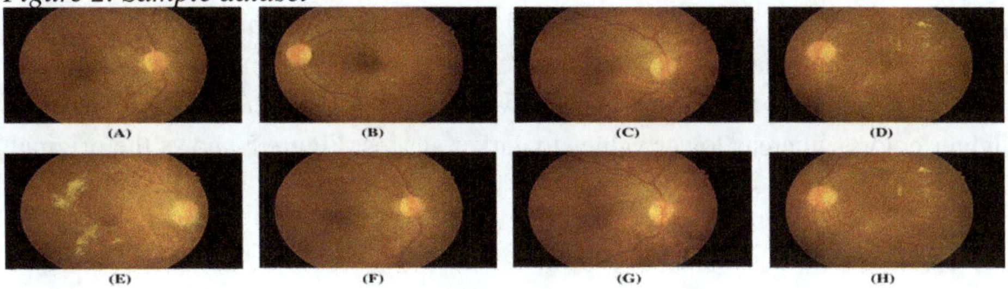

Figure 3. Type 1, Type 2 Diabetic and normal retina images

1. Type 1 2. Type 2 3. Normal Eye

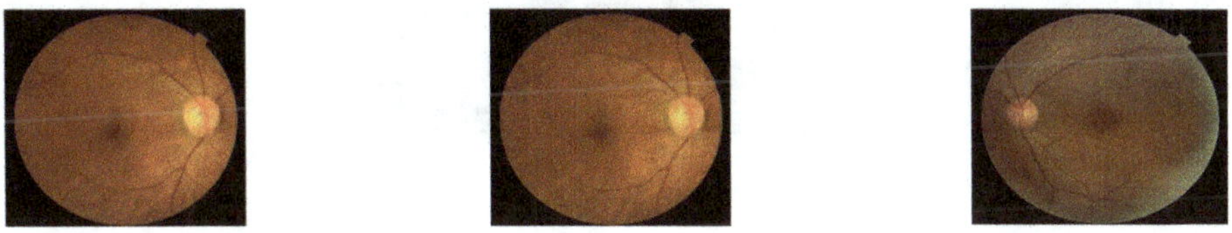

2.2. Data Preprocessing

Due to the sensitivity of the human eye to external light and interference, which can significantly reduce image quality, image pre-processing is essential. For this study, the dataset underwent pre-processing to ensure consistency and eliminate extraneous features. This phase not only reduces the effort required for subsequent procedures but also enhances image quality. To improve and sharpen retinal fundus images, a median filter was applied to highlight edges and remove noise. The pre-processing steps included the removal of the black border, gamma adjustment to account for variations in illumination, a Gaussian filter to eradicate noise, grayscale conversion for algorithm simplicity, and median filtering to retain edge features while removing noise. Together, these steps work to enhance image quality before model training, leading to accurate learning and reliable experimental results.

2.2.1. Gray Scale Conversion

Grayscale refers to a situation in which each pixel in a digital image solely contains information about the light's intensity. It contains an intensity range from deepest black to brightest white which is visible in photos. In other words, the only colors present in the image are black, white, and grey, the latter of which includes several shades. The outcome for grayscale images is a two-dimensional array with equal row and columns as the image's pixel rows and columns. Higher numbers links to lighter colors, whereas lower values to darker shades. Figure.5 shows the original image, and Figure.4 shows the converted grayscale image.

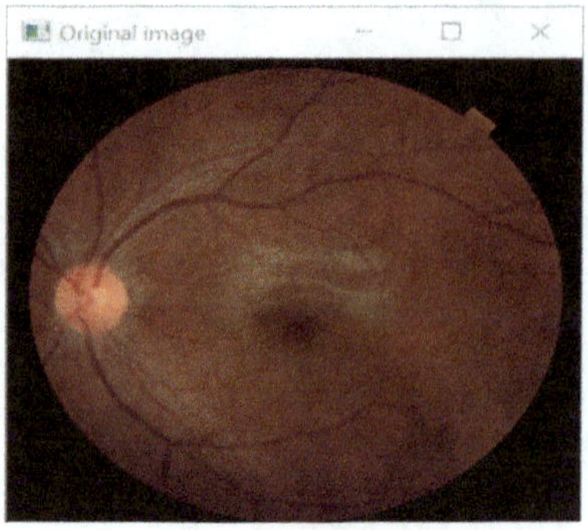

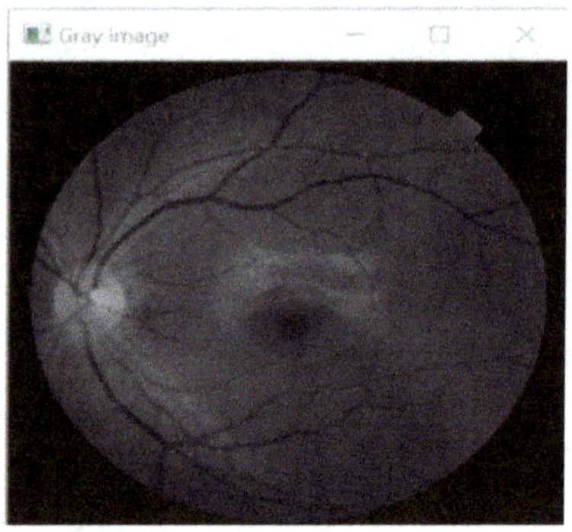

The combination of eight binary values, or “8 bits,” indicates a pixel’s pixel value, which is how grayscale images are typically represented. With 256 grayscale levels, the value range of each pixel is therefore 0-255 (0b00000000-0b11111111) 0b indicates binary format. To get a range of 0 to 1, we divide by 255.

The average approach and the weighted method are two frequently used techniques for converting RGB images to grayscale images.

· Average Approach

The average of Red, Green, and Blue is the result of the grayscale conversion by the Average technique.

Grayscale = (R + G + B) / 3

This approach is straightforward but performs less effectively than anticipated. The explanation is that RGB causes distinct reactions in human eyes. Green light is the most sensitive to eyes, whereas red light and blue light are less sensitive. As a result, the distribution of the three weights should be varied. We now arrive at the weighted technique.

· Luminosity method or weighted method

Red, Green, and Blue are given different weights based on their wavelengths in the weighted technique, also known as the luminosity method. The revised equation is as follows

Grayscale = 0.299R + 0.587G + 0.114B

Compared to RGB, grayscale photographs are less informative. However, they are frequently used in image processing because doing so is quicker and uses less space when dealing with complex computations.

2.2.2. Noise Removal

Noise is often caused by the technical restrictions of the image gathering sensor or by unfavorable environmental conditions. Noise is typically characterized as a random variation in brightness or color information. Image noise is a prevalent problem which has to be addressed through the proper denoising methods. Image noise may be created by various intrinsic and extrinsic factors that are impossible to avoid in practical scenarios.

Noise Sources

Noise may enter the image during picture acquisition and transmission. There could be a number of reasons why noise appears in the image. The number of injured pixels count in the image determines how much noise is present.

The main factors that contribute to noise in digital photographs are as follows: -

· Environmental factors could have an impact on the sensor.
· Low light and sensor defects can also produce noise in the image.
· Noise caused by tiny particles in the scanner.
· Channel interference during transmission.

Various types of noise

The various noise types include

- · Gaussian
- · speckle
- · poison
- · salt and pepper and
- · Impulse noise.

To reduce noise from photos while maintaining the nuances of the images, filtering is a procedure employed in practically every image processing system (Behera et al., 2020; Luo et al., 2017b). The type of data and filter behavior influence the selection (Noise Filtering in Digital Image Processing | by Anisha Swain | Medium, n.d.). Filtering improves image clarity and allows us to clearly discern the finer elements. Although it doesn't directly alter the image's brightness or contrast, the elimination of noise may make the final image appear brighter. The Figure.6 shows the original image from which the noise is removed, shown in Figure.7.

Figure 6. Original Image

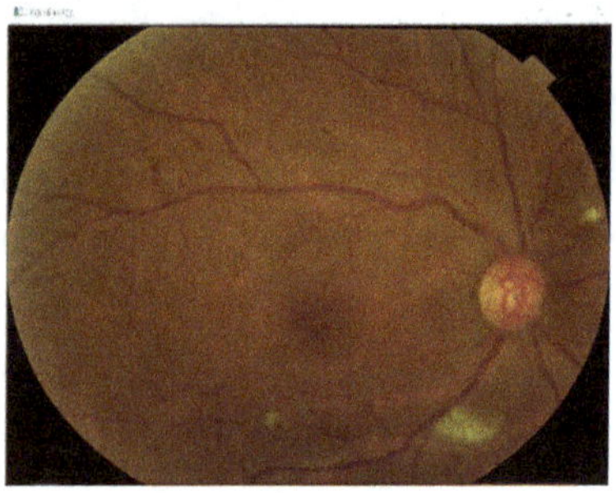

Figure 7. Noise Removed Image

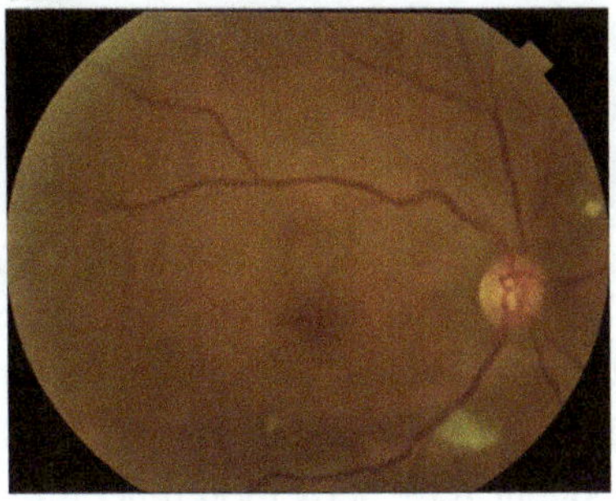

2.3. Feature Extraction

Image analysis features such as ridges, corners, edges, and points of interest contribute in the identification of image-oriented patterns. A dimension reduction phase, feature extraction, condenses original data into digestible parts, simplifying processing (Costaner et al., 2024). Massive datasets contain multiple aspects that necessitate a significant amount of processing resources to evaluate. Feature extraction picks and classifies variables quickly, extracting relevant characteristics from large datasets (Das et al., 2021). This precise classification simplifies data processing, making it both accurate and simple.

2.4. CNN Algorithm

The Convolutional Neural Network (CNN) is a Deep Learning technique specifically created for working with images(Govindarajan, Abhishek, et al., 2024) and videos(Alyoubi et al., 2020b). It uses photographs as input data, extracts feature from them and, learns the image's attributes, then categorizes the images using the learned features. It is a type of ANN utilized for picture recognition and processing that was created with the purpose of handling data (pixels). With enough training, CNN(*Convolutional Neural Network with Implementation in Python*, n.d.) can automatically learn these filters and properties(Srivastava et al., 2017). When arranged in our suggested CNN framework, each initial set of ocular data can yield many features.

The CNN model has two steps(Devi D et al., 2024)(Govindarajan et al., 2024)

· Feature extraction – this is a phase in which the photos are subjected to various filters and levels to collect their details and features. Once this phase is complete, the images are then moved on to the following phase.

· Classification is the process of classifying data according to the problem's goal variable.

Layers in CNN

1. Input Layer: The raw image input is handled in this layer.
2. Convolution Layer: This layer calculates the output using the dot product between each filter and image patch (Sangeetha & Govindarajan, 2023).
3. Activation function layer: In this layer, the output of the convolution will be subjected to the component-wise activation function layer.
4. Pooling Layer: The main goal of this layer is to reduce the size and quantity of output images in order to speed up the calculation, conserve memory, and prevent overfitting. Two common types of pooling - max and average pooling.
5. Fully-Connected Layer: It is a conventional network that uses the input from the layer before to calculate the output values and outputs a 1-D array with the same number of classes.

Algorithm

The first step is to get the retinal image dataset. Then pre-process it by performing operations like grayscale conversion, noise filtering, etc. After pre-processing, perform feature extraction by repeatedly applying convolution, ReLU, and pooling(Al Mamari et al., 2023). Then train the samples. Optimize the trained samples. Test the samples and classify the tested and trained samples to get the desired output. At last, display the classified output along with the accuracy rate.

The steps of the algorithm

- Step 1: Get the retinal image dataset.
- Step 2: Preprocess the images by performing operations like grayscale conversion, noise filtering etc.
- Step 3: Perform feature extraction by repeatedly applying convolution, ReLU, and pooling.
- Step 4: Train the samples.
- Step 5: Optimize the trained samples.
- Step 6: Test the samples.
- Step 7: Classify the tested and trained samples to get the desired output.
- Step 8: Display the classified output along with the accuracy rate.

Convolutional Layer

The term "convolutional neural network" denotes the use of a mathematical operation known as "convolution," which is a specific type of linear operation. They are basic networks with at most 1 layer that employs convolution instead of conventional matrix multiplication. Each image is represented as an array of values during the convolution phase, which requires matrix arithmetic operations (pixels). In order to extract or analyze features from the input image, the filters are applied to the convolution layer, as shown in Figure.8. Multiple filtering operations are performed on the image to produce a feature map that aids in categorizing the input image(Liu et al., 2021). A feature map is obtained after applying a filter with information about the input.

Figure 8. Convolutional Layer Operation

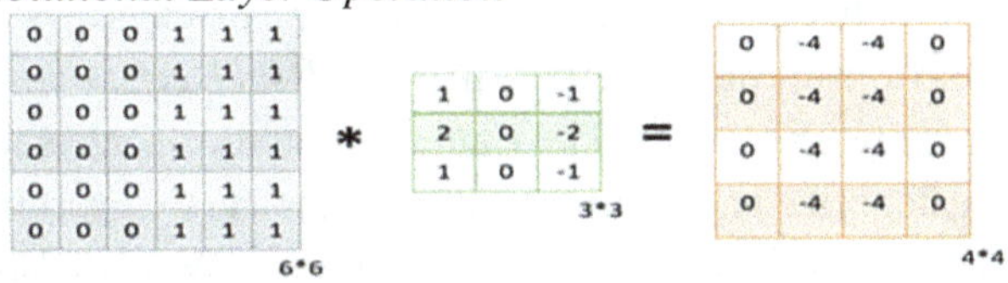

Activation Function

The activation function is called the Rectified Linear Unit, which is not linear. If the input is positive, the input is output; otherwise, it is zero. All negative values in the filtered images are eliminated and switched out for zeros in this layer(*Convolutional Neural Network (CNN) | TensorFlow Core*, n.d.). This process prevents the sum values from becoming zero after adding up. Since it is simpler to train and solves the vanishing gradient problem, it is the most popular activation function for many different neural networks. This enables models to learn more quickly and perform better. The result is a rectified feature map.

Pooling Layer

Pooling layer, reduces the feature map's size, aiding in the preservation of the input image's key details or features while speeding up the computation. The large or significant portions of the input image are still in the lower-resolution version of the input produced by pooling. Overfitting is avoided by lowering the dimensionality because there are only fewer weights for the network to calculate. Furthermore, it helps in training the system by letting and finding the dominating characteristics images.

Fully Connected Layer

The input image is classified into a label using the fully connected layer. This layer links the data that was extracted in the earlier phases to the output layer, ultimately labeling the input according to the classification. The input is multiplied by a weight matrix before being added by a fully linked layer. The convolutional layers are followed by one or more fully connected layers. When a layer of neurons is fully linked, every neuron in that layer is connected to all layers.

The results of the last layers are passed to the fully connected layer, where it is flattened before being applied. The working prototype categorizes images via the Softmax Classification method across a number of epochs by identifying dominant and specific low-level features. The resultant two-dimension arrays are flattened to single, long vectors from the pooled feature maps(*CNN in Deep Learning: Algorithm and Machine Learning Uses*, n.d.). The flattened output is sent as feed to the next layer in order to categorize and obtain the results depicts the working of the CNN algorithm with an example(*Image Classification Using CNN : Python Implementation - Analytics Vidhya*, n.d.). The image of size 32x32x3 with 6 filters is given as input to convolutional layer 1, which reduces the input size by 28x28x6 for stride = 1. It is then passed to the max pool layer, where its dimension is reduced o half for stride = 2 by 14x14x6. The same process is repeated for the second layer, and it is then passed to the hidden layer where it is flattened to 400, then by 120, and finally, it is given to the output layer where it is applied with the softmax function to get the predicted result.

3. RESULTS AND DISCUSSION

3.1. Train the dataset

Algorithms play a crucial role in deep learning by extracting knowledge from datasets. They identify patterns, gain insights, make judgments, and evaluate those judgments. The deep learning algorithm is sophisticated and utilizes iterative training on each image to recognize features, shapes, and even objects such as people or animals. As the model processes the data, it continually assesses its performance to gain a better understanding of how to behave, making modifications along the way to achieve its goals. This iterative training process is essential for the system's development. Typically, the size of the training dataset is larger than the testing dataset, as the model requires as much data as possible to detect and learn useful patterns. Once trained with the data, the model applies the patterns it has learned to make informed decisions.

The steps taken to train the model are as follows (Mateen et al., 2020)

1. Upload Data image
2. Input layer processing
3. Convolutional layer processing
4. Pooling layer processing
5. Dense layer processing
6. Output Layer gives the result

3.2. Test the dataset

Once the model has been created, it is essential to test it using unobserved data. The testing data helps evaluate the performance of the algorithms and the effectiveness of their training. Based on these assessments, adjustments can be made to improve the algorithms for better outcomes. It is vital that none of the observations in the test set come from the training set.

There are two primary criteria for testing data:

1. It should reflect the characteristics of the real dataset.
2. It must be large enough to produce accurate predictions.

When the testing dataset is prepared, the results from the original dataset are removed. The trained model is then tested with this new data. The predictions generated by the model are compared with the actual results. This comparison allows us to evaluate the model's performance based on its results with the testing dataset.set.

3.3. Classification

Classification is crucial for grouping data into predefined categories by comparing visual patterns with target patterns. The process begins by determining the class of supplied data, with classes referred to as targets or labels. The objective is to assign new data to a specific class based on the relationship between independent and dependent variables. In predicting diseases for diabetes patients, a CNN classifier is employed, distinguishing between type 1 diabetes, type 2 diabetes, and normal individuals (Ramasamy et al., 2021). Pre-processed images undergo feature extraction and are trained with 100 epochs using a 7-layer model. Testing yields a high accuracy of 98.8%, showcasing the effectiveness of the classification model in predicting diabetic conditions.

3.4. Evaluation metrics analyses and discussion

The effectiveness of the deep learning model is assessed using evaluation measures. It is crucial for every project to evaluate deep learning models or algorithms. It is essential to gauge how well a model predicts the desired outcome as it is being developed.

A model can be tested using a wide variety of evaluation criteria. These consist of

- Classification accuracy – typically, what we mean when we use the term accuracy is the ratio of a number of accurate predictions concerning total input samples.
- Logarithmic loss - commonly known as log loss, functions by penalizing the incorrect classifications.
- A confusion matrix - produces a matrix and summarizes the overall functionality of the model.

When testing a model or method, evaluation metrics require combining these evaluation metrics. The objective is to develop and choose a model that performs well on the dataset. It is essential to evaluate the model using a variety of evaluation metrics since a model might perform well when one evaluation metric's measurement is used but poorly when another evaluation metric's measurement is used (Fan et al., 2021).

3.5. Confusion matrix

An error or confusion matrix is a table that displays the kind of errors being made as well as the percentage of wrong and right predictions of the model in relation to the actual result of the classification. It is described as a table which frequently illustrates a classification system's efficiency when applied to test data.

These are the important terminologies of the confusion matrix(*Confusion Matrix - Clearly Explained | Towards Data Science*, n.d.)

- TP- True Positive: The output coincides with the actual result, concluding that both values are true.
- TN- True Negative: The output coincides with the actual result, concluding that both values are negative.

- FP- False Positive: This type 1 error occurs when the estimated value is wrongly predicted as positive when it is negative.
- FN- False Negative: This Type 2 error occurs when the estimated value is incorrectly estimated to be negative when the actual value is positive.

The Confusion Matrix provides us with 5 classification metrics

- **Accuracy:** The percentage of all predictions that were accurate. It is employed to evaluate system effectiveness. The total number of accurate predictions the classifier made is taken into consideration.
- **Precision:** It accurately identifies positive instances. The percentage of True Positives to every positive result the model predicted. The precision decreases as the model predicts more false positives. Precision indicates the proportion of correctly anticipated cases that really resulted in positive results.
- **Recall/Sensitivity:** The percentage of genuinely positive cases that are accurately identified. It is the proportion of actual positives to total dataset positives. It gauges how well the model can identify positive samples. The recall decreases as the model predicts more false negatives.

· **Specificity:** The percentage of correctly detected true negative cases.

3.5.1. Evaluation metrics for CNN prototype

The confusion matrix - the trained CNN prototype is shown in Figure.9

Figure 9. Confusion Matrix

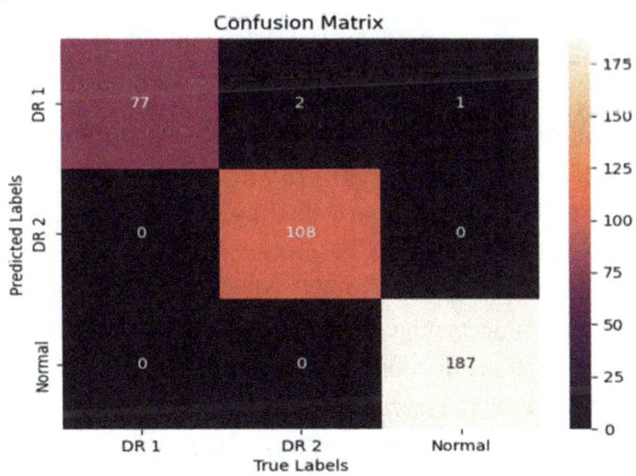

From the figure, the accuracy of the model can be seen as 98.8%. The confusion matrix can be interpreted as

- 77 retinal images are correctly classified as DR 1.
- 108 retinal images are correctly classified as DR 2 and
- 187 retinal images are correctly classified as normal.
- Only 2 retinal images are incorrectly classified as DR 1, which is very less when compared to the overall prediction accuracy.

Table 1 provides a detailed analysis of the precision, sensitivity, and specificity calculations for each of the three classes evaluated in the model. Precision reflects the proportion of true positive identifications among all positive predictions, thereby indicating the accuracy of the model's positive outcomes. Sensitivity, also known as recall, quantifies the model's capacity to correctly detect actual positive cases, emphasizing its effectiveness in identifying true positives. In contrast, specificity measures the model's ability to accurately recognize negative cases, thereby illustrating its proficiency in minimizing false positive rates. Collectively, these metrics furnish essential insights into the model's performance, facilitating a thorough assessment of its overall efficacy across the various classes.

Table 1. The evaluation metrics of CNN with perspective to DR severity after setting epoch to 100

Severity of DR	Precision	Sensitivity	Specificity
DR 1	1.00	0.96	0.98
DR 2	0.98	1.00	0.99
Normal	0.99	1.00	1.00

The detection of diabetic retinopathy (DR) has been explored through various models, including the Deep Residual Network with a deep transfer learning approach using the Inception v3 network, bilinear pooling neural networks, support vector machines (SVM), and MobileNetV3 based on neural networks. However, these models typically achieve an accuracy of 97% or lower. Each of these models has its limitations, particularly concerning the selection of parameters and their accuracy rates. Accuracy is crucial in any model, as it impacts the correctness of the output. In contrast, the proposed model has demonstrated an impressive accuracy of nearly 99%. After classification, the accuracy of this model stands at 98.8%, surpassing that of other prediction models. Table 2 provides a comparison of various models alongside their evaluation metrics, clearly indicating that the convolutional neural network (CNN) prototype proposed here achieves the highest accuracy of 98.8%.

This is significantly better than the other existing models. Figures 10 through 27 illustrate the detailed process and accuracy results.

Table 2. Results of CNN compared with other DR prediction models

Models	Accuracy	Precision	Sensitivity	Specificity
CNN	98.8%	99%	98.6%	99%
GENet	95.6%	95.6%	95.6%	98.9%
ResNet-50	86%	86.3%	86%	96.5%
DenseNet-121	92.1%	92.4%	92.1%	98%
GoogLeNet	90%	90.1%	90%	97.5%

3.6. Real-time working model and its projection

Figure 10. Home Page

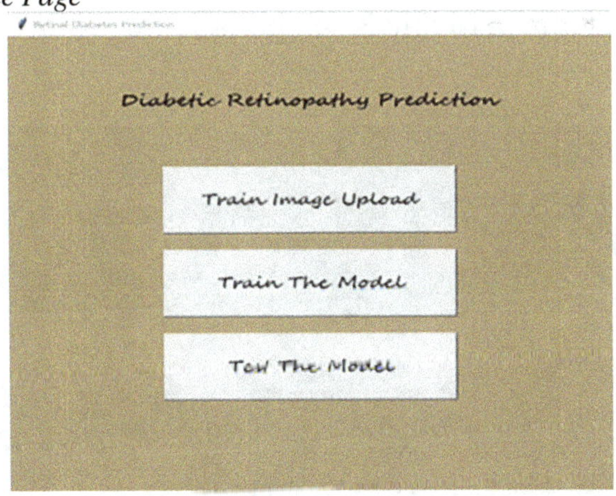

Figure 11. Upload Input Image

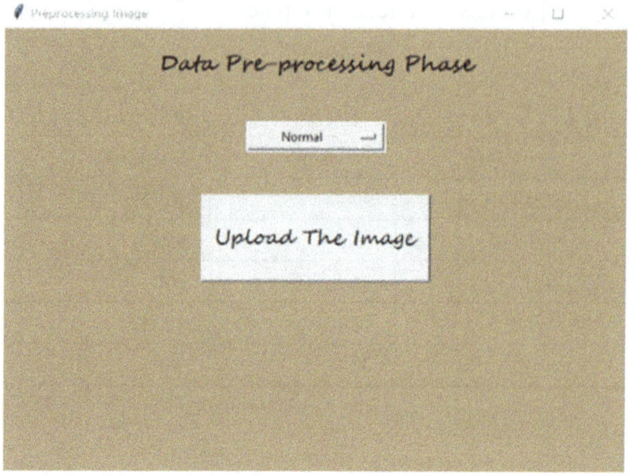

Select the input image of any 3 categories

Figure 12. Select the input image

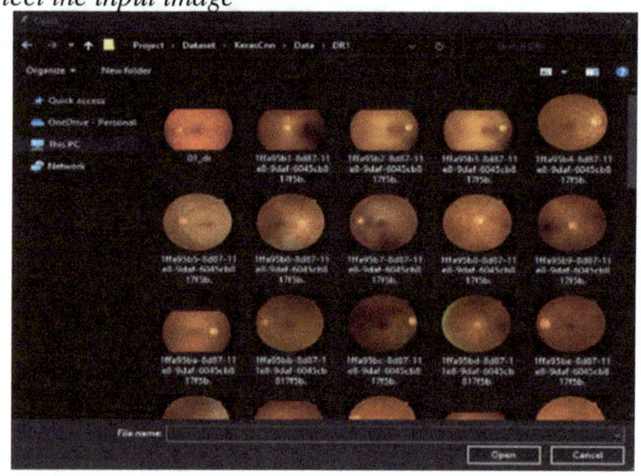

Pre-processing the input image

Figure 13. Original Input Image

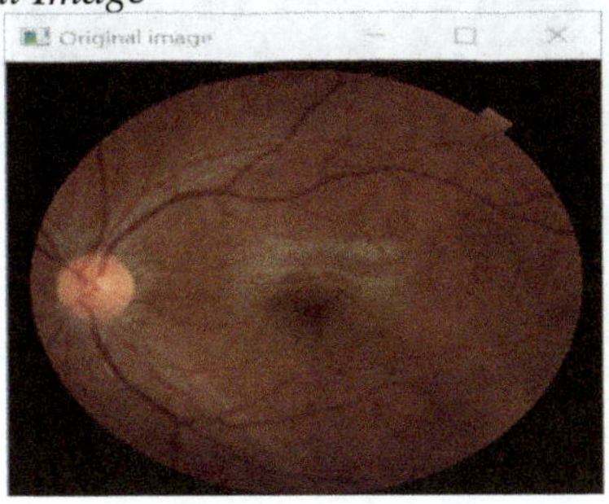

Figure 15. Inverted Input Image

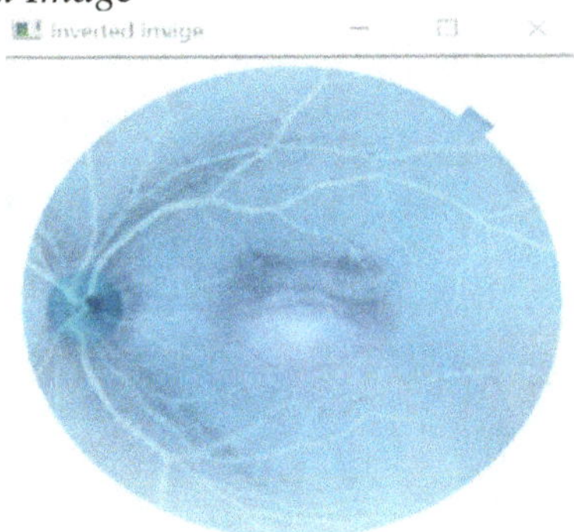

Figure 14. Grey Scale Input Image

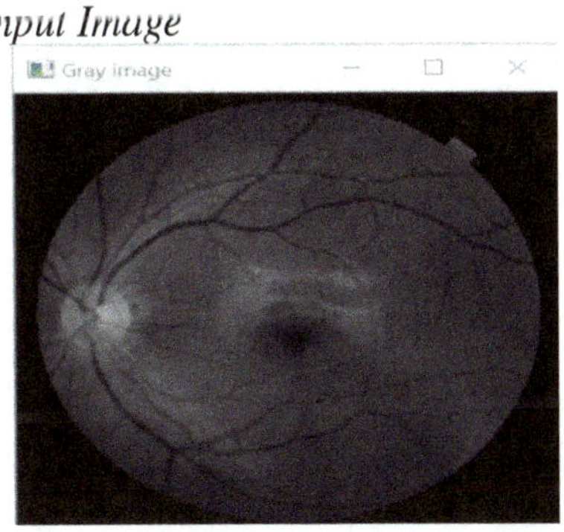

Figure 16. Noise Remove Input Image

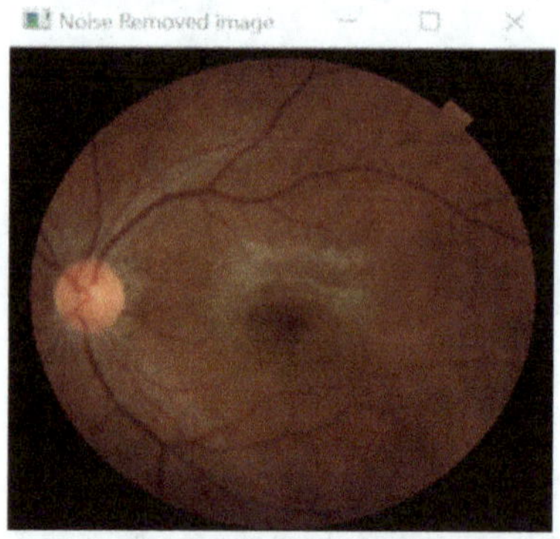

Training Accuracy for 100 epochs-98.8%

Figure 17. Training Accuracy

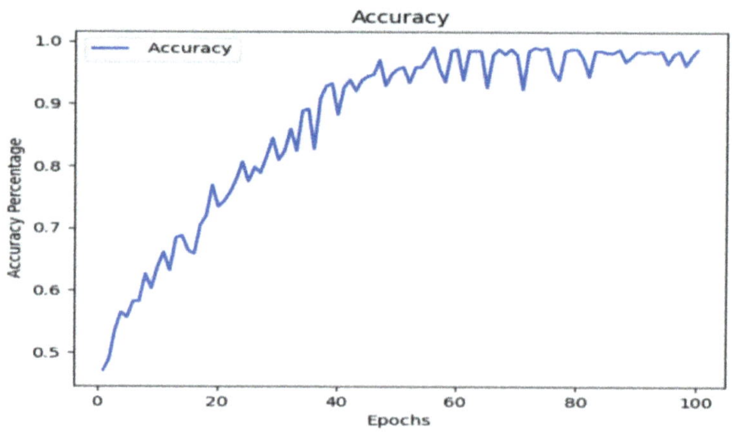

Figure 18. Training Loss

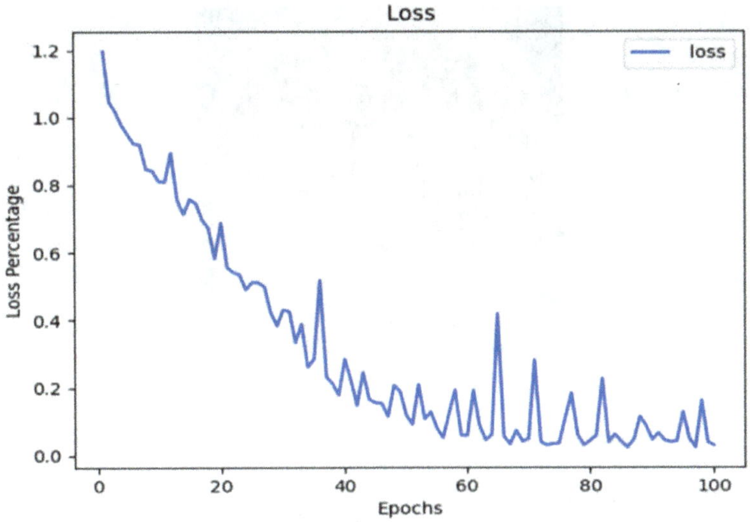

Test image is pre-processed

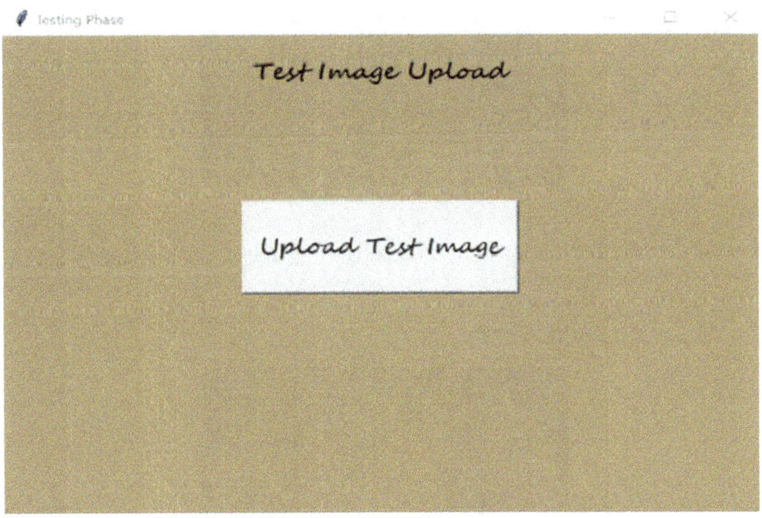

Figure 20. Original Test Image

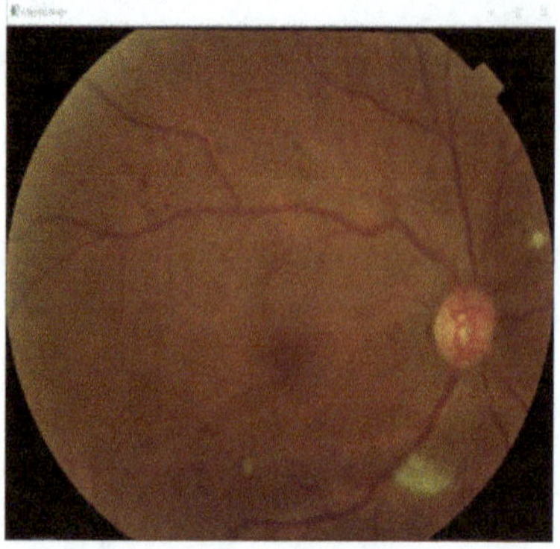

Figure 21. Gray Test Image

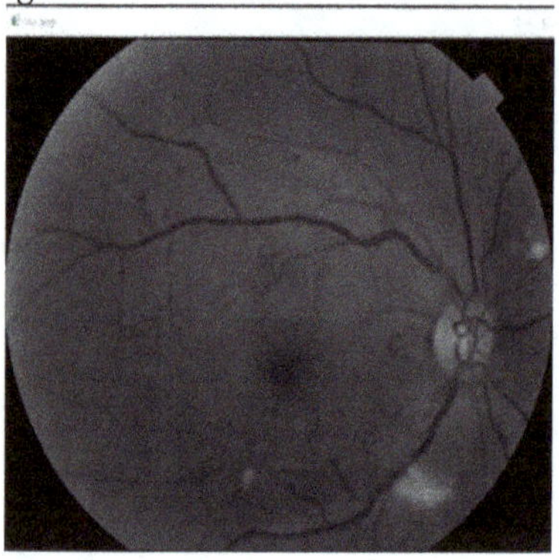

Figure 22. Noise Removed Test Image

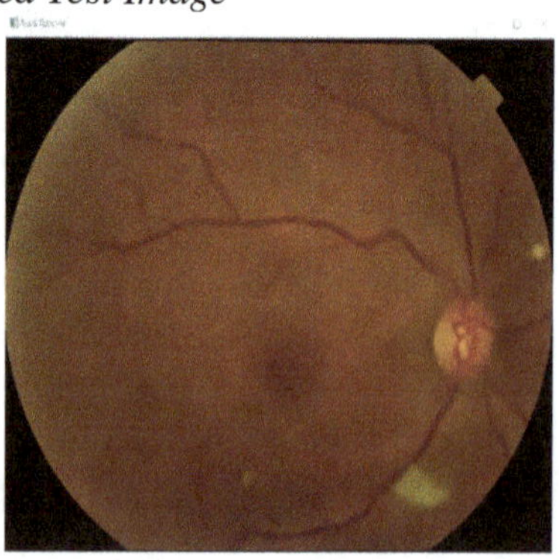

Classification of images:

Images are classified into 3 categories as Type 1, 2 and Normal. The prescription for the disease will be in any of the two modes, like "Short-acting (regular) insulin" or "Diabetic medication such as Metformin".

Figure 23. Result Type 1 Diabetics

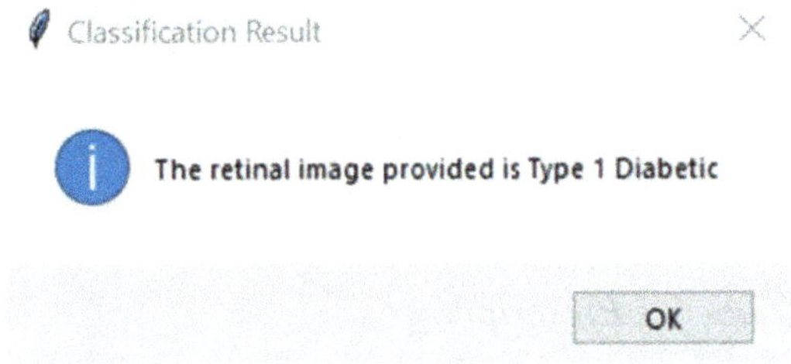

Figure 24. Result Type 2 Diabetics

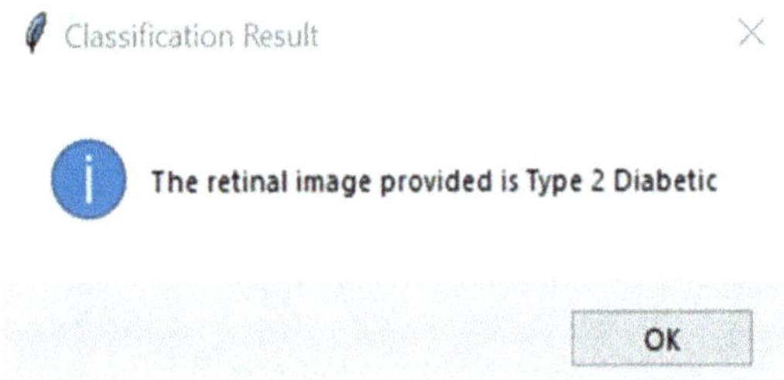

Figure 25. Result- Normal Patient

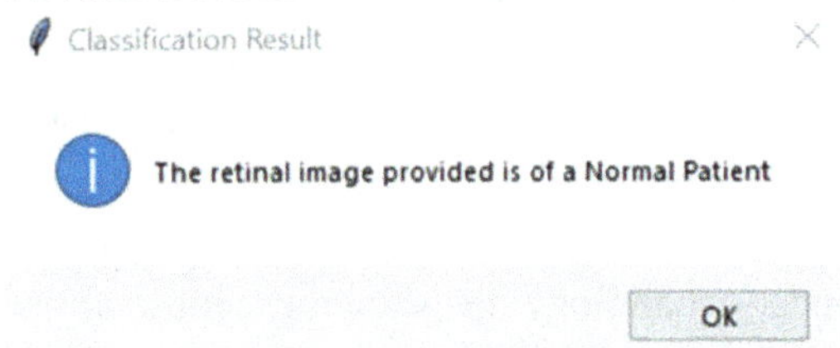

Prescription is displayed for the disease as

Figure 26. Type 1 Diabetics Prescription

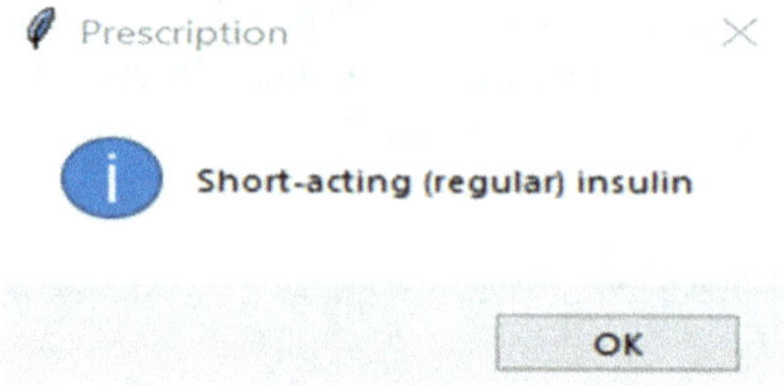

Figure 27. Type 2 Diabetics Prescription

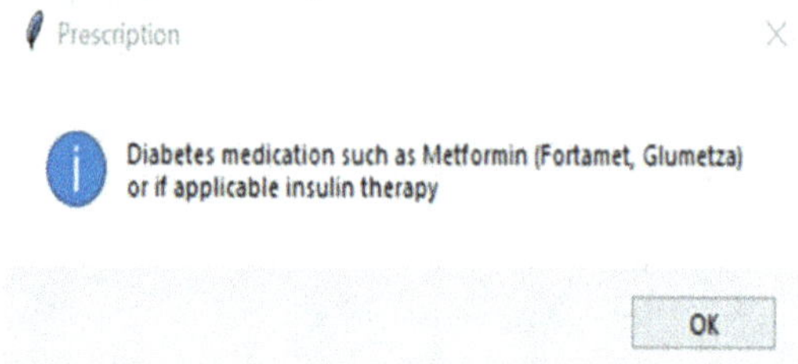

CONCLUSION

Diabetic retinopathy is a critical health issue for individuals living with diabetes, posing a significant risk of vision impairment and potential blindness. This condition arises from damage to the blood vessels in the retina, necessitating regular and thorough health screenings to facilitate early detection and treatment. Traditional manual detection methods, while valuable, can be labor-intensive and costly, leading to lengthy delays in obtaining results and subsequent treatment. In response to these challenges, researchers have developed an innovative automatic retinal image processing technique that leverages the power of Convolutional Neural Networks (CNNs). This advanced technology has shown exceptional performance with an impressive accuracy rate of 98.8%. Compared to other existing detection methods, this CNN model stands out for its superior reliability and efficiency. The automated system offers several advantages, including significantly reduced processing times that allow for prompt analysis of retinal images. By delivering results quickly, healthcare providers can initiate timely interventions, mitigating the progression of diabetic retinopathy and improving patient outcomes. Moreover, this system alleviates the workload on healthcare professionals, enabling them to focus on direct patient care rather than time-consuming analysis. Overall, this CNN-based method represents a groundbreaking advancement in the fight against diabetic retinopathy, serving as a vital preventative measure that enhances both diagnostic accuracy and treatment accessibility, ultimately safeguarding patients from the threat of irreversible vision loss.

Future Work

The model has the potential for future enhancements that could enable it to classify diabetic retinopathy into two specific categories: proliferative and non-proliferative. This advancement would allow for more precise treatment responses based on the severity of the condition. Furthermore, the model could be fine-tuned to identify a wider range of eye diseases, such as glaucoma and age-related macular degeneration, while also being capable of processing large volumes of data without compromising its outstanding accuracy. However, it is essential to note that increasing the number of parameters in the model might introduce challenges related to standardization, which could affect its reliability across different applications. The development of a real-time prototype is particularly exciting, as it could provide immediate results through user-friendly interfaces such as mobile applications or websites. This innovation has the potential to significantly transform current diagnostic practices, leading to timely interventions that could prevent vision loss and blindness in a vast population worldwide.

REFERENCES

Abbas, Q., Fondon, I., Sarmiento, A., Jiménez, S., & Alemany, P. (2017a). Automatic recognition of severity level for diagnosis of diabetic retinopathy using deep visual features. *Medical & Biological Engineering & Computing*, *55*(11), 1959–1974. DOI: 10.1007/s11517-017-1638-6 PMID: 28353133

Abbasi-Sureshjani, S., Dashtbozorg, B., ter Haar Romeny, B. M., & Fleuret, F. (2018). Exploratory Study on Direct Prediction of Diabetes Using Deep Residual Networks. *Lecture Notes in Computational Vision and Biomechanics*, *27*, 797–802. DOI: 10.1007/978-3-319-68195-5_86

Al Mamari, H. I. B., Al Washahi, N. A. A., Al Busaidi, M. H. K., & Hajamohideen, F. (2023). Deep neural network based composting processing technology: A solution for municipality and fertilizer companies. *IET Conference Proceedings,* 2022(26), 422–430. DOI: 10.1049/icp.2023.0642

Alyoubi, W. L., Shalash, W. M., & Abulkhair, M. F. (2020a). Diabetic retinopathy detection through deep learning techniques: A review. *Informatics in Medicine Unlocked*, *20*, 100377. DOI: 10.1016/j.imu.2020.100377

Barriga, E. S., Murray, V., Agurto, C., Pattichis, M., Bauman, W., Zamora, G., & Soliz, P. (2010). Automatic system for diabetic retinopathy screening based on AM-FM, partial least squares, and support vector machines. *2010 7th IEEE International Symposium on Biomedical Imaging: From Nano to Macro, ISBI 2010 - Proceedings*, 1349–1352. DOI: 10.1109/ISBI.2010.5490247

Behera, M. K. (2020). Prediction of different stages in Diabetic retinopathy from retinal fundus images using radial basis function based SVM. *Indian Journal of Science and Technology*, *13*(20), 2030–2040. DOI: 10.17485/IJST/v13i20.322

NN in Deep Learning: Algorithm and Machine Learning Uses. (n.d.). Retrieved August 5, 2025, from https://www.simplilearn.com/tutorials/deep-learning-tutorial/convolutional-neural-network

Confusion Matrix - Clearly Explained | Towards Data Science. (n.d.). Retrieved August 5, 2025, from https://towardsdatascience.com/confusion-matrix-clearly-explained-fee63614dc7/

Convolutional Neural Network (CNN) | TensorFlow Core. (n.d.). Retrieved August 5, 2025, from https://www.tensorflow.org/tutorials/images/cnn

Convolutional Neural Network with Implementation in Python. (n.d.). Retrieved August 5, 2025, from https://www.analyticsvidhya.com/blog/2021/08/beginners-guide-to-convolutional-neural-network-with-implementation-in-python/

Costa, P., Galdran, A., Smailagic, A., & Campilho, A. (2018). A Weakly-Supervised Framework for Interpretable Diabetic Retinopathy Detection on Retinal Images. *IEEE Access : Practical Innovations, Open Solutions*, *6*, 18747–18758. DOI: 10.1109/ACCESS.2018.2816003

Costaner, L., Informatika, T., Ilmu Komputer, F., & Lancang Kuning -Riau, U. (2024). Feature Extraction Analysis for Diabetic Retinopathy Detection Using Machine Learning Techniques. *SISTEMASI, 13*(5), 2268–2276. DOI: 10.32520/stmsi.v13i5.4600

Das, S., Kharbanda, K., M, S., Raman, R., & D, E. D. (2021). Deep learning architecture based on segmented fundus image features for classification of diabetic retinopathy. *Biomedical Signal Processing and Control*, *68*, 102600. DOI: 10.1016/j.bspc.2021.102600

Devi, D. (2024). Towards real-time earthquake forecasting in Chile: Integrating intelligent technologies and machine learning. *Computers & Electrical Engineering*, *117*, 109285. DOI: 10.1016/j.compeleceng.2024.109285

Diabetic Retinopathy Columbus | Diabetes Norfolk | Eye Physicians P.C. (n.d.). Retrieved August 5, 2025, from https://www.eyephysicianspc.com/ocular-disease-treatments-columbus/diabetic-retinopathy/

Dutta, S., Manideep, B. C. S., Basha, S. M., Caytiles, R. D., & Iyengar, N. C. S. N. (2018). Classification of diabetic retinopathy images by using deep learning models. *International Journal of Grid and Distributed Computing*, *11*(1), 89–106. DOI: 10.14257/ijgdc.2018.11.1.09

Fan, R., Liu, Y., & Zhang, R. (2021). Multi-scale feature fusion with adaptive weighting for diabetic retinopathy severity classification. *Electronics (Basel)*, *10*(12), 1369. Advance online publication. DOI: 10.3390/electronics10121369

Govindarajan, P., Abhishek, M., Niharika, K., & Tesfahun, A. (2024). Lungcanary-Pioneering Early Lung Cancer Detection using Machine Learning Algorithms. *8th IEEE International Conference on Computational System and Information Technology for Sustainable Solutions, CSITSS 2024*. DOI: 10.1109/CSITSS64042.2024.10816854

Govindarajan, P., Shreya, N. S., Tesfahun, A., & Amrithavarshini Bhargava, S. (2024). Computing Approach to Detect the Factors and their Impact in Prevalence of Thyroid. *Proceedings of the 18th INDIAcom; 2024 11th International Conference on Computing for Sustainable Global Development, INDIACom 2024*, 1493–1500. DOI: 10.23919/INDIACom61295.2024.10498625

Image Classification using CNN : Python Implementation - Analytics Vidhya. (n.d.). Retrieved August 5, 2025, from https://www.analyticsvidhya.com/blog/2021/06/image-classification-using-convolutional-neural-network-with-python/

Kanungo, Y. S., Srinivasan, B., & Choudhary, S. (2017). Detecting diabetic retinopathy using deep learning. *RTEICT 2017 - 2nd IEEE International Conference on Recent Trends in Electronics, Information and Communication Technology, Proceedings, 2018-January*, 801–804. DOI: 10.1109/RTEICT.2017.8256708

Khan, Z., Khan, F. G., Khan, A., Rehman, Z. U., Shah, S., Qummar, S., Ali, F., & Pack, S. (2021). Diabetic Retinopathy Detection Using VGG-NIN a Deep Learning Architecture. *IEEE Access : Practical Innovations, Open Solutions*, *9*, 61408–61416. DOI: 10.1109/ACCESS.2021.3074422

Lam, C., Yi, D., Guo, M., & Lindsey, T. (n.d.). *Automated Detection of Diabetic Retinopathy using Deep Learning*.

Li, F., Liu, Z., Chen, H., Jiang, M., Zhang, X., & Wu, Z. (2019). Automatic detection of diabetic retinopathy in retinal fundus photographs based on deep learning algorithm. *Translational Vision Science & Technology*, *8*(6), 4. Advance online publication. DOI: 10.1167/tvst.8.6.4 PMID: 31737428

Liu, P., Yang, X., Jin, B., & Zhou, Q. (2021). Diabetic retinal grading using attention-based bilinear convolutional neural network and complement cross entropy. *Entropy (Basel, Switzerland)*, *23*(7), 816. Advance online publication. DOI: 10.3390/e23070816 PMID: 34206941

Luo, T., Gast, T. J., Vermeer, T. J., & Burns, S. A. (2017b). Retinal Vascular Branching in Healthy and Diabetic Subjects. *Investigative Ophthalmology & Visual Science*, *58*(5), 2685. DOI: 10.1167/iovs.17-21653 PMID: 28525557

Mateen, M., Wen, J., Hassan, M., Nasrullah, N., Sun, S., & Hayat, S. (2020). Automatic Detection of Diabetic Retinopathy: A Review on Datasets, Methods and Evaluation Metrics. *IEEE Access : Practical Innovations, Open Solutions*, *8*, 48784–48811. DOI: 10.1109/ACCESS.2020.2980055

Mekala, V. K., Vadlamudi, G., Firdaus, A., Vemuru, N., Aramandla, K., & Rajeswara Rao, D. (2021). Early Detection of Diabetic Retinopathy. *International Journal for Research in Applied Science and Engineering Technology*, *9*(IX), 429–435. Advance online publication. DOI: 10.22214/ijraset.2021.37918

Nayak, J., Bhat, P. S., Acharya, U. R., Lim, C. M., & Kagathi, M. (2008). Automated identification of diabetic retinopathy stages using digital fundus images. *Journal of Medical Systems*, *32*(2), 107–115. DOI: 10.1007/s10916-007-9113-9 PMID: 18461814

Nguyen, H. T., Butler, M., Roychoudhry, A., Shannon, A. G., Flack, J., & Mitchell, P. (1996). Classification of diabetic retinopathy using neural networks. *Annual International Conference of the IEEE Engineering in Medicine and Biology - Proceedings*, *4*, 1548–1549. DOI: 10.1109/IEMBS.1996.647546

Noise filtering in Digital Image Processing | by Anisha Swain | Medium. (n.d.). Retrieved August 5, 2025, from https://medium.com/@anishaswain/noise-filtering-in-digital-image-processing-d12b5266847c

Orujov, F., Maskeliūnas, R., Damaševičius, R., & Wei, W. (2020). Fuzzy based image edge detection algorithm for blood vessel detection in retinal images. *Applied Soft Computing*, *94*, 106452. DOI: 10.1016/j.asoc.2020.106452

Priya, R., & Aruna, P. (2012). SVM and Neural Network based Diagnosis of Diabetic Retinopathy. *International Journal of Computer Applications*, *41*(1), •••. DOI: 10.5120/5503-7503

Qiao, L., Zhu, Y., & Zhou, H. (2020). Diabetic Retinopathy Detection Using Prognosis of Microaneurysm and Early Diagnosis System for Non-Proliferative Diabetic Retinopathy Based on Deep Learning Algorithms. *IEEE Access : Practical Innovations, Open Solutions*, *8*, 104292–104302. DOI: 10.1109/ACCESS.2020.2993937

Quellec, G., Charrière, K., Boudi, Y., Cochener, B., & Lamard, M. (2017). Deep image mining for diabetic retinopathy screening. *Medical Image Analysis*, *39*, 178–193. DOI: 10.1016/j.media.2017.04.012 PMID: 28511066

Ramasamy, L. K., Padinjappurathu, S. G., Kadry, S., & Damaševičius, R. (2021). Detection of Diabetic Retinopathy Using a Fusion of Textural and Ridgelet Features of Retinal Images and Sequential Minimal Optimization Classifier. *PeerJ. Computer Science*, *7*, 1–21. DOI: 10.7717/peerj-cs.456 PMID: 34013026

Roychowdhury, S., Koozekanani, D. D., & Parhi, K. K. (2014). DREAM: Diabetic Retinopathy Analysis Using Machine Learning. *IEEE Journal of Biomedical and Health Informatics*, *18*(5), 1717–1728. DOI: 10.1109/JBHI.2013.2294635 PMID: 25192577

Sangeetha, J., & Govindarajan, P. (2023). Prediction of agricultural waste compost maturity using fast regions with convolutional neural network(R-CNN). *Materials Today: Proceedings*. Advance online publication. DOI: 10.1016/j.matpr.2023.01.112

Santhakumar, R., Tandur, M., Rajkumar, E. R., Geetha, K. S., Haritz, G., & Rajamani, K. T. (2017). Machine learning algorithm for retinal image analysis. *IEEE Region 10 Annual International Conference, Proceedings/TENCON*, 1236–1240. DOI: 10.1109/TENCON.2016.7848208

Santoso, A. S., & Nelloh, L. A. M. (2017). *Hasil Peer Reviewer Juril Elsevier2-LN*. https://doi.org/DOI: 10.1016/J.PROCS

Soares, J. V. B., Leandro, J. J. G., Cesar, R. M., Jelinek, H. F., & Cree, M. J. (2006). Retinal vessel segmentation using the 2-D Gabor wavelet and supervised classification. *IEEE Transactions on Medical Imaging*, *25*(9), 1214–1222. DOI: 10.1109/TMI.2006.879967 PMID: 16967806

Soomro, T. A., Afifi, A. J., Zheng, L., Soomro, S., Gao, J., Hellwich, O., & Paul, M. (2019). Deep Learning Models for Retinal Blood Vessels Segmentation: A Review. In *IEEE Access* (Vol. 7, pp. 71696–71717). Institute of Electrical and Electronics Engineers Inc. DOI: 10.1109/ACCESS.2019.2920616

Srivastava, R., Duan, L., Wong, D. W. K., Liu, J., & Wong, T. Y. (2017). Detecting retinal microaneurysms and hemorrhages with robustness to the presence of blood vessels. *Computer Methods and Programs in Biomedicine*, *138*, 83–91. DOI: 10.1016/j.cmpb.2016.10.017 PMID: 27886718

Srivastava, R., Wong, D. W. K., Duan, L., Liu, J., & Wong, T. Y. (2015). Red lesion detection in retinal fundus images using Frangi-based filters. *Proceedings of the Annual International Conference of the IEEE Engineering in Medicine and Biology Society, EMBS, 2015-November*, 5663–5666. DOI: 10.1109/EMBC.2015.7319677

Teo, Z. L., Tham, Y. C., Yu, M., Chee, M. L., Rim, T. H., Cheung, N., Bikbov, M. M., Wang, Y. X., Tang, Y., Lu, Y., Wong, I. Y., Ting, D. S. W., Tan, G. S. W., Jonas, J. B., Sabanayagam, C., Wong, T. Y., & Cheng, C. Y. (2021). Global Prevalence of Diabetic Retinopathy and Projection of Burden through 2045: Systematic Review and Meta-analysis. *Ophthalmology*, *128*(11), 1580–1591. DOI: 10.1016/j.ophtha.2021.04.027 PMID: 33940045

Usman Akram, M., Khalid, S., Tariq, A., Khan, S. A., & Azam, F. (2014). Detection and classification of retinal lesions for grading of diabetic retinopathy. *Computers in Biology and Medicine*, *45*(1), 161–171. DOI: 10.1016/j.compbiomed.2013.11.014 PMID: 24480176

Wu, L. (2013). Classification of diabetic retinopathy and diabetic macular edema. *World Journal of Diabetes*, *4*(6), 290–296. DOI: 10.4239/wjd.v4.i6.290 PMID: 24379919

Xiaohui, Z., & Chutatape, O. (2004). Detection and classification of bright lesions in color fundus images. *Proceedings - International Conference on Image Processing, ICIP*, *1*, 139–142. DOI: 10.1109/ICIP.2004.1418709

Yang, B., Li, T., Xie, H., Liao, Y., & Chen, Y. P. P. (2022). Classification of Diabetic Retinopathy Severity Based on GCA Attention Mechanism. *IEEE Access : Practical Innovations, Open Solutions*, *10*, 2729–2739. DOI: 10.1109/ACCESS.2021.3139129

Chapter 6
Generative AI Approaches for Synthetic Health Data Generation:
Methods, Applications, and Challenges

V. Vanitha
https://orcid.org/0000-0003-1010-3241
Sri Ramachandra Faculty of Engineering and Technology, India

M. Srivani
Sri Ramachandra Faculty of Engineering and Technology, India

ABSTRACT

Generating realistic synthetic health data using Artificial Intelligence models offers a powerful solution to privacy restrictions and data scarcity in healthcare. Modern generative frameworks such as Generative Adversarial Networks, Variational Autoencoders, diffusion models, and transformer-based language models enable the synthesis of diverse clinical data, including structured EHR tables, time-series vitals, unstructured clinical notes, and medical images. These models are evaluated on fidelity, utility, and privacy, with applications ranging from data augmentation to privacy-preserving data sharing. GANs excel at learning joint distributions, VAEs capture smooth latent structures, diffusion models yield high-fidelity samples, and transformers produce coherent medical text. Challenges remain in ensuring clinical validity, diversity, and robust privacy protection while avoiding biases and mode collapse. Emerging research explores multimodal generation, promising richer, more integrated synthetic patient records that can transform healthcare research and AI model development.

DOI: 10.4018/979-8-3373-5641-9.ch006

1. INTRODUCTION

Synthetic health data have surged in importance due to privacy regulations and the high cost of collecting large medical datasets. Modern healthcare relies on large-scale electronic health records (EHRs), imaging archives, and genomic databases, but sharing these data is often restricted by laws (e.g., HIPAA, GDPR) or institutional policies. At the same time, many medical applications—such as developing AI models for disease prediction—require abundant, diverse, and richly annotated data.

By mimicking the statistical properties of real data, synthetic datasets enable broader data sharing, data augmentation, and fairness in analysis. Ibrahim et al. (2025) note that synthetic data facilitate sharing while protecting privacy, augment existing datasets, and promote fairness in AI applications. Similarly, Goncalves et al. (2020) emphasize that the scarcity of patient data has slowed progress in medicine, making high-quality synthetic data critical when real data are difficult, expensive, or limited to acquire.

Synthetic datasets can help address the lack of representative samples (e.g., for rare diseases) and accelerate the development of diagnostic models and statistical studies. By mirroring the statistical structures of real data while severing links to individuals, they allow researchers to access realistic datasets without exposing actual patient information. In practice, carefully generated synthetic data support broad sharing, foster algorithm development, and serve as benchmarks—all with minimal privacy risk.

1.1 The Importance of Synthetic Health Data

The key benefits of synthetic health data include:

1. **Data augmentation** – Expanding scarce datasets, especially for rare conditions or under-represented populations. For instance, synthetic images of rare tumors or EHR records of uncommon comorbidities can improve model training and reduce overfitting. Techniques such as Variational Autoencoders and GANs have successfully generated medical images (e.g., pneumonia in chest X-rays) and clinical signals, improving performance on minority classes.
2. **Privacy preservation** – High-quality synthetic EHRs can be shared between institutions without leaking Protected Health Information (PHI). The records mimic real data but are decoupled from real individuals, minimizing re-identification risk, (Nikolentzos et al., 2023).
3. **Fairness promotion** – By oversampling or simulating data for vulnerable or under-represented groups, synthetic datasets can help mitigate bias and improve the fairness of AI models.

1.2 The Role of Generative AI in Generating Synthetic Health Data

Generative AI models are central to creating realistic synthetic health data. Frameworks such as GANs, VAEs, diffusion models, and large language models learn complex data distributions and can produce new examples resembling real patient records or medical images.

GANs and VAEs have been widely applied to synthesize structured patient data and medical imagery, while recent work leverages diffusion processes and transformer-based architectures to generate clinical text and multimodal datasets. Importantly, generative AI can create new data from scratch—preserving statistical realism while decoupling it from actual individuals—offering stronger privacy protection than traditional anonymization.

1.3 Overview of the Paper

This paper is organized as follows. Section 2 reviews major generative AI frameworks (GANs, VAEs, diffusion models, and Transformer-based LLMs), explaining their operation and discussing their strengths and weaknesses in healthcare contexts. Section 3 examines applications to different health data modalities: structured EHR and time-series data, unstructured clinical text, and medical imaging, highlighting model choices in each domain. Section 4 discusses core challenges in synthetic health data generation, including ensuring clinical validity, maintaining diversity, and protecting privacy. Section 5 surveys key use cases – from addressing data scarcity to enabling software testing and benchmarking – where synthetic data provide concrete benefits. Finally, Section 6 summarizes the paper and outlines future research directions.

2. GENERATIVE FRAMEWORKS FOR SYNTHETIC HEALTH DATA

2.1 Generative Adversarial Networks

2.1.1 How GANs Work

Generative Adversarial Networks are a powerful class of generative models introduced by Goodfellow *et al.* (2014). A GAN consists of two neural networks – a generator (G) and a discriminator (D) – trained in tandem through an adversarial process as shown in figure 1. The generator takes random noise as input and attempts to produce realistic synthetic data, while the discriminator receives either real data samples or generator outputs and learns to distinguish between them. During training, G and D play a minimax game: the generator tries to fool the discriminator by producing ever more realistic samples, and the discriminator tries to catch the fakes. Over many iterations, the generator ideally learns the true data distribution, enabling it to create novel samples that the discriminator cannot easily distinguish from real data.

Figure 1. Synthetic data Generation using GAN.

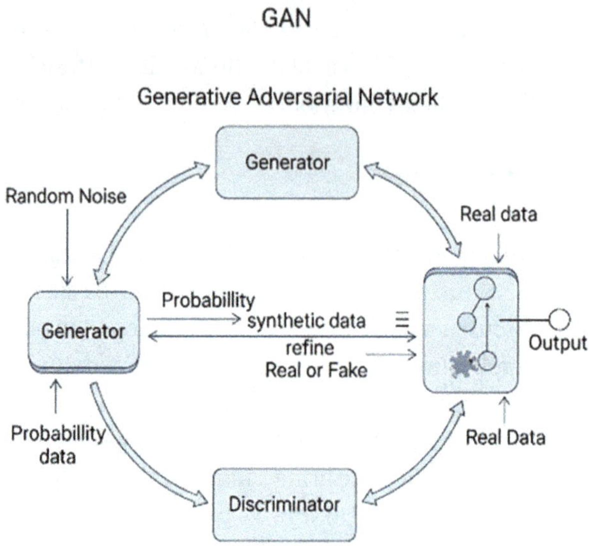

Mathematically, GAN training optimizes the generator G to minimize and the discriminator D to maximize the following objective:

$$\min_G \max_D E_{\{x \sim p_{\{data\}(x)}\}}[\log D(x)] + E_{\{z \sim p_{z(z)}\}}[\log(1 - D(G(z)))] \quad (1)$$

Informally, the discriminator tries to assign high probability to real samples and low to fake ones, while the generator aims to generate samples that maximize the discriminator's error. Well-known variants (e.g. Conditional GANs or CGANs) allow conditioning generation on labels or attributes; Wasserstein GANs (WGANs) improve stability by using Wasserstein distance; and many other architectures (e.g. CycleGAN, StyleGAN) have been developed for specific tasks. In healthcare, GANs have been applied to generate images (MRI, X-ray), time-series (ECG), and even tabular records.

2.1.2 Strengths and Weaknesses for Health Data

Strengths. GANs are celebrated for producing sharp, high-quality samples (especially images) that closely resemble real data. GANs have emerged as a powerful tool in AI, particularly for unsupervised learning. They can capture complex, high-dimensional distributions without explicit modeling of domain features, making them flexible across modalities. For example, synthetic medical images generated by GANs (such as MRI or ultrasound scans) have been used effectively for data augmentation and anonymity. In tabular or EHR data, GANs like MedGAN and CTGAN can reproduce joint patterns of diagnoses, medications and demographics, (Ashrafi et al., 2023). Importantly, GANs do not directly copy training samples; by design they output novel combinations of learned features, enabling data privacy through abstraction. Studies show that GAN-generated records can mimic patient cohorts without revealing identifiable details.

Weaknesses. Despite their power, GANs face several challenges. The adversarial training is notoriously unstable and can suffer from mode collapse, where the generator produces limited varieties of outputs. In mode collapse, G converges to a limited set of patterns, failing to capture the full diversity of real patient data, (Ahmed, 2024). For instance, a GAN trained on chest X-rays might repeatedly produce images of healthy lungs and miss rare pathologies. This is especially problematic in healthcare, where minority conditions are important to capture. Furthermore, GANs lack straightforward metrics for assessing output quality, making it hard to quantify how realistic or diverse the synthetic data are. Training can also be sensitive to hyperparameters and large datasets; GANs often require careful tuning to avoid convergence to suboptimal equilibria, (Yan et al., 2024). Finally, conventional GANs do not inherently guarantee privacy: without modifications, a GAN can sometimes memorize and reproduce aspects of individual training records, risking leakage. In summary, while GANs excel at generating realistic synthetic data, they must be used with care to avoid mode collapse, training instability, and privacy risks.

2.2 Variational Autoencoders (VAEs)

2.2.1 How VAEs Work

Variational Autoencoders are probabilistic generative models that learn a continuous latent representation of data. A VAE consists of an encoder neural network that maps input data (e.g. an image or patient record) to parameters of a latent distribution (typically a Gaussian), and a decoder network that reconstructs data from a sample drawn from this latent distribution. Crucially, VAEs impose a prior (e.g. a standard normal) over the latent space and train the encoder–decoder pair to maximize a variational lower bound on the data likelihood. This involves two loss terms: a reconstruction loss (making decoded outputs similar to inputs) and a KL-divergence penalty (pushing the latent distribution toward the prior). During training, the reparameterization trick is used to allow gradient descent through the sampling step.

The result is that the latent space becomes a smooth, structured representation of the data. In practice, VAEs are learned so that samples drawn from the latent distribution are passed to the decoder to reconstruct the input, enabling generation of new data, (Teli, 2025). Figure 2 shows the latent space as a bottleneck through which features are compressed, and new samples are generated by sampling this bottleneck distribution. After training, one can produce synthetic data by sampling z from the prior (e.g. N(0,1)) and feeding it through the decoder. VAEs thus approximate the true data distribution with a parametric model that is easy to sample from.

Figure 2. Variational Autoencoder (VAE) Architecture

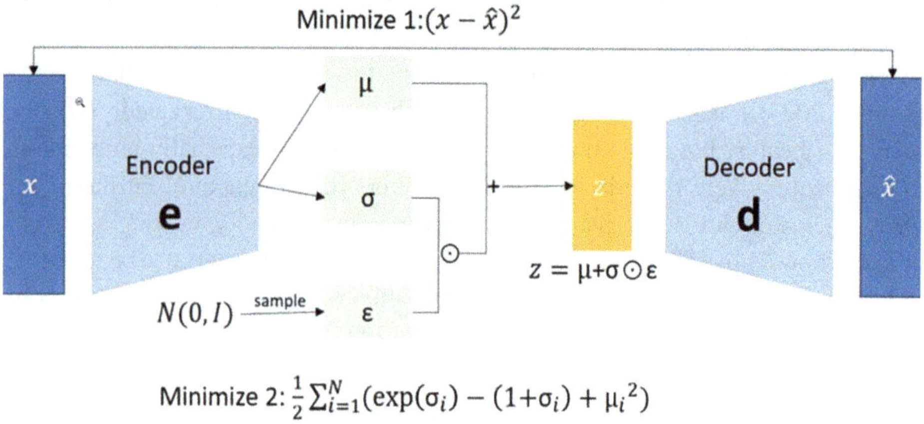

2.2.2 Strengths and Weaknesses for Health Data

Strengths. VAEs offer a number of advantages for synthetic health data. The latent space is explicitly probabilistic, providing a principled way to quantify uncertainty in generation. The smooth latent representation can capture meaningful variation in data (e.g. disease stages or demographic factors) and can be interpolated between for new combinations. Importantly, VAEs tend to be more stable to train than GANs, since they optimize a well-defined objective and do not involve adversarial games. In practice, VAEs have been used to generate synthetic medical images (e.g. X-rays, histopathology) that maintain global structure. They are also naturally extensible:

for instance, graph-based VAEs can model patient trajectories, and conditional VAEs can incorporate labels. VAEs learn a probabilistic representation of the data, enabling image generation and have been applied to augment datasets of clinical images, including those of rare diseases.

Weaknesses. However, vanilla VAEs often produce blurrier outputs compared to GANs. Because the VAE objective averages over all possible outputs to minimize reconstruction error, fine details can be smoothed out. A limitation of VAEs is their tendency to generate blurry image reconstructions, which can be problematic in medical imaging where sharp edges matter. VAEs also may underfit complex data if the latent space is too small or the model insufficiently expressive. In structured/tabular data, VAEs can struggle with discrete or heterogeneous variables without specialized architectures. Nonetheless, many recent works have combined VAEs with other techniques (e.g. coupling with GANs, or using vector quantization) to improve fidelity while retaining the stability of training. For health data, VAEs provide a reliable way to capture distributional structure, at the cost of sometimes sacrificing realism of individual samples.

2.3 Diffusion Models

2.3.1 How Diffusion Models Work

Denoising diffusion models (also known as Score-Based Generative Models) are a newer class of generative models that have shown great promise in image and signal generation. The basic idea is to start with data and gradually add noise in a forward diffusion process, turning a data sample into pure noise over many small steps as shown in figure3. Then, a neural network is trained to reverse this process: given a noisy input, the model predicts and removes the noise, step by step, until a clean sample is recovered. Sampling a new synthetic example thus starts from a random noise vector and iteratively denoises it into a data sample. Kreis *et al.* have shown that diffusion models produce exceptionally high-fidelity images when enough denoising steps are used, (Kreis et al., 2022).

Figure 3. Architecture of diffusion model

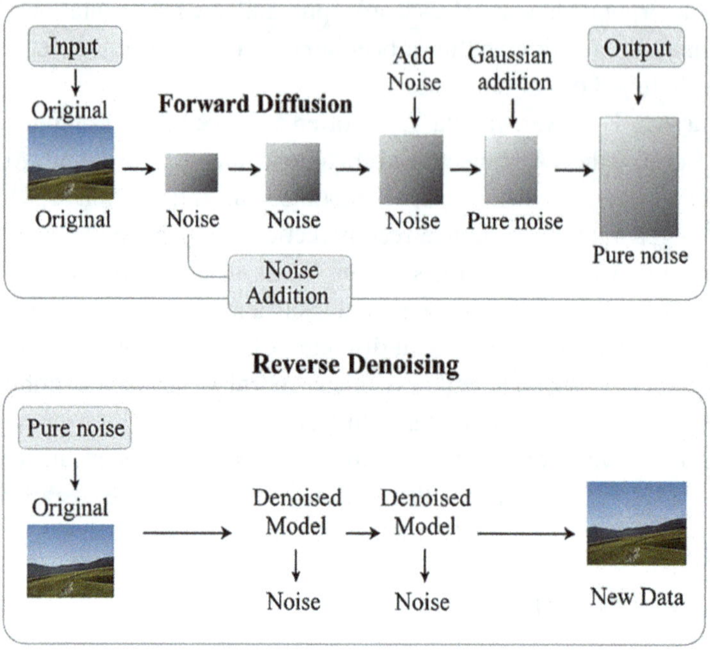

In summary, a diffusion model is trained to minimize the difference between the original clean data and the denoised output at each noise level. A key strength is that this generative process covers the data manifold thoroughly: because it essentially performs a sequence of small refinements, it avoids jumping between modes and thus captures diverse modes of the data. Recent surveys note that diffusion models have emerged as powerful generative model offering strong sample diversity and faithful mode coverage. In other words, diffusion models often outperform GANs in covering all variations of the data, though at the expense of more computation.

2.3.2 Strengths and Weaknesses for Health Data

Strengths. For medical data generation, diffusion models' main advantage is sample quality and diversity. They achieve very high-fidelity outputs (often surpassing GANs) for complex distributions like images or high-frequency signals. This makes them attractive for synthesizing medical images (e.g. MRI, CT) and potentially complex time series. The iterative nature also provides flexibility: diffusion models can be conditioned on class labels or segmentations (e.g. denoise with condition: tumor present) and extended to tasks like super-resolution or inpainting. Importantly, they inherently avoid the mode collapse problem of GANs – as the literature notes, diffusion models have strong mode coverage, meaning they can generate examples from rare subpopulations that GANs might miss.

Weaknesses. The primary drawback of diffusion models is computational cost. Because generation requires hundreds or thousands of sequential denoising steps, sampling from a diffusion model is much slower than a one-shot generator in a GAN. As diffusion experts note, slow sampling has been the main weakness of these models. In a medical context, generating a large synthetic dataset via diffusion can thus be resource-intensive. There is also added complexity in tuning the noise schedule and training the score network. Additionally, diffusion models have been studied less extensively for non-image modalities: adapting them to structured EHR or text data is still an active research area. In summary, diffusion models promise higher-quality synthetic medical images (and potentially time-series), but they require heavy computation and careful engineering to be practical on large health datasets.

2.4 Transformer-based Language Models

2.4.1 How Transformers Work

Transformer models are the foundation of modern large language models like GPT. At their core is the self-attention mechanism: each token in an input sequence (e.g. a word or clinical code) attends to every other, allowing the model to capture long-range dependencies. Transformers stack multiple layers of self-attention and feed-forward networks, processing sequences in parallel rather than sequentially. In the generative setting (e.g. autoregressive models), the transformer is trained to predict the next token given previous ones, learning to generate coherent text or token sequences.

For synthetic health data, transformer-based models can be used in several ways. The most obvious is text generation: clinical notes, discharge summaries, or physician reports can be generated by feeding seed prompts into a medical LLM (such as GPT-based models). But transformers can also be repurposed for structured data: for instance, tabular EHR or time-series data can be serialized (e.g. as sequences of tokens or events), and a transformer can be trained or fine-tuned to generate such sequences. This approach leverages the model's ability to learn complex joint distributions. Recent studies have explored GPT-like generation of synthetic patient records, (Miletic & Sariyar, 2024).

2.4.2 Strengths and Weaknesses for Health Data

Strengths. Transformer-based models excel at capturing rich contextual dependencies, especially in text data. They can generate highly fluent and contextually appropriate clinical narratives. For clinical notes, modern Large Language Models (LLM) produce text that often reads very realistically. In other modalities, transformers offer flexibility: by treating EHR features as tokens, an LLM can model correlations among diverse medical attributes. Miletic and Sariyar show that even moderately sized transformer models can match or exceed GANs in synthesizing tabular health data: larger LLMs outperformed a CTGAN baseline on synthetic EHR generation. Also, using pre-trained models (e.g. BERT, GPT) means benefiting from huge prior knowledge; fine-tuning or prompting such a model on a hospital's data can yield high-quality outputs with relatively little task-specific data. Transformer models, being feed-forward at generation time, can produce samples more quickly than diffusion models.

Weaknesses. However, transformer generative models also have challenges in healthcare. First, they are data-intensive: training or fine-tuning an LLM requires large corpora and significant compute. As one review observes, generating synthetic clinical notes with LLMs has demonstrated significant improvements but at the cost of massive resources (one LLM took 560 A100 GPUs for 20 days to train). Second, LLMs can suffer from hallucination: they may generate plausible-sounding but clinically incorrect or inconsistent information, especially for complex multi-step reasoning tasks (Loni et al., 2025). This is a risk for synthetic medical text, where subtle errors can have major implications. Third, while transformers can model diversity, they might over-represent frequent patterns learned during pretraining, and controlling for underrepresented patient subgroups can be non-trivial. Finally, like GANs, LLMs have privacy concerns: they can memorize training texts and inadvertently regurgitate sensitive fragments (Nahid & Hasan, 2024). In summary, transformer-based generative models are powerful (especially for text) but require careful handling to ensure clinical accuracy, computational feasibility, and privacy.

Table 1 presents a comparative matrix of generative model. This matrix illustrates the suitability of various generative AI models—GANs, VAEs, Diffusion Models, and Transformer-based LLMs for different types of healthcare data: structured data (e.g., EHRs), clinical text, and medical images. Color intensity and symbols indicate the relative effectiveness of each model across these modalities, with GANs and VAEs excelling in image generation, while Transformer LLMs show high compatibility with clinical text generation.

Each framework has complementary uses: GANs/VAE hybrids are popular for structured/tabular data, diffusion models excel in image and some tabular tasks, and transformers dominate text generation. Table 1 summarizes key properties of these generative families.

Table 1. Comparison of generative model families for synthetic data. Key features, data modalities, strengths, and limitations are listed. Citations illustrate each model's use in healthcare synthetic data.

Model Type	Mechanism	Example Medical Use	Strengths	Limitations
GAN	Adversarial training (generator vs. discriminator).	Synthetic EHR vectors, imaging (PGGAN for X-rays)	High-quality samples; models joint distributions; good for continuous data	Training instability, mode collapse (may miss rare cases); struggles with discrete tokens without workarounds
VAE	Probabilistic encoder–decoder. Learns latent distribution.	EHR record generation, structured timelines (graph VAEs)	Smooth latent space (interpolation, diversity); principled likelihood.	Often blurrier outputs; less realistic detail than GANs; continuous output by design (can discretize labels).
Diffusion	Forward noising + reverse denoising Markov chain.	High-res medical images (e.g. radiology, dermatology); tabular data (TabDDPM)	State-of-art fidelity; stable training; handles various modalities (images, 3D); naturally multi-step.	Heavy computation; slow sampling; requires many steps.
Transformer (LLM)	Autoregressive or encoder-decoder seq2seq.	Clinical text generation (notes, reports), tokenized EHR sequences (CEHR GPT)	Captures long-range context; produces coherent text; flexible with modalities (text, tokens)	Extremely data- and compute-hungry; prone to hallucination; ensuring factual/clinical accuracy is challenging.

3. APPLICATIONS TO HEALTH DATA MODALITIES

3.1 Structured EHR and Time-Series Data

3.1.1 GAN-based Approaches

Structured EHR data consist of tables of patient demographics, diagnoses, medications, lab results, and time-stamped events. GANs have been widely applied to such data. For static, tabular EHR records, architectures often combine an autoencoder with a GAN. MedGAN (Ashrafi et al., 2023) is a classic example: it uses a multilayer perceptron generator to synthesize patient records, and an autoencoder to handle discrete variables. Other tabular GANs include CTGAN (Ince et al., 2024) for mixed numerical/categorical data, and TableGAN for general tables. For *longitudinal* or time-series data, recurrent GANs have been developed. Models like RCGAN and TimeGAN (Liu et al., 2024) generate sequential trajectories of patient visits or vital sign time series. In addition, research like DoppelGANger and EHR-M-GAN synthesize multi-dimensional patient timelines, combining GANs with sequence models.

These GAN-based methods have shown they can capture many statistical patterns of EHR data. For example, generative models accurately capture the statistical properties of real EHR data while inducing low privacy risks. They produce realistic distributions of diagnoses and correlations, often evaluated by training a predictor on synthetic data and testing on real data. However, limitations remain: GANs tend to struggle with rare events and low-prevalence concepts. GAN synthetic EHRs can under-represent rarely observed conditions, since the generator prefers high-density regions. Stability is also a concern – GAN training on tabular data can be unstable (just as in imaging). Overall, GANs offer a potent tool for EHR synthesis, but achieving clinical fidelity for longitudinal trajectories can require careful architectures and tuning. Privacy-conscious variants (e.g. adding differential privacy) have been proposed to safeguard the output.

3.1.2 Hybrid Models (VAEs, Graph-based Autoencoders, Diffusion Processes)

Hybrid generative models combine elements of VAEs, graph networks, and other approaches to better handle EHR complexity. For instance, Variational Graph Autoencoders (VGAEs) treat each patient's record as a graph (nodes = events, edges = temporal/semantic links) and learn to generate entire clinical trajectories. Mami *et al.* (2022) used a VGAE to synthesize patient records and found that the generated trajectories were realistic and privacy-preserving. This approach captures the rich structure of EHRs, including long-range dependencies between visits. Other methods incorporate probabilistic graphical models or Bayesian networks to ensure medical plausibility. For example, early synthetic EHR systems combined population statistics and clinical guidelines (manually encoded knowledge) with generative sampling to produce realistic records. While fully data-driven models (GANs, VAEs) are disease-agnostic, blending in expert constraints or epidemiological priors can improve validity.

Diffusion processes have also been explored: one can apply score-based models to time-series data, gradually noising patient trajectories and learning to denoise them. Although less common today, such diffusion-based generative processes could benefit from the diversity advantages discussed above. In sum, hybrid approaches attempt to merge the flexibility of deep models with the structure of statistical domain knowledge. As an example of VAE usage, a study by Bassani et al. (2025) highlights how synthetic data generated by VAEs has been used for rare disease imaging and can similarly be applied to sparse EHR scenarios. Continued research explores combinations (e.g. VAE-GAN hybrids) to get the best of each model.

3.1.3 Transformer-based Approaches

Transformer-based models are now being applied to structured EHR data. In one line of work, researchers tokenize tabular records and treat rows or sequences of medical codes as text. Large pre-trained language models (like GPT) are then fine-tuned to generate new patient profiles. Miletic and Sariyar (2025) show that even relatively small transformer models can perform on par with specialized GANs: as the number of parameters increases, LLMs outperform the reference GAN (CTGAN); even the smallest LLM (14M parameters) performs comparably to CTGAN. This suggests that LLMs can capture complex feature interactions in EHR. Moreover, transformer architectures can directly model event sequences over time – for example, each hospital visit can be a token sequence including diagnoses, labs, and treatments. These sequence models can then generate synthetic patient histories.

The main strength of transformers here is leveraging pretraining on large biomedical corpora or EHR text, which imparts rich contextual knowledge. However, weaknesses include the need for substantial computing and the potential for medically incorrect outputs if not constrained. Overall, transformer-based generation of EHR is an emerging area, with initial results showing promise for data augmentation and sharing.

3.2 Unstructured Clinical Text

3.2.1 Transformer-based Language Models

Clinical text (discharge summaries, progress notes, radiology reports) is inherently suited to Transformer-based LLMs. Models like GPT, BioGPT, or specialized medical LMs can be fine-tuned on clinical corpora to generate plausible new notes. Current literature shows that large language models are the dominant approach for synthetic clinical text. A recent scoping review observes that generative adversarial and VAE methods are rarely used for free text; instead LLMs have been well-received mainly for generating synthetic texts. Indeed, transformer LLMs (such as GPT-3 or ChatGPT derivatives) can produce coherent patient narratives when prompted appropriately. For example, one may fine-tune a GPT model on anonymized pathology reports and then sample new reports by conditioning on patient demographics or preliminary findings. These LLMs capture medical terminology and formatting remarkably well, often creating realistic note structures and reasoning.

However, these models require careful handling: training or fine-tuning large LMs demands massive compute resources. As one review notes, generating synthetic clinical notes with modern LLMs involved 560 A100 GPUs for 20 days in one case. Moreover, LLMs can hallucinate or produce inconsistent details. Unlike structured outputs, evaluating the realism of generated text is challenging and often relies on expert review or downstream task performance. Despite this, transformer LLMs currently achieve the best fluency and context in synthetic text generation, outperforming older methods like RNN-based language models.

3.2.2 Challenges and Recent Techniques

Synthetic clinical text poses unique challenges. The first is clinical plausibility and coherence. A note must be factually consistent (e.g. medications should align with diagnoses, chronology of events should make sense). LLMs can sometimes fail on such logical consistency, generating contradictory or medically unsound statements. Recent work has explored advanced prompting strategies (e.g. Chain-of-Thought prompting) to improve reasoning in generated notes, but no solution is perfect.

Second, privacy leakage is a concern: a large language model fine-tuned on actual patient notes may inadvertently reproduce snippets of original text, thus risking disclosure. Rigorous filtering and anonymization of training text is essential.

Third, evaluation metrics for synthetic clinical text are still in development. Standard NLP metrics (BLEU, perplexity) do not fully capture clinical validity. Recent reviews note that evaluation metrics currently available for generic LLMs lack an understanding of medical and health-related concepts. Some works propose clinical-domain scores or use retrieval-based metrics, but evaluation remains a moving target.

Recent advances to address these challenges include reinforcement learning from human feedback (RLHF) to align LLM outputs with medical correctness, applying factuality classifiers to post-edit output, and incorporating medical knowledge graphs to constrain generation. For example, one can force the model to check drug–disease interactions against a knowledge base before finalizing a note. Ongoing research also uses differential privacy techniques (see Section 4.3) to mitigate memorization. Overall, while transformer-based text generation is powerful, it requires domain-specific tuning and careful safeguards to ensure quality and safety.

3.3 Medical Imaging

3.3.1 GANs and Diffusion Models

Medical imaging (MRI, CT, X-ray, ultrasound, etc.) has been a prime target for generative models. GANs, in particular, have a long history in this area. The systematic review by Akpinar et al. (2024) finds that the majority of recent GAN applications in healthcare focus on imaging: cGAN (conditional GAN) and CycleGAN are among the most popular architectures. cGANs are often used when labels are available (e.g. generating an X-ray given a disease label), while CycleGANs are used for unsupervised image-to-image translation (e.g. converting CT scans to MRI domain). GANs have been used to create synthetic brain MRI slices, chest X-rays with various pathologies, retinal fundus images, and many other types. These GANs allow flexible conditional generation: for example, one can train a GAN to produce images of pneumonia vs. healthy lungs, or even generate images with specified tumor size.

More recently, diffusion models have been applied to medical imaging. Given their high sample fidelity, diffusion models can generate very realistic and detailed images. In practice, conditional diffusion models are being explored (e.g. to enhance resolution or fill missing slices). For instance, a diffusion model trained on brain MRIs can generate synthetic MR images that preserve subtle anatomical variability. Diffusion models offer strong mode coverage and quality in image generation, suggesting they can better capture the range of normal and pathological variations than GANs alone.

3.3.2 Data Augmentation and Conditional Generation

One of the main uses of synthetic imaging data is augmentation of limited datasets. In computer vision, adding GAN- or diffusion-synthesized images has been shown to improve the performance of classifiers, especially in regimes with few real examples. In medical imaging, this often takes the form of augmenting rare cases (e.g. small tumors, uncommon fractures). Researchers also generate images under controlled conditions: e.g. varying a parameter like tumor size or image contrast.

Conditional generation is widely used. In GAN-based pipelines, one often feeds a class label or segmentation mask into the generator, so that the output image has those characteristics. For example, Conditional GANs have been used to generate MRIs with and without Alzheimer's plaques given a patient age input. Similarly, diffusion models can be conditioned on text prompts (text-to-image) or clinical metadata to steer the generation.

Overall, in medical imaging the combination of GANs and diffusion models provides a toolkit: GANs offer fast one-shot generation suitable for large-scale augmentation, while diffusion models deliver the highest visual fidelity for critical imaging tasks. Both approaches have enabled conditional synthesis (class- or label-driven), which is valuable for creating synthetic datasets labeled by disease or modality.

3.4 Evaluation metrics

Synthetic data used in the field of healthcare must be evaluated, in order to be representative of real-world data and not to violate the privacy of patients. Unless assessed carefully, synthetic data can cause statistical biases, fail to generalize to clinical knowledge, or even accidentally reveal confidential material. The metrics used within fidelity, utility, privacy and fairness criteria indicate whether the synthetic data is sufficiently trustworthy to be used during model training, research or decision making. Since healthcare decisions hold a big stake, the assessment of synthetic data assures safe, ethical, and effective application of the data; ultimately, regulatory compliance, reproducibility, and equitable health outcomes can be achieved. This is strong evaluation that lends confidence in the application of synthetic data in life-saving applications.

Table 2 summarizes common evaluation metrics. It outlines key evaluation metrics for synthetic healthcare data, covering fidelity, utility, privacy, and fairness. Also, highlights how well synthetic data mimics real data, supports model performance, protects patient privacy, and maintains demographic fairness. These metrics are critical to ensure that synthetic data is both safe and effective for real-world medical research and applications.

Table 2. Evaluation metrics for synthetic health data.

Parameter	Metric (Healthcare Example)	Interpretation	Desired Behavior
Fidelity	MMD between real/ synth labs; Discriminative accuracy	How similar are distributions?	Low MMD, low classification accuracy (real vs fake indistinguishable)
	Correlation heatmap (vitals)	Are feature correlations preserved?	Synthetic correlations ≈ real (high Pearson r)
	Medical rule checks (e.g. no contradictory codes)	Does data obey clinical logic?	Zero violations (realistic combinations)

continued on following page

Table 2. Continued

Parameter	Metric (Healthcare Example)	Interpretation	Desired Behavior
Utility	TSTR (train on synth, test on real)	Model performance on real data	Performance ≈ model trained on real only
	TSRTR (train on real+synthetic)	Data augmentation effect	Model improves vs using real only
Privacy	Membership inference accuracy	Can an attacker detect real vs. synthetic?	Low attack accuracy (near random)
	Nearest neighbor distance	Are synthetic points far from any real?	High average distance (no copy)
	Differential privacy ε	Formal privacy guarantee	Smaller ε means stronger privacy
Fairness	Group representation parity	Does synthetic data reflect demographics?	Matches real-world proportions or desired rebalancing
	Outcome balance (e.g., disease rates by group)	Maintains fairness metrics	No undue bias transfer or amplified disparity

3.5. Application of Synthetic Data

3.5.1 Key Use Cases of Synthetic Data in Healthcare AI

Synthetic data unlocks several high-impact use cases in healthcare and is summarised in Table 3.

- **Data Augmentation for Machine Learning**: Enriching scarce classes. For instance, generating extra examples of rare cancers, drug interactions, or adverse events can boost classifier performance. In the NeurIPS 2024 SynthEHR challenge, transformer-generated synthetic patient sequences for rare outcomes led to significantly better rare-event prediction. Augmentation is especially valuable in imbalanced datasets (e.g. underrepresented demographics or uncommon diagnoses).
- **Privacy-Preserving Data Sharing**: Organizations can share synthetic cohorts instead of real records. A hospital could release a fully synthetic EHR dataset to external researchers, preserving statistical patterns while protecting individuals. This enables multi-site studies and federated research without PHI. For example, synthetic patient data have been proposed for public release when real data sharing is legally or ethically constrained. Even commercial entities (e.g. pharmaceutical companies) explore generating simulated trial cohorts to collaborate without disclosing proprietary data.

- **Algorithm Testing and Benchmarking**: Synthetic cases can test clinical decision support tools under controlled scenarios. Developers can evaluate their models on simulated patients with extreme or unusual presentations that might be hard to find in reality. Synthetic data also allow reproducible benchmarks (see Table 4 for examples).
- **Clinical Trial Simulation and Planning**: Synthetic cohorts can model what-if scenarios. For instance, one could simulate treatment effects by applying alternative interventions to synthetic patients, helping to design studies or explore hypotheses. Synthetic data serve as input for virtual trials or simulations of disease progression under different policies.
- **Fairness and Bias Mitigation**: Synthetic generation can deliberately oversample minority groups or adjust demographic proportions, mitigating biases in original data. For example, if black or rural patients are underrepresented in an EHR, a generative model can be conditioned or steered to produce more of those profiles. This enriched data, when used in training, can improve equity of downstream AI models.
- **Education and Software Development**: Synthetic health records provide safe data for training medical students or testing new software without risking privacy. Hospitals can use synthetic EHRs and images to train staff or validate new EHR systems, ensuring functionality before live deployment.

Table 3. Key use cases of synthetic health data with examples.

	Description & Examples	Benefits
Augmentation	Generate cases for rare diseases (e.g. diabetic retinopathy images) or outcomes (neonatal deaths). Example: adding synthetic pulmonary embolism cases to an X-ray dataset improves classifier recall.	Increases model robustness; addresses class imbalance; reduces need for expensive data collection.
Data Sharing	Release synthetic EHR for research consortia. Example: a hospital syndicate published fully synthetic patient data to allow algorithm benchmarking.	Enables multi-center studies; respects privacy regulations; fosters collaboration.
Testing/ Benchmarking	Synthetic unusual cases for stress-testing diagnostics. Example: creating synthetic cardiac MRI scans with rare congenital anomalies to test analysis software.	Safe, reproducible testing environment; standardized benchmarks across labs.
Simulation/Trials	Virtual clinical trial cohorts. E.g., simulating 10,000 synthetic patients to evaluate trial designs or treatment strategies.	Cost-effective trial planning; explore what-if scenarios without risk.
Fairness Improvement	Oversample demographic groups or conditions. E.g., generating more female patients with certain cardiology cases to balance training data.	Reduces bias; improves model generalizability to underserved groups.

3.5.2 Synthetic Data Deployment in Healthcare Institutions

Table 4 presents real-world examples of how synthetic health data is being actively deployed across healthcare institutions and organizations to support a wide range of use cases. Institutions such as Beth Israel Deaconess Medical Center have used synthetic ICU records derived from MIMIC datasets to develop and validate early warning systems, improving clinical decision support tools while safeguarding patient privacy. The UK's National Health Service (NHS) has released synthetic hospital datasets through initiatives like OpenSAFELY to facilitate research and innovation while complying with stringent privacy regulations.

In digital health, the SMART on FHIR sandbox provides developers with synthetic electronic health records in FHIR format to test applications under realistic clinical scenarios without access to real patient data. Similarly, Stanford's biomedical informatics center has employed synthetic patient cohorts to simulate clinical trial scenarios, optimizing trial design and eligibility criteria.

Pharmaceutical companies like Roche and Genentech use synthetic genomic and EHR data to enable secure collaboration with external partners while protecting intellectual property. Within government systems, the U.S. Department of Veterans Affairs (VA) uses synthetic patient records for EHR software validation and staff training, minimizing risks associated with using real data.

Table 4. Examples of Synthetic Data Deployment in Healthcare Institutions

Institution / Organization	Purpose	Synthetic Data Type	Outcome
Beth Israel Deaconess Medical Center	Model Development & Testing	Synthetic ICU EHR (MIMIC-derived)	Improved early warning systems using GAN-generated ICU data
NHS (UK) – NHS Digital	Public Data Sharing	Synthetic Hospital Records	Released datasets for research and innovation under privacy mandates
SMART on FHIR Sandbox	App Development & Interoperability	Synthetic EHR (FHIR format)	Used by developers to test health apps in realistic scenarios
Stanford Center for Biomedical Informatics	Simulation of Clinical Trials	Synthetic EHR cohorts	Simulated different enrollment criteria for trial planning
Roche / Genentech	Data Collaboration with Partners	Synthetic Genomic & EHR Data	Shared synthetic patient cohorts to preserve proprietary data
U.S. Veterans Affairs (VA)	Training and Software Validation	Synthetic Patient Records	Used for internal EHR testing and staff training

These examples underscore the growing adoption of synthetic data as a practical, privacy-preserving tool that enhances research, supports AI model development, and ensures safe, scalable innovation across healthcare ecosystems.

4. CHALLENGES IN SYNTHETIC HEALTH DATA GENERATION

Generating synthetic health data is technically challenging. We focus on three interlinked issues: clinical validity, diversity, and privacy. A synthetic dataset is only useful if it is (a) medically plausible, (b) sufficiently diverse to cover population variability, and (c) privacy-preserving. Each of these brings specific obstacles.

4.1 Clinical Validity

4.1.1 Ensuring Medical Logic and Variability

Synthetic health records must adhere to medical logic. A synthetic patient data should not have impossible or contradictory features (e.g. a male patient receiving ovarian cancer treatment). More subtly, correlations between variables (like lab values rising with disease severity) should be preserved. This is often difficult, since generative models optimize statistical similarity, not explicit medical rules. For example, synthesizing a patient's longitudinal trajectory requires capturing temporal consistency (e.g. diagnoses should follow plausible sequences). Without constraints, a model might generate a patient with inconsistent vital sign patterns or improbable medication combinations.

To illustrate, some synthetic EHR generators incorporate domain knowledge to enforce validity. Dube and Gallagher's approach uses public health statistics, clinical guidelines, and medical code standards to assemble realistic patient records. By contrast, purely data-driven models rely on the training data alone. If the training set has biases or missing patterns, the synthetic data will replicate those flaws. Thus, ensuring variability (so that the synthetic data spans the range of real-world cases) and avoiding unrealistic outliers are active concerns. A high-quality synthetic data should preserve the original data's statistical properties, yet respecting confidentiality; striking this balance is nontrivial.

4.1.2 Techniques for Improving Validity

Researchers have proposed various strategies. One approach is conditional generation with domain constraints: e.g. encode known relationships (if age<18, omit certain drugs) and either train the model with these labels or post-filter outputs.

Hybrid models using explicit domain knowledge (e.g. knowledge graphs of medical concepts) can be used in tandem with neural generators to correct anomalies. Another idea is to use a multi-objective loss that rewards both statistical fidelity and domain consistency; for instance, adding a term that penalizes medically impossible records.

Active evaluation by clinicians is also key. Some groups involve human experts to review generated samples and iteratively refine the model. Debugging the generator by analyzing where it violates medical rules can guide adjustments (e.g. adding more examples of rare events into the training data). Ultimately, robust evaluation metrics that capture clinical plausibility are needed – this remains an open research area. For now, integrating expert knowledge (as in) and building interpretable latent spaces are among the best practices for improving validity.

4.2 Diversity

4.2.1 Preventing Mode Collapse

Diversity in synthetic data means covering all relevant subpopulations and conditions. Mode collapse (from Section 2.1) directly undermines diversity by producing repetitive, narrow outputs. Preventing mode collapse is therefore critical.

Techniques include using GAN variants like WGAN or Unrolled GANs that stabilize training, adding minibatch discrimination layers to promote output variance, or explicitly clustering and encouraging diversity in the loss. For example, clustering real data into subgroups and training the generator to sample from each cluster can help cover rare patterns. Also, one can over-sample underrepresented cases in the training phase to balance the generator's attention. In practice, detecting and combating mode collapse often involves monitoring sample diversity metrics (e.g. coverage of classes or value ranges). Mode collapse causes the generator to fail to capture the full variability of the data – careful training and monitoring are needed to mitigate this.

4.2.2 Balancing Quality and Variety

There is an inherent trade-off between individual sample quality and overall variety. A model can be tuned to produce extremely realistic outputs, but if it sees only the most common modes of data, it will lack diversity. Conversely, pushing a model to produce every possible variation (even outliers) can degrade the fidelity of any given sample. Achieving balance requires hyperparameter tuning and possibly using ensembles of models. Some works train multiple generators, each specializing in different subgroups. Others interpolate between different generative approaches:

for instance, using GANs for majority modes (high quality on frequent cases) and simpler models (like variational or copula-based generators) for rare events.

Using diffusion models can help this balance: as noted, diffusion models excel in mode coverage. One can even combine GAN and diffusion outputs to blend quality and diversity. Ultimately, evaluating the diversity of synthetic datasets requires domain-specific metrics (e.g. coverage of diagnoses, patient demographics). There is no one-size-fits-all solution, and work in this area remains ongoing.

4.3 Privacy

4.3.1 Preventing Leakage of Real Patient Information

A paramount goal is that synthetic data should *not* reveal individual patient information. However, generative models can sometimes memorize training samples, risking leakage. For example, Foomani *et al.* (2022) demonstrate that classical GANs can recall training samples, making re-identification possible. Similarly, LLMs trained on EHR text can regurgitate exact phrases or rare identifiers (as shown in studies of GPT memorization). To mitigate this, one must rigorously check generated data for traces of real records. Techniques include auditing the model with membership inference attacks: if an attacker can reliably distinguish whether a specific patient was in the training set, the synthetic generator leaks information. Privacy-enhancing training algorithms (e.g. differentially private SGD) can be applied during model training to limit memorization (see below).

Empirically, researchers often blend synthetic and real data and test whether a classifier can spot real vs. fake, or use human review to detect copied content. Adversarial testing (trying to reconstruct training examples from the generator) is another audit method. It has been found that even medical generators aren't immune: Sharing data sets is difficult because de-identified data can often be re-identified by linking attributes. Thus, preventing leakage requires strict mechanisms and ongoing assessment in any deployment.

4.3.2 Integrating Differential Privacy and Evaluating Re-identification Risk

A leading method to guard against leakage is Differential Privacy (DP). DP provides a formal guarantee that the inclusion or exclusion of any one individual in the training data has limited effect on the output distribution. Concretely, DP is often implemented via adding noise to gradients during training (DP-SGD) or injecting noise into the outputs. In the generative context, DP-GANs or DP-VAEs Incorporate carefully calibrated noise during training so that the resulting model satisfies differential privacy. For large language models, recent work has shown that DP can be enforced even during inference: Xiao et al. (2025) presents a framework of differential privacy to protect sensitive data in the training of Large Language Model. Its feature including dynamic privacy budget allocation, adaptive noise injection, and performance optimization, offer robust privacy guarantees, small utility loss, and decrease in computational overhead, setting new standards of secure LLM deployment.

Beyond technique, rigorous evaluation is crucial. Privacy risk is often assessed by membership inference attacks, which attempt to guess if a record was in the training set given synthetic data. A strong synthetic generator should fool such an attack (output synthetic data indistinguishable from some held-out real data in terms of membership). Other metrics include *k*-anonymity-like measures on the synthetic outputs. In all cases, combining DP with these assessments yields the most confidence. Ultimately, deploying synthetic healthcare data requires both model-level defenses (DP training) and data-level audits (re-identification testing) to ensure patient privacy.

5. USE CASES FOR SYNTHETIC HEALTH DATA

Synthetic health data unlock many practical applications. Below we outline key use cases: enabling AI development, preserving privacy in sharing, software testing, and more.

5.1 Alleviating Data Scarcity for AI Model Development

One of the most immediate benefits of synthetic data is addressing limited data. In machine learning, performance often hinges on abundant, diverse training samples. In many healthcare applications, the real datasets are small or imbalanced. Synthetic data can augment training sets, effectively rescuing underpowered tasks. For example, VAEs have been used to synthesize examples of rare pathologies (like uncommon cancers) in medical images, significantly improving classifier training. Similarly, synthetic EHR records for minority patient groups can help a predictive model learn features of those groups, reducing bias and improving generalization.

Beyond augmentation, synthetic data can allow development of models where no real data are available at all. Research on completely synthetic patients (with no corresponding real-world counterpart) can be used to pre-train models or prototype algorithms. Since synthetic data preserve the statistical structure of real data (Jävergård et al., 2024), AI models trained on synthetics often perform well when later fine-tuned on real data. In essence, synthetic data expansion boosts data quantity (and sometimes quality) for model building.

5.2 Privacy-Preserving Data Sharing

Synthetic datasets enable broader data sharing without compromising patient privacy. Institutions that cannot share raw EHRs or images can instead release high-quality synthetic versions. For example, a hospital could generate a synthetic cohort matching its patient demographics and disease incidence and make that publicly available for research. This was the intent behind projects like N3C's synthetic COVID data or the UK CRPD synthetic sets. As suggested by Giuffrè and Shung (2023), synthetic data can be safely shared among healthcare providers, academics, and private stakeholders without leaking sensitive or personally identifiable information.

Practically, many organizations are using synthetic data in this way. For instance, the SMART on FHIR sandbox provides synthetic clinical records for app developers, and synthetic Medicare claims have been used in policy research. Because the synthetic data mimic real data formats, analysts can develop queries and algorithms as if working with actual patient data, but with zero risk of re-identifying individuals. In summary, synthetic health data serve as a privacy-preserving stand-in for real patient data, facilitating research collaboration, public releases, and data accessibility.

5.3 Pre-release Testing of Medical Software

Synthetic data are invaluable for developing and validating healthcare software. In regulatory settings or software development, one often needs large test datasets before real-world deployment. For example, a new medical imaging algorithm can be validated on synthetic scans of tumors before a clinical trial. Likewise, health IT applications (EHR software, data exchange platforms, decision support tools) use synthetic patient records to test functionality. As the federal Health IT and other bodies have recognized, synthetic data provide realistic test data for intended test cases at much lower cost. The SMART sandbox (SMART Health IT, 2017) mentioned above is an example: it contains synthetic patient records for developers to test FHIR-compatible apps.

Synthetic data also support *in silico* clinical trials and device testing. For instance, synthetic cohorts can be used in computer simulations to evaluate a drug's effect or a device's performance under a wide range of conditions. The narrative review notes that synthetic data have been used for testing the safety and/or efficacy of new drugs and new medical devices through simulated trials. In essence, before deploying to real patients, developers can stress-test algorithms on comprehensive synthetic datasets that reflect potential clinical scenarios.

5.4 Creating Challenge Benchmarks

Academic and industry challenges often require public data. When real clinical datasets are proprietary or sensitive, organizers may release synthetic data as stand-ins. Synthetic benchmarks allow the community to compare methods on equal footing. For example, a challenge to predict ICU outcomes might provide participants with a synthetic EHR dataset mirroring a real ICU population. Using synthetic data avoids privacy hurdles and allows unlimited sharing of challenge data. Furthermore, synthetic benchmarks can be designed to include a known ground truth structure or rare events, enabling objective evaluation. While references specifically citing such contests are scarce, this is a natural extension of data sharing: synthetic releases can seed competitions in medical AI.

5.5 Facilitating Simulation Studies

Synthetic patient data are also used for simulations in public health and policy research. Simulation studies often require large synthetic populations with realistic health trajectories. For instance, public health researchers studying disease progression might generate a cohort of synthetic patients with diabetes, including longitudinal lab trends, to model outcomes. The narrative review Gonzales et al. (2023) highlights that synthetic Medicare claims data have been used to simulate healthcare financing strategies. Synthetic populations can also test epidemiological models under hypothetical scenarios (e.g. pandemic spread models with synthetic infection histories). In short, any study that benefits from what-if analysis on patient cohorts can leverage synthetic data for cost-effective and rapid simulation.

5.6 Mitigating Real-World Biases

Finally, synthetic data can mitigate biases present in original datasets. Real-world health data often under-represent minorities or certain conditions. By generating targeted synthetic examples, one can rebalance the dataset. For example, if Black patients are underrepresented in a heart failure dataset, synthetic records of Black patients with heart failure can be added to the training set. As Draghi *et al.* (2024) observed, synthetic health data have been used to address such bias, noting scenarios like Black patients were less likely to be admitted to cardiology in original data. By amplifying minority profiles synthetically, models become fairer and less skewed towards majority groups. Care must be taken to represent realistic outcomes for those groups, but synthetic augmentation is a powerful tool against data bias.

In summary, synthetic health data serve many practical functions: they enlarge datasets for AI training, enable sharing and collaboration under privacy constraints, support software and policy testing, and provide benchmarks. These use cases are already being realized in healthcare research and industry.

6. CONCLUSION

6.1 Summary of the Paper

This paper surveyed generative AI methods for creating synthetic health data, covering both technical frameworks and applications. We reviewed four classes of generative models – GANs, VAEs, diffusion models, and transformer LLMs – explaining how each works and its strengths and weaknesses for healthcare data. GANs and VAEs are versatile for images and tables, diffusion models offer high diversity in image synthesis, and transformers excel at generating clinical text and sequential data. We then examined how these models apply to different modalities: structured EHR and time-series, free-text notes, and medical imaging. For each modality, we discussed representative approaches (GAN-based, hybrid, transformer-based) and current research trends.

The paper also identified key challenges in synthetic health data generation. Ensuring clinical validity means that synthetic samples must obey medical logic; techniques such as incorporating domain knowledge or hybrid architectures can help. Maintaining diversity requires combating mode collapse and balancing fidelity with coverage; diffusion models and advanced GAN variants can improve mode coverage. Protecting privacy is essential: generative models must not leak real patient information. Strategies like differential privacy and rigorous re-identification testing are being integrated into model training.

We also highlighted concrete use cases: synthetic data help overcome data scarcity for AI development, enable privacy-preserving data sharing, support software testing (e.g. the SMART FHIR sandbox), provide benchmarks for challenges, and facilitate simulation studies in public health. All these applications underscore the practical value of synthetic health data across the healthcare ecosystem. The summary is depicted in figure 4.

Figure 4. Synthetic data in healthcare: A snapshot

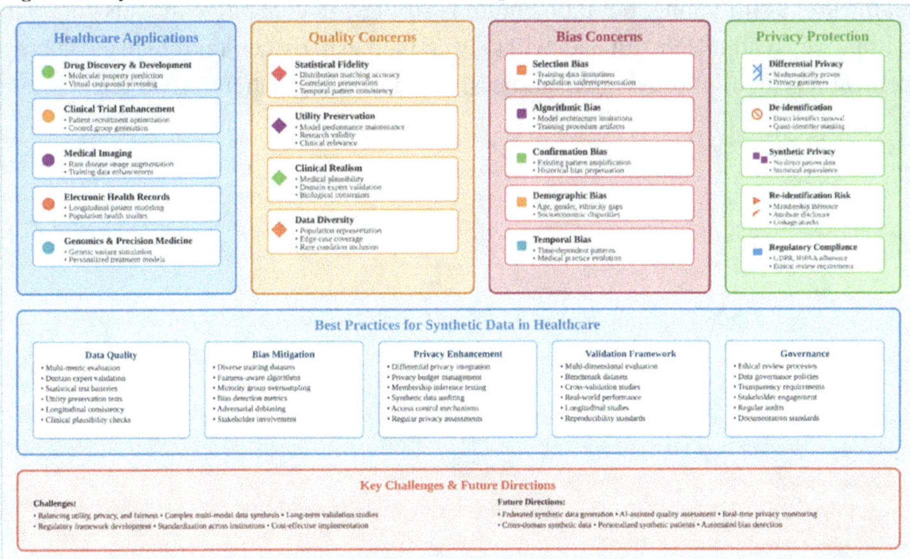

6.2 Future Directions for Research and Practice

Looking forward, the field is rapidly evolving. One clear direction is multi-modal generation: combining imaging, text, and EHR data in one synthetic patient profile. Early work on multi-modal generative models (e.g. GANs that take both image and tabular inputs) suggests that coherent integration of modalities can yield richer synthetic data. Developing such models could enable fully synthetic patient records that include chart notes, lab values, and scans simultaneously.

Improving evaluation metrics is another priority. As the reviews note, existing metrics often fail to capture medical nuance. Research must create healthcare-specific quality measures (e.g. event plausibility scores, multi-attribute distribution tests) and standard benchmarks for synthetic data. Better benchmarks would aid in comparing generative methods and ensuring reproducibility.

In model development, combining generative frameworks with domain expertise will be important. For example, integrating clinical ontologies, treatment guidelines, or physiological models into the learning process could yield data that are both statistically realistic and medically sound. On the practical side, further work on privacy-preserving training (e.g. DP-LM techniques) and post-generation auditing will help bring synthetic data into regulatory compliance.

Finally, real-world adoption will require guidelines and best practices. Initiatives such as the Health Level Seven (HL7) or the FDA might in future provide standards for synthetic data quality, privacy, and usage. The shift toward generative AI in healthcare is still young, but momentum is strong. As generative models continue to improve, synthetic health data will play an increasingly central role in advancing medical research, improving AI fairness, and protecting patient privacy.

REFERENCES

Ahmed, H. S. (2024). Uncover this tech term: Generative adversarial networks. *Korean Journal of Radiology, 25*(5), 493. DOI: 10.3348/kjr.2023.1306 PMID: 38627875

Akpinar, M. H., Sengur, A., Salvi, M., Seoni, S., Faust, O., Mir, H., Molinari, F., & Acharya, U. R. (2024). Synthetic data generation via generative adversarial networks in healthcare: A systematic review of image- and signal-based studies. *IEEE Open Journal of Engineering in Medicine and Biology, 6*, 183–192. DOI: 10.1109/OJEMB.2024.3508472 PMID: 39698120

Ashrafi, N., Schmitt, V., Spang, R. P., Möller, S., & Voigt-Antons, J. N. (2023, June). Protect and extend-using GANs for synthetic data generation of time-series medical records. In *2023 15th International Conference on Quality of Multimedia Experience (QoMEX)* (pp. 171-176). IEEE. DOI: 10.1109/QoMEX58391.2023.10178496

Ashrafi, N., Schmitt, V., Spang, R. P., Möller, S., & Voigt-Antons, J. N. (2023, June). Protect and extend-using GANs for synthetic data generation of time-series medical records. In *2023 15th International Conference on Quality of Multimedia Experience (QoMEX)* (pp. 171-176). IEEE. DOI: 10.1109/QoMEX58391.2023.10178496

Bassani, T., Cina, A., Galbusera, F., Cazzato, A., Pellegrino, M. E., Albano, D., & Sconfienza, L. M. (2025). Feasibility of generating sagittal radiographs from coronal views using GAN-based deep learning framework in adolescent idiopathic scoliosis. *European Radiology Experimental, 9*(1), 11. DOI: 10.1186/s41747-025-00553-6 PMID: 39881022

Draghi, B., Wang, Z., Myles, P., & Tucker, A. (2024). Identifying and handling data bias within primary healthcare data using synthetic data generators. *Heliyon, 10*(2), e24178. DOI: 10.1016/j.heliyon.2024.e24164 PMID: 38288010

Foomani, F. H., Anisuzzaman, D. M., Niezgoda, J., Niezgoda, J., Guns, W., Gopalakrishnan, S., & Yu, Z. (2022). Synthesizing time-series wound prognosis factors from electronic medical records using generative adversarial networks. *Journal of Biomedical Informatics, 125*, 103972. DOI: 10.1016/j.jbi.2021.103972 PMID: 34920125

Giuffrè, M., & Shung, D. L. (2023). Harnessing the power of synthetic data in healthcare: Innovation, application, and privacy. *npj. Digital Medicine, 6*(1), 186. DOI: 10.1038/s41746-023-00927-3 PMID: 37813960

Goncalves, A., Ray, P., Soper, B., Stevens, J., Coyle, L., & Sales, A. P. (2020). Generation and evaluation of synthetic patient data. *BMC Medical Research Methodology, 20*(1), 108. DOI: 10.1186/s12874-020-00977-1 PMID: 32381039

Gonzales, A., Guruswamy, G., & Smith, S. R. (2023). Synthetic data in health care: A narrative review. *PLOS Digital Health*, *2*(1), e0000082. DOI: 10.1371/journal.pdig.0000082 PMID: 36812604

Goodfellow, I., Pouget-Abadie, J., Mirza, M., Xu, B., Warde-Farley, D., Ozair, S., Courville, A., & Bengio, Y. (2014). Generative adversarial nets. In *Advances in Neural Information Processing Systems* (Vol. 27, pp. 2672-2680).

Ibrahim, M., Al Khalil, Y., Amirrajab, S., Sun, C., Breeuwer, M., Pluim, J., & Dumontier, M. (2025). Generative AI for synthetic data across multiple medical modalities: A systematic review of recent developments and challenges. *Computers in Biology and Medicine*, *189*, 109834. DOI: 10.1016/j.compbiomed.2025.109834 PMID: 40023073

Ince, V., Bader-El-Den, M., & Sari, O. F. (2024, August). Enhanced dataset synthesis using CTGAN for metagenomic dataset. In *2024 IEEE 12th International Conference on Intelligent Systems (IS)* (pp. 1-6). IEEE. DOI: 10.1109/IS61756.2024.10705275

Jävergård, N., Lyons, R., Muntean, A., & Forsman, J. (2024). Preserving correlations: A statistical method for generating synthetic data. *arXiv preprint arXiv:2403.01471*. https://doi.org//arXiv.2403.01471DOI: 10.48550

Kreis, K., Gao, R., & Vahdat, A. (2022, June). Denoising diffusion-based generative modeling: Foundations and applications. In *Proceedings of the IEEE/CVF Conference on Computer Vision and Pattern Recognition (CVPR)* (Tutorial).

Liu, Z. G., Ji, T. Y., Chen, J. W., Zhang, L. J., Zhang, L. L., & Wu, Q. H. (2024). Conditional-TimeGAN for realistic and high-quality appliance trajectories generation and data augmentation in nonintrusive load monitoring. *IEEE Transactions on Instrumentation and Measurement*, *73*, 1–15. DOI: 10.1109/TIM.2024.3381263

Loni, M., Poursalim, F., Asadi, M., & Gharehbaghi, A. (2025). A review on generative AI models for synthetic medical text, time series, and longitudinal data. *npj. Digital Medicine*, *8*(1), 281. DOI: 10.1038/s41746-024-01373-1 PMID: 40374917

Mami, C. A., Coser, A., Medvet, E., Boudewijn, A. T., Volpe, M., Whitworth, M., Crook, D. W., Walker, A. S., Peto, T. E. A., & Saccani, S. (2022). Generating realistic synthetic relational data through graph variational autoencoders. *arXiv preprint arXiv:2211.16889*. https://doi.org//arXiv.2211.16889DOI: 10.48550

Miletic, M., & Sariyar, M. (2024). Large language models for synthetic tabular health data: A benchmark study. In Ugon, A., Karlsson, D., Klein, G. H., & Moen, A. (Eds.), *Digital Health and Informatics Innovations for Sustainable Health Care Systems* (pp. 963–967). IOS Press., DOI: 10.3233/SHTI240571

Miletic, M., & Sariyar, M. (2025). Synthetic data generation methods for longitudinal and time series health data. In *Global Healthcare Transformation in the Era of Artificial Intelligence and Informatics* (pp. 367–371). IOS Press. DOI: 10.3233/SHTI250740

Nahid, M. M. H., & Hasan, S. B. (2024). SafeSynthDP: Leveraging large language models for privacy-preserving synthetic data generation using differential privacy. *arXiv preprint arXiv:2412.20641*. https://doi.org//arXiv.2412.20641DOI: 10.48550

Nikolentzos, G., Vazirgiannis, M., Xypolopoulos, C., Sarrah, H., & Chatzianastasis, M. (2023). Synthetic electronic health records generated with variational graph autoencoders. *npj. Digital Medicine*, *6*(1), 83. DOI: 10.1038/s41746-023-00822-x PMID: 37120594

SMART Health IT. (2017). *SMART on FHIR sandbox*. https://docs.smarthealthit.org/

Teli, A. (2025). Uncover this tech term: Variational autoencoders. *Korean Journal of Radiology*, *26*(6), 616. DOI: 10.3348/kjr.2025.0073 PMID: 40341889

Xiao, X., Zhang, Y., Chen, H., Ren, W., Zhang, J., & Xu, J. (2025). A differential privacy-based mechanism for preventing data leakage in large language model training. *Academic Journal of Sociology and Management*, *3*(2), 33–42. DOI: 10.70393/616a736d.323732

Yan, C., Zhang, Z., Nyemba, S., & Li, Z. (2024). Generating synthetic electronic health record data using generative adversarial networks: Tutorial. *JMIR AI*, *3*, e52615. DOI: 10.2196/52615 PMID: 38875595

Chapter 7
AI in Modern Health Services: Synthetic Data Approach

Bobur Raximov
Mamun University, Uzbekistan

Hamza Iftikhar
National University of Science and Technology, Pakistan

Abdullaeva Dilbar Ubaydullaevna
National Pedagogical University of Uzbekistan, Uzbekistan

Munir Ahmad
https://orcid.org/0000-0003-4836-6151
Survey of Pakistan, Pakistan

Babaqul Khudayqulov
Termez University of Economics and Service, Uzbekistan

ABSTRACT

Synthetic data is rapidly emerging as a transformative enabler of artificial intelligence in healthcare, addressing long-standing challenges of privacy, accessibility, and data scarcity. By generating realistic yet non-identifiable datasets, it supports innovation in clinical research, diagnostics, precision medicine, and public health planning. Emerging trends, including hybrid real-synthetic models, federated learning, and cross-border collaborations, highlight its growing role in building scalable and equitable AI systems. To maximize impact, policymakers must establish clear regulations. Institutions should integrate synthetic data into their digital health

DOI: 10.4018/979-8-3373-5641-9.ch007

strategies, and developers must ensure transparency and fairness. As adoption expands, synthetic data remains a cornerstone of ethical and sustainable AI-driven healthcare services.

INTRODUCTION

Artificial Intelligence (AI) has emerged as one of the most transformative forces in modern healthcare, with the potential to revolutionize the way we diagnose, treat, monitor, and manage our health systems (Garg et al., 2025; Rashid et al., 2025). From predictive analytics that forecast disease progression to intelligent imaging tools that improve diagnostic accuracy, AI-powered applications are gradually becoming a part of clinical workflows. From individualised medicine to macro-scale public health planning, these developments not only promise better patient outcomes but also bring efficiency improvements to healthcare offerings.

At the heart of this transformation is data, the fuel that fuels AI algorithms. Electronic Health Records (EHRs), diagnostic imaging, wearable devices, genomic sequences, and real-time monitoring systems create an enormous amount of medical data (Rani et al., 2025; Shen et al., 2025; Tong et al., 2023). When appropriately applied, these data can enable machine learning models to identify patterns, guide decision making, and provide individualized interventions. However, the performance of AI depends critically on the availability, quality, and representativeness of such data.

Healthcare is a data-rich field, but there are major obstacles to using the data. Patient privacy has always been and will continue to be a top priority, and the strict regulations like HIPAA in the United States (Lutkevich, 2019) and GDPR in Europe (Francesca, 2019; Li et al., 2019) have provided necessary but constraining controls for access and sharing of sensitive information. In addition, there are often problems with the availability of real-world medical datasets due to fragmented health systems and unequal access to digitized health records. Incomplete data: The presence of biases in existing data - such as under-representation of minority groups, rare conditions, or certain geographic areas - further undermines the validity of AI models and may potentially perpetuate health inequalities.

Because of these challenges, researchers and practitioners have considered synthetic data a promising solution. Synthetic data is a term to refers to artificially created datasets that reproduce the statistical properties and structure of real-world data, but do not reveal any real patient information. Generative modeling techniques, such as GANs (Generative Adversarial Networks) (Bengesi et al., 2024) and Variational Autoencoders (VAEs), have been heavily applied to generate highly realistic health datasets. This approach provides a pathway to overcome the silos of privacy, scarcity, and bias, facilitating broader collaboration, accelerating AI development, and ensuring safer and more equitable innovation in today's health services.

In this context, the synthetic data approach is gaining increasing recognition not only as a technical development, but as a strategic enabler of trusted and scalable AI in healthcare. This chapter illustrates the concepts, applications, benefits, challenges, and future directions of synthetic data in present-day health services, with attention to the transformative potential of synthetic data on the way health systems produce knowledge, provide care, and maintain ethical standards.

SYNTHETIC DATA FOR HEALTHCARE: CONCEPTS AND METHODS

Introduction to Synthetic Data

Synthetic data are artificially generated data produced from algorithms to mimic the statistical characteristics, distributions, and structural relationships in real-world data (Dankar & Ibrahim, 2021; Giuffrè & Shung, 2023; Umer & Adnan, 2024). Unlike conventional anonymization or de-identification approaches, which generally involve masking, removal, or encryption of personal identifiers from real patient records, synthetic data is created from the ground up. This implies that, although it maintains the analytical integrity and representativeness of the original data, it is intrinsically privacy-preserving (and does not reveal any real individual information).

For example, an anonymized patient record dataset may retain latent identifiers that, for example, are unusual combinations of age, location, or diagnosis that may be able to be linked back to an individual when combined with external datasets. In contrast, in synthetic data, we generate the data based on mathematical and generative models that reproduce population-level trends without any real patients. For instance, if a synthetic cohort were capable of reflecting the age, sex, comorbidity, and treatment outcome distributions of the diabetes patients at a given hospital, it would include no patient record whatsoever, in a real sense.

This distinction is very important in healthcare, where patient confidentiality is not only a legal requirement (as mandated by regulations like HIPAA in the United States and GDPR in Europe) but also an ethical one. By severing the direct connection between data and actual individuals, synthetic datasets enable the safe sharing of data across institutions, provide collaborative research opportunities, and drive the development of AI models without compromising trust or compliance. In addition, synthetic data can augment underrepresented populations and simulate rare clinical cases, further increasing its utility over traditional anonymization.

Synthetic Health Data Generation Methods

Synthetic healthcare data generation is based on a set of statistical, machine learning, and simulation methods, all of which are suitable for different data types and use cases, and each offering a different benefit. The four leading approaches are:

Generative Adversarial Networks (GANs)

GANs are one of the most commonly applied frameworks for the creation of synthetic data (Biswas et al., 2023; Saxena & Cao, 2021). They are composed of two rival neural networks, a generator that creates synthetic samples, and a discriminator that tries to tell real data from synthetic. With a process of training, the generator homes in on its outputs until it can no longer distinguish them from real data. In the healthcare context, GANs have been used to create synthetic medical images, including MRIs, CT scans, and X-rays, and tabular datasets like electronic health records (EHRs).

GANs are particularly powerful for learning complex high-dimensional distributions of data, but can suffer from issues such as mode collapse, in which the generator only generates a small number of variations, and training instability. Despite these issues, GANs are still a mainstay for synthetic image generation, making it possible for AI models to identify nuanced pathological patterns and rare conditions that can be underrepresented in real datasets.

Variational Autoencoders (VAEs)

VAEs encode and decode the real data into a latent representation of lower dimensionality and perform reconstruction as synthetic outputs (Papadopoulos & Karalis, 2023; Wei et al., 2020). Unlike GANs, VAEs use a more stable non-adversarial training methodology and can be readily used for the generation of tabular or time-series healthcare data such as patient vitals, lab reports, or wearable device readings.

VAEs give researchers the ability to control the variability of synthesized data in a way that's important when generating datasets for a particular subgroup or clinical condition. For instance, VAEs can be used to simulate the variability of heart rate in elderly patients of different medical treatments, which offer AI systems with realistic and varied training scenarios. VAEs are robust against different noises and are relatively interpretable, making them suitable for applications that need synthetic datasets that are structured, robust, and reproducible.

Diffusion Models

Diffusion-based generative models (DGMs) are a recent development in synthetic data generation, especially in high-fidelity image synthesis (Cao et al., 2024; Yang et al., 2024). These models learn the inverse diffusion process, using random noise as input and converting it into structured data, in an iterative process. In healthcare, diffusion models are becoming used for radiology and pathology imaging, where synthetic datasets are generated that contain complex anatomical details and rare presentations of diseases.

Compared to GANs, diffusion models generally result in better mode coverage, that is, they are less likely to miss rare but clinically important cases. This makes them particularly useful in training diagnostic AI systems from small or imbalanced imaging datasets, in such a way that models are exposed to the full range of possible presentations without depending on large volumes of real patient images.

Rule-Based and Simulation Procedures

Apart from deep learning, synthetic data can be created with rule-based or simulation approaches, which are based on predefined statistical rules or domain-specific knowledge. For example, synthetic patient populations are generally developed from simulations of clinical trials using known prevalence of disease, distributions of demographics, and treatment responses.

While less flexible than generative models, rule-based methods are highly interpretable and reproducible, making them amenable to regulatory testing, controlled experiments, and hypothesis testing. For example, it can be useful to simulate age groups of cardiovascular risk profiles or to model synthetic responses to a new drug without access to sensitive patient data.

Characteristics of High Quality Synthetic Data

To be effective in healthcare, synthetic datasets should fulfill three key requirements:

- Synthetic data should be representative of real data in terms of statistical distributions, correlations, and variability. For instance, artificial chest X-rays should be realistic enough to replicate anatomical structures, tissue densities, and pathological patterns that can be used as training data for developing diagnostic AI systems. High realism means that models trained on synthetic data perform as well as models trained on real-world data.

- In addition to visual or structural similarities, synthetic data should maintain analytical value. The synthetic data should be able to create a predictive model that mimics the performance of a model trained on real data (accuracy, sensitivity, specificity). This is important for disease classification, patient risk stratification, resource allocation, and clinical decision support, among other things.
- The most important attribute of synthetic data is that it protects individual privacy. Synthetic data is used to counter this and ensures there is no single-to-single mapping between the synthetic and real patients to allow for residual re-identification risks that might remain with anonymization. These synthetic datasets are essentially safe to share within hospitals, research institutes, and international collaborations, while staying within privacy regulations like HIPAA and GDPR.

Synthetic data is the paradigm shift in healthcare AI, promising to unleash the power of diverse datasets while upholding patient privacy. Through the use of cutting-edge generative models (e.g., GANs, VAEs, diffusion methods, etc.) and more traditional rule-based simulations, synthetic data can closely mimic the richness and variability of the medical data while preserving strong analytical utility and ethical validations. This ability will enable responsible innovation by researchers, clinicians, and AI developers, speed discovery, and improve inter-institutional collaboration to make AI-enabled healthcare solutions safer, more inclusive, and better at delivering. Table 1 shows a summary of synthetic data usage in healthcare, covering methods, properties, advantages, and examples.

Table 1. Synthetic Data for Healthcare

Aspect	Description / Role	Key Advantages	Healthcare Examples / Use Cases
Defining Synthetic Data	Artificially generated data that replicates statistical patterns and structures of real data without exposing real patient records.	Strong privacy protection, eliminates re-identification risks, and allows sharing across institutions.	Simulated patient cohorts for research, synthetic EHRs, and anonymized imaging datasets for AI training.
Distinction from Anonymized/De-identified Data	Unlike anonymization, synthetic data is fully generated and not derived from actual patients.	Avoids latent identifiers, stronger privacy guarantees, and easier compliance with HIPAA/GDPR.	Synthetic cohorts for clinical trial design, privacy-preserving multi-center research collaborations.
Generative Adversarial Networks (GANs)	Two neural networks (generator and discriminator) compete to produce highly realistic data.	Captures complex, high-dimensional distributions; excellent for images; supports realistic variability.	Synthetic MRIs, CT scans, X-rays; synthetic EHRs; rare disease pattern simulation.
Variational Autoencoders (VAEs)	Probabilistic encoding/ decoding to generate structured outputs from a latent space.	Stable training, controllable variability, suitable for tabular and time-series data.	Synthetic vitals from wearables, lab test simulations, and structured patient datasets.
Diffusion Models	Iteratively transform noise into structured data by reversing a diffusion process.	Produces high-fidelity images, better mode coverage than GANs; captures rare cases.	Radiology imaging, pathology slides, training diagnostic AI for rare conditions.
Rule-Based / Simulation Approaches	Generate data using predefined statistical rules or domain-specific models.	Highly interpretable, reproducible, ideal for controlled experiments and regulatory testing.	Clinical trial simulations, synthetic cardiovascular risk profiles, treatment outcome modeling.
Realism (Key Property)	Synthetic data should reflect real-world statistical distributions, correlations, and variability.	Ensures AI models trained on synthetic data generalize well to real-world tasks.	Chest X-rays with realistic anatomical structures, lab test distributions, and disease progression patterns.
Utility (Key Property)	Data must preserve analytical value, allowing AI models to achieve comparable performance to real data.	Supports predictive modeling, risk stratification, and clinical decision support.	Disease classification, patient risk prediction, and resource planning models.
Privacy Preservation (Key Property)	No one-to-one mapping between synthetic and real patients; strong regulatory compliance.	Safe to share across institutions and countries, mitigates ethical and legal concerns.	Multi-institution research collaboration, international AI development, federated learning with synthetic datasets.

APPLICATIONS OF SYNTHETIC DATA IN HEALTH SERVICES

The advent of synthetic data into healthcare is a tipping point that changes how medical research, clinical practice, and health system planning are done. By generating high-quality, privacy-preserving datasets, synthetic data can help researchers and practitioners overcome limitations related to real-world medical records and facilitate the safe and ethical development of AI-driven innovations. Its uses are extensive in clinical research, imaging, decision support, telemedicine, and population health fields.

Clinical Trials and Research

Clinical research and trials are basic to medical innovation, and they suffer from age-old problems such as difficulty in capturing patients, incomplete data, high cost, and ethical apprehensions with exposing actual patient data (Azizi et al., 2021). Generalizability of results is limited by the fact that many studies do not include enough subjects who represent different demographics, comorbidities, and disease severities. Synthetic data is a powerful tool to simulate patient populations that reflect real-world variability (e.g., age distributions, genetics, disease prevalence, treatment responses, etc.).

For instance, synthetic cohorts could be generated to test drug efficacy, safety profiles, or the progression of a disease without having to commit to costly and time-consuming clinical trials (Ayilara et al., 2023; Pasculli et al., 2025). Synthetic data enables scenario modeling (e.g., rare adverse events or interventions of interest for underrepresented sub-populations), which would otherwise be impossible due to a small sample size. By increasing the diversity of the population, synthetic data can enhance the inclusivity and generalizability of trial results.

Beyond the design of a trial, synthetic data can speed the research cycle by allowing for iterative testing and hypothesis refinement. Researchers can test different approaches to recruitment, modify inclusion criteria, and identify potential confounding factors in silico before recruiting any real participants. This possibility is becoming recognized by regulatory agencies, though some are tentatively considering a set of guidelines to allow the inclusion of synthetic data in clinical trial submissions-they say this should be considered especially for early-stage or rare disease trials. This growing realisation highlights the transformative impact of synthetic data in accelerating clinical research, making it safer and more equitable, while minimising the logistical burdens and ethical risks that often derive from using patient records.

Medical Imaging

Synthetic data is one of the most mature applications in medical imaging. In order to train AI systems to do complicated tasks, such as the detection of tumors in CT scans, fractures in X-rays, or pneumonia in chest radiographs, high-quality imaging datasets are needed. However, obtaining, annotating, and sharing large amounts of imaging data is expensive, time-consuming, and limited by patient privacy issues. In many cases, clinical repositories under-represent rare diseases, and hence the model AI cannot reliably identify rare pathologies (Paproki et al., 2024; Thambawita et al., 2022).

Synthetic imaging data - generated with techniques such as GANs, VAEs, and diffusion models - enables the creation of extensive libraries of realistic medical images. These datasets can be specifically curated to incorporate rare diseases, subtle anatomical variations, or complex co-occurring conditions that would otherwise be missed by the AI model. In addition to model training, synthetic images are useful for algorithm testing, allowing you to create controlled testing situations in which AI performance can be rigorously tested before deployment into clinical practice.

Furthermore, synthetic imaging datasets promote multi-institution collaboration, because investigators can share large, annotated image repositories without concern for patient privacy. For example, tumor detection algorithms can be trained jointly by international research groups, or imaging-based diagnostic challenges simulated for AI competition platforms. By delivering scalable, privacy-preserving, and versatile imaging data, synthetic techniques improve diagnostic accuracy, mitigate bias, and expedite the deployment of AI tools in radiology and pathology.

Electronic Health Records (EHRs)

EHRs are a wealth of information about patients, including demographics, medical histories, lab results, prescriptions, treatment plans, and outcomes. However, access to EHRs is extremely limited by privacy regulations and the risk of re-identification, limiting their utility for research, AI training, and cross-institutional collaboration. Synthetic EHRs provide a privacy-preserving alternative by mimicking the structure of real-world records with the same statistical distributions and correlations without disclosing actual patient data (Bietsch et al., 2023; Yoon et al., 2023).

Synthetic records are increasingly being used as a platform for testing and developing predictive analytics and decision support applications. For instance, synthetic EHR data can be employed to train risk stratification models for chronic disease management, forecast hospital readmissions, or build AI-aided triage systems in emergency care. By creating a more accessible foundation of representative data, synthetic EHRs enable hospitals, universities, and technology companies to collaborate to expedite innovation while adhering to ethical and legal requirements.

In addition, synthetic EHRs allow institutions to test new algorithms in a setting that mimics real-world complexity, where there are variable comorbidity profiles, missing data, and heterogeneities in treatment patterns. We're able to trial interventions, fine-tune workflow, and predict patient outcomes for diverse cohorts, with less reliance on sensitive real-world datasets. Ultimately, synthetic EHRs strike a balance between data access and privacy, enabling healthcare providers and developers to unlock the full potential of AI while still safeguarding the trust of patients.

Telemedicine

The advent of telemedicine and wearable health devices has created ongoing streams of sensitive data, such as heart rate monitoring, glucose levels, sleep patterns, and video consultation records. While this wealth of information can significantly improve patient care, its heterogeneity and high sensitivity complicate information sharing for AI testing or algorithm development, or system validation. An alternative is to use synthetic datasets that can simulate telehealth encounters and remote monitoring artifacts without revealing patient-identifiable data (Apellaniz et al., 2025; Cascella et al., 2023).

For example, AI-based diagnostic chatbots can be trained and validated with synthetic conversations, including a wide range of patterns, descriptions of symptoms, and patient questions. Similarly, data recorded from wearable sensors can be synthetically generated to represent a wide range of activity levels, physiological responses, and health conditions. This work enables remote monitoring algorithms to be stress-tested with different scenarios, providing robustness, accuracy, and adaptability to different populations.

Synthetic data is also able to assist infrastructure testing and emergency preparedness. In addition, hospitals and telehealth platforms can create simulated high-demand scenarios, such as unexpected increases in patient consultations during pandemics, and test system performance without affecting real patient data. Through a combination of privacy preservation and realistic variability, synthetic datasets empower telemedicine providers to build, validate, and deploy AI solutions that are both scalable and ethically sound, increasing confidence and trust in remote healthcare.

Public Health Modeling

Synthetic data plays a key role in public health planning and policy modelling, especially when real-time data is incomplete, slow, or inconsistent across regions (Gonzales et al., 2023; Murtaza et al., 2023). In the context of pandemics and outbreaks or health emergencies on a larger scale, decision-makers often experience gaps in reporting, delayed laboratory confirmation, and disparate quality of data that can prevent effective interventions. Synthetic datasets enable modeling disease dynamics, testing interventions, and predicting resource allocation in a safe and controlled environment.

For instance, in the COVID-19 pandemic, synthetic data was used to simulate infection curves, hospital bed occupancy, ICU demand, and vaccination strategies to provide actionable insights even when real-world data were scarce or inconsistent. In addition to infectious disease modeling, synthetic data can power long-term simulations of chronic disease burden, the planning of the healthcare workforce, and the effects of demographic change on service demand. These datasets can be used to enable policymakers to run 'what-if' scenarios, predict the impact of possible health interventions, and prioritize resources while respecting patient privacy.

Further, the use of synthetic data enables international collaboration and comparative research, as countries can exchange modeled data without breaching local privacy laws. This allows the public health trends, epidemic responses, and population-level interventions to be analysed globally. By providing safe, scalable, and shareable datasets, synthetic data reinforces evidence-based policymaking, increases preparedness for future health crises, and enables cross-border data-driven public health response. Table 2 provides a summary of the applications of synthetic data in healthcare, including detailed descriptions, benefits, and examples for each subdomain.

Table 2. Applications of Synthetic Data for Healthcare

Application Area	Description / Role of Synthetic Data	Benefits / Advantages	Examples / Use Cases
Clinical Research and Trials	Simulates patient populations with realistic variability in demographics, disease prevalence, and treatment responses.	Accelerates research cycle, enables hypothesis testing, improves trial inclusivity, and reduces reliance on real patient data.	Modeling synthetic cohorts to test drug safety, simulate rare disease progression, augment underrepresented groups, and perform early-phase trial simulations.
Medical Imaging	Generates realistic imaging datasets (X-rays, MRIs, CT scans) using GANs, VAEs, or diffusion models.	Provides large, annotated datasets for AI training, includes rare or subtle pathologies, supports algorithm validation while protecting privacy.	Tumor detection in CT scans, pneumonia diagnosis from X-rays, rare condition imaging, and multi-institution AI competitions.
Electronic Health Records (EHRs)	Produces privacy-preserving synthetic patient records with realistic statistical distributions and correlations.	Enables predictive model development, facilitates cross-institutional collaboration, preserves regulatory compliance, and allows testing of complex analytics tools.	Risk stratification for chronic diseases, decision support for emergency care, development of hospital-wide predictive models, and multi-center research.
Telemedicine and Remote Monitoring	Simulates remote health interactions, wearable sensor data, and patient-provider communication.	Allows AI system testing, stress-testing of telehealth platforms, and ensures robustness and adaptability to diverse populations.	Training AI chatbots, validating monitoring algorithms, simulating sensor data for heart rate or glucose monitoring, and emergency scenario testing.
Public Health Modeling	Generates population-level datasets for disease spread simulation, resource planning, and policy evaluation.	Supports timely, evidence-based decisions, fills gaps in incomplete or delayed real-world data, and facilitates international collaboration.	COVID-19 pandemic simulations, hospital bed and ICU demand forecasting, vaccination strategy modeling, chronic disease burden projections, and workforce planning.

BENEFITS AND ADVANTAGES OF THE SYNTHETIC DATA APPROACH

In healthcare, the synthetic data are used for several benefits that go beyond technical efficiency: It offers a basis for developing trusted, scalable, and equitable AI systems, while at the same time tackling some of health data management's most intractable obstacles. Four key advantages are highlighted: privacy, access, collaboration, and equity.

Maintaining Patient Privacy and Regulatory Compliance

Patient confidentiality is one of the greatest issues in the ongoing digitalization of healthcare. With the rise of electronic health records, telemedicine platforms, wearable devices, and AI-based diagnostic tools, a massive amount of sensitive personal health information is constantly being generated and processed (Giuffrè & Shung, 2023; Mendes et al., 2025). Laws like the Health Insurance Portability and Accountability Act (HIPAA) in the United States and the General Data Protection Regulation (GDPR) in Europe have strict guidelines for how patient data is collected, stored, and shared. These frameworks are built to safeguard patient privacy while enabling responsible use of medical data. However, even anonymized or de-identified datasets are subject to re-identification risks when combined with external data sources, such as publicly available databases, social media, or genomic data. Such threats of re-identification are a major ethical and legal risk and may deter institutions from releasing data for research or AI development.

Synthetic data overcomes these challenges by generating entirely new datasets that are representative of the statistical properties of real patient populations, but without duplicating individual records. Unlike simple anonymization that may leave residual identifiers, synthetic data ensures that the underlying correlations, distributions, and relationships are preserved and that individual identities are protected. For instance, a synthetic patient cohort can replicate the distribution of hypertension, diabetes, and cardiovascular risk factors of a hospital population, without disclosing any real patient data. This approach greatly minimizes the privacy risks and enhances adherence to legal frameworks, empowering researchers and AI developers to safely utilize high-quality datasets. In addition, synthetic data improves privacy-preserving data sharing, which in turn builds trust between patients, clinicians, and regulators, enabling the wider use of AI technologies in healthcare without undermining patient confidence.

Overcoming Scarcity and Imbalance of Real-World Medical Data

A serious bottleneck in developing AI for healthcare is the lack of good-quality datasets, particularly for rare diseases, minority populations, or uncommon clinical settings. Many machine learning models need thousands or millions of samples to give strong performance, but more and more often this is not so because real-world medical notes aren't sufficiently permissive, for example, because of the rarity of diseases or the lack of representation of certain demographic groups. For instance, predictive models for pediatric diseases will likely perform poorly if the training data are collected almost exclusively from adult populations, or diagnostic AI for rare genetic disorders will not have enough case examples to learn meaningful patterns.

Synthetic data is a powerful answer because it allows the creation of large, varied, statistically representative datasets. Using model-based methods like generative adversarial networks (GANs) or variational autoencoders (VAEs), synthetic datasets can be generated to simulate rare disease cases, augment underrepresented demographic groups, and even out otherwise biased data distributions. For example, synthetic EHRs can be used to simulate cohorts of patients with rare autoimmune conditions or complex comorbidities, which will give AI models enough training examples to learn nuanced patterns of symptoms or clinical data. Apart from enhancing model performance, this feature improves research productivity as investigators can experiment with hypotheses, validate algorithms, and experiment with treatment strategies in silico prior to conducting expensive or lengthy clinical studies. Synthetic data can help address both scarcity and imbalance, ensuring that AI applications in healthcare are robust, inclusive, and generalizable across different patient populations.

Facilitating Cross-Institutional Collaboration

Healthcare data is inherently fragmented, existing in hospitals, clinics, research laboratories, public health databases, and national health systems. These silos, together with strict legal, ethical, and institutional constraints, frequently make cross-institutional data sharing difficult. The lack of access to extensive datasets often impedes or delays the development of AI models that can be generalized across populations or the conduct of collaborative research and multi-center clinical studies.

Synthetic data is a safe and efficient alternative. By creating realistic but non-identifiable data sets, institutions can release important information without revealing real patient data. This ensures that researchers, clinicians, policymakers, and AI developers can work together more transparently, compare results across regions, and come up with models that are useful to a wide variety of people. For instance, hospitals across countries could co-train AI models for early detection of cancer on synthetic datasets that match the demographics of their local populations in a privacy-compliant way. In addition, synthetic data allows international collaborations, resulting in a situation where research is conducted in countries with different regulatory requirements. By allowing organizations to break down data silos whilst preserving confidentiality, synthetic data helps to create a more connected, collaborative, and innovation-friendly healthcare ecosystem, and put us on the path to accelerating medical research and AI-driven patient care.

Enhancing Fairness and Reducing Bias in AI Models

Bias in AI models has become a well-identified issue in healthcare with potentially serious implications for patient safety and equity. While models trained on incomplete data, skewed data, or imbalanced data may perform poorly for some populations, these models can further exacerbate current health disparities. For example, diagnostic algorithms trained mostly on one ethnic group's data may not perform well when tested on other racial or socioeconomic groups, resulting in misdiagnoses or disparities in access to care. Similarly, predicated chronic illness risk models may not be able to predict risk for underrepresented age groups or in regions where their data are not well represented.

Synthetic data offers a mechanism to reduce the impact of these biases by synthetically increasing the representation of underrepresented populations, rare diseases, and uncommon clinical scenarios in training data. Through careful design, synthetic datasets can help add heterogeneity that reflects real-life heterogeneity, ensuring exposure of AI models to a broader range of patient cases. For instance, synthetic data may complement minority population samples in studies of cardiovascular disease or rare genetic mutations in oncology datasets to enable AI models to learn patterns that would otherwise be underrepresented. By taking a proactive stance on imbalance, synthetic data boosts algorithmic fairness, eliminates systemic bias, and supports better clinical outcomes across patient populations. Moreover, this approach is consistent with ethical principles of healthcare equity, encouraging the creation of AI solutions that are inclusive, principled, and able to benefit all patients, not just a subset of the population. Table 3 provides details on benefits along with examples, implications, and mitigation strategies.

Table 3. Benefits of Synthetic Data for Healthcare

Benefit / Advantage	Description	Implications for Healthcare AI	Examples / Applications	Mitigation / Best Practices
Preserving Patient Privacy and Regulatory Compliance	Synthetic data protects individual identities while maintaining the statistical properties of patient populations, enabling compliance with HIPAA, GDPR, and other privacy regulations.	Reduces risk of re-identification, protects patient trust, and allows safe sharing of health data across institutions and platforms.	Generating synthetic EHRs for multi-center research, anonymized imaging datasets for AI diagnostics, or wearable health data for remote monitoring.	Validate synthetic data against privacy standards, use strong generative models, audit for potential re-identification risks, and ensure transparency in data generation.
Overcoming Scarcity and Imbalance of Real-World Data	Allows generation of large, diverse, and balanced datasets where real-world cases are limited, rare, or underrepresented.	Improves model performance, robustness, and generalizability, particularly for rare diseases or minority populations.	Synthetic cohorts for rare pediatric diseases, expanding underrepresented ethnic groups in cardiovascular studies, or simulating rare drug reactions.	Use hybrid models combining synthetic and real data, carefully monitor statistical fidelity, and perform bias checks to avoid introducing artificial distortions.
Enabling Cross-Institutional Collaboration Without Raw Data Sharing	Facilitates sharing of synthetic datasets that retain statistical richness without exposing real patient data.	Promotes collaborative research, multi-center AI model development, and international studies while respecting privacy laws.	Hospitals in different countries are collaboratively training AI for early cancer detection, federated learning with synthetic data, or cross-regional public health simulations.	Maintain metadata describing synthetic dataset characteristics, enforce secure transfer protocols, and document validation methods to ensure trustworthiness.
Enhancing Fairness and Reducing Bias	Introduces diversity into datasets, expanding underrepresented populations and rare conditions to mitigate model bias.	Increases equity of AI predictions across different demographic, genetic, and socioeconomic groups; reduces systemic health disparities.	Augmenting minority population samples in predictive models for diabetes, simulating rare genetic variants in oncology datasets, and balancing age groups in pediatric AI tools.	Implement fairness metrics during model evaluation, continuously monitor model performance across subgroups, and ensure synthetic augmentation reflects clinical realities.

continued on following page

Table 3. Continued

Benefit / Advantage	Description	Implications for Healthcare AI	Examples / Applications	Mitigation / Best Practices
Accelerating Innovation and Model Development	Synthetic data enables faster experimentation, model training, and validation without the legal and logistical delays of accessing real-world patient data.	Speeds up AI development, testing, and deployment, particularly in rapidly evolving areas like pandemic response or emerging therapies.	Pandemic simulations for resource allocation, virtual clinical trial simulations, and AI-based diagnostic tool development using synthetic imaging datasets.	Combine synthetic datasets with real-world validation, maintain documentation of generation and assumptions, and establish iterative testing pipelines for model refinement.
Supporting International and Cross-Jurisdictional Research	Synthetic data circumvents legal and privacy barriers across borders, enabling global collaboration.	Broadens the scope of research, allows diverse population inclusion, and improves the generalizability of AI models across regions.	Multi-country epidemiological studies, AI-driven global health policy simulations,	Ensure adherence to local and international privacy regulations, harmonize validation protocols, and maintain traceable audit logs of data use.

CHALLENGES, LIMITATIONS, AND ETHICS

While there is great promise in the use of synthetic data in healthcare, there are some serious challenges. As with any new technology, there are technical, regulatory, and ethical challenges associated with its use, which need to be carefully considered to ensure responsible implementation. These challenges may be categorized broadly as those of representation, validation, regulation, ethics, and security.

Representing Real-World Complexities

A key risk with synthetic data is that it may not reflect the complex variability of real-world health conditions. Indeed, unlike traditional datasets, which naturally embed rare anomalies and subtle correlations that are present in patient populations, synthetic datasets are created by generative models that are trained on existing data (Houston & Cosma, 2023; Poucin et al., 2021). While such models are highly effective at replicating common patterns, they may not be able to capture rare disease states, unexpected drug interactions, or outliers that are critical to clinical decision-making. Such edge cases are everywhere in health care, whether it's that rare autoimmune disease, the uncommon presentation of a common disease, or that treatment side effect that only happens in a small fraction of patients. If these signals are left out of synthetic data, AI systems trained on them will show high performance in controlled tests, but don't hold up when they are subjected to the uncontrolled conditions of clinical practice.

For example, a synthetic dataset may correctly simulate conditions such as diabetes or hypertension and may produce enough data for predictive modeling for the general population's health. However, it may underestimate the occurrence of diabetes together with rare genetic disorders or the special effect of multi-drug resistance in infectious diseases. This leaves AI training, therefore, incomplete, and models can generalize poorly when faced with the full variety of patient presentations. This limitation underlines the risk of depending only on synthetic data, without further validation with real-world data.

In addition, health care systems exist in a variety of demographic, socioeconomic, and geographic settings. Generative models run the risk of encoding biases present in their training data, resulting in synthetic data that is underrepresented in marginalized groups or over-represented in trends that result from more data-rich populations. Not only does this put at risk the equity of AI applications, but it also creates clinical blind spots where underserved patient communities may be less accurately identified or less effectively treated by AI-driven interventions. Building models to mitigate these risks necessitates thoughtful design and ongoing validation, as well as hybrid solutions that use a mix of synthetic and real data inputs.

Quality Assurance and Validation Challenges

Another major issue in implementing synthetic data in healthcare is to guarantee its quality, accuracy, and reliability. Unlike real-world data, for which there might be a direct reference to a clinical record or medical evidence, synthetic data does not have a clear benchmark for authenticity. As a result, institutions need new, specialized frameworks and metrics to assess whether the data "looks" statistically correct, but also maintains the nuanced relationships between clinical variables. Without such rigor, synthetic datasets may unknowingly bias relevant associations, such as the relationship between patient age and treatment efficacy or the association between comorbidity and disease progression.

Consider, for instance, a synthetic electronic health record (EHR) dataset. It can be loaded with age, gender, and diagnosis codes that match actual hospital data to create the illusion of high quality. However, on further inspection, it may become apparent that relationships among conditions (for example, the interaction of diabetes with chronic kidney disease or the interaction of age with surgical risk) are not well preserved. Such distortions can be misleading for predictive models, leading to outputs that seem correct during initial testing but are wrong in production.

This calls into question the utility of synthetic data and may jeopardize the clinical outcomes if these diagnostic or therapeutic decisions are used to inform decisions.

The more general problem is that we have no standard way of validating things. While a number of techniques have been suggested, including statistical similarity tests, machine learning performance benchmarks, and expert-driven clinical evaluations, there is not yet universal adoption of any approach. This lack of consensus results in inconsistencies among institutions and impedes trust in synthetic data. Furthermore, validation must not only be done for technical correctness, but also with respect to fairness, bias detection, and alignment with clinical realities. Strategic, multi-layered validation processes (integration of statistical, ethical, and clinical) will be required to ensure that synthetic data can be used to support reliable AI applications in healthcare.

Regulatory Uncertainty and Lack of Standardization

The regulatory environment surrounding synthetic data is fragmented and uncertain, which creates major challenges for its use in healthcare. While the technology has the potential to be used as a privacy-preserving substitute for real patient data, the legal and ethical status of the technology has yet to be entirely defined in any jurisdiction. At the moment, there is no established standard for synthetic data generation, validation, and clinical research and product development. Lack of clarity makes it hard for institutions to trust synthetic data for functions that are critical to their institutions, such as clinical trials, drug safety assessments, or regulatory filings with agencies like the FDA or EMA.

For example, the European Union's General Data Protection Regulation (GDPR) identifies synthetic data as a possible tool to mitigate privacy risks, but it does not specifically define a set of criteria for its conformity in research settings. In contrast, U.S. regulatory authorities such as the FDA have been conservative and often require high levels of transparency and validation before synthetic datasets are considered acceptable for regulatory filings. This lack of consensus makes a dataset considered acceptable in Europe potentially more stringent in the United States, which will impair international collaborations and hinder innovation.

The lack of standardization also has wider implications for cross-border research and data-sharing activities. Synthetic data has frequently been put forward as a way to overcome global barriers to health data by enabling researchers in different countries to collaborate in a way that does not break local privacy regulations. However, the absence of harmonized standards leaves uncertainty about what is considered truly 'anonymous' synthetic data, how its provenance should be captured, and what degree of validation is needed to be acceptable for regulatory approval. Until such standards are in place on a global scale, synthetic data is unlikely ever to be fully exploited in a high-stakes healthcare setting, although the potential for synthetic data to speed up research and innovation is evident.

Ethical Dilemmas

The ethical dilemmas within the context of synthetic data use are as complex as the technical and regulatory challenges. While synthetic data are not direct copies of real patient data, they are frequently created from real data, raising important questions about transparency, consent, and trust. For example, should patients be notified that their health records were used to construct synthetic datasets that are used in research or commercial applications? If so, do their original consent to share data apply to the creation of derivative synthetic versions? Most of these questions are left unanswered, creating a void that could jeopardize patient confidence in data-driven healthcare efforts.

Equally important is the issue of transparency of the process around synthetic data creation and application. Many generative models are "black boxes," where little insight is provided into the mechanisms by which synthetic records are generated. Without transparent disclosure, it may be hard for healthcare providers, regulators, and even patients to determine if the data used in AI development is valid, unbiased, and safe. A lack of transparency risks eroding trust in not only synthetic data but also the broader application of AI in healthcare. Ethical best practices: The principles of explainability, accountability, and transparent communication are essential for fostering trust among stakeholders.

However, ethical concerns reach far beyond patient consent to the wider societal implications of synthetic data. "If companies producing these synthetic datasets, which are healthcare institutions or technology firms, adopt these datasets without clear labeling, then it can be seen as an attempt to circumvent the existing protection mechanisms surrounding privacy and consent." However, an overzealous approach that imposes such strict constraints can stifle innovation and hinder the realization of synthetic data's potential as a safe, scalable alternative to conventional datasets. Balanced policies that respect patient autonomy while promoting innovation, coupled with a heavy emphasis on building public trust through transparency and accountability, can help navigate this tension in a balanced manner.

Potential Abuse and Security Issues

The same properties that give synthetic data its utility-realism, scalability, and shareability-are what prevent it from being used without prejudice and open up serious security implications. Synthetic data can be used to create fraudulent medical records, allowing malicious actors to make fraudulent insurance claims or create fake medical records. Similarly, adversarial AI systems can be trained to mimic clinical patterns that deceive diagnostic tools using synthetic data, which represents a potential threat to patient safety. In addition to fraud, synthetic datasets could be used as a tool to strain healthcare IT systems and potentially identify weaknesses in electronic health record systems, hospital networks, or medical devices.

There is also the risk of sensitive data leaking. The generation of synthetic data is often used to ensure the protection of patient privacy; however, the improper generation of synthetic data or a lack of safeguards may inadvertently recreate patterns that can be linked back to individual patients. For example, if generative models overfit to the training data, rare cases such as a patient with a unique combination of conditions may be partially reconstructed in the synthetic output. This compromises the very privacy safeguards that synthetic data is supposed to provide, and it raises questions of accountability in the event of a breach.

Reinforcing governance frameworks and implementing proactive security measures are essential to mitigate these risks. Secure generation pipelines include the need for audit trails, monitoring systems, and occasional reviews for vulnerabilities or accidental disclosures. Institutions should adopt the principles of "defense in depth" and use multiple layers of safeguards to help ensure that synthetic data is protected against malicious misuse and unintentional disclosure. At the same time, international cooperation is required to establish best practices to prevent misuse and, at the same time, allow for legitimate research. By acknowledging and addressing these concerns proactively, synthetic data can realize its potential to become a safe, ethical, and innovative facilitator of AI-driven healthcare. Table 4 summarizes challenges of synthetic data in healthcare, including the concern, its implications, and possible mitigation strategies.

Table 4. Challenges of Synthetic Data for Healthcare

Challenge	Description / Concern	Implications for Healthcare AI	Mitigation Strategies
Representation & Real-World Complexity	Synthetic data may fail to capture rare anomalies, subtle correlations, and complex interactions in real-world medical data.	AI models may generalize poorly in clinical settings, miss rare disease cases, and provide inaccurate predictions for underrepresented patient groups.	Use hybrid models combining real and synthetic data, incorporate domain knowledge into generative models, and validate outputs against real datasets.
Quality Assurance & Validation	Difficulty in confirming that synthetic data maintains clinical relevance, statistical accuracy, and fairness.	Distorted correlations or inaccurate distributions could mislead predictive models, reducing trust and clinical utility.	Develop standardized validation frameworks, employ statistical similarity tests, involve clinical experts, and implement multi-level evaluation (accuracy, fairness, utility).
Regulatory Uncertainty & Standardization	Lack of globally accepted rules for generating, validating, and using synthetic data in research and clinical applications.	Hesitancy to adopt synthetic data in regulated contexts (e.g., clinical trials, FDA submissions) and barriers to international collaboration.	Advocate for clear regulatory guidelines, harmonize standards across jurisdictions, and maintain detailed documentation of generation and validation processes.
Ethical Dilemmas: Transparency, Trust, Consent	Questions around patient consent, disclosure of synthetic data use, and transparency in generative methods.	Risk of eroding trust among patients, clinicians, and regulators; potential misuse could violate ethical norms.	Ensure informed consent policies include synthetic data, provide transparent reporting on data generation methods, and implement accountability measures.
Potential Misuse & Security Concerns	Realistic, shareable synthetic data could be exploited for fraud, adversarial AI training, or accidental leakage of sensitive patterns.	Patient privacy may be compromised; AI systems may be manipulated; institutional liability increases.	Apply secure generation pipelines, audit trails, periodic security reviews, defense-in-depth measures, and governance frameworks to prevent misuse.

CONCLUSION

Synthetic data is set to emerge as an enabling technology in the field of artificial intelligence in healthcare, bridging the gap between innovation and the challenges of privacy, accessibility, and fairness. With the data-driven healthcare ecosystem, the capability to create realistic yet privacy-preserving datasets is transforming the way clinical research, diagnostics, and public health planning are done. Despite synthetic data being a niche tool now, the trajectory follows the view that it will become a mainstream resource for AI-enabled health services.

Synthetic data in healthcare is emerging as a powerful force that can drive innovation and protect privacy, and the future of synthetic data is particularly promising. One of the major developments is the emergence of hybrid models that integrate real patient data along with the synthetic datasets to ensure accuracy, scalability, and clinical relevance, forming balanced solutions where purely synthetic data may fail to capture intricate nuances. Another major trend is the incorporation of synthetic data into federated learning frameworks, where institutions can effectively jointly train AI models without actually sharing sensitive records, increasing data usefulness while protecting privacy. Furthermore, synthetic data is helping to unlock data collaborations between different jurisdictions, allowing researchers to share data and further medical research without breaking local data protection laws in the process. Together, these new trends underscore synthetic data's potential to fuel innovation while adhering to ethical and legal boundaries.

Synthetic data will play an important role in driving precision medicine, which is the practice of tailoring treatment and prevention efforts to the different ways people vary in genetics, environment, and lifestyle. By supplementing limited data on rare diseases, underserved populations, or specific genetic profiles, synthetic data ensures a more inclusive and equitable approach to personalised healthcare solutions. It is empowering predictive models to better identify treatment responses, optimize clinical pathways, and improve patient outcomes at the individual and population level.

To fully leverage the potential of synthetic data in healthcare, it's crucial to have a concerted effort among various stakeholders. Regulatory landscape: Policymakers should define clear regulatory frameworks and validation standards that govern the use of synthetic data in clinical and research settings, ensuring patient safety while promoting innovation. In order to facilitate the use of synthetic data in research, diagnostics, and decision support, healthcare institutions need to integrate it into their overall digital plans by investing in infrastructure, personnel training, and system integration. At the same time, AI developers should make principles of transparency, fairness, and explainability a primary focus when creating and using synthetic data sets, making sure that resulting models are both clinically relevant and trustworthy.

Synthetic data is not just a technical solution; it's a pillar of ethical, scalable, and innovative healthcare AI. By bridging the gap between data-driven innovation and the ethical imperative of patient privacy, it paves the way for a future where medical AI is both potent and responsible. As the field evolves, synthetic data will not just expedite innovation but also ensure that the advantages of AI are distributed equitably, further bolstering the resilience, inclusiveness, and sustainability of contemporary health services.

REFERENCES

Apellaniz, P. A., Galende, B. A., Jim, A., Parras, J., & Zazo, S. (2025). Advancing Cancer Research with Synthetic Data Generation in Low-Data Scenarios. *IEEE Journal of Biomedical and Health Informatics*, 1–15. DOI: 10.1109/JBHI.2025.3595371 PMID: 40758491

Ayilara, O. F., Platt, R. W., Dahl, M., Coulombe, J., Ginestet, P. G., Chateau, D., & Lix, L. M. (2023). Generating synthetic data from administrative health records for drug safety and effectiveness studies. *International Journal of Population Data Science*, *8*(1). Advance online publication. DOI: 10.23889/ijpds.v8i1.2176 PMID: 38414538

Azizi, Z., Zheng, C., Mosquera, L., Pilote, L., & El Emam, K. (2021). Can synthetic data be a proxy for real clinical trial data? A validation study. *BMJ Open*, *11*(4), e043497. Advance online publication. DOI: 10.1136/bmjopen-2020-043497 PMID: 33863713

Bengesi, S., El-Sayed, H., Sarker, M. K., Houkpati, Y., Irungu, J., & Oladunni, T. (2024). *Advancements in Generative AI: A Comprehensive Review of GANs, GPT, Autoencoders, Diffusion Model, and Transformers*. IEEE., DOI: 10.1109/ACCESS.2024.3397775

Bietsch, D., Stahlbock, R., & Voß, S. (2023). Synthetic Data as a Proxy for Real-World Electronic Health Records in the Patient Length of Stay Prediction. *Sustainability (Basel)*, *15*(18), 13690. Advance online publication. DOI: 10.3390/su151813690

Biswas, A., Md Abdullah Al, N., Imran, A., Sejuty, A. T., Fairooz, F., Puppala, S., & Talukder, S. (2023). Generative Adversarial Networks for Data Augmentation. In *Data Driven Approaches on Medical Imaging*. DOI: 10.1007/978-3-031-47772-0_8

Cao, H., Tan, C., Gao, Z., Xu, Y., Chen, G., Heng, P. A., & Li, S. Z. (2024). A Survey on Generative Diffusion Models. *IEEE Transactions on Knowledge and Data Engineering*, *36*(7), 2814–2830. Advance online publication. DOI: 10.1109/TKDE.2024.3361474

Cascella, M., Scarpati, G., Bignami, E. G., Cuomo, A., Vittori, A., Di Gennaro, P., Crispo, A., & Coluccia, S. (2023). Utilizing an artificial intelligence framework (conditional generative adversarial network) to enhance telemedicine strategies for cancer pain management. *Journal of Anesthesia, Analgesia and Critical Care*, *3*(1), 19. Advance online publication. DOI: 10.1186/s44158-023-00104-8 PMID: 37386680

Dankar, F. K., & Ibrahim, M. (2021). Fake It Till You Make It: Guidelines for Effective Synthetic Data Generation. *Applied Sciences 2021, Vol. 11, Page 2158, 11*(5), 2158. DOI: 10.3390/app11052158

Francesca, T. (2019). *Comparing privacy laws: GDPR v. CCPA*. https://futurium.ec.europa.eu/en/european-ai-alliance/open-library/comparing-privacy-laws-gdpr-v-ccpa

Garg, P. P., Jayashree, J., & Vijayashree, J. (2025). Revolutionizing healthcare: The transformative role of artificial intelligence. In *Responsible and Explainable Artificial Intelligence in Healthcare* (pp. 1–23). Elsevier. DOI: 10.1016/B978-0-443-24788-0.00001-7

Giuffrè, M., & Shung, D. L. (2023). Harnessing the power of synthetic data in healthcare: Innovation, application, and privacy. *NPJ Digital Medicine*, *6*(1), 1–8. DOI: 10.1038/s41746-023-00927-3 PMID: 37813960

Gonzales, A., Guruswamy, G., & Smith, S. R. (2023). Synthetic data in health care: A narrative review. *PLOS Digital Health*, *2*(1), e0000082. Advance online publication. DOI: 10.1371/journal.pdig.0000082 PMID: 36812604

Houston, A., & Cosma, G. (2023). A genetically-optimised artificial life algorithm for complexity-based synthetic dataset generation. *Information Sciences*, *619*, 540–561. Advance online publication. DOI: 10.1016/j.ins.2022.11.015

Li, H., Yu, L., & He, W. (2019). The Impact of GDPR on Global Technology Development. In *Journal of Global Information Technology Management* (Vol. 22, Issue 1). DOI: 10.1080/1097198X.2019.1569186

Lutkevich, B. (2019). What is HIPAA (Health Insurance Portability and Accountability Act)? In *WhatIs.com*.

Mendes, J. M., Barbar, A., & Refaie, M. (2025). Synthetic data generation: A privacy-preserving approach to accelerate rare disease research. *Frontiers in Digital Health*, *7*, 1563991. DOI: 10.3389/fdgth.2025.1563991 PMID: 40171526

Murtaza, H., Ahmed, M., Khan, N. F., Murtaza, G., Zafar, S., & Bano, A. (2023). Synthetic data generation: State of the art in health care domain. In *Computer Science Review* (Vol. 48). DOI: 10.1016/j.cosrev.2023.100546

Papadopoulos, D., & Karalis, V. D. (2023). Variational Autoencoders for Data Augmentation in Clinical Studies. *Applied Sciences (Basel, Switzerland)*, *13*(15), 8793. Advance online publication. DOI: 10.3390/app13158793

Paproki, A., Salvado, O., & Fookes, C. (2024). Synthetic data for deep learning in computer vision & medical imaging: A means to reduce data bias. *ACM Computing Surveys*, *56*(11), 1–37. DOI: 10.1145/3663759

Pasculli, G., Virgolin, M., Myles, P., Vidovszky, A., Fisher, C., Biasin, E., Mourby, M., Pappalardo, F., D'Amico, S., Torchia, M., Chebykin, A., Carbone, V., Emili, L., & Roeshammar, D. (2025). Synthetic Data in Healthcare and Drug Development: Definitions, Regulatory Frameworks, Issues. *CPT: Pharmacometrics & Systems Pharmacology*, *14*(5), 840–852. DOI: 10.1002/psp4.70021 PMID: 40193292

Poucin, F., Kraus, A., & Simon, M. (2021). Boosting Instance Segmentation with Synthetic Data: A study to overcome the limits of real world data sets. *Proceedings of the IEEE International Conference on Computer Vision, 2021-October*. DOI: 10.1109/ICCVW54120.2021.00110

Rani, S., Kumar, R., Panda, B. S., Kumar, R., Muften, N. F., Abass, M. A., & Lozanović, J. (2025). Machine Learning-Powered Smart Healthcare Systems in the Era of Big Data: Applications, Diagnostic Insights, Challenges, and Ethical Implications. *Diagnostics (Basel)*, *15*(15), 1914. DOI: 10.3390/diagnostics15151914 PMID: 40804880

Rashid, Z., Ahmed, H., Nadeem, N., Zafar, S. B., & Yousaf, M. Z. (2025). The paradigm of digital health: AI applications and transformative trends. *Neural Computing & Applications*, *37*(17), 1–32. DOI: 10.1007/s00521-025-11081-0

Saxena, D., & Cao, J. (2021). Generative Adversarial Networks (GANs). In *ACM Computing Surveys* (Vol. 54, Issue 3). DOI: 10.1145/3446374

Shen, Y., Yu, J., Zhou, J., & Hu, G. (2025). Twenty-five years of evolution and hurdles in electronic health records and interoperability in medical research: Comprehensive review. *Journal of Medical Internet Research*, *27*, e59024. DOI: 10.2196/59024 PMID: 39787599

Thambawita, V., Salehi, P., Sheshkal, S. A., Hicks, S. A., Hammer, H. L., Parasa, S., de Lange, T., Halvorsen, P., & Riegler, M. A. (2022). SinGAN-Seg: Synthetic training data generation for medical image segmentation. *PLoS ONE, 17*(5 May). DOI: 10.1371/journal.pone.0267976

Tong, L., Shi, W., Isgut, M., Zhong, Y., Lais, P., Gloster, L., Sun, J., Swain, A., Giuste, F., & Wang, M. D. (2023). Integrating multi-omics data with EHR for precision medicine using advanced artificial intelligence. *IEEE Reviews in Biomedical Engineering*, *17*, 80–97. DOI: 10.1109/RBME.2023.3324264 PMID: 37824325

Umer, F., & Adnan, N. (2024). Generative artificial intelligence: synthetic datasets in dentistry. In *BDJ Open* (Vol. 10, Issue 1). DOI: 10.1038/s41405-024-00198-4

Wei, R., Garcia, C., El-Sayed, A., Peterson, V., & Mahmood, A. (2020). Variations in Variational Autoencoders - A Comparative Evaluation. *IEEE Access : Practical Innovations, Open Solutions*, *8*, 153651–153670. Advance online publication. DOI: 10.1109/ACCESS.2020.3018151

Yang, L., Zhang, Z., Song, Y., Hong, S., Xu, R., Zhao, Y., Zhang, W., Cui, B., & Yang, M. H. (2024). Diffusion Models: A Comprehensive Survey of Methods and Applications. *ACM Computing Surveys*, *56*(4), 1–39. Advance online publication. DOI: 10.1145/3626235

Yoon, J., Mizrahi, M., Ghalaty, N. F., Jarvinen, T., Ravi, A. S., Brune, P., Kong, F., Anderson, D., Lee, G., Meir, A., Bandukwala, F., Kanal, E., Arık, S., & Pfister, T. (2023). EHR-Safe: Generating high-fidelity and privacy-preserving synthetic electronic health records. *NPJ Digital Medicine*, *6*(1), 141. Advance online publication. DOI: 10.1038/s41746-023-00888-7 PMID: 37567968

Chapter 8
AI for Early Diagnosis and Risk Prediction of Neurodegenerative Diseases

Chenchu Swetha
https://orcid.org/0009-0005-1835-0679
SR University, India

Chiranjeevi Manike
https://orcid.org/0000-0002-7831-6916
SR University, India

ABSTRACT

Multiple sclerosis, Parkinson's disease, and Alzheimer's disease are difficult to manage because there are no accurate treatments available and they worsen over time. It is very important to identify these illnesses early and observe their progression over time. Traditional methods for diagnosing these diseases usually rely on the subjective evaluation of medical professionals and different symptoms that emerge later. Recently, AI, particularly machine learning (ML) and deep learning (DL), are developing into a powerful tool for to treat these illnesses. This paper looks at how AI can be used to study different types of brain scans, such as MRI, PET, and EEG. By combining these types of data, AI can help doctors make more accurate diagnoses of brain-related diseases. This chapter highlights how important it is to keep working on testing, improving, and using these technologies in the right way so they can have the best possible impact in real medical practice.

DOI: 10.4018/979-8-3373-5641-9.ch008

1. INTRODUCTION

Neurodegenerative diseases are long-term health conditions that slowly damage the brain and nervous system over time. Diseases and they cannot grow back, once these cells are gone, . That is the reason neurodegenerative diseases are treated as permanent and there is no cure. Moreover, today medical treatments can help and manage the symptoms and, in some cases, slow down the spread of these diseases. the examples include Huntington's disease, Motor Neuron Disease (MND), Amyotrophic Lateral Sclerosis (ALS),Parkinson's disease, and Alzheimer's disease, Among these, Alzheimer's and Parkinson's are the most common, especially in older people. No of cases are expected to rise as people live longer (Galal et al., 2024).

Parkinson's disease makes hard to move the body which is caused by slowly loss of brain cells that produce dopamine, which is chemical that helps control movement in the body. Very Common symptoms in human are speech, difficulty with balance, tremors, and stiffness. More ever, the exact cause of the disease isn't fully known, an integration of genetics and environmental factors is believed to major a role. On the other hand, Alzheimer's disease affects memory behavior and thinking. It is related to the build-up of abnormal protein in the brain which interferes with normal functions of brain. Symptoms generally start with confusion and memory loss and get worse over time. The rare one is Huntington's disease, which affects a person's ability to move, think, and control emotions. It the disease starts between the ages of 30 and 50 and gets worse over time. ALS, also known as Lou Gehrig's disease, it is a kind of disease that weakens the muscles as the nerve cells that control them begin to die (Huang G et al.,2023)

As these symptoms becomes As Motor Neuron Disease (MND) worsens everyday activities like eating, walking, speaking or even breathing can become very difficult. MND is not just one condition it is a group of similar diseases, including Amyotrophic Lateral Sclerosis (ALS), that totally damage the nerve cells which are responsible for controlling movement. As the condition worsens, it may lead to muscle weakness and loss of coordination (Uyanik, H., et al., 2025). Amyotrophic Lateral Sclerosis (ALS) is a deadly brain and nerve disease that causes the gradual loss of motor neurons, which control muscle movement. Because ALS affects people in very different ways and we don't fully understand what causes these differences, and since it is a rare disease, using artificial intelligence (AI) to study or predict it is especially challenging.

To understand better and diagnose these diseases the doctors are using multimodal biomarkers to understand better and diagnose these diseases. Instead of depending on a single test they integrate information from different tests like spinal fluid analysis, brain scans, and genetic testing. When they are used all together, these tools offer a clearer picture of the disease how far it has advanced, and how the treatments are working. This systematic approach is helping researchers and clinicians to develop more effective ways to treat and manage and mostly prevent these conditions in the future (Galal et al., 2024)..

2. LITERATURE SURVEY

Recent progress in Artificial Intelligence (AI) have opened up new possibilities for detecting neurodegenerative diseases like Alzheimer's (AD) and Parkinson's (PD)in an early stage. This section highlights knowledge from around 30 key studies and reviews, focusing on the different methods used, types of data involved, major takeaways, and current challenges researchers are facing .

2.1. Systematic Reviews & Surveys

2.1.1 Borchert et al. (2021)

In this PRISMA-based review, the researches worked over 250 machine learning studies that used brain imaging to diagnose different types of neurodegenerative diseases like Alzheimer's, Parkinson's, vascular dementia and frontotemporal dementia, . Most of the research is depended heavily on data from the Alzheimer's Disease Neuroimaging Initiative (ADNI) and used models like Convolutional Neural Networks (CNNs) and Support Vector Machines (SVMs). These models were good at differentiating between various conditions. Moreover, a general weakness was that most of them were not tested on datasets which are from. The deficiency in testing raises concerns about how well these tools would perform in real-world clinical settings(chenchu et al.,2025)

2.1.2 AI in Neurological Disease Diagnosis (2021)

This comprehensive review explored AI's application in diagnosing a broad spectrum of neurological disorders—including ALS, Huntington's, and Multiple System Atrophy using diverse data types such as EEG, sleep patterns, and neuroimaging. It proposed a structured taxonomy of symptoms and computational approaches for analysis .

2.1.3 Deep Learning for Alzheimer's Using Structural MRI (2024)

Focusing on ~130 studies, this paper reviewed deep learning models aimed at predicting progression from Mild Cognitive Impairment (MCI) to AD. Regions of interest like the hippocampus were frequently analyzed using architectures such as U-Net and region-based ensemble models, which achieved high classification accuracy (85–99%) and AUC scores (~94%).

2.1.4 Review on ML/DL for Alzheimer's Prediction (2024)

This review examined 100 studies applying ML and deep learning to predict AD using MRI, PET, genetic markers (like APOE), and CSF biomarkers. CNN-based models occasionally reached 100% accuracy(Huang G et al.,2023)

2.1.5 Rudroff et al. (2024)

This narrative review compared single-modality (e.g., MRI or PET alone) with multimodal approaches in Alzheimer's prediction It explains how it is important to know about the symptoms and how they worse along the time the AI system should be easy to understand .

2.1.6 Koksalmis et al. (2025)

A forward-looking survey covering patient-specific disease modeling, this work highlighted the use of recurrent neural networks (RNNs), graph neural networks (GNNs), and generative models like GANs and VAEs.

2.1.7 Rao et al. (2024)

This survey focused on gait-based AI diagnostics across multiple NDs, particularly PD. It examined 169 studies that utilized motion capture, wearable sensors, and video data. It proposed a framework for evaluating dataset quality and encouraged future work in 3D skeleton tracking and lightweight models for real-world deployment (Galal et al., 2024)..

2.2 Application Studies by Data Modality

2.2.1 Neuroimaging (MRI, PET) and Multimodal Approaches

2.2.1.1 Brain Informatics Review (2023) This review analyzed deep learning applications for classifying individuals into normal, MCI, or AD categories using MRI and PET data. Many studies focused on early-stage diagnosis and tracking MCI-to-AD progression using CNNs and autoencoders (Huang G et al.,2023)

2.2.1.2 AI Review (2024) A meta-analysis covering deep learning in neuro-imaging, this study reported up to 99% diagnostic performance. However, it pointed out that most models were limited in scope and lacked external validation, making them less generalizable.
2.2.1.3 ADNI-Based Analyses Numerous studies based on the ADNI dataset achieved diagnostic accuracies exceeding 95% for AD and over 82% for classifying MCI. Deep learning models have also demonstrated >90% accuracy in predicting future conversion from MCI to AD years in advance (chenchu et al.,2025).

2.2.2 Gait and Biomechanical Data for Parkinson's Disease

2.2.2.1 Gait-Based Studies Studies by Setiawan & Lin (2021), Erdaş & Sümer (2024), Guarín et al. (2024), and Muñoz-Mata et al. (2024) explored gait analysis using CNNs and time–frequency features derived from wearable or video sensors. These models showed promising results in identifying early PD symptoms and disease severity.
2.2.2.2 Yin et al. (2024) This study applied machine learning techniques to detailed gait dynamics, confirming that subtle movement irregularities could serve as early indicators of Parkinson's, even before clinical diagnosis (Uyanik, H., et al., 2025).
2.2.2.3 **Wang et al. (2024)** By combining signal processing and ML, this study achieved effective early-stage PD classification and staging using hybrid feature sets from gait signals.
2.2.2.4 Meng et al. (2023) This work highlighted the diagnostic importance of "turning phase" gait metrics, captured using inertial sensors, in improving the accuracy of early PD detection.
2.2.11 Zhao et al. (2023) IoT-integrated wearable anklets were developed to continuously monitor gait and tremor activity, enabling real-time PD symptom tracking through a smart AI system.

2.2.3 Ocular Imaging and EHR-Based Prediction

2.2.3.1 Ophthalmic Imaging for AD/PD (2025) AI-based analysis of retinal images can detect microvascular and nerve fiber abnormalities linked to both AD and PD. This approach offers a low-cost, non-invasive screening method with potential for widespread deployment.
2.2.3.2 Nureyev Dementia Tool (Scotland) This AI tool analyzed nearly one million optometry scans to identify patterns suggesting dementia risk.

Its real-world applicability makes it promising for early public screening and trial recruitment.

2.2.3.3 Monash Health AI (Australia, 2025) A novel tool developed from EHR data analyzed subtle behavioral and cognitive changes to flag potential dementia risks. Though not diagnostic, it performed well in real-world clinical flagging scenarios.

2.2.3.4 UCSF AI-EHR Study (2023) This study mined seven years of anonym zed health records to identify both established (e.g., cardiovascular disease) and novel (e.g., osteoporosis in women) risk factors predictive of AD. AI models could predict AD onset up to seven years in advance with ~72% accuracy.

2.2.3.5 Neurodegeneration Proteomics Consortium (2025) Utilizing an enormous proteomic dataset with over 250 million biomarker measurements, AI was used to uncover novel protein signatures associated with AD and PD risk, creating an open resource for future research (Uyanik, H., et al., 2025).

2.3 Key Insights and Trends

- Dominant Techniques: CNNs and deep learning dominate across neuroimaging tasks. RNNs and GNNs are increasingly used in personalized disease progression models.
- Most Common Datasets: ADNI remains the primary benchmark for imaging-based studies. EHR and wearable data are gaining prominence for scalability (chenchu et al., 2025).
- Accuracy Benchmarks: Many models report AUCs of 90–99% and MCI→AD conversion accuracy around 85–95%, though most lack external validation.
- Emerging Modalities: Non-invasive diagnostics using eye imaging and wearable devices are rapidly evolving.
- Challenges: A major gap remains in the generalizability of models due to homogeneous datasets. There's also a pressing need for interpretable AI models and robust ethical governance .

2.4 Research Gaps

- External Validation: Most studies are trained and tested on single datasets (often ADNI), limiting real-world application.
- Multimodal Integration: Combining imaging, genetics, clinical notes, and behavior data in unified models is an emerging but underdeveloped area.
- Explainability: Interpretability of AI decisions remain limited, impeding clinical adoption.

- Diversity and Bias: Datasets lack demographic diversity, which risks bias in predictions.
- Deployment Readiness: Ethical concerns around privacy, explainability, and AI governance need more structured solutions.

Neurodegenerative diseases like Parkinson's disease (PD) and Alzheimer's disease (AD) are generally known for causing brain cell damage, which leads to problems in brain like thinking and body movements

Generally, people with Alzheimer's will walk slowly, they will take shorter steps, and show irregularities in the walking pattern you may find irregularities the People who are suffering with Parkinson's generally experience problem in movements they cannot move freely, stifness all the steps affects in body movement(chenchu et al., 2025).

With recent technology these movement changes are tracked by using the wearable devices .Throughout the day and night continuously the devices use accelerometers to measure movement

At first, researchers used these devices just to study general physical activity. They found that people who are more active and spend less time sitting have a lower risk of developing dementia and other brain diseases.

As technology and research improved, the focus shifted to more detailed information, like walking patterns, daily activity changes, and sleep behavior. This has been especially helpful in studying Parkinson's disease, which has distinct movement symptoms. How the disease is progressed overtime is detected by these wearable devices(Huang G et al.,2023)

Researchers have also started using machine learning a type of AI to analyze the data from these devices. For example the disease detection percentage is 85% by using support vector machine to analyze data from wrist devices(Uyanik, H., et al., 2025)

To get these results, researchers used advanced techniques to extract important features from the movement data. In a larger study using data from the UK Biobank, scientists found that combining different types of movement data (such as walking patterns and periods of low activity) improved diagnostic accuracy. They used a model called a Gaussian mixed model and found it could detect Parkinson's with good performance—an AUC (area under the curve) of 0.85 when combining different activity types.

Another study in 2023 by Schalkamp and his team showed that wearable data—analyzed with more advanced machine learning techniques like random forests and Markov models—was more accurate at predicting Parkinson's disease than traditional methods such as genetics, lifestyle habits, or even blood tests.

More recently, these techniques have also been applied to Alzheimer's detection. A 2024 study again using UK Biobank data showed that movement patterns like daily rhythm, activity consistency, and how active someone is during their most active hours can predict the development of both Alzheimer's and Parkinson's.

3. OVERVIEW: THE NEED FOR AI IN NEURODEGENERATIVE DISEASE CARE

Neurodegenerative diseases like Alzheimer's, Parkinson's, ALS (amyotrophic lateral sclerosis), and multiple sclerosis are becoming more common, especially in aging populations. According to the World Health Organization, these conditions are expected to overtake cancer as one of the leading causes of death in developed countries by 2040. These diseases gradually damage the brain and nervous system, leading to memory loss, movement issues, and a decline in the ability to live independently. Since there are no known cures and current treatments have limited effectiveness, it's urgent that we find better ways to diagnose and treat these conditions earlier and more accurately . This is where Artificial Intelligence (AI) is showing great promise (Huang G et al.,2023)

3.1 Why Artificial Intelligence Matters

- In healthcare AI is becoming important because it can identify diseases much faster than traditional methods. Generally, disease like Alzheimer's are diagnosed only after damage has already happened in the brain. To find small and early changes AI can look at brain scans, genetic information, and other medical data often before any symptoms even show up. For example,93% accuracy is seen in some AI systems that analyze MRI scans and genetic data to detect Alzheimer's in its early stages w . There's also research using AI to examine images of the eye to find signs of Alzheimer's, offering a innovative way to screen for the disease
- Another main strength of AI is its ability to integrate different types of medical data like genetic profiles, brain images, blood tests,, and even lifestyle habits into one model. This kind of integration will help researchers to understand the disease more appropriately. AI-based radio genomics, for example, can connect brain scan patterns with genetic changes, provide ideas how can the disease starts and spreads .
- AI also helps to predict how a disease will develop in different patients. Machine learning algorithms can analyze past data to estimate how quickly a person's symptoms will worsen or how they might respond to a specific treatment. Some models are able to predict Alzheimer's up to seven years in advance by learning and analyzing electronic health records. In Parkinson's,

AI is being used to identify blood protein markers that can trace the disease years before diagnosis.

- Smart sensors and wearable devices play a major role. These tools will collect the data on a patient speech, walking patterns and movements by which AI can track regularly to detect early changes. This allows doctors alter or adjust treatment methods without any frequent hospital visits for treatment. For example, in ALS and Parkinson's, AI can detect difference in voice to detect early motor symptoms. This kind of tracking can improve quality of life and reduce the burden on care givers

One main area is brain imaging. AI-powered tools can now read MRI and PET scans with more accuracy sometimes even better than human experts. They're able to identify small changes in the brain's structure that may suggest the early stages of Alzheimer's or other neurological diseases (Bhavana et al., 2025).

AI is also detecting how we analyze brainwaves, like those seen in EEG (electroencephalogram) tests. Generally, doctors have to observe at these recordings by hand, which can take more time and can be tricky. But new AI systems can automatically recognize patterns that point to dementia, making the process faster and more dependable .

Another main use of AI is in identifying new biomarkers signals in the body that can help detect or track diseases. For example, platforms like Insilco's Panda Omics uses deep learning to search for molecules that could be used to diagnose or treat conditions like ALS. AI also helped scientists to discover certain blood proteins that might reveal Alzheimer's earlier than current tests can .

In the field of radio genomics, AI is helping connect the dots between what's seen in medical scans and a person's genetic makeup. This helps researchers understand how genes and brain changes are linked, opening the door to perform more accurate and personalized treatments.

Lastly, AI is improving telehealth in different ways. Voice assistants and digital companions are being used to talk with older adults, offering mental exercises, conversation, and even spotting early signs of memory loss all over a simple phone call, with no internet needed. These tools help seniors to maintain mentally activeness and give assist doctors helpful about cognitive changes early on (Huang G et al.,2023).

- In health care even though AI has developed a lot, in real time still we are facing challenges. One of the major problems is the lack of huge, high-quality datasets. Neurodegenerative diseases are generally rare and complicated, so we don't have enough data available to train reliable AI models. other thing is hospitals often collect and store data in different ways, which makes us difficult to create AI tools that work well across all situations.

- Trust is another issue. Many AI models are considered "black boxes" because even the developers don't always understand how they work. This makes it difficult for doctors and patients to trust the results. That's why researchers are now working on explainable AI systems that can show how they arrive at a decision.
- Ethical issues need to be addressed. For other populations it may not work if AI is trained mostly on data from certain groups (for example, mostly from Western countries). Maintaining fairness and equity in AI tools is critical so that everyone can benefits fairly.
- There are also regulatory and practical barriers. To use AI tools in clinics, they must be tested thoroughly. That process can be slow and tough. Many hospitals especially from low-income areas may not have the proper infrastructure or trained staff to use advanced AI systems.

3.2 Why AI Is Needed Now More Than Ever

Now it is correct time to invest in AI for detecting neurodegenerative diseases, and there are several good reasons why. First, the number of people affected by these disorders are increasing faster especially as people are living longer. This puts more stress on already formatted healthcare systems. AI can help to reduce the burden by making it faster and easier to detect and diagnose and treat patients. Second, these diseases are are very complex. They impact the brain in many ways from tiny molecular changes to how a person thinks and behaves and they change over time. AI is great at integrating together all this data, something that's far too intense for a human doctor to do alone. Third, early detection is very important the earlier we can catch these diseases, the better the chance of slowing them down. AI tools can detect early warning signs, giving patients more time to make lifestyle changes, join clinical trials, or start treatments that might delay the disease (chenchu et al., 2025).

3.3 Looking Ahead: Building an AI-Powered Future for Neurodegenerative Care

In healthcare we use AI, especially for neurodegenerative diseases, the use of AI is highly encouraging. With the more availability of large research datasets like ADNI and international biobanks, AI can have the access to the kind of detailed, multi-layered information it needs to make predictions accurately. The new technologies like remote monitoring tools, wearable devices, and even retinal scans are making it easier to collect health data passively and continuously giving a clearer idea of a person's condition over time. we can also see the progress in AI methods, like federated learning. This approach allows hospitals and research centers to train

AI models together without having to share sensitive patient information. It's a major big step for building powerful tools while still protecting privacy. Governments and health organizations are also taking AI seriously Initiatives like the Milken Institute's SPARC program are helping by creating clear guidelines and offering funding to bring AI into real-world clinical settings more quickly and safely (Uyanik, H., et al., 2025).

4. AI TECHNIQUES FOR DIAGNOSIS

To detect brain related diseases the AI is having a major role in . One main area is brain imaging. To detect early signs of brain damages the techniques and methods like machine learning and deep learning, are used to estimate scans from MRI, PET, and CT Deep learning models those developed to recognize patterns in images are mainly good at tracking changes in brain structure. AI is also being used to integrate brainwave data from EEG recordings[4]. Instead of focusing on just a few regions or frequencies, AI looks at the full picture, making it easier to detect early signs of that can find the conditions like Alzheimer's or dementia. Another major use of AI is predicting how a person's brain health might change based on time . These predictive tools can estimate when cognitive problems might begin, giving doctors a head start in planning early interventions. AI is helping doctors make decisions. The tools which are powered by AI can consider the complex data and give predictions for the treatment. This helps us to take care of patients more unique manner (Bhavana et al., 2025)..

4.1 Review on case studies of successful AI implementation in neurodegenerative care:

From the Alzheimer's Disease Neuroimaging Initiative (ADNI) the most IMPORTANT applications of AI in neurodegenerative care comes In this case, The deep learning models is developed by the researchers mainly convolutional neural networks (CNNs), to analyze an estimate from MRI scans and clinical data to predict whether patients with (MCI) will have the Alzheimer's disease (AD). the model has achieved over 90% accuracy in detecting disease development up to six years in advance, providing doctors with a tools for early planning to overcome.

IBM Research, in collaboration with the Michael J. Fox Foundation, For Parkinson's Progression Markers Initiative the researchers used machine learning the. Their AI models is able to identify the sub version of the disease. By predicting motor and non-motor symptom evolution the researcher enhanced understanding of how Parkinson's progresses across different patients but also supported more personalized treatment decisions .

Another case for the early detection of dementia researchers used machine learning to analyze EEG data. The researches demonstrated that their AI-based approach can identify the various changes in brainwave patterns, including the conditions like Alzheimer's and Lewy body dementia (Bhavana et al., 2025)..

Neuroreader™, developed by Brainreader, is one of the few AI tools in this domain to receive FDA clearance. Highlighting structural changes It offers automated volumetric analysis of MRI brain scans, in regions commonly affected by Alzheimer's disease. To support the assessments Radiologists and neurologists use the tool to, especially in early-stage dementia cases helping to confirm diagnoses more quickly and consistently (Uyanik, H., et al., 2025).

DeepMind, in partnership with University College London Hospitals (UCLH), developed an AI model to predicting cognitive decline before clinical symptoms become worsen. The patients at risk are identified by By combining all the data deep learning system maintaining earlier monitoring and the possibility of initiating preventive measures before cognitive deficits emerge.

Aiforia® is a great example of how AI is transforming neuropathology. In brain tissue Their platform to automatically measure amyloid plaques and tau tangles the methods are implemented two key features of Alzheimer's disease. This technology has sped up the work of neuropathologists and made tissue evaluations more consistent, especially in research settings and post-mortem diagnoses. Another promising example comes from ReMYND, a biotech company that has created an AI-driven platform combining blood-based proteomics and cerebrospinal fluid (CSF) data. It's designed to predict whether someone is amyloid-positive—an important early marker of Alzheimer's. Because it uses non-invasive blood samples, this tool can help with early screening and identify individuals who might need further testing or qualify for clinical trials (Bhavana et al., 2025)..

QMENTA is a platform that involves AI to combine different kinds of brain-related data and cognitive test scores to support both patient care and research (Uyanik, H., et al., 2025).

Enlitic's BrainScreen™ is another promising tool that uses AI to scan brain MRIs and highlight cases that may show signs of cognitive disorders, such as dementia. The iDASH Challenge showcased the power of federated learning in protecting patient privacy during AI development. In this case, researchers developed Alzheimer's prediction models that could be trained on sensitive medical data across multiple hospitals without transferring the data itself. This privacy-preserving approach supports large-scale collaboration while maintaining strict data security standards (Bhavana et al., 2025).

Cognetivity's Integrated Cognitive Assessment (ICA) is an FDA-approved AI-powered visual test that assesses cognitive performance in under five minutes. It uses rapid image recognition tasks and analyzes performance using AI algorithms to detect signs of mild cognitive impairment. The tool is now being used in clinics and research settings as a fast, scalable screening tool for dementia risk.

In multiple sclerosis care, the AIMS project applied AI for accurate lesion segmentation on brain MRIs. The tool improved diagnostic accuracy and significantly reduced the time radiologists spent on manual segmentation. Although the focus was MS, the underlying AI framework has implications for broader neuroimaging applications in dementia and neurodegeneration.

At University College London, researchers built an AI model that uses natural language processing (NLP) to analyze clinical notes and speech patterns to identify early signs of dementia. The model could flag at-risk patients based on how they describe their symptoms or behave in conversation, showing promise as a non-invasive screening technique within primary care or telehealth.

The DREAM Challenge in ALS research focused on stratifying patients by disease progression. Machine learning algorithms were trained on clinical and genetic data to identify patient subgroups with distinct progression patterns. This work has helped design better-targeted clinical trials by selecting participants based on expected disease trajectories .

An Israeli research team created an AI model using electronic health record data and cognitive scores to predict Alzheimer's onset up to three years before clinical diagnosis. The model achieved 91% accuracy and has sparked interest in using routine health data to proactively identify at-risk individuals for early intervention.

Finally, pharmaceutical companies like Amgen have turned to AI to integrate multi-omics data—combining genomics, proteomics, and imaging biomarkers—to discover novel indicators of neurodegenerative disease. These models are being used to accelerate drug discovery and stratify patients more effectively for personalized treatment approaches

5. EXPLORATIVE AI ALGORITHMS IN NEURODEGENERATIVE DISEASE RESEARCH – A SIMPLE EXPLANATION

Artificial Intelligence (AI) is changing how we understand and treat neurodegenerative diseases like Alzheimer's, Parkinson's, Huntington's, and ALS. These diseases are hard to diagnose early and manage because they progress slowly and involve multiple complex biological systems. Explorative AI helps by uncovering patterns and insights from large amounts of data that would be too difficult or time-consuming for humans to analyze manually.

In this overview, we'll explain in simple terms how different AI algorithms—ranging from traditional machine learning to advanced deep learning and bio-inspired models—are used in this field.

5.1. Classical Machine Learning Algorithms

These are the more traditional models that have been widely used before deep learning became popular. They are still very useful, especially when the dataset is small or structured.

5.1.1 Support Vector Machines (SVM)

SVM is like drawing a line (or plane) to separate different disease categories. For example, it can help separate patients with Alzheimer's from healthy people by analyzing brain scan data. It's effective in small datasets and often used with MRI or EEG features.

5.1.2 Decision Trees and Random Forests

Decision trees split data based on simple yes/no questions, like "Is this brain volume above a certain level?" They are easy to understand. Random forests are like a team of decision trees working together, which makes them more accurate and less prone to errors. They're useful in diagnosing Parkinson's or finding gene markers for diseases (Uyanik, H., et al., 2025).

5.1.3 K-Nearest Neighbors (KNN)

KNN looks at similar past cases to make predictions. It's useful in small datasets where you want to see which known cases are "closest" to the new one. It's been used in EEG and protein data for early detection.

5.1.4 Naïve Bayes

This algorithm works by calculating probabilities. It assumes each feature (like age, brain volume, or memory score) is independent, which isn't always true, but it makes the model fast and simple. It's used for predicting dementia risk.

5.1.5 Gradient Boosting and XGBoost

These algorithms build one model after another, each learning from the mistakes of the last. XGBoost is an improved version and is very powerful for predicting disease progression or identifying key biomarkers from blood or genetic data (Uyanik, H., et al., 2025).

5.1.6 PCA (Principal Component Analysis)

PCA isn't a classifier—it's a tool to simplify data. It reduces the number of features by keeping only the most important ones. This helps make models faster and more accurate, especially when analyzing noisy data like EEG signals.

5.2. Deep Learning Algorithms

These are more advanced models that learn directly from large, complex data. They're especially good at analyzing images and time-series data

5.2.1 Convolutional Neural Networks (CNNs)

CNNs are very good at analyzing images, like brain scans. They can identify patterns in 2D EEG plots or 3D MRI images that might signal early disease. Some models combining MRI and PET data have achieved over 90% accuracy in classifying Alzheimer's and MCI patients.

5.2.2 Recurrent Neural Networks (RNNs), LSTM, and GRU

These models are designed to handle time-series or sequential data. They're ideal for tracking disease progression over time using patient history, wearable sensor data, or repeated EEG recordings. LSTM and GRU are modified versions that can have over a long period of time, making them useful for forecasting future symptoms.

5.2.3 Hybrid and Attention-Based Models

Hybrid models combine CNNs with RNNs by this it helps the model focus on the most important features in the data. For example, one model used CNN + Bi-GRU + attention layers to classify Parkinson's from EEG data with very high accuracy.

5.2.4 Graph Convolutional Neural Networks (GCNN)

GCNNs are used when data is structured like a network for example, connections between brain regions. These models help capture how different parts of the brain are functionally connected, improving disease classification

5.3. Explorative and Evolution-Inspired AI Approaches

These algorithms are inspired by biological processes like evolution or the human immune system. They are still developing but show trust in complex scenarios.

5.3.1 Neuro evolution

Neuroevolution uses evolutionary strategies (like mutation and selection) to design the best neural networks without needing a lot of labeled training data. This approach is helpful when there's not enough data, which is often the case in rare neurodegenerative diseases (Bhavana et al., 2025)..

5.3.2 Artificial Immune System (AIS) Algorithms

AIS algorithms mimic how the immune system detects harmful invaders. They're useful for spotting unusual patterns or outliers in data—such as early, rare disease markers. Examples include the clonal selection algorithm and dendrite cell algorithms, which help detect hidden abnormalities in biomarker data (Uyanik, H., et al., 2025).

5.3.3 Genetic Algorithms

These simulate natural selection to find the best solution among many possibilities. They've been used to optimize models that combine genetic and brain activity data, giving insights into the biological causes of neurodegenerative changes.

5.4. Feature Extraction and Preprocessing Techniques

Before feeding data into an algorithm, we often need to extract meaningful features.

5.4.1 Spectral and Time-Frequency Analysis

For EEG data, it's common to analyze brain wave frequencies. Tools like power spectral density (PSD), fuzzy entropy, and wavelet transforms help quantify changes in brain activity linked to disease.

5.4.2 Transform-Domain Techniques

Sometimes, EEG or imaging data is transformed into another domain (like frequency space) to make it easier for AI models to learn from. Combining PCA and Karhunen–Loève transforms helps reduce noise while preserving useful information.

5.5. Real-World Applications

Here are some examples of how these AI methods are used in practice:

- MRI-based Alzheimer's detection: 3D CNNs trained on brain scans can detect early-stage Alzheimer's with around 90% accuracy.
- EEG-based Parkinson's diagnosis: Hybrid models like CNN + Bi-GRU + attention have achieved near-perfect accuracy (close to 100%) in distinguishing patients from healthy individuals.
- Disease progression forecasting: RNNs and LSTMs help predict how mild cognitive impairment (MCI) will evolve into full Alzheimer's
- Biomarker discovery: XGBoost and gradient boosting models help identify genes or proteins strongly linked to neurodegeneration.
- Radio genomic models: These systems connect brain scan data with genetic risk factors to provide personalized predictions.

5.6. Pros and Cons of Major Algorithm Types

Table 1.

Algorithm Type	Strengths	Limitations
SVM	Great for small datasets, clear boundaries	Struggles with large or unbalanced data
Random Forest	Easy to interpret, robust to noise	Can overfit noisy data
XGBoost / Gradient Boost	Very accurate, handles missing data well	Needs tuning, can be slow
KNN	Simple, good for small data	Sensitive to noise, slow for large data
Naïve Bayes	Fast, works well with imbalanced classes	Assumes independence among features
CNN	Great for image data	Requires lots of data, doesn't handle time well
RNN / LSTM / GRU	Good for sequences and time-series	Can be hard to train, memory issues
Hybrid Models	Combines best of both worlds (spatial + temporal)	Complex to design and train

continued on following page

Table 1. Continued

Algorithm Type	Strengths	Limitations
GCNN	Understands relationships between data points	Requires graph structure
Neuroevolution	Doesn't need labeled data	Very computationally expensive
Immune-inspired Models	Good at detecting rare or unusual patterns	Still experimental in this field

6. DATA TYPES USED FOR EARLY DETECTION OF BRAIN DISEASES

To catch neurodegenerative diseases early — like Alzheimer's or Parkinson's — scientists and doctors are now using many different types of information. These include brain scans, genetic details, and health check-up results. When this information is combined, it helps machine learning (ML) systems detect patterns that could mean something is going wrong in the brain — even before a person starts to feel sick. This approach, known as **multimodal data integration**, makes early diagnosis more accurate and opens the door for better treatment options tailored to each individual (Uyanik, H., et al., 2025).

6.1 Brain Scans: MRI, PET, and fMRI

Magnetic Resonance Imaging (MRI)

MRI helps doctors see if the brain has changed in shape or size. In people who may be developing brain diseases, small parts of the brain might shrink or change shape early on.

Machine learning can look at many MRI scans and learn what early signs of diseases like Alzheimer's look like. For example, a trained ML model can notice small changes in brain volume or the shape of specific brain areas — things that a human doctor might miss at first glance. Functional MRI (fMRI) goes a step further. It tracks brain activity by measuring blood flow, helping researchers understand which brain regions are active or inactive. ML algorithms can use this data to identify unusual patterns of brain activity that happen before symptoms show up (Bhavana et al., 2025)..

6.2 Positron Emission Tomography (PET)

PET scans are a special type of imaging that show how the brain is working at a chemical level. Patients are given a small amount of a radioactive substance, which travels through the blood and shows how different parts of the brain are using energy.

In Alzheimer's disease, PET scans can detect harmful proteins like beta-amyloid, while in Parkinson's disease, they can show if there is a lack of dopamine, a chemical that helps with movement. Machine learning helps analyze these scans by spotting patterns that are linked to specific diseases. This helps doctors figure out what disease might be starting and begin treatment earlier. It can also help tell the difference between diseases that look similar.

6.3 Functional MRI (fMRI)

FMRI is a type of MRI that focuses on brain activity. It works by detecting changes in blood flow, which increase when a part of the brain is active. This scans shows how different parts of the brain "talk" to each other — this is called functional connectivity.

In the early stages of brain diseases, this communication between brain areas often becomes weaker or disrupted. Machine learning can spot these subtle changes in how the brain networks are working. By catching these changes early, it becomes possible to plan interventions or therapies before the disease gets worse.

6.4 Genetic Information: Biomarkers and Risk Factors

6.4.1 Genetic Biomarkers

Genes play a big role in determining a person's risk of developing a neurodegenerative disease. Certain small changes in the DNA, called single nucleotide polymorphisms (SNPs), can increase the chances of getting diseases like Alzheimer's or Huntington's.

Machine learning tools can look at thousands of genetic profiles and find common patterns in people who later develop these diseases. This helps scientists create risk profiles, which doctors can use to identify people who may need early monitoring or preventive care. By catching the signs early, people may be able to make lifestyle changes or take treatments to delay disease onset.

6.4.2 Risk Factors

In real life, it's not just genes that matter — your environment and lifestyle also play a role. Things like smoking, pollution, diet, and stress can interact with your genes and raise your risk even more.

Machine learning can study how different factors — both genetic and environmental — work together to influence disease development. This is useful because it gives a more complete picture of a person's health. ML models that include both types of data can more accurately predict who might be at higher risk, allowing for early preventive actions and more personalized healthcare.

6.5 Clinical Assessments: Cognitive and Movement Tests

6.5.1 Cognitive Tests

Cognitive tests check how well a person's brain is working — especially memory, attention, language, and problem-solving. These tests are often the first tools doctors use when they suspect a brain disease.

Machine learning can look at test scores over time and find very small changes that may not be obvious at first. It can compare results with thousands of other cases to see if a person's scores match early signs of diseases like Alzheimer's. This helps in quicker diagnosis and helps doctors suggest treatments specific to the patient's condition.

6.5.2 Motor Function Assessments

Some diseases, like Parkinson's, start with changes in how people move. A person might not notice it, but small changes in walking, hand movements, or posture can be early warning signs.

Today, wearable devices like smartwatches or motion sensors can track how someone moves throughout the day. These devices collect data like walking speed or hand tremors. Machine learning can study this data to catch subtle changes that could mean early-stage Parkinson's or another movement disorder. This is especially helpful because movement changes often start before a diagnosis is made (Haocong Rao et al., 2025).

6.6 Structural MRI brain parameters as imaging biomarkers for neurogenerative diseases

In the last 20 years, neuroimaging techniques have become very important for detecting and tracking neurodegenerative diseases. MRI is one of the most popular tools used by doctors and researchers. There are different types of MRI scans, like structural MRI, functional MRI, diffusion tensor imaging, and neuromelanin-sensitive MRI. Among these, structural MRI is the most common because it's easier to perform and has strong support from research.

Structural MRI is great at showing patterns of brain shrinkage (atrophy) that happen in different diseases. For example, people with Alzheimer's disease (AD) often show significant shrinkage in parts of the brain like the temporal lobe and the medial parietal cortex. Key areas like the hippocampus, amygdala, and other nearby regions in the medial temporal lobe tend to shrink as Alzheimer's progresses. The size of the hippocampus is especially important — smaller hippocampal volume is a reliable sign of AD and is linked to how severe the disease is. This shrinking also relates to the build-up of harmful proteins and worse memory performance.

In frontotemporal dementia (FTD), the shrinking is mostly seen in the frontal, insular, and anterior temporal lobes. Parkinson's disease (PD) patients show less consistent brain shrinkage, usually only in some regions like the parahippocampal gyrus, temporal gyrus, and occipital lobe when the disease is severe. However, newer studies with larger groups of patients found that even early on, Parkinson's can cause shrinkage in many parts of the brain, including deep brain areas like the basal ganglia and various parts of the cortex.

Besides looking at brain volume, measuring the thickness of the brain's cortex is also useful. For example, thinner cortex in the entorhinal cortex is a sensitive sign of mild cognitive impairment and Alzheimer's. People with moderate to severe Parkinson's also show overall thinning of the cortex, especially after 5 years of having the disease. Cortical thickness can even help tell Alzheimer's apart from FTD, since Alzheimer's patients usually have more thinning.

Another important feature seen on MRI is white matter hyperintensities (WMHs). These are bright spots on certain MRI scans that often indicate small blood vessel problems in the brain. They may be caused by poor blood flow, damage to the blood-brain barrier, or even inflammation. WMHs have been linked to many neurodegenerative diseases like mild cognitive impairment, Alzheimer's, Parkinson's, Lewy body dementia, and FTD. The amount of WMHs also seems to be related to how severe a person's cognitive and psychiatric symptoms are.

While structural MRI is very helpful there are some challenges. Different MRI machines and scanning methods can affect how well these brain changes are detected. Sometimes, it's necessary to do multiple scans over time to really see disease progression. Also, many patients have other health issues or more than one brain disease, which can make interpreting the scans harder. For example, WMHs are also seen in people who've had strokes, so not every MRI finding points only to neurodegenerative diseases (Huang G et al.,2023).

7. A GROWING CRISIS: UNDERSTANDING AND TACKLING NEURODEGENERATIVE DISEASES

As the U.S. population gets older, more and more people are developing neurodegenerative diseases (NDDs), especially those that cause dementia. Dementia is a group of symptoms that affect memory, thinking, and daily functioning. The risk of developing dementia after age 55 is very high — nearly 48% for women and 35% for men. Experts predict that by 2060, the number of new dementia cases in the U.S. will double, reaching about 1 million people each year. This increase will put enormous pressure on the healthcare system, with total yearly costs for care expected to soar to \$1 trillion by 2050 (Chenchu et al., 2025)..

Detecting dementia early and giving a clear diagnosis is very important. Early detection helps patients get the care they need and qualify for new treatments that might slow the disease. It also supports research to find better therapies. Sadly, over half of dementia cases in the U.S. are diagnosed late — only after symptoms become moderate or severe. This delay is even worse in racial and ethnic minority communities. There are also many mistakes in diagnosing different types of dementia, which means some patients do not receive the right care.

Catching dementia early can uncover causes of memory and thinking problems that might be reversible. It helps keep patients safe and allows them to plan ahead for their care and legal decisions. Early detection also connects patients and their families to special programs that improve their quality of life and reduce healthcare costs.

Recently, new treatments approved by the FDA are available to modify the course of Alzheimer's disease (AD) and other neurodegenerative diseases. These treatments work best in the early stages and are not effective for advanced illness. Identifying patients early also helps find suitable candidates for clinical trials, which are essential for developing better future treatments.

Diagnosing these diseases is very hard. Many primary care doctors feel they don't have enough time or confidence to diagnose dementia properly. They often prefer to send patients to specialists, but there are not enough dementia specialists to meet the demand, and this shortage is growing. Many neurologists and geriatricians hesitate to take complex dementia cases and instead refer them to specialized centers. The waiting time to see a dementia specialist is expected to be over 40 months by 2027, and the delay is even worse in rural areas, where wait times can be three times longer than in cities.

The diagnosis process is complicated because it involves collecting a lot of information and carefully analyzing it, which takes a lot of time. After diagnosis, managing these diseases is becoming more difficult as new treatments require intensive monitoring. Many primary care providers struggle to keep up with the fast pace of research and treatment options. New care models suggested by Centers for Medicare and Medicaid Services (CMS) also require resources that the current healthcare workforce cannot fully support (Galal et al., 2024)..

7.1 Collecting High-Quality Data: The First Step to Better Diagnosis

Collecting detailed and reliable data is the foundation for diagnosing dementia accurately and quickly. High-quality, standardized data helps doctors create personalized care plans and supports research efforts. It also allows Artificial Intelligence (AI) systems to learn and improve continuously (Haocong Rao et al., 2025).

In areas like brain imaging, genetic testing, and some biomarker tests, standard ways to organize and share data already exist. For example, brain MRI scans use a system called Brain Imaging Data Structure (BIDS) to keep data organized. Genetic data follows standards like VCF and HGVS, and biomarkers have formats like MIAME and MIAPE. However, other important data types, like results from cognitive tests or speech assessments, don't have widely accepted standards yet. This lack of standards makes it hard to compare and combine data from different research centers.

It's important that data collection methods are easy for patients and their caregivers, increase access to care, and don't add extra burden to healthcare providers. Experts should come together to create and update these standards. A national group like the National Institutes of Health (NIH) could help lead this effort, although other models for managing AI and data collection have also been considered.

7.2 Prioritizing Useful Clinical Data

The data collected should first focus on what doctors currently use to diagnose neurodegenerative diseases. This includes:

* Patient history (what symptoms started, when, and how they changed)
* Physical examination findings
* Cognitive test results
* Brain imaging like MRI scans
* Biomarkers (tests that measure disease indicators in blood or spinal fluid)

In the future, AI might also use data gathered automatically from wearable devices, sensors, and electronic health records (EHRs) to detect early signs of dementia. AI could review old medical records and notes to find important clues and generate questions for doctors to ask during patient visits.

Passive data, collected continuously through devices that monitor sleep, speech, typing, and walking, shows promise in spotting subtle changes months or years before symptoms become obvious. However, this kind of data is mostly used in research right now, not in everyday clinical care.

7.3 Collecting the Patient's History: The Starting Point

Right now, diagnosing dementia depends on patients or their caregivers noticing changes and telling their primary care doctor. More people are using the internet and online tools to learn about their symptoms, which could help identify dementia earlier.

To support early detection, we need tools that can capture symptoms as soon as possible, either during healthcare visits or at home. These tools should fit into routine doctor visits, like the Medicare annual wellness visit, using short screening questions to spot cognitive problems. If the patient seems at high risk, a more detailed assessment should be available (Haocong Rao et al., 2025) .

Because older patients may find writing or typing difficult, these tools should allow patients to talk naturally, like having a conversation with a caring doctor. Conversational agents—computer programs that can talk with people—show promise for collecting medical histories. So far, most have used text only and for simple cases, but new large language models (LLMs) can power voice-based conversational agents that speak naturally and adapt explanations to a patient's language and education level. These tools could help reduce disparities by serving patients who speak different languages or have limited access to care. However, some studies show these tools don't always work well for non-English speakers, so more work is needed.

Because doctor visits are short, it is hard for doctors to get a complete history from patients who may be confused or upset. Patients often see many specialists, leading to repeated questions and delays in diagnosis. Incomplete notes also limit the data available for AI support.

A conversational agent with an LLM, given enough time, could collect a detailed history like a specialist would. It could ask focused questions that help distinguish different types of dementia, such as Alzheimer's, frontotemporal dementia, or Lewy Body disease. Voice-based agents could be used over the phone, improving access for people with lower income, language barriers, or mobility issues.

These agents could be used at many points in the care pathway. For example, when a patient calls to schedule an appointment mentioning memory problems, or when a nurse calls before the visit, they could connect the patient to the conversational agent to gather information before seeing the doctor. This approach would save valuable time during the appointment, letting doctors focus on discussing results and care plans.

An LLM can also help by summarizing the patient's history into clear notes for the doctor, highlighting key symptoms and patterns. It can include relevant past information from previous visits. This summary can then be used by AI tools to support the doctor's decision-making, reducing their workload and encouraging adoption of these tools.

Meanwhile, many healthcare centers are using "ambient AI scribes," which listen to doctor-patient conversations and automatically write notes in real time. This technology is a first step toward comprehensive AI help in documentation and could improve diagnosis support in the future. However, these scribes still miss some early details, such as how the illness first appeared.

7.4 Cognitive Testing: Objective Measures of Brain Function

When symptoms are concerning, doctors need objective tests to measure thinking and memory problems. These tests should be easy to give, scalable, and able to identify which brain functions are affected, helping doctors understand the pattern of impairment and make an accurate diagnosis.

Currently, cognitive tests take time, require trained staff, and can be less accurate for underserved minorities. In the past, doctors usually recorded only a total score, without noting which specific abilities were weak. AI could help interpret these tests better.

Luckily, new digital cognitive tests are being developed. Some can be done at home or in clinics by medical assistants with little training. For example, the TabCAT Brain Health Assessment (BHA) used at UCSF has been widely adopted in primary care clinics. It showed higher sensitivity for detecting dementia and mild cognitive impairment (MCI) than older tests like the MoCA.

Research into digital cognitive tests is growing, and AI is being incorporated to improve them further.

After collecting history and cognitive test results, AI tools could generate a list of possible diagnoses, explain them, and suggest next steps, such as lab tests or brain scans. The doctor would get this information before the visit, verify details with the patient, and discuss the results and plans during the appointment.

Collecting history and test results beforehand frees up the doctor's time to build trust and make shared decisions with the patient and family. AI can also help explain things clearly and empathetically.

7.5 Physical Examination Still Matters

Physical exams remain important for diagnosing some dementia types. For example, motor symptoms like tremors, balance problems, or speech issues may indicate diseases like Lewy body dementia, corticobasal syndrome, or amyotrophic lateral sclerosis. Conversely, Alzheimer's disease usually lacks these motor signs.

While in-person exams are best, video visits can reveal many physical signs, helping patients who can't travel to specialists. AI models are getting better at analyzing video for speech and movement patterns, which could support diagnosis.

7.6 Neuroimaging: Brain Scans

MRI brain scans are more widely available now, including mobile scanners that bring imaging closer to patients. Although brain scans are less often a bottleneck, their diagnostic value is sometimes overlooked in traditional reports.

Integrating AI to interpret MRI scans spotting patterns of brain shrinkage or damage—will help doctors diagnose dementia more accurately (Haocong Rao et al., 2025).

Biomarkers: Disease Indicators in Blood and Fluid

Biomarkers have become valuable for diagnosing Alzheimer's and other dementias. Tests like amyloid PET scans or cerebrospinal fluid (CSF) analysis are less accessible, but new blood tests show great promise and are becoming available in clinics.

These tests provide structured data that AI can interpret easily. Still, they must be considered alongside patient history, cognitive tests, and imaging to be accurate.

In summary, collecting standardized, detailed, and high-quality data from many healthcare systems is key to using AI successfully in dementia diagnosis and management. Good data improves AI's diagnostic accuracy now and allows it to learn and improve over time.

As new diagnostic tests become better and easier to use, the data needed may change. For example, a very accurate blood test for Alzheimer's might simplify history taking.

To make this happen, we need a strong, inclusive system across many institutions to gather data and continuously refine what is collected. Doing so will unlock the full power of AI to help doctors interpret patient information and provide better care for people with neurodegenerative diseases.

8. CHALLENGES IN IMPLEMENTING AI-DRIVEN ND DIAGNOSTICS

While AI has shown great promise in diagnosing neurodegenerative diseases, its implementation in real-world healthcare settings is fraught with a number of complex challenges. These issues span data limitations, technical hurdles, ethical concerns, and broader institutional and societal barriers.

The challenge is to get access to correct dataset to build the AI tool we require all different types of data without losing accuracy and on other hand sharing the sensitive data should maintain the privacy Before the AI model is used it should be tested properly Many doctors and patients may feel uncomfortable putting too much trust in AI especially when it comes to serious medical decisions. Fairness is other challenge AI model should work for all the data Not every healthcare facility has the resources These systems often need powerful computers, fast internet, and skilled professionals to operate and maintain them (Haocong Rao et al., 2025).

9. FUTURE DIRECTIONS AND EMERGING TRENDS IN NEURODEGENERATIVE DISEASES

9.1 Personalized Medicine Through Genetics:

we should be very thankful to new genetic research and scientists because they are able to find certain genes that can increase a person's risk of getting brain diseases like Alzheimer's or Parkinson's. This can helps doctors to treat considering specifically each person's uniquc genes.

9.2 Easier Diagnosis with Blood Tests:

In olden days, to find brain diseases doctors had to do some painful tests like spinal taps or brain scans to find brain diseases. But now, new signs in the blood like p-Tau217 and PSD-95 are making it easier. With the help of simple blood or plasma tests, doctors are able to detect these diseases earlier and more safely.

9.3 AI and Big Data Working Together:

The new technology Artificial Intelligence is helping doctors to find early signs of brain diseases. It can learn and study from brain scans, blood tests, and even EEG results. AI can also gather and combine information from different sources like images, genetic tests, and medical records to give a clearer idea of patient health. By tracking symptoms over time the Wearables and health apps can also help .

9.4 New Treatments for Brain Diseases:

Instead of treating the warning signs and symptoms, researchers are now dealing to find the ways to reduce or treat brain damage. Newly introduced methods like gene therapy, RNA-based drugs, and stem cell treatments are tested. These may help to treat diseases more effectively.

9.5 Better Diagnoses with Multiple Tools:

Doctors are now using a integration of tests to get more accurate and faster results. For example, they may combine PET scans, blood tests, and AI tools. These methods and technologies are used in real hospitals to enhance how brain diseases are diagnosed.

9.6 Using Digital Tools for Healthier Habits:

To stay healthy Apps and smart devices are helping people. They can track every action like sleep, exercise, and eating habits. Based on this data, the app will suggest the different ideas to improve daily routines, which may help to reduce brain diseases.

9.7 Worldwide Long-Term Studies:

over many years, Large studies around the world are tracking people by collecting data on genetics, lifestyle, blood tests, and digital tools, scientists are learning more about how brain diseases start and how to treat them better.

9.8 Making AI Fair and Easy to Understand:

Researchers are working hard to make AI tools more accurate and easier to understand. Researchers want doctors and patients to trust these tools and make sure they work equally well for people of all backgrounds.

9.9 Rules to Use AI Safely in Real Life:

In hospitals to utilize safely this new technology, government agencies and researchers are p framing some rules. These rules will help us that know that AI tools are properly tested and used in a safely and accurate way in healthcare.

9.10 Exploring the Power of AGI (Artificial General Intelligence):

Some scientists are beginning to look into how a more advanced type of AI, called Artificial General Intelligence will help to treat brain diseases. In the future, AGI may look at different kinds of information like brain scans, genetic data, and patient behavior all at the same time. This will help doctors understand the disease better to make smarter choices and give treatment and care that's more suited to each patient (Haocong Rao et al., 2025).

10 CONCLUSION: EXPLORATIVE AI IN NEURODEGENERATIVE DISEASES

Artificial Intelligence is playing a major role in understanding and how to treat neurodegenerative diseases. AI has the ability to study and gain information from large and various types of data, such as genetic tests, brain scans and also life style habits and it is helping researchers and doctors to detect the early signs of diseases. Generally, exploratory AI will be useful for identifying the hidden patterns and spotting the warnings that might be missed,, which can lead to early and more accurate diagnoses.

By knowing the data of all types of information regarding medical AI can help to create personalized plans for treatment a to detect how a disease will develop over the time. This will help doctors to take appropriate actions as early as possible and give the patients better treatment and care. Moreover, implementing AI in healthcare can have some challenges. challenges may include maintaining privacy for patient records and making sure AI tools are more accurate. Helping healthcare systems adapt to new technologies. Despite these obstacles, AI offers a better future where neurodegenerative diseases can be detected in early stages and handled more effectively, giving patients a better quality of life.

REFERENCES

Bhavana, S., Akula, A., Rao, V. N., & Swetha, C. (2025). Advanced AI Approaches in Education. In *Supporting Personalized Learning and Students' Skill Development With AI* (pp. 1–16). IGI Global Scientific Publishing. DOI: 10.4018/979-8-3693-8965-2.ch001

Chenchu, S., Kandem, V., Dattaram, T., & Rao, T. V. N. (2025). The convergence of artificial intelligence and graphical user interface. In *Supply Chain Transformation Through Generative AI and Machine Learning* (pp. 69–102). IGI Global Scientific Publishing. DOI: 10.4018/979-8-3693-4433-0.ch004

Erdaş, Ç. B., & Sümer, E. (2024). CNN-Based Neurodegenerative Disease Classification Using QR-Represented Gait Data. *Brain and Behavior*, *14*(10), e70100.

Galal, A., Moustafa, A., & Salama, M. (2024), Transforming Neurodegenerative Disorder Care with Machine Learning: Strategies and Applications. Available at *SSRN*: https://ssrn.com/abstract=5114443 or http://dx.doi.org/DOI: 10.2139/ssrn.5114443

Huang, G., Li, R., Bai, Q., & Alty, J. (2023, July 22). Multimodal learning of clinically accessible tests to aid diagnosis of neurodegenerative disorders: A scoping review. *Health Information Science and Systems*, *11*(1), 32. DOI: 10.1007/s13755-023-00231-0 PMID: 37489153

Muñoz-Mata, B. G., Dorantes-Méndez, G., & Piña-Ramírez, O. (2024). Classification of Parkinson's disease severity using gait stance signals in a spatiotemporal deep learning classifier. *Medical & Biological Engineering & Computing*, *62*(11), 3493–3506.

Rao, H., Zeng, M., Zhao, X., & Miao, C. (2025). A survey of artificial intelligence in gait-based neurodegenerative disease diagnosis, Neurocomputing, Volume 626,, 129533, ISSN 0925-2312, DOI: 10.1016/j.neucom.2025.129533

Setiawan, F., & Lin, C. W. (2021). Identification of neurodegenerative diseases based on vertical ground reaction force classification using time–frequency spectrogram and deep learning neural network features. *Brain Sciences*, *11*(7), 902.

Uyanik, H., Sengur, A., Salvi, M., Tan, R. S., Tan, J. H., & Acharya, U. R. (2025). Automated Detection of Neurological and Mental Health Disorders Using EEG Signals and Artificial Intelligence: A Systematic Review. *Wiley Interdisciplinary Reviews. Data Mining and Knowledge Discovery*, *15*(1), e70002. DOI: 10.1002/widm.70002

Wang, M., Ma, C., Liu, A., Xiao, H., Ren, Y., Li, Z., Wang, Z., Xia, Q., Dou, P., Li, B., & Chen, P. (2024). A bibliometric analysis of acupuncture for Parkinson's disease non-motor symptoms from 2003 to 2023. *Complementary Therapies in Medicine*, *87*, 103111. DOI: 10.1016/j.ctim.2024.103111 PMID: 39542379

ABBREVIATIONS

AD- Alzheimer's Disease:
ADNI- Alzheimer's Disease Neuroimaging Initiative:
AI- Artificial Intelligence:
ALS- Amyotrophic Lateral Sclerosis:
CNNS- Convolution Neural Networks:
GNN- Graph Neural Networks:
MCI- Mild Cognitive Impairment:
MND- Motor Neuron Disease:
PD- Parkinson's Disease:
RNN- Recurrent Neural Networks:
SVM- Support Vector Machines:

Chapter 9
A Novel Stacking-Based Sustainability-Driven Machine Learning for COVID-19 Prediction

P. Umamaheswari
https://orcid.org/0000-0003-2007-697X
SASTRA University, India

ABSTRACT

The role of machine learning is no longer limited to the field of computation. Machine learning has a huge potential in every possible field. The field of medicine is not an exception. Machine learning can be used to predict if a person is affected by COVID-19 or not as well as predict the number of cases of COVID-19 on a given day. The existing solutions give the result based on a particular machine learning model and other statistical models. This has many disadvantages, as the single machine learning model chosen, say for example logistic regression, to predict if a person is affected by the disease or not and to predict the number of cases may or may not give accurate results. This is where the importance of our solution comes in. Here the proposed solution is a hybrid model, which is the combination of machine learning models such as Naive Bayesian, logistic regression, random forest, etc. The results demonstrate that hybrid ML models can provide reliable and scalable tools for aiding clinical decision-making and public health policy.

DOI: 10.4018/979-8-3373-5641-9.ch009

1 INTRODUCTION

The Coronavirus disease is an emergency that started its development in the end of 2019 and quickly turned into the global health crisis that impacted human life, economy, and healthcare systems around the world significantly. The introduction of the new virus and the unparalleled spread with the resulting impact raised the significance of effective prediction, early detection, and real-time decision-support mechanisms. The traditional epidemiological models, however, useful, were not able to withstand the dynamicity and non-linearity of the pandemic process, huge influx of heterogeneous data, and the dynamism of the social and environmental environment affecting the spread of the disease.

Here, machine learning (ML) has become a revolutionary solution that can be used to model intricate relationships and derive meaningful trends when working with huge and multidimensional datasets. Using the data provided by the clinical records and laboratory tests, imaging modalities, mobility patterns, and even social media trends, the ML algorithms can help predict the rates of infection, anticipate the outcomes of the patient, and allocate healthcare resources efficiently. Their ability to combine a wide range of data sources, constantly learn new information and provide highly accurate predictions due to their adaptability makes them invaluable resources in the intelligence of pandemics.

Machine learning algorithms, including classical methods like decision trees, support vector machines, and random forests and deep learning models like convolutional neural networks and recurrent neural networks, have been adequately utilized to a wide range of COVID-19-related problems. They are the early detection of medical images (CT scans, X-rays), the identification of patients with high risks according to demographic and clinical data, the forecast of mortality and recovery rates, and the forecast of the infection trends by region.

Furthermore, the predictive analytics that is driven by ML has been of critical importance in aiding policymakers and authorities in health. Governments have been in a position to evaluate the efficiency of the containment efforts, forecast the healthcare needs, and formulate intervention strategies based on the data through predictive modeling and real-time surveillance. The combination of artificial intelligence, analytics of big data and cloud computing has also made it possible to install predictive models in practical scenarios at a scale and quickly.

Nonetheless, there are difficulties with the integration of ML in the prediction of pandemics. The question of data quality, imbalance, privacy, model interpretability, and regional generalizability are some of the issues that should be handled with caution to achieve reliable results. Nevertheless, even with these shortcomings, the pandemic has further spurred digitalization in the healthcare sector and highlighted the critical role of smart systems in addressing international health crises. The disease caused by Coronavirus is a significant threat and pandemic with a footprint in more than 212 countries.

The need of the hour is to look into the parameters of space to control and prevent the pandemic which as on 14th of June 2020 had taken the lives of over 4,32,902 people and affected over 78,98,442 people all over the world. The objective is to find the crucial factors that affect the spread of COVID-19 in Iran and present the results so that they can be useful in the decision-making of competent authorities. Nowadays, the hybrid deep learning model developed by the authors by combining a Convolutional neural network and a recurrent neural network. The main focus of combining these two models was that they required good results. Since these are bio-inspired algorithms, they have very good computational power. Since this is a classification problem, the major problem was overcoming and bridging the gap created due to a lack of thorough investigation and combinations of deep learning models built to predict COVID-19.

The SARS-CoV-2 virus, which is the cause of the COVID-19 pandemic, has impacted approximately 507 million people worldwide. Medical practitioners now use imaging to improve diagnostic accuracy for conditions that were first diagnosed with real-time RT-PCR assays. However, deciphering COVID-19 (Shoeibi et al., 2024) from these pictures takes a lot of work and is prone to human mistakes. Deep learning (DL) models, in particular, are a type of artificial intelligence (AI) that can produce consistently high-performing outcomes. An extensive overview of the use of DL methods for COVID-19 diagnosis using medical imaging is presented in this publication. To diagnose COVID-19, the study explores crucial areas of Computer-Aided Diagnosis Systems (CADS) based on DL techniques, including segmentation, classification, explainable AI (XAI), and predictive research. In light of COVID-19, it also examines rehabilitation technologies like the Internet of Medical Things (IoMT).

Research on uncertainty quantification (UQ) is presented, with a particular emphasis on DL models for Covid-19 diagnosis. According to a study looking at the prevalence of the Hepatitis A virus (HAV) among men who have sex with men (MSM) in Amsterda (Alberts et al., 2019), the Netherlands, the incidence rose in 2016–17 following a four-year hiatus and peaked in MSM at the age of 35. The HAV seroprevalence among MSM who visited the STI clinic was 37%; this prevalence rose with age and was consistent from 2006 to 2017. In multivariable analysis, older age, nationality from a HAV endemic country, and HBV seropositivity were determinants of HAV seropositivity. When the HAV immunization was available for free instead of a fee, MSM opted-in more frequently (89% versus 11%, respectively; $p<0.001$). When payment was necessary for vaccination, younger MSM were less likely to get the shot ($p= 0.010$). According to post-hoc analysis, whether the HAV vaccination was provided for free or for 75 euros, respectively, 98% versus 46% of

MSM who visited the Amsterdam STI clinic would be protected against contracting the virus. The study found that the Amsterdam MSM population is susceptible to another HAV outbreak and strongly advised that MSM be provided with free hepatitis A vaccinations.

2 LITERATURE SURVEY

This literature review has covered the relevant research on COVID-19 prediction techniques, providing an overview of several models, their uses, and comparative evaluations of their advantages and disadvantages.

This study adds to the above in a number of ways. Authors (Aviv-Reuven & Rosenfeld, 2021) focused on both COVID-19 and non-COVID-19 papers, providing an assessment of how the effects of the pandemic differ concerning these two types of papers; (3) their study analyzes time to acceptance for COVID-19 and non-COVID-19 publications as well as international collaboration by the diversity of the countries that are collaborating; (1) their study gives a wider perspective in which the influence of the pandemic on current research can be observed; (2)Due mostly to an increase in COVID-19 articles, there were fewer COVID-19 papers published in January, which resulted in a higher SEM. From February onward, the SEM gradually increased. In contrast to non-COVID-19 publications in 2020 and publications in 2016–2019, COVID-19 papers appear to "enjoy" a quicker time to acceptance period, notwithstanding the trend that has been noticed.

Their data and analyses support the previous hypothesis that a correlation exists between non-COVID-19 status and a longer acceptance time. To fully comprehend the implications of the short time to acceptance for COVID-19-related studies, more research is necessary, both about post pandemic publications in general and other, non-COVID-19 publications published at the time of the pandemic. Due to the rapid spread of COVID-19, a prompt and precise diagnosis method is now required. The chest X-ray scan (Elaraby et al., 2024) is a reliable and effective viral identification method. Based on chest X-ray scans, this study suggests a hybrid intelligent model for COVID-19 patient identification. Preprocessing X-ray pictures, extracting robust features using five different methods, classifying the scans using a deep convolutional neural network (DCNN), and creating an IoT platform with a mobile client application and backend system are the five steps of the model.

The COVID-19 epidemic has spread over the world, and no effective treatment or vaccine has yet been created. Experts in healthcare are attempting to provide early detection and prompt treatment strategies. The goal of their work(Atta-ur-Rahman et al., 2021) is to present a thorough analysis of the function that AI and machine learning play in examining virus prediction methods.

To assess and identify possible threats, a mathematical model has been developed. The model that has been suggested is a cloud-based smart detection technique that makes use of support vector machines (CSDC-SVM). A 15-fold cross-validation approach was used to attain an accuracy of 98.4% in the experimental results. Comparing the suggested CSDC-SVM model to comparable cutting-edge techniques, the former has higher accuracy and efficiency.

Another study(Moulaei et al., 2022) focuses on how artificial intelligence (AI) and machine learning are being used to investigate COVID-19 pandemic prediction methods. Comparing machine learning techniques for COVID-19 mortality prediction utilizing patient data at the time of initial admission was the goal of the research. To forecast COVID-19 mortality, the researchers trained multiple machine learning algorithms using data they took out of the Ayatollah Taleghani Hospital registry in Abadan, Iran. Among the 1500 patients that took part in the trial, men made up the majority. The study identified 38 characteristics, and the three most significant predictors of COVID-19 death were dyspnea, ICU admission, and oxygen therapy. The three least significant predictors were platelet count, aminotransferase, and smoking. With accuracy, sensitivity, precision, specificity, and receiver operating characteristic (ROC) values of 95.03%, 90.70%, 94.23%, 95.10%, and 99.02%, respectively, Random Forest (RF) outperformed other machine learning (ML) methods in terms of performance. Instead of using susceptible-infected-recovered (SIR) and susceptible-exposed-infectious-removed (SEIR)(Ardabili et al., 2020) models to predict the COVID-19 epidemic, this paper compares the efficacy of machine learning and soft computing methods.

Promising outcomes were demonstrated by two models: the adaptive network-based fuzzy inference system (ANFIS) and the multi-layered perceptron (MLP). The highly complex nature of the COVID-19 epidemic and its variance in behavior across nations lead the study to propose machine learning as a viable approach to simulate the outbreak.

In addition to suggesting that combining machine learning and SEIR models can result in a true novelty in outbreak prediction, the work offers preliminary benchmarks to illustrate the potential of machine learning for future research. Having access to precise models for outbreak prediction is crucial to gain an understanding of the potential transmission and outcomes of infectious illnesses.

The novel coronavirus disease, known as COVID-19, has shown itself to be nonlinear and complex, with many known and unknown factors contributing to its propagation and the intricate behavior of its population across multiple geographical zones. Global population has been greatly affected by COVID-19, especially vulnerable populations like diabetic patients. Studies on the topic have multiplied exponentially, although their bibliometric properties are unknown. The purpose of this article is to describe the global research output on diabetes and COVID-

19 that is indexed in Scopus. The scientific production comprised a total of 1956 documents with 35086 citations and an h-index of 67. Publications from Diabetes and Metabolic Syndrome: Clinical Research and Reviews (n¼127) and American researchers (n¼498) dominated the literature. The most influential articles (n¼314) were written by Chinese authors, as indicated by the citations they earned (n¼21757).

Leading nations in terms of research participation include China, India, and Spain. Leading the way in this broad international scientific collaboration are Italy, the United States, and China (Prakash, 2020). The number of papers on COVID-19 and diabetes as well as their influence on science demonstrate the motivation that these diseases' research provides to the world's scientific community. Nations in Europe, China, and the United States mostly contribute to publications.

Surgical and emergency care guidelines, viral etiology, and international responses to the COVID-19 pandemic are the most often discussed subjects. Research strategies to address COVID-19 issues varied throughout nations based on affluence and degree of transmission. (Tran et al., 2020) The necessity of international research cooperation between high- and low-/middle-income nations in the various phases of pandemic prevention and control was brought to light by the findings.

As of February 10, 2020, information is available regarding the current understanding of the transmission of SARS-CoV, MERS-CoV, and SARS-CoV-2 through blood products. Pathogen inactivation techniques for coronaviruses are also covered. (Chang et al., 2020) Humans developed severe respiratory illness as a result of two further coronavirus infections: Middle East Respiratory illness (MERS) in 2012 and SARS in 2002–2003. The three newly discovered infectious diseases that are spreading over the world are all brought on by β-coronaviruses.

Coronaviruses often affect the upper or lower respiratory tract but can also shed their virus into the serum or plasma. Thus, the transfusion of labile blood products carries a theoretical risk of coronavirus transmission. Concerns regarding blood safety and coronaviruses have emerged, particularly in endemic locations, since an increasing number of asymptomatic infections are being discovered among COVID-19 cases. Healthcare institutions desperately need decision-making systems to combat this infection and assist them in receiving appropriate recommendations in real-time to stop its spread (Vaishya et al., 2020). Artificial Intelligence functions effectively to emulate human intelligence. It might also be extremely important in comprehending and recommending the creation of a COVID-19 vaccine. Proper screening, analysis, prediction, and tracking of existing patients and possible future patients are done with the help of this result-driven technology.

The important apps track data on instances that have been confirmed, recovered from, and died.

In the end, 36 patients received a COVID-19 pneumonia diagnosis. At the time of presentation, 35 individuals had abnormal CT results, and 1 patient had a normal CT.

Thirty patients tested positive for rRT-PCR, with six cases initially missing. These six patients showed results from the first two rRT-PCR assays (after two, two, and three days, respectively), whereas the other three patients did not show results until the third round of rRT-PCR testing (after five, six, and eight days, respectively). [12] Consequently, the initial rRT-PCR sensitivity was only 83.3%, while the CT sensitivity at presentation was 97.2%. In summary, rRT-PCR could result in an initial false negative result. Severe (Cao, 2020) coronavirus disease 2019 (COVID-19) symptoms include lymphopenia, pneumonia, worn-out lymphocytes, and a cytokine storm. There is a noticeable increase in antibody production, however it is unclear if this is pathogenic or protective. Determining the immunopathological alterations in COVID-19 patients is crucial for clinical care and offers possible targets for medication development. The leading funding organizations that (Akintunde et al., 2021) promoted mental health research and provided assistance for over 180 papers were the National Institutes of Health in the United States, the National Institutes of Health in the United States, and the National Natural Science Foundation of China.

The United States of America accounted for the largest share of COVID-19 Pandemic papers on mental health, contributing 1157 (21.23%), closely followed by China with 741 (13.60%). The research offers valuable insights into the worldwide research outlook for scientific advancements regarding the COVID-19 Pandemic public health emergency and mental health concerns. This can have a substantial impact on and support interventions aimed at enhancing individuals' mental health following the pandemic. The severity level among COVID-19 patients admitted to the hospital was determined by the requirement for mechanical ventilation and the 30-day mortality (30DM) rates.

Outcomes There were 1795 patients in this sizable COVID-19 cohort from a single institution.

The age distribution was heterogeneous, with a mean of 59.7 years. 156 patients (8.6%) passed away within 30 days of admission, while 236 patients (13%) needed mechanical ventilation. The 10-CV approach was used to validate each prediction model's predicted accuracy. With 192 sub-trees, the Random Forest classifier for the 30DM model produced results of 0.72 sensitivity, 0.78 specifcity, and 0.82 AUC. The 64 sub-trees in the model used to predict MV (Raman et al., 2023) yielded 0.81 AUC, 0.75 sensitivity, and 0.75 specifcity. (Assaf et al., 2020) to better prioritize medical resources, and to enhance COVID-19 pandemic management in general. Based on 14 clinical variables, the researchers used six distinct classifiers (i.e., BaileysNet, Logistic, IBk, CR, PART, and J48) (Arpaci et al., 2021) to build six predictive models for COVID-19 diagnosis.

Existing studies examined 114 cases from the Zhejiang Province's Taizhou Hospital in China. With an accuracy of 84.21%, the results demonstrated that the CR meta-classifier is the most accurate classifier for predicting positive and negative

COVID-19 cases. The findings may aid in the early detection of COVID-19, particularly when RT-PCR kits are insufficient for detecting the virus. They may also support developing nations beset by a lack of specialist laboratories and RT-PCR test kits.(Khanday et al., 2020) in the future for increased accuracy. These are the findings from the work of a few researchers.

Initially, verification data was used to confirm that the deep learning-based economic effect prediction model (Devaraj et al., 2021), which was developed using historical data on infectious diseases, could forecast inflation rates with 77% accuracy. Second, the COVID-19 trend and the findings of the economic impact prediction model for the next year were provided by the author. This model is based on the deep learning-based infectious disease. Currently, the majority of research on COVID-19 that has been published focuses on using statistical mathematical calculations to anticipate the spread of the disease. Using deep learning technology and historical infectious diseases data, this study is expected to serve as an empirical reference for effective and proactive decision-making by forecasting the economic conditions and illness propagation associated with COVID-19.

3 PROPOSED FRAMEWORK

This part describes the process flow of the proposed system. The proposed system has been implemented in the following steps. First, the datasets- genuine and fake are read. Now, each of these datasets is added to a target column and fill it with "True" and "Fake" in their respective datasets. Both of these datasets are concatenated. After that, datasets are shuffled for better accuracy. In the Second step, the input data are preprocessed. Here, the "Date" column is dropped, followed by the drop of the "Title" column. Then, all the data is converted to lowercase, followed by the removal of all. The workflow of the proposed system is shown in the Figure.1

Figure 1. Block Diagram of the Proposed Framework

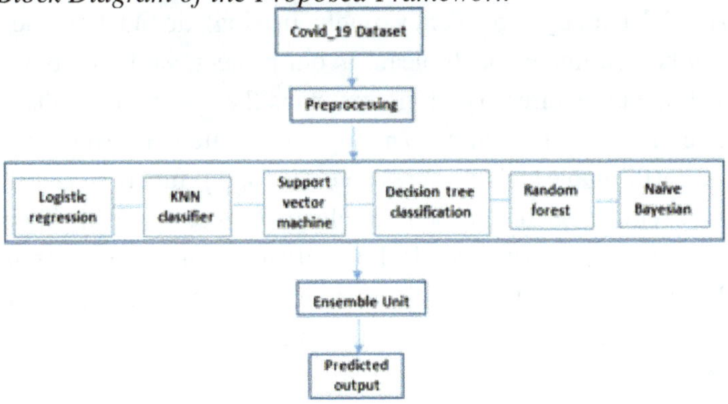

The dataset is first preprocessed which is per- formed by dropping the id column, filling null values by Nan Object for better processing runtime, replacing the empty age values with the average of the age column, label encoding gender and symptoms, converting dates into date-time objects, converting date time objects into ordinal values and dropping location and country columns, in the order specified. Next, the data is split into 80 percent training and 20 percent testing data. This is followed by subjecting the training data to the six machine learning models. Logistic regression is applied with a random state of 99. Next, KNN classification is done in a loop for various values of 'k'. The optimal value obtained for both training and testing data is k=11. Hence, the value of k was assigned to 11 with a random state of 99. Next, SVM was run with a random state of 1 followed by DTC with the same random state and with a depth of 1 for maximum accuracy. This was followed by RFC, with the number of estimators at 200 for optimality.

At last NB classification was performed with a random state of 99. Now that all the model have been trained with the 80 percent training data, all of them are subject to evaluation with the 20 percent testing data. Now, the ensemble algorithm is applied to the output obtained from all of the models mentioned above under the maximum voting parameter, and followed by this output is generated.

The proposed methodology is that instead of relying entirely on one particular machine learning algorithm, relying upon a hybrid model is much better.

3.1 Logistic Regression

In this model, we use the logistic function to model the occurrence of a particular class in the result column of a data set, which is generally Boolean in nature. In our project, it is either positive or negative. This can also be generalized to problems that don't have Boolean output. In that case, the output will be mapped to any value between a zero and a one. It is a model in Mathematics that is based on a logistic equation to model a binary dependent variable. In a logistic function, the dependent variables may be continuous or Boolean. In our project, we have both Boolean as well as non-Boolean features. The function maps the logarithm of the odds to the result variable or the target column. The log-odds scale is measured using a logit unit; hence, it got the name logistic regression. Analogous functions can also be used.

The logistic regression model itself actually models outcome likelihood in terms of input and does not perform statistical classification (it is not a classifier), but it can be used to create a classifier, e.g., by selecting a cut-off value and by classifying inputs with a probability more significant than the cut-off as one class, below the cut-off as the other; this is a typical way to make a binary class. This is how we have used this in our project. Here we use logistic regression to classify if a person has COVID-19 or not based on the data set we have which is obtained from Kaggle. With a random state of 99, LR was performed on the dataset, giving an accuracy of 89.5 percent, as seen in Figure 2.

Figure 2. Logistic regression (a) Confusion Matrix (b) Evaluation Metrics

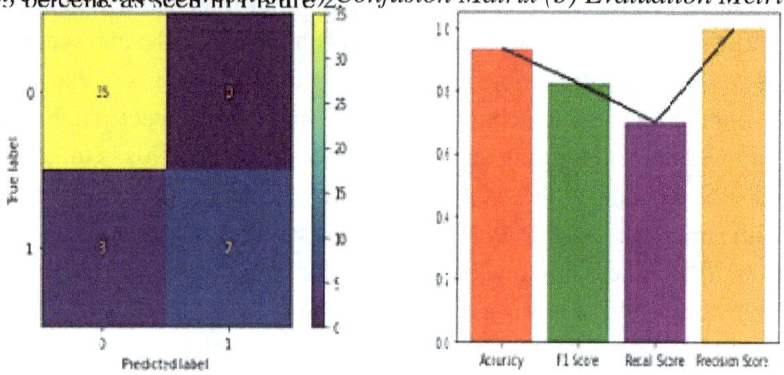

3.2 KNN algorithm

The KNN algorithm is based upon the fact that if two objects are similar, they will be placed near each other. There is a famous saying that if one tells his/her friends, we can tell his/her character.

The principle behind the KNN algorithm is also the same. This algorithm classifies the data points into clusters, and we can see that within each cluster, the distance between the points is lesser than the distance between a point in the current cluster and a point in the nearby or far cluster.

One of the key parameters this algorithm considers is the number of neighbors. With a random state 99, the algorithm was executed. It was run from 1 to 99 to find the optimal value of ‘k’. It was observed that at k=11, the best accuracy was obtained for both training as well as testing data. Hence, k was fixed to be 11. As

Figure 5. KNN Classifier (a) Confusion Matrix (b) Evaluation Metrics

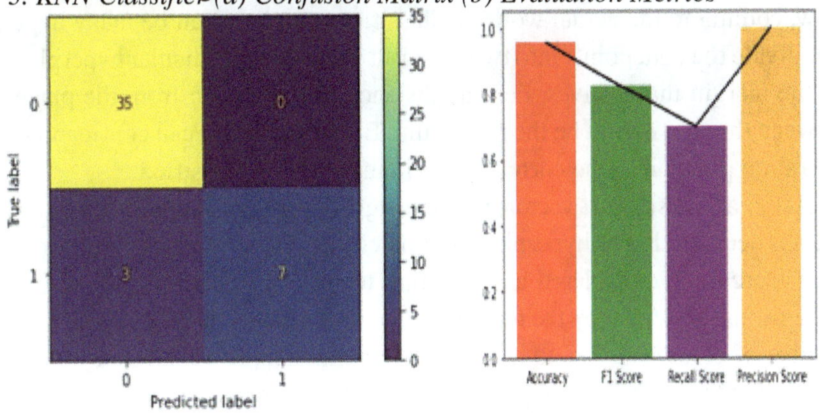

The KNN Algorithm

1. The first step is to get the data loaded.
2. The second step is to set the value of 'k', the number of neighbors to be taken into consideration (the optimal value of k is 11)
3. The third step is a loop to be performed for every data point present.
   - The first step in the loop is to find the distance between the data under the query and the current data.
   - The second step in the loop is to add this example and its distance to a collection which is ordered in nature.
4. The fourth step is to subject the ordered collection of indices and distances in increasing order based on the distance
5. The fifth step is picking up the first 'k' rows from the sorted collection.
6. The sixth step is to obtain the selected rows' labels
7. The last step is the return of 'k' labels' most occurring element

3.3 Support Vector Machine

With less computation power, if we need a machine learning model, we first need to consider the support vector machine. Though support vector machines can be utilized for both classification and regression, the general purpose or the most widely used purpose is classification.

This is why we chose this as a classification model in our project. The main theme of the support vector machine algorithm is to label sets of points in their respective classes based on a plane called a hyperplane which parameters of the data given to the model. Now, the parameters that are present in the data are called dimensions. Now, coming to the actual work of Classification, there can be many hyperplanes that divide the data points into two sets. But we select a particular hyperplane based on the margin that it gives, i.e., the distance of separation from the plane or that between the sets should be the maximum. By doing so, we can confidently classify the future points into the correct set of points already classified.

As far as the support vector machine algorithm is concerned, the boundary that takes a decision is the hyperplane that is chosen. The points that fall on a particular side can be considered as belonging to that particular class. The number of dimensions is decided by the number of features present in the data set or the actual number of columns given to the model. For example, if we have only two features to be considered, then the hyperplane of separation is just a line. Now, consider the number of features

Or columns we have is 3, in this case we get a 2-D plane as a hyperplane. The hyperplane will be plane with one or many bents or curves when the number of features we have is greater than 3, as in our case. Now, there are many points on either side of the hyperplane. There will be points that have an influential character because they are near the hyperplane, and they are even capable of altering the hyperplane itself! These points are called support vectors. If we add or delete one or more of these support vectors, we can alter the hyperplane. The intention is maximizing the margin to the highest extent possible. If the output of the SVM is 1, then it means that the data point belongs to one class, and if it is -1, it belongs to another. In our case, it is positive or negative. SVM was executed with a random state of 1, and it got an accuracy of 89 percent, as seen in Figure 7

Figure 4. Support vector machine (a) Confusion Matrix (b) Evaluation Metrics

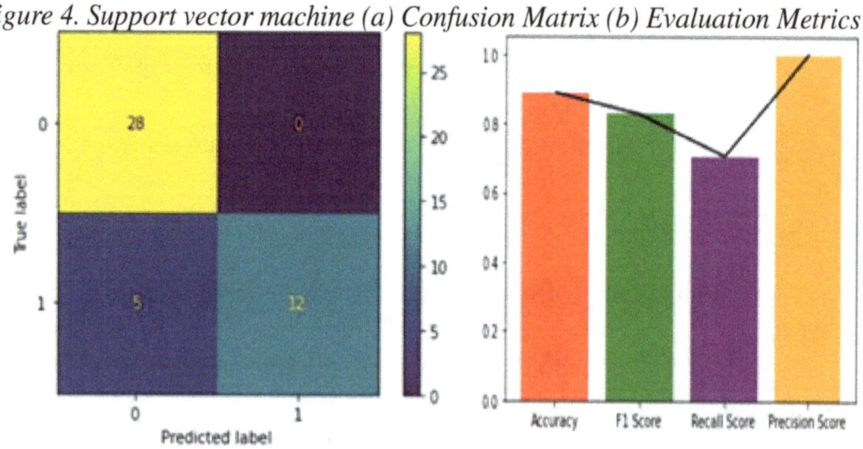

3.4 Decision Tree Classifier

This machine learning model works by asking queries and getting the answers. The queries are based on the data set we have. If it gets an answer, then following that particular answer, a series of questions is asked. This is done until and unless a target column is achieved, thereby building a tree. Now we define a decision tree to be a data structure that is hierarchical in nature. Just like a tree in data structures, here too we have a set of nodes and a set of edges that are directed. So, we can also define this to be a tuple containing a set of nodes and another set of edges, each having a direction.

Now, the following are the fundamental units of the decision tree: 1) Root node is the first and foremost node of the tree. As it is the root node, it strictly doesn't have any incoming edge and may or may not have one or more edges going out of it. 2) Internal nodes are the nodes that are internal to the tree, meaning that they have precisely one edge that is incoming and at least one or more edges going out from them. If they don't have any outgoing edge, they fall under the third category.3)Leaf or terminal nodes are the nodes that have one incoming node, just like any internal node, but strictly don't have any edge going out from them. We assign a class label to each leaf node of a decision tree.

Figure 5. Decision tree classifier (a)Confusion Matrix (b) Evaluation Metrics

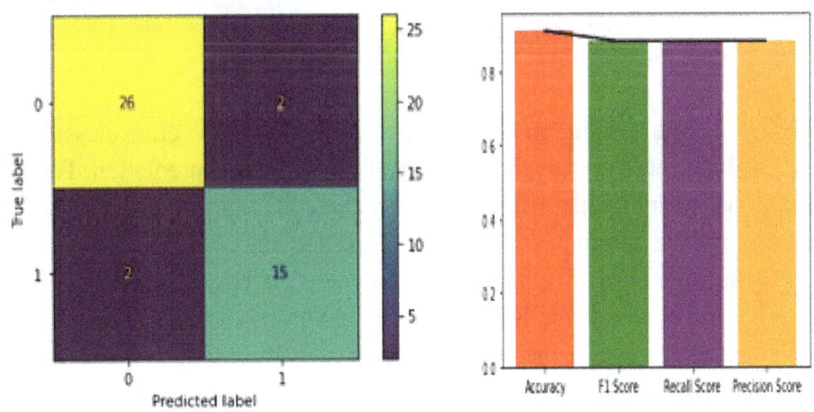

All the other non-terminal nodes, the root node, and other internal nodes are used for decision-making. They act as conditional determiners for deciding which part of its children the current data belongs to. The impurity degree of the child nodes is considered when selecting the split that best fits our data. The class distribution will be skewed if the impurity chosen is less. To find whether a test condition performs well or not, we will compare the parent node's impurity degree before the split and the child nodes' impurity degree after the split. We say that a test condition is reasonable based on the difference observed. If it is high, it means that the test condition or the split is good else it is poor.

Another factor to be determined is the depth of the tree and in our project for the best accuracy, we limited the depth to 1. As seen in Figure. 6, DTC, with a depth of 1, got an accuracy of 93 percent. Random forest classifier A Random forest classifier, by itself, is an ensemble of many decision trees that are already built based on various parameters.

Figure 6. Random forest (a) Confusion Matrix (b) Evaluation Metrics

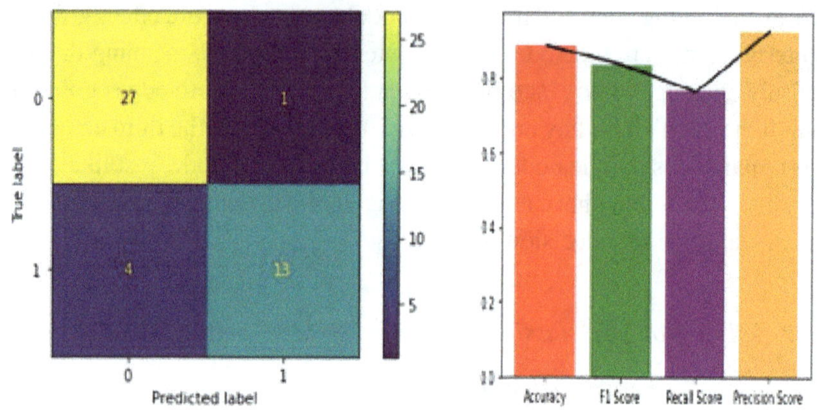

This machine learning model itself acts as a maximum voting classifier- it takes the class that is predicted by the majority of the trees as its prediction. The main idea behind this model is that instead of considering a single tree's output, it is always better to give the output based on many trees. It is one of the best models available: "A large number of relatively uncorrelated models (trees) operating as a committee will outperform any of the individual constituent models." The statistically basic logic behind this is that the correlation between the fundamental units (trees) is very low; hence, each fundamental unit is independent of anything else in the pool of trees. It can be seen that the ensemble model's predictions are much better than any of the individual predictions. Since all the trees don't err in the same direction, they protect each other.

This is the core reason this is such a good model. Let us assume 'I' trees produce the wrong result. This means that the remaining 'n-I' trees have given the correct output and it is clear that 'I' will always be strictly less than 'n/2'. The above also becomes a part of the prerequisites of this model: One or many of our features must signal so that it is much better than simply giving the output based on randomness. The correlation between the individual trees must be low so that each tree performs work as an independent unit. To get the maximum accuracy, the number of estimators was fixed to 200, and it achieved an accuracy of 90 percent, as seen in Figure. 8.

Naive Bayesian Classifier Bayes' Theorem was based on independent events and hence gave rise to a set of classification algorithms referred to as Naıve Bayes Classifiers. Every classification made in this set of classifiers is independent of classification made by any other classifier and hence they constitute a family of Naive Bayesian Classifiers. Our data set consists of many features like age, gender, place, etc. Consider our dataset, which describes the details of a person under the COVID probe. Given the details, each row is classified as Positive ("Yes"). or Negative("No") for COVID positivity. This set of classifiers divides the data into two major components – the response vector and the feature matrix. The matrix contains all the parameter values or the rows of the data set, and hence, it is treated as a matrix as far as Naiıve Bayesian Classifiers are concerned. In the above dataset, features are 'Hospital visited,' 'Symptom1', 'Visited COVID Places' and 'From COVID Places,' 'Age,' 'Gender' etc. The response vector is the collection of all values present in the target column or feature of the dataset. In our dataset, the class variable name is 'Result'.

The prerequisites of these set of classifiers is that each parameter makes an independent contribution and an equal contribution to the result of the model As far as our dataset is concerned, this can be said as follows: No two features are dependent on each other. For example, the "Symptom1" parameter being 'Fever' has nothing to do with the parameter "From COVID Places" being 1 or the parameter "Visited COVID Places" being '0' has no effect on 'Age'. It is therefore clear that each feature is independent of each other. The other notable thing in these classifiers is that each input parameter is given the same weightage. Also, no feature is completely irrelevant to the outcome, and each parameter is equally accountable for the outcome.

There are two Naive Bayes classifiers as follows: Multinomial Naive Bayes Classifier: In a multinomial distribution, if we represent the frequencies with which events are generated as feature vectors, it comes under the multinomial Naive Bayesian Classifier. This type is used in document classification problems. Bernoulli Naive Bayes: In this classifier, the features are either a '1' or a '0'. This can be used in problems where we need, say for example, the frequencies of each word in a document. In our project with a random state of 99, it got an accuracy of 92 percent as seen in Figure. 8.

At last, the ensemble model is built which takes the maximum votes from each of the above said models and gives the output as positive or negative.

Figure 7. Naive Bayesian Classifier (a) Confusion Matrix (b) Evaluation Metrics

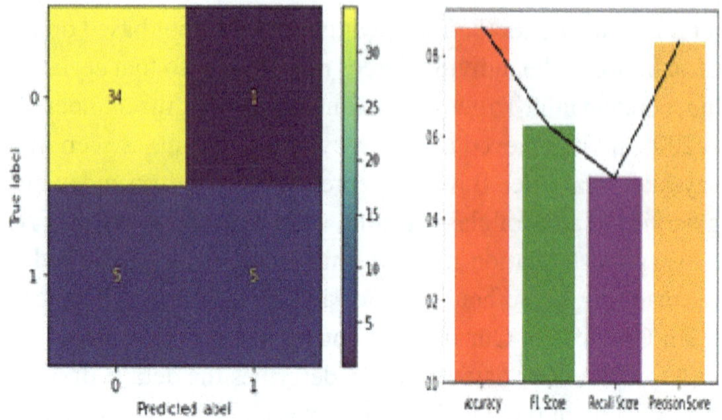

4 EVALUATION BY COMPARING OF ALL THE MACHINE LEARNING MODELS

Comparative analysis and evaluation of machine learning models plays an important role in determining the most appropriate algorithm to use in the COVID-19 prediction problems. Because both models possess their advantages, assumptions, as well as performance features, objective analysis can make sure that forecasting is not only correct but also applicable to the unknown data. The process of evaluation is based on the training of various models, e.g. decision trees, support of machine learning (SVM) and neural networks on the same dataset and the evaluation of their predictive ability based on the usual metrics of performance. Such a comparative analysis can contribute to identifying the most suitable model that could be used to characterize the multifaceted relationships between demographic, clinical, and imaging characteristics of patients with COVID-19. The initial part of model evaluation is dividing the given data into training and testing to avoid overfitting. The training set is used to train models and the testing set is used to test the models to determine their ability to generalize. Accuracy, precision, recall, F1-score, and area under the ROC curve (AUC) are some of the most commonly used performance measures. To give an example, in the forecasting of the COVID-19 infection or its severity, a high-precision model will reduce the number of false positives, whereas a high recall rate will ensure that most of the true cases are correctly detected. An equal F1-score means that the performance is good in terms of sensitivity and specificity, which is necessary in medical prediction tasks where false alarms and missed detections are both serious consequences.

Various models have varied performance characteristics with respect to the data complexity and structure. Decision trees can be readily interpreted and work well in smaller datasets and might overfit. Support vector machines have high classification boundaries and can effectively deal with nonlinear data but it has to be used with great care on tuning of hyperparameters. Neural networks especially deep learning models are capable of modelling large and high-dimensional data such as CT or X-ray images, although they require a great deal of computing power and large training sets to prevent bias.

Figure 8. Comparison of all classifier model

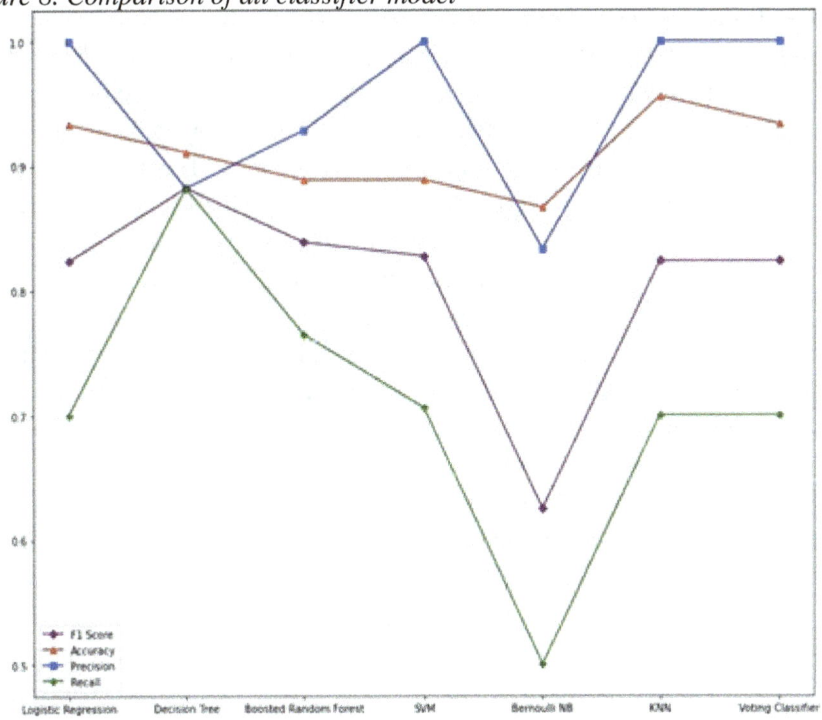

Through comparison, the researchers will be able to determine trade-offs between interpretability, accuracy, and computational efficiency by comparing these models under comparable experimental conditions. Lastly, another useful tool in the evaluation process is to make use of the statistical validation and visualization tools like cross-validation and ROC curves in addition to confusion matrices. These tools are able to give more information about the behavior of models at various thresholds and data divisions.

In addition to numerical measures, model interpretability and clinical relevance are equally critical - particularly when predictions are used to make medical decisions in the real world. Therefore, the evaluation process will not only be used to benchmark models according to technical performance, but also identify how applicable in practice the models would be in healthcare systems in predicting pandemics, patient triage, and decision support. With the comparison, researchers will be able to propose the best balanced and reliable machine learning model to inform evidence-based responses to the COVID-19 crisis.

5 CONCLUSION AND FUTURE PLANS

Overall, the use of machine learning methods has already shown itself as a promising strategy in terms of causing and predicting COVID-19 cases. These smart models can not only aid in detecting infections but also provide the best management of patients because they can be matched and even customized to monitor and treat at the individual level of the progression of the disease. The machine learning will result in a quicker, data-driven decision-making in the healthcare setting by using a variety of datasets, including clinical parameters and imaging, as well as epidemiological data. Nonetheless, to guarantee clinical utility and validity of these predictive systems, it is necessary to validate them further using large and real-world datasets. The strong testing of various populations and healthcare environments will improve the generalizability and accuracy of the models. To apply in practice, the suggested application may be applied to end-user systems to enable individuals or healthcare practitioners to input the necessary data and get instant predictions or risk assessment.

This is a convenient design that makes it easy to access and use by a diverse population. Although the discussed machine learning-based COVID-19 prediction system has a great potential to help healthcare practitioners and the general population, there are multiple ways in which its functioning and application can be improved. Further studies need to be dedicated to the enhancement of the model dataset with more demographic, clinical, and genomic variables, which would allow making more accurate and personalized predictions. The model can also be enhanced with the inclusion of the data of different geographical areas and the transformation of the virus types, which would increase the flexibility and stability of the model to the emergence of new patterns of the disease. The other trend worth following is integration of the Internet of Things (IoT) and cloud computing technologies to establish an intelligent and connected prediction ecosystem.

REFERENCES

Akintunde, T. Y., Musa, T. H., Musa, H. H., Musa, I. H., Chen, S., Ibrahim, E., Tassang, A. E., & Helmy, M. S. E. D. M. (2021). Bibliometric analysis of global scientific literature on effects of COVID-19 pandemic on mental health. *Asian Journal of Psychiatry*, *63*, 102753. DOI: 10.1016/j.ajp.2021.102753 PMID: 34280888

Alberts, C. J., Boyd, A., Bruisten, S. M., Heijman, T., Hogewoning, A., Rooijen, M. V., Siedenburg, E., & Sonder, G. J. B. (2019). Hepatitis A incidence, seroprevalence, and vaccination decision among MSM in Amsterdam, the Netherlands. *Vaccine*, *37*(21), 2849–2856. DOI: 10.1016/j.vaccine.2019.03.048 PMID: 30992222

Ardabili, S., Mosavi, A., Ghamisi, P., Ferdinand, F., Varkonyi-Koczy, A., Reuter, U., Rabczuk, T., & Atkinson, P. (2020). COVID-19 Outbreak Prediction with Machine Learning. *Algorithms*, *13*(10), 249. DOI: 10.3390/a13100249

Arpaci, I., Huang, S., Al-Emran, M., Al-Kabi, M. N., & Peng, M. (2021). Predicting the COVID-19 infection with fourteen clinical features using machine learning classification algorithms. *Multimedia Tools and Applications*, *80*(8), 11943–11957. DOI: 10.1007/s11042-020-10340-7 PMID: 33437173

Assaf, D., Gutman, Y., Neuman, Y., Segal, G., Amit, S., Gefen-Halevi, S., Shilo, N., Epstein, A., Mor-Cohen, R., Biber, A., Rahav, G., Levy, I., & Tirosh, A. (2020). Utilization of machine-learning models to accurately predict the risk for critical COVID-19. *Internal and Emergency Medicine*, *15*(8), 1435–1443. DOI: 10.1007/s11739-020-02475-0 PMID: 32812204

Atta-ur-Rahman, , Sultan, K., Naseer, I., Majeed, R., Musleh, D., Abdul Salam Gollapalli, M., Chabani, S., Ibrahim, N., Yamin Siddiqui, S., & Adnan Khan, M. Atta-ur-Rahman. (2021). Supervised Machine Learning-Based Prediction of COVID-19. *Computers, Materials & Continua*, *69*(1), 21–34. DOI: 10.32604/cmc.2021.013453

Aviv-Reuven, S., & Rosenfeld, A. (2021). Publication patterns' changes due to the COVID-19 pandemic: A longitudinal and short-term scientometric analysis. *Scientometrics*, *126*(8), 6761–6784. DOI: 10.1007/s11192-021-04059-x PMID: 34188333

Cao, X. (2020). COVID-19: Immunopathology and its implications for therapy. *Nature Reviews. Immunology*, *20*(5), 269–270. DOI: 10.1038/s41577-020-0308-3 PMID: 32273594

Chang, L., Yan, Y., & Wang, L. (2020). Coronavirus Disease 2019: Coronaviruses and Blood Safety. *Transfusion Medicine Reviews*, *34*(2), 75–80. DOI: 10.1016/j.tmrv.2020.02.003 PMID: 32107119

Devaraj, J., Madurai Elavarasan, R., Pugazhendhi, R., Shafiullah, G. M., Ganesan, S., Jeysree, A. K., Khan, I. A., & Hossain, E. (2021). Forecasting of COVID-19 cases using deep learning models: Is it reliable and practically significant? *Results in Physics*, *21*, 103817. DOI: 10.1016/j.rinp.2021.103817 PMID: 33462560

Elaraby, M. E., Ewees, A. A., & Anter, A. M. (2024). A robust IoT-based cloud model for COVID-19 prediction using advanced machine learning technique. *Biomedical Signal Processing and Control*, *87*, 105542. DOI: 10.1016/j.bspc.2023.105542

Khanday, A. M. U. D., Rabani, S. T., Khan, Q. R., Rouf, N., & Mohi Ud Din, M. (2020). Machine learning based approaches for detecting COVID-19 using clinical text data. *International Journal of Information Technology : an Official Journal of Bharati Vidyapeeth's Institute of Computer Applications and Management*, *12*(3), 731–739. DOI: 10.1007/s41870-020-00495-9 PMID: 32838125

Moulaei, K., Shanbehzadeh, M., Mohammadi-Taghiabad, Z., & Kazemi-Arpanahi, H. (2022). Comparing machine learning algorithms for predicting COVID-19 mortality. *BMC Medical Informatics and Decision Making*, *22*(1), 2. DOI: 10.1186/s12911-021-01742-0 PMID: 34983496

Prakash, K. B. (2020). Analysis, Prediction and Evaluation of COVID-19 Datasets using Machine Learning Algorithms. *International Journal of Emerging Trends in Engineering Research*, *8*(5), 2199–2204. DOI: 10.30534/ijeter/2020/117852020

Raman, G., Ashraf, B., Demir, Y. K., Kershaw, C. D., Cheruku, S., Atis, M., Atis, A., Atar, M., Chen, W., Ibrahim, I., Bat, T., & Mete, M. (2023). Machine learning prediction for COVID-19 disease severity at hospital admission. *BMC Medical Informatics and Decision Making*, *23*(1), 46. DOI: 10.1186/s12911-023-02132-4 PMID: 36882829

Shoeibi, A., Khodatars, M., Jafari, M., Ghassemi, N., Sadeghi, D., Moridian, P., Khadem, A., Alizadehsani, R., Hussain, S., Zare, A., Sani, Z. A., Khozeimeh, F., Nahavandi, S., Acharya, U. R., & Gorriz, J. M. (2024). Automated detection and forecasting of COVID-19 using deep learning techniques: A review. *Neurocomputing*, *577*, 127317. DOI: 10.1016/j.neucom.2024.127317

Tran, B. X., Ha, G. H., Nguyen, L. H., Vu, G. T., Hoang, M. T., Le, H. T., Latkin, C. A., Ho, C. S. H., & Ho, R. C. M. (2020). Studies of Novel Coronavirus Disease 19 (COVID-19) Pandemic: A Global Analysis of Literature. *International Journal of Environmental Research and Public Health*, *17*(11), 4095. DOI: 10.3390/ijerph17114095 PMID: 32521776

Vaishya, R., Javaid, M., Khan, I. H., & Haleem, A. (2020). Artificial Intelligence (AI) applications for COVID-19 pandemic. *Diabetes & Metabolic Syndrome*, *14*(4), 337–339. DOI: 10.1016/j.dsx.2020.04.012 PMID: 32305024

Chapter 10
Diabetic Retinopathy Detection at Early Stage Using DRNET13 With Attention Mechanism

M. Kamaladevi
https://orcid.org/0000-0001-8486-5092
SASTRA University, India

V. Venkataraman
SASTRA University, India

A. Sumathi
https://orcid.org/0000-0003-4700-5573
SASTRA University, India

ABSTRACT

Diabetic Retinopathy (DR) is a diabetes complication that affects the eyes and damaged blood vessels in the retina which can lead to vision loss and even blindness. Machine learning algorithms for DR detection have some limitations, such as lagging in feature extraction and selection. Data are taken from the Diabetic retinopathy detection dataset, which is available at www.kaggle.com for training and evaluate the model. Deep Learning methods, such as Diabetic Retinopathy Network 13 (DRNet13), a CNN-based architecture model performed exceptionally well, attaining the best result. But not concentrate on retinal images that have mild DR-related abnormalities may be less resilient to minor alterations in the appear-

DOI: 10.4018/979-8-3373-5641-9.ch010

ance of the lesion or differences in image quality. In proposed technique combining the novel DRNet13 architecture with an attention mechanism to enhance diagnostic performance. Proposed technique outperform the existing methods,

1.INTRODUCTION

Diabetic Retinopathy (DR) is one of the leading causes of blindness among working-age adults globally. Preventing serious vision loss requires early diagnosis of this microvascular consequence of diabetes that affects the retina. Conventional manual screening procedures are subjective, time-consuming, and mostly rely on ophthalmologists' knowledge. Artificial intelligence has been transformed by deep learning, and two of the most popular architectures are Convolutional Neural Networks (CNNs) and Recurrent Neural Networks (RNNs). The main purpose of a Convolutional Neural Network (CNN) is to handle input that has a grid-like structure, like photographs. CNNs automatically extract spatial information like edges, textures, and forms by using convolutional layers. CNNs lower dimensionality while keeping important information by using filters and pooling procedures. Because of this, they perform exceptionally well in activities like computer vision applications, object identification, image classification, and medical imaging. They eliminate the need for human feature engineering by learning hierarchical features straight from raw data.

A Recurrent Neural Network (RNN), on the other hand, is designed especially to manage sequential or time- A Recurrent Neural Network (RNN), on the other hand, is designed especially to process sequential or time-series data, where the input order is important. RNNs can retain "memory" of past inputs because, in contrast to conventional feedforward networks, their connections create directed cycles. RNNs are therefore ideally suited for machine translation, speech recognition, natural language processing (NLP), and stock market forecasting. By efficiently handling long-term dependencies, variants such as Long Short-Term Memory (LSTM) and Gated Recurrent Unit (GRU) overcome the drawbacks of conventional RNNs. When combined, CNNs and RNNs offer strong solutions for a variety of real-world issues involving sequential and spatial data. Automated deep learning algorithms have demonstrated great promise in supporting the early detection and categorization of diabetic retinopathy. Globally Many working people loss their vision the reason behind this scenario due to chronic diabetic.

The early stages of DR are marked by the presence of microaneurysms (MAs), small red dots in the retina caused by the weakening of capillary walls. Identifying the early indicators of diabetic retinopathy is crucial to prevent its advancement into severe non-proliferative or proliferative stages. Qiao et al. (2020) developed a deep learning–based diagnostic model capable of detecting microaneurysms (MAs) and assessing the severity of non-proliferative diabetic retinopathy (NPDR) through semantic segmentation and convolutional neural networks (CNNs). Similarly, Goel et al. (2021) explored deep learning methods for stage-wise classification of DR severity using color fundus images. Their study showed that CNNs surpass traditional machine learning techniques by automatically extracting key features and delivering high accuracy. In addition, hybrid CNN models such as CNN-ResNet and CNN-DenseNet have been employed for automated DR stage classification. Yasashvini et al. (2022) reported that among these, the hybrid CNN-DenseNet model achieved superior results with an accuracy of 96.22%, reinforcing the effectiveness of deep learning models in analyzing fundus images.Rapid developments in deep learning have made automated diagnosis with retinal fundus images a dependable and effective method. A 13-layer deep convolutional neural network called DRNet13 was presented as a specific architecture designed for the identification of diabetic retinopathy in order to overcome the difficulties associated with precise classification and feature extraction in DR. In order to detect mild symptoms like microaneurysms, hemorrhages, and exudates early on, DRNet13 is made to extract hierarchical spatial features from retinal pictures.Nevertheless, not every extracted feature makes an equivalent contribution to classification in conventional CNNs. The attention mechanism is incorporated into DRNet13 to get around this restriction, improving the model's capacity to concentrate on the most pertinent retinal regions.

Attention enhances interpretability and diagnostic precision by giving clinically important features greater weights and suppressing irrelevant ones. Better sensitivity in identifying early-stage DR and greater robustness in differentiating between severity levels are guaranteed by this combination of DRNet13 and attention. In the end, the integration facilitates computer-aided detection of diabetic retinopathy that is more accurate, dependable, and clinically significant.

Convolutional Neural Networks (CNNs) have become the standard choice for medical image analysis since they can automatically extract hierarchical features directly from raw image data. Using publicly available datasets such as MESSIDOR, Kaggle DR, and IDRID, many CNN-based models have achieved impressive accuracy in detecting, grading, and segmenting diabetic retinopathy (DR).

Pinedo-Diaz et al. (2022) highlighted the importance of assessing retinal image quality in DR screening. They noted that real-world clinical images often suffer from issues like noise, blurriness, or poor lighting, which can significantly reduce the performance of deep learning models trained on high-quality datasets. To address this, the authors developed a lightweight CNN for classifying image quality into binary categories, achieving an outstanding AUC of 98.6%. Their findings emphasize that integrating image quality assessment with DR detection models enhances both the robustness and generalizability of automated screening systems in real clinical environments.

The accuracy of DR classification has seen significant improvement with the adoption of transfer learning using pre-trained models such as DenseNet, ResNet, InceptionV3, and AlexNet. Among these, DenseNet has demonstrated superior performance in distinguishing between various stages of diabetic retinopathy and predicting disease progression, achieving an impressive classification accuracy of 98%.

In a recent study, Bhimavarapu and Battineni (2023) proposed an enhanced activation function to improve DR detection using CNNs. Their experiments, which compared different CNN architectures across datasets like DIARETDB0, DRIVE, CHASE, and Kaggle, revealed that ResNet-152 achieved an outstanding accuracy of 99.41% on Kaggle images. Their approach effectively combined deep convolutional neural networks with GPU acceleration, enabling efficient and high-speed analysis of retinal fundus images with minimal processing delay. Semantic segmentation enables detailed pixel-level analysis of retinal images, allowing even small microaneurysms (MAs) to be accurately detected. This fine-grained approach greatly improves the ability to categorize diabetic retinopathy (DR) severity across different stages—early, moderate, and severe non-proliferative DR (NPDR).. The study further incorporates feature extraction strategies such as Maximum Matching Filter Response (MFR), Mutual Information (MI), and Laplacian of Gaussian (LoG) filters, optimized using Differential Evolution techniques. This combination enables a robust framework for the detection of retinal lesions that surpasses traditional image processing methods. Comparing with other literature, several studies reinforce the efficacy of CNNs in DR detection and classification.. Their model incorporated transfer learning to handle the limited availability of labeled data and showed notable improvement in classifying DR stages from early to proliferative phases.

In this article, proposed an advanced solution using custom convolution neural network architecture named DRNet13, integrated with a Convolution Block Attention Module (CBAM) to enhance feature extraction and classification accuracy. Motivated by the success of architectures such as VGG, ResNet, and DenseNet, researchers have explored customized lightweight networks for specialized applications in medical imaging. Within this context, DRNET13 is introduced as a novel deep CNN framework specifically designed for the detection and classification of diabetic retinopathy (DR) from retinal fundus images.

Thirteen convolutional layers make up the DRNET13 architecture, which is thoughtfully arranged to strike a compromise between computing efficiency and depth. In contrast to conventional networks that prioritize incredibly deep hierarchies, DRNET13 concentrates on progressive feature refinement. This means that while deeper layers extract higher-level pathological features like microaneurysms, exudates, and hemorrhages, low-level layers capture basic retinal structures like blood vessels. The goal of this architecture was to reduce the computational burden of overly deep models while simultaneously increasing the sensitivity of DR detection, especially in the early phases.

The flexibility of DRNET13 for attention integration is one of its unique features. Standard CNNs might not be able to capture the discriminative relevance of DR lesions since they are frequently tiny and poorly dispersed. In order to overcome this restriction, DRNET13 incorporates attention modules that direct the network to minimize unimportant background patterns and highlight clinically significant retinal regions. CBAM attention mechanism is used. Convolutional neural networks benefit from the lightweight and effective CBAM attention mechanism, which improves feature learning. It uses attention in two dimensions in a sequential manner:By giving various feature channels weights and highlighting the most instructive ones, Channel Attention establishes what is significant.By emphasizing particular spatial areas in the image that are most crucial to the prediction (such as retinal lesions), spatial attention helps identify what is significant.

The model can better predict diabetic retinopathy by focusing on important features in retinal fundus pictures, such as microaneurysms, hemorrhages, and exudates, thanks to CBAM, which combines channel and spatial attention.The network is guaranteed to learn global representations as well as fine-grained information that are crucial for precise early diagnosis thanks to its selective focus mechanism.

Model training and evaluation are the initial steps in the system's extensive pipeline, which begins with dataset collection and preprocessing (CLAHE enhancement, noise removal, and augmentation). Fundus pictures are classified into five DR phases by the model: No_DR, Mild, Moderate, Severe, and Proliferate_DR. Incorporating sophisticated image enhancement techniques and attention processes, the proposed system seeks to increase detection accuracy, decrease false diagnoses, and support rapid decision-making by medical experts.

2. LITERATURE REVIEW

Diabetic retinopathy (DR) remains one of the leading causes of preventable blindness, and its effective management largely depends on early diagnosis. In recent years, machine learning (ML) and deep learning (DL) approaches have been extensively explored for the automated detection of DR from retinal fundus images. These studies have focused on enhancing diagnostic accuracy, reducing computational cost, and addressing challenges related to image quality and dataset limitations.

According to Das et al. (2022), DR detection methods have evolved from traditional ML models to more advanced DL architectures. Earlier ML techniques such as Support Vector Machines (SVM) and Decision Trees, which relied on manually engineered features, showed some potential in classifying fundus images. However, they often struggled to capture the complex hierarchical patterns associated with retinal abnormalities like microaneurysms, hemorrhages, and exudates. In contrast, deep learning models—particularly Convolutional Neural Networks (CNNs) and transfer learning frameworks such as VGGNet and ResNet—have achieved superior results by automatically learning multi-level features directly from raw image data.. The analysis does, however, highlight enduring issues that impede the clinical application of these models, such as overfitting, data imbalance, and inadequate explainability.

(Keerthi et al., n.d.)created a CNN-based approach that can classify the severity of DR into five groups, from proliferative DR to no DR. Using VGG-16 and VGG-19, their model demonstrated 82% accuracy, a sensitivity of 80%, a specificity of 82%, and an area under the curve (AUC) of 0.904. The potential of CNN architectures in clinical decision assistance is demonstrated by this performance. Notably, their study also underlined how crucial it is to preprocess fundus photos, such as by adjusting contrast and brightness, in order to improve model performance. In difficult real-world datasets, the system demonstrated robust classification by identifying small features like microaneurysms and exudates under various lighting conditions.

When taken as a whole, these results show a distinct direction for DR research: away from feature-based ML models and toward end-to-end DL frameworks that combine classification, feature extraction, and preprocessing into cohesive systems. Class imbalance can be addressed using sophisticated resampling techniques, model interpretability can be enhanced, and algorithms can be validated on a variety of clinical datasets to guarantee generalizability. Reviews and empirical research indicate that hybrid models that integrate explainable AI techniques with the advantages of machine learning and deep learning have great potential for DR screening and early intervention in the real world.

(Fayyaz et al., 2023)when effective screening is used, early detection of DR can prevent up to 90% of cases of visual loss. Ant colony optimization was used for feature selection in their study, which presented a hybrid DL-based system that combines AlexNet and ResNet101 feature extraction with support vector machine (SVM) classification. The model's 93% accuracy rate on 750 features shows how well convolutional neural networks (CNNs) operate in conjunction with conventional machine learning classifiers. Crucially, they emphasized the use of data augmentation and preprocessing methods like resizing and k-means clustering to solve class imbalance, which is still a major problem in DR datasets.

Building on prior research, Thanki (2023) proposed a computer-aided triage system for classifying retinal fundus images that integrates traditional machine learning classifiers—such as logistic regression, random forests, and k-nearest neighbors—with deep neural network features. The experimental findings revealed that combining logistic regression with deep features extracted from fundus images outperformed existing glaucoma triage systems, achieving higher sensitivity and specificity. This study also highlighted the versatility of fundus imaging in diagnosing multiple eye diseases, including glaucoma and diabetic retinopathy. Moreover, it emphasized that ensemble methods and transfer learning approaches, particularly those using architectures like VGGNet, ResNet, and DenseNet, can significantly enhance model performance. Further extending this line of research, Mohanty et al. (2023) conducted an in-depth analysis of deep learning models for DR detection by comparing a hybrid VGG16-XGBoost classifier with a DenseNet-121 architecture on the APTOS 2019 Blindness Detection dataset.

. The hybrid VGG16-XGBoost model achieved an accuracy of 79.5%, while the DenseNet-121 architecture demonstrated superior performance, reaching an impressive accuracy of 97.3%. The study also emphasized the critical importance of addressing class imbalance in DR datasets, as unequal representation of severity levels can lead to biased model predictions and reduced diagnostic reliability. Their findings imply that the modest retinal characteristics suggestive of early-stage DR are better captured by deeper designs with dense connectivity

Concurrently, thorough evaluations of DR detection methodologies offer insightful information about patterns and potential paths forward. Because CNN-based models can automatically extract hierarchical features from raw fundus images, removing the need for manual feature engineering, numerous studies consistently show that they perform better than classical ML models. However, when combined with deep feature extraction, conventional classifiers like SVM and random forests continue to be useful and provide good results in hybrid systems ((Fayyaz et al., 2023); (Mohanty et al., 2023)).

Because severe and proliferative DR cases are underrepresented in comparison to normal or mild DR photos, imbalanced datasets are a recurrent problem in the literature. Advanced resampling techniques, data augmentation, and the creation of synthetic images through the use of Generative Adversarial Networks (GANs) have all been used extensively to address issue. Interpretability is still a major issue as well. Despite their excellent accuracy, deep networks' "black-box" nature prevents widespread clinical use. Hybrid ML-DL techniques, according to researchers like (Thanki, 2023), can increase transparency by integrating interpretable features including lesion identification, vessel segmentation, and cup-to-disc ratios.

The use of transfer learning, in which pretrained models like InceptionV3, ResNet50, and VGGNet—which were first trained on big datasets like ImageNet—are refined on DR-specific datasets like EyePACS, Messidor, and APTOS, is another new trend. This approach enhances generalization while lowering computational expenses. Research has demonstrated that CNNs based on transfer learning attain cutting-edge performance, with area under the curve (AUC) values occasionally surpassing 0.94 (Thanki, 2023; Mohanty et al., 2023).

As a whole these studies demonstrate how end-to-end DL systems with excellent classification precision are replacing handcrafted features and conventional ML. The development of explainable AI systems, generalizability across populations, and the requirement for big annotated datasets are still obstacles, nevertheless. To further increase diagnostic accuracy, future studies are probably going to concentrate on interpretable DL frameworks, hybrid and ensemble models, and the incorporation of multimodal data (such as fundus pictures and clinical history).The works under consideration show that automated DR detection and classification could greatly benefit from the use of DL and hybrid ML-DL techniques. The field is moving closer to therapeutically acceptable solutions with DenseNet-121 and hybrid systems demonstrating outstanding results and logistic regression combined with deep features providing interpretability advantages.

(Vij & Arora, 2023) The shift from conventional machine learning (ML) techniques to end-to-end deep learning frameworks is one of the main issues in DR research. Handcrafted characteristics, such as vessel segmentation, microaneurysm recognition, and exudate localization, were necessary for traditional machine learning approaches including support vector machines (SVM), k-nearest neighbors (KNN), and random forests. Although these techniques worked well on some controlled datasets, they were not very generalizable or scalable when used on a variety of populations. On the other hand, it has been shown that convolutional neural networks (CNNs) and transfer learning models are better at automatically extracting hierarchical features from fundus images, which has resulted in notable performance gains .

In DR detection, CNN-based models like AlexNet, VGGNet, ResNet, and DenseNet have been used extensively. Because of their capacity to tackle vanishing gradient issues and identify more profound visual patterns, the ResNet and DenseNet architectures stand out among the others. One especially successful method is transfer learning, which involves fine-tuning models that have already been trained on large-scale datasets like ImageNet on DR-specific datasets like Messidor and EyePACS. This method enhances performance on comparatively smaller medical datasets while significantly lowering training expenses. These models' clinical promise is highlighted by reported accuracies that frequently surpass 90%, with some obtaining area under the curve (AUC) values exceeding 0.95 .

In most DR datasets, images representing mild or normal stages are far more common than those depicting severe or proliferative stages, leading to a significant class imbalance problem. This imbalance often causes models to favor majority classes, thereby reducing their ability to detect early, subtle signs of the disease that are clinically important. To address this issue, researchers have explored various strategies such as cost-sensitive learning, the use of Generative Adversarial Networks

(GANs) to generate synthetic samples, and data augmentation techniques. However, class imbalance continues to pose a challenge, particularly in ensuring that models maintain consistent performance across all levels of DR severity.

Image quality assessment and preprocessing also play a crucial role in achieving reliable model performance. Retinal fundus images often suffer from issues such as noise, blurriness, or uneven lighting, which can hinder accurate feature extraction. To overcome these challenges, preprocessing methods like Gaussian filtering, histogram equalization, and contrast enhancement are commonly used to normalize and improve image quality before inputting them into deep learning models. Additionally, some recent studies suggest incorporating image quality evaluation modules at the initial stage of DR detection pipelines to enhance robustness when dealing with real-world clinical data.

Despite their high accuracy, CNNs and other deep learning architectures often function as "black boxes," providing limited transparency about how decisions are made. This lack of interpretability can reduce clinicians' confidence in automated systems and remains a key barrier to their broader adoption in routine clinical practice.. To address this, researchers have introduced visualization techniques such as class activation maps (CAMs) and heatmaps, which highlight regions of interest in fundus images. By increasing transparency, these techniques allow ophthalmologists to confirm that the model is concentrating on pertinent retinal lesions.The review concludes by highlighting the significance of hybrid and ensemble models, which mix handmade features with deep features or combine the advantages of several classifiers. Hybrid methods have demonstrated superior generalization, as they leverage the precision of DL with the interpretability of traditional ML.

A wide variety of DR detection research are synthesized in which divides them into three categories: hybrid frameworks, deep learning models, and classical machine learning techniques. Support vector machines (SVM), k-nearest neighbors (KNN), random forests (RF), logistic regression, and naive Bayes were among the traditional machine learning techniques that mostly depended on manually created features taken from fundus photos. These characteristics frequently included textural descriptors, exudate location, microaneurysm detection, and vessel segmentation. Although these methods had some success, their scalability and adaptability across a variety of datasets were limited by variations in feature representation and image quality

These drawbacks were resolved by the move toward deep learning, especially convolutional neural networks (CNNs), which made it possible to automatically extract hierarchical features straight from fundus photos. In DR detection and grading tasks, CNN-based architectures like AlexNet, VGGNet, ResNet, DenseNet, and InceptionNet have continuously outperformed their ML counterparts. For example, it has been demonstrated that multitask learning models that integrate regression and classification outputs enhance agreement with clinical grading scales, with some research achieving kappa scores above 0.8 (Systematic Review, 2023). Transfer learning has been a particularly effective technique, lowering computational costs and enhancing model generalizability. This involves fine-tuning pretrained models on big datasets, such as ImageNet, on medical image datasets, such as EyePACS, Messidor, and APTOS.

Despite the significant progress in DR detection, challenges related to dataset composition remain. One of the most persistent issues is class imbalance, where datasets tend to contain a much larger number of images representing mild or normal DR compared to those showing severe or proliferative stages. This imbalance causes models to become biased toward the majority classes, reducing their ability to accurately detect vision-threatening cases. Techniques such as data augmentation, cost-sensitive loss functions, and the use of Generative Adversarial Networks (GANs) to generate synthetic samples have been explored to address this problem. Nevertheless, achieving balanced and reliable diagnostic performance across all DR severity levels continues to be a major challenge.

In *The Lancet Digital Health*, Li et al. (2021) emphasized the importance of AI explainability and regulatory pathways for safe deployment in healthcare. These studies form the foundation for clinical-grade AI, bridging computer vision research and medical diagnostics. The proposed DRNet13 with attention mechanism builds upon these principles by combining interpretability and computational efficiency, aiming to deliver both technical and clinical value.

Nahiduzzaman et al. (2023) made a noteworthy contribution to this area by proposing a novel framework that integrates a Parallel Convolutional Neural Network (PCNN) for feature extraction with an Extreme Learning Machine (ELM) classifier. The effectiveness and robustness of their PCNN-ELM approach were validated using two benchmark datasets—APTOS 2019, comprising 3,662 images, and Kaggle DR 2015, which includes 34,984 images.In both balanced and imbalanced data settings, the suggested system outperformed numerous cutting-edge CNN-based classifiers with accuracies of 91.78% and 97.27%, respectively. Furthermore, the approach worked well with both small and large datasets, solving a significant problem in practical medical applications where the availability of annotated data can fluctuate

(Vij & Arora, 2023)The significance of explainability in clinical AI adoption is further emphasized by the systematic review. Deep learning models are sometimes derided as "black boxes" despite their excellent accuracy. By emphasizing areas of interest in fundus pictures, visualization methods like heatmaps and class activation maps (CAMs) have been used to make these models easier to understand. In addition to fostering clinician trust, this explainability makes ensuring that models base their judgments on medically significant characteristics such as exudates, hemorrhages, and microaneurysm.

Computer-aided diagnostic (CAD) systems that employed handcrafted features including vessel segmentation, exudate detection, and microaneurysm identification were a major component of early DR research . CAD techniques were typically divided into two categories: unsupervised techniques, which used morphological processes and deformable models, and supervised techniques, which used classifiers such as Support Vector Machines (SVMs) trained with labeled data Although these methods demonstrated potential, their reliance on feature engineering and susceptibility to noise in fundus pictures hindered their effectiveness.

An important turning point in DR research was the transition from feature engineering to deep learning architectures. The capacity of Convolutional Neural Networks (CNNs) to automatically extract hierarchical characteristics made them a popular choice. For instance, segmented vessels using CNN and Random Forests, albeit at the price of computational efficiency. Similar to this, some researched showed increased accuracy in retinal vascular recognition by using an ensemble of autoencoders with a softmax classifier. In DR classification tasks, CNN-based frameworks like GoogleNet and ResNet have lately demonstrated impressive performance, frequently over 90% accuracy

The shortcomings of individual CNN models have led to the popularity of hybrid and ensemble techniques. To increase generalization, these techniques mix CNN feature extraction with additional classifiers or combine many networks. This method is demonstrated in a bi-layer deep learning model by (Phridviraj et al., 2023). Using CNN-based models, the first layer of their framework extracts features, and the second layer improves classification by combining features from several models to increase robustness. By capturing both local and global retinal characteristics, this layered technique improves classification accuracy.

Deep learning models are frequently criticized for being “black boxes” despite their excellent predictive capabilities. Clinical adoption is hampered by this lack of interpretability, which also reduces clinician trust. Class activation maps (CAMs), a visualization approach, have been created to solve this issue by highlighting image regions that influence model predictions (Omer, 2024). Bi-layer models may become even more effective as ophthalmologists' decision-support tools if explainability is added.

(Rom et al., 2024)Recent studies have advanced the field by showing that, using fundus images of people without diabetes, AI models can identify diabetes itself—even before retinal problems appear. With an AUC of 0.86 per patient visit and an AUC of 0.83 per image, a convolutional neural network trained on extensive datasets such as EyePACS demonstrated that diabetes can be non-invasively diagnosed from retinal scans. These results demonstrate AI's capacity to identify systemic disease-related subclinical microvascular alterations.

(Shivappriya et al., 2024) proposed Unbalanced distributions of DR severity levels are frequently seen in public datasets. To lessen this problem, methods like picture augmentation (rotation, flipping horizontally and vertically) are frequently used. Proactive patient management is facilitated by deep learning models that not only categorize DR phases but also forecast development timetables. Based on feature similarity percentages, studies have developed algorithms to assess the probability and duration of transition from NPDR to PDR.

(Mishra et al., 2024)By making it possible to automatically extract features from fundus images, deep learning—in particular, Convolutional Neural Networks, or CNNs—revolutionized the diagnosis of DR. showed how transfer learning with VGGNet may improve classification accuracy while addressing the problems of sparse annotated datasets. To improve interpretability and clinical relevance, multi-stage frameworks that integrate lesion segmentation and classification have also been developed. A multi-stage deep learning pipeline for DR grading was presented by who achieved state-of-the-art results on benchmark datasets.Finding important areas of interest (ROI) such hemorrhages, exudates, and microaneurysms requires segmentation. Before deep model training, fundus images are often improved using methods like Otsu thresholding, Contrast Limited Adaptive Histogram Equalization (CLAHE), and morphological procedures.

Although there is no cure for DR, early detection through retinal exams is crucial to halting or preventing vision loss. In order to assist ophthalmologists, a computer-supported diagnostic system that combines ensemble learning, feature extraction, and image segmentation. Multi-level Otsu thresholding for fundus image segmentation, a tried-and-true method for boosting picture contrast and identifying pertinent retinal regions, is the first step in the methodology. Advanced feature extraction techniques, especially the Gray-Level Co-occurrence Matrix (GLCM), which detects textural patterns suggestive of disease severity, are subsequently used to evaluate the segmented pictures. The feature selection and extraction procedure is further strengthened by the addition of dynamic Flemingo optimization, which guarantees that only the most discriminative traits are kept.

(Taifa et al., 2024) reported that the diversity in retinal pictures hindered the use of handmade features with classifiers such as SVM in early investigations. With transfer learning reducing data scarcity, deep learning—in particular, CNNs—improved automatic feature extraction and classification accuracy. Lesion visibility was improved by segmentation methods like CLAHE and Otsu thresholding, while robustness was increased using ensemble models like ResNet and VGG. For increased accuracy, recent studies combine attention processes with hybrid optimization. Despite advancements, issues with generalizability across clinical contexts, imbalanced datasets, and interpretability still exist.

(Prathibha & Siddappaji, 2024) highlights the multifaceted signs and symptoms of DR, such as retinal detachment, exudates, hemorrhages, and microaneurysms. The variability of retinal fundus images—spatiotextural diversity and complicated vascular structures—combined with these changes makes automated detection very difficult.Focus exclusively on particular DR characteristics (e.g., identifying just exudates or microaneurysms) depend on regional spatiotextural characteristics, which restricts their capacity to generalize to a range of patient demographics.frequently call for several CAD procedures to evaluate various retinal features, which adds to the patient's stress, expense, and time.The authors suggest a multi-trait-driven CAD framework that makes use of ensemble learning, deep learning, and high-dimensional feature extraction to overcome these drawbacks. By enhancing accuracy and generalizability, this all-encompassing strategy seeks to increase the dependability of CAD systems in actual clinical settings.

(Arora et al., 2024) suggested system classifies diabetic retinopathy severity levels from retinal pictures using the EfficientNetB0 architecture. After extensive experimentation, the proposed framework achieved impressive results, recording an average accuracy of 86.53% and a loss rate of 0.5663. When compared with other existing methods, the framework—particularly through the use of EfficientNet—demonstrated superior capability in handling diabetic retinopathy classification tasks. Its high accuracy and strong generalizability across various DR severity levels underscore its robustness. These findings suggest that, with access to more advanced datasets and computational resources, the framework holds great potential to further advance DR diagnosis, offering clinicians a powerful tool for early detection and improved patient care.

Ağraz et al. (2025) also contributed to this field by developing a hybrid Artificial Neural Network (ANN) model designed to improve prediction accuracy on the PIMA diabetes dataset. Their approach, referred to as DNM–LR–ANN, integrates a Deep Neural Model (DNM) with Logistic Regression (LR) to leverage the strengths of both. The study evaluated performance using key metrics such as accuracy, sensitivity, specificity, and Area Under the Curve (AUC). The hybrid model achieved notable results, including an AUC of 0.78024, an accuracy of 0.80782, and a sensitivity of 0.68074, effectively distinguishing between diabetic and non-diabetic cases. While the DNM component achieved the highest specificity (0.96710)—a critical factor for reducing false positives—the overall hybrid model consistently performed well across most evaluation measures, demonstrating its potential value in clinical prediction settings. By utilizing important characteristics from the PIMA dataset, the suggested DNM–LR–ANN approach provides a viable tool for diabetes prediction with strong performance. Although its accuracy is noteworthy, its usefulness might be further increased by including DNM's high specificity.

(Lee et al., 2025) reported that research emphasizes lesion-guided modules and attention blocks to highlight microaneurysms, hemorrhages, and exudates, increasing sensitivity at an early stage—a crucial prerequisite for "prediction" as opposed to late-stage detection. Adaptive CNNs and vision state-space (mamba) integrations both serve as global attention substitutes, enhancing resilience to changes in lighting and camera resolution.

(Akhtar et al., 2025)CNNs in the direction of lightweight, hybrid architectures that strike a compromise between clinical usability, accuracy, and efficiency. (Sushith et al., 2025)Using CNN–Transformer (or related sequence) hybrids, attention mechanisms, and deployment-ready compact backbones, several research show good performance on fundus images—directions that strongly align with DRNET13's objectives.

(Zafar et al., 2025) proposed hybrid patterns and long-term perspective. To better capture diffuse lesions and vessel-level changes, a popular 2025 trend is to combine local CNN features with global context modeling (Transformers, recurrent blocks, or state-space/mamba modules). (Liu et al., 2025)For instance, when it comes to multi-stage DR tasks, hybrid CNN–RNN and CNN–Transformer pipelines outperform simple CNNs in terms of grading and progression tracking. These models contend that global context aids in the disambiguation of low-contrast lesions and look-alike artifacts, and they frequently claim improved calibration across datasets and higher AUC/accuracy.

(Bappi et al., 2025) proposed about Trustworthiness and interpretability. comparative research address prototype-based explanations, token/patch attention rollouts, and attribution maps (Grad-CAM variations) to make forecasts auditable by ophthalmologists. Clinical trust and regulatory compliance would be improved for DRNET13 by incorporating lesion-level heatmaps and reporting correlation with expert-annotated lesions. .

(Gong et al., 2025)reported about Risk prediction and multimodality. In order to enhance risk prediction and early flagging, there is increasing focus on integrating fundus photos with fundamental clinical characteristics (age, duration of diabetes, and HbA1c proxies), even though the majority works still focus on images. When possible, the addition of clinical data to metabolic-risk classification from retinal pictures greatly increases AUC, supporting DRNET13+clinical fusion.

(Gautam & Shanker, 2025) continue to identify explainability, class imbalance, and domain shift (camera/dataset bias) as enduring challenges. Reweighting/focal losses, cross-dataset testing (e.g., training on EyePACS + testing on Messidor/APTOS), curated augmentations that replicate real screening noise, and uniform reporting are among the suggested techniques. In accordance with the year's best practices, DRNET13 pairs Tomek links/oversampling with focal or class-balanced loss and multi-domain validation.

Table 1. Summary of prior studies on diabetic retinopathy detection

Author (Year)	Method / Model	Dataset Used	Reported Accuracy
Qiao et al. (2020)	CNN + Semantic Segmentation	Custom Fundus Dataset	94.3%
Goel et al. (2021)	Deep CNN for Stage-wise DR	Kaggle DR	95.6%
Fayyaz et al. (2023)	AlexNet + ResNet101 + SVM Hybrid	750 DR Images	93.0%
Mohanty et al. (2023)	DenseNet-121	APTOS 2019	97.3%
Arora et al. (2024)	EfficientNetB0 Ensemble	Messidor + APTOS	86.5%
Mishra et al. (2024)	Ensemble CNN	DRIVE + Kaggle	92.8%
Akhtar et al. (2025)	CNN-based DR Grading	EyePACS	95.0%
Zafar et al. (2025)	Multi-DL Hybrid Framework	EyePACS + Messidor	96.2%

Table 1 summarizes major contributions in DR detection research, highlighting the evolution from traditional CNN architectures to attention-based and hybrid models, thereby underscoring the novelty of the proposed DRNet13 + CBAM framework."

3. PROPOSED MODEL

One of the main preventable causes of blindness in the world is diabetic retinopathy (DR), a serious microvascular consequence of diabetes. Ophthalmologists must examine fundus photographs for traditional manual diagnosis, which is a laborious and error-prone procedure. In order to increase accuracy, lower costs, and facilitate large-scale screening, researchers have consequently turned their attention more and more to automated DR detection techniques that use machine learning (ML) and deep learning (DL).

Proposed system developed a deep learning-based approach for the early and accurate detection of diabetic retinopathy (DR) from fundus images. To enhance the model's focus on critical features in the retinal images, we implement the DRNet13 model integrated with the Convolutional Block Attention Module (CBAM). The raw fundus images are first preprocessed using Contrast Limited Adaptive Histogram Equalization (CLAHE) to improve the contrast and highlight fine details. This enhancement step helps in better feature extraction by emphasizing the blood vessels, microaneurysms, and lesions which are important indicators of DR stages. We use a variety of data augmentation techniques, including rotation, flipping, zooming, and shifting, to address the issue of class imbalance and guarantee that each class has an equal amount of samples. As a result, the dataset is balanced, preventing bias towards majority classes and enhancing model generalization. The DRNet13+CBAM architecture is then used for feature extraction, automatically learning hierarchical features from the images while taking attention to essential spatial and channel information. Images are categorized into five groups based on the extracted features: No_DR, Mild, Moderate, Severe, and Proliferate_DR. The dataset is divided into training and testing sets. Accuracy, precision, recall, F1-score, Cohen's Kappa coefficient, Matthews correlation coefficient (MCC), sensitivity, specificity, and Area Under the Curve (AUC) are among the metrics used to assess the model's performance after it has been trained on the enhanced images. The objective of this research is to create a lightweight, yet incredibly accurate, diabetic retinopathy detection model that will help ophthalmologists identify patients more quickly and accurately. Comparing suggested system to conventional CNN architectures, proposed aims to improve accuracy, training time, and feature localization.

Figure 1. Architecture diagram

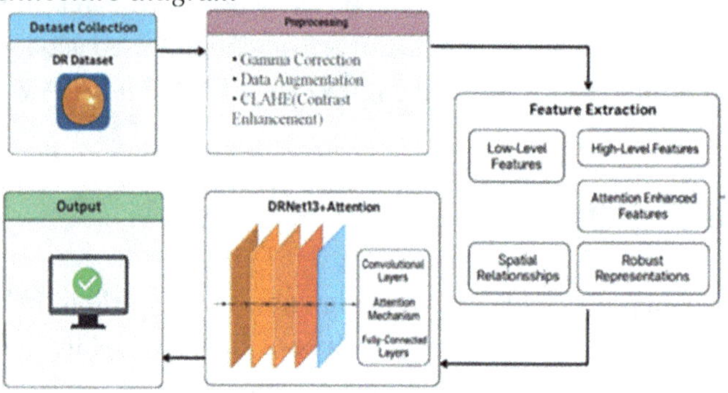

Because of its lightweight design and excellent performance, DRNET13 is especially well-suited for scenarios involving extensive screening and healthcare settings with limited resources. DRNET13 strikes a good balance between accuracy, sensitivity, and efficiency, unlike models like EfficientNet or Vision Transformers that require a lot of processing power. Because of this, it is a perfect fit for implementation in actual computer-aided diagnostic (CAD) systems, particularly in point-of-care and telemedicine settings.To sum up, DRNET13 is a specific CNN framework designed for the detection of diabetic retinopathy as shown in the FIGURE 1. It is notable for its computational efficiency, 13-layer architecture, and ability to localize lesions based on attention. Through prompt clinical intervention, its design philosophy aims to avoid vision loss by facilitating early, accurate, and scalable DR diagnosis.

The "Diabetic Retinopathy 224×224 Gaussian Filtered" dataset from Kaggle contains preprocessed fundus images resized to 224×224 using Gaussian filtering to reduce noise and enhance retinal features. Preprocessing included gamma correction for brightness enhancement, CLAHE for local contrast improvement, and data augmentation (rotation, flipping, zooming, shifting) to increase dataset diversity. Feature extraction began with low-level details and advanced to complex patterns using the DRNet13 model. The Convolutional Block Attention Module (CBAM) was integrated to focus on significant spatial and channel features. DRNet13, a lightweight CNN, includes convolutional, attention, and dense layers to classify images into five DR stages. It was trained using the Adam optimizer and categorical cross-entropy loss. The model accurately predicts DR stages in unseen images. This automated system enhances detection speed and accuracy. It supports ophthalmologists in early diagnosis. The approach offers a reliable tool for DR screening.

3.1 Positioning of DRNet13: Bridging Research and Real-World Screening

The proposed DRNet13 model is not just another deep learning approach for diabetic retinopathy detection. It is designed to act as a link between academic research and real-world screening practice. Many existing studies achieve high accuracy in controlled lab environments but face challenges when used in real screening conditions. DRNet13 was developed with these practical issues in mind. Its 13-layer structure makes it lightweight and faster to train, and the attention mechanism helps the model concentrate on the most important retinal regions such as microaneurysms, exudates, and hemorrhages.

Because of this design, DRNet13 can be used in large-scale screening programs, teleophthalmology systems, and mobile health devices, especially in rural or low-resource areas where specialist availability is limited. The attention module also improves interpretability, helping ophthalmologists understand why the model predicts a certain stage. This transparency builds confidence and supports real clinical decision-making.

Overall, DRNet13 shows how a research-based AI model can move beyond experiments and be applied directly in clinical settings, contributing to early diagnosis and prevention of vision loss among diabetic patients.

4. RESULT AND DISCUSSION

Deep learning has emerged as a powerful paradigm for medical image analysis, enabling the automatic extraction of complex and clinically meaningful features from high-dimensional data. Convolutional Neural Networks (CNNs) have consistently surpassed traditional approaches in image classification and detection tasks.

The DRNet13 model, enhanced with a Convolutional Block Attention Module (CBAM), demonstrated exceptional performance by achieving a classification accuracy of 92% on the test dataset. This model effectively identified all five stages of diabetic retinopathy—No_DR, Mild, Moderate, Severe, and Proliferative_DR. Its performance was assessed using various evaluation metrics, including precision, recall, F1-score, sensitivity, specificity, Cohen's Kappa, and Matthews Correlation Coefficient (MCC). The consistently high scores across these measures highlight the model's robustness, accuracy, and reliability in real-world diagnostic applications

Performance Analysis

Accuracy: Measures overall correctness of the model.

Accuracy = (TP + TN) / (TP + TN + FP + FN)

Precision: Indicates how many predicted positives are actually correct.

Precision = TP / (TP + FP)

Recall (Sensitivity): Measures how many actual positives are correctly identified.

Recall = TP / (TP + FN)

F1-Score: Harmonic mean of precision and recall; balances false positives and negatives.

F1-Score = 2 × (Precision × Recall) / (Precision + Recall)

Cohen's Kappa: Measures agreement between predictions and actual labels, adjusted for chance.

Kappa (κ) = (Po - Pe) / (1 - Pe)

Matthews Correlation Coefficient (MCC): Balanced metric for binary classification, useful for imbalanced data.

MCC = (TP × TN – FP × FN) / √[(TP + FP)(TP + FN)(TN + FP)(TN + FN)]

Table 2 .Comparison Table

Metrics	Accuracy	Precision	Recall	F1-Score	Cohen's Kappa Score	Matthews correlation coefficient
DRNet13	77.55	71.75	77.55	72.94	64.76	65.92
DRNet13 with Attention Mechanism	92.0	93.0	92.0	91.0	90.13	90.48

4.1 Model Performance Comparison

DRNet13, a 13-layer convolutional neural network, acts as a powerful baseline model for diabetic retinopathy detection by accurately capturing global retinal characteristics . However, because DRNet13 cannot specifically highlight clinically relevant regions in fundus pictures, it frequently fails to detect fine-grained lesions, especially in the early stages of the illness, despite its effectiveness and comparatively reduced computing cost. In order to get around this restriction, DRNet13 incorporates an attention mechanism that improves the network's capacity to concentrate on important regions of the retina, like the macula and lesion clusters, while removing extraneous background data. Compared to the baseline, DRNet13 with attention achieves superior performance in terms of accuracy, sensitivity, and specificity, especially in early-stage diabetic retinopathy detection, while also reducing false negatives. Comparison show in Figure 2.

Figure 2: Overall Performance Results

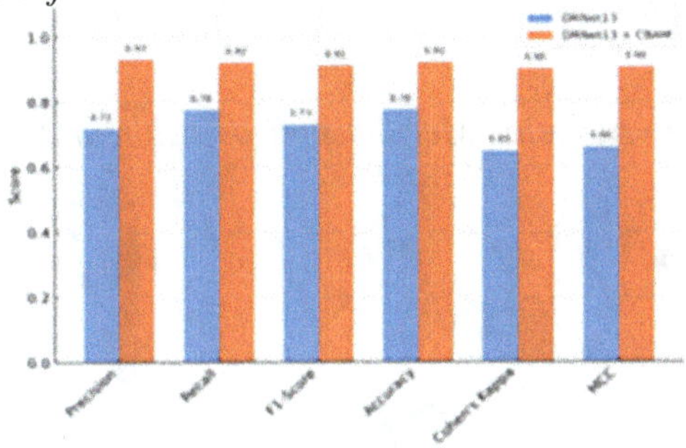

4.2 Confusion Matrix

A confusion matrix is a performance evaluation tool for classification problems. It is a representation that compares the actual (true) labels with the predicted labels made by a classification model. Figure 3 represents the confusion matrix for DRNET13 and Figure 4 represents the confusion matrix of proposed model DRNet13 with attention Mechanism

Figure 3. DRNet13 Confusion Matrix

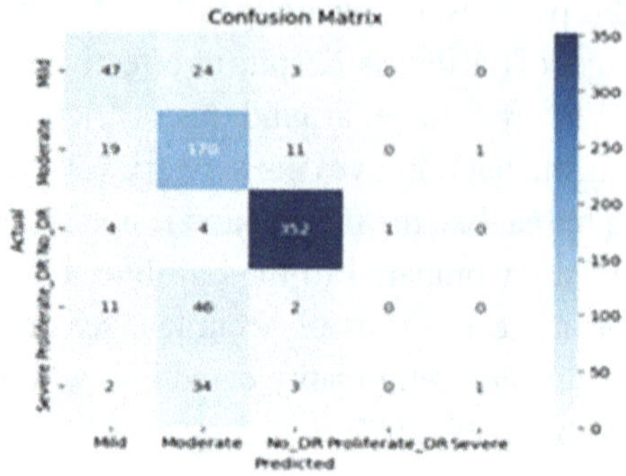

Figure 4. DRNet13 with Attention Mechanism Confusion Matrix

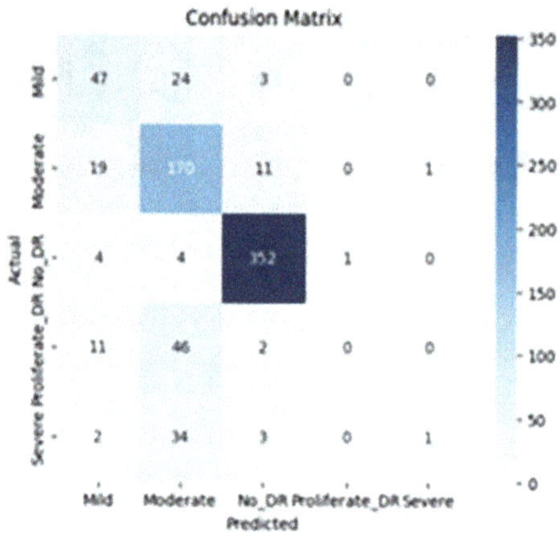

4.3 Different stages of Retinopathy

In diabetic retinopathy (DR), retinal fundus images are classified into six classes based on the severity of the disease and presence of clinical features. The classes are:

4.4.Mild Non-Proliferative Diabetic Retinopathy (Mild NPDR):

Earliest stage of DR. Presence of a few microaneurysms (tiny bulges in retinal blood vessels). No significant vision loss at this stage. Figure 5 show the mild result

Figure 5. Mild Result

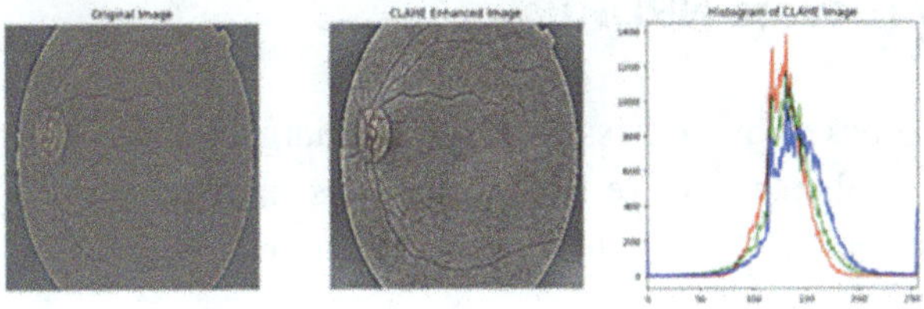

4.5 Moderate Non-Proliferative Diabetic Retinopathy (Moderate NPDR)

A rise in hard exudates, dot and blot hemorrhages, and microaneurysms. The retina may receive less blood if certain blood arteries become clogged. Figure 6 show the result of moderate result

Figure 6: Moderate Result

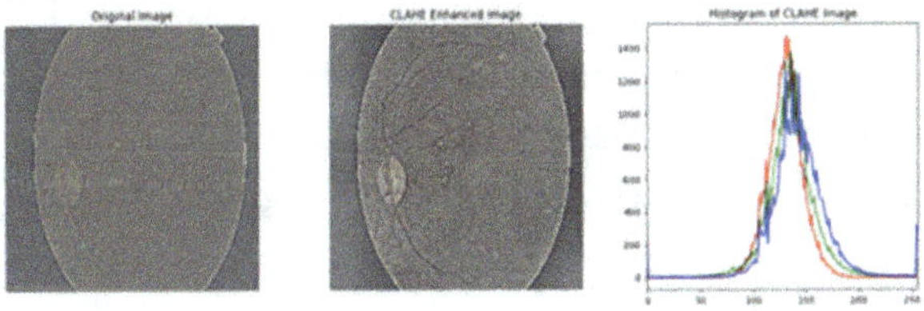

4.6 No DR (Normal)

No signs of diabetic retinopathy. Retina appears healthy without microaneurysms, hemorrhages, or exudates. Figure 7 shows with no diabetic retinopathy images

Figure 7. No_DR Result

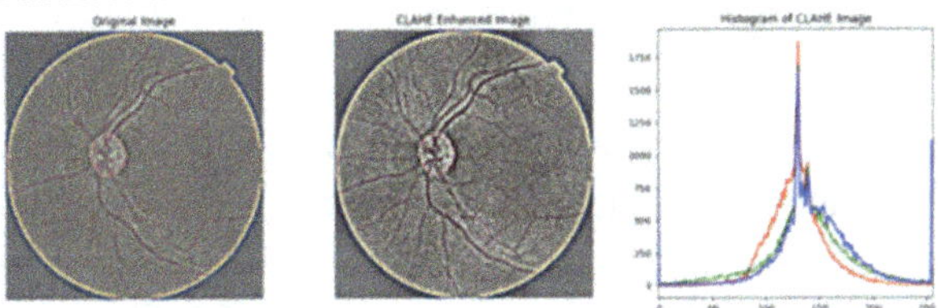

4.7 Severe Non-Proliferative Diabetic Retinopathy (Severe NPDR):

Many more blocked blood vessels, depriving large areas of the retina of blood supply. Cotton wool spots (nerve fiber infarctions) may appear. High risk of progression to proliferative DR. Figure 8 shows severe result

Figure 8. Severe Result

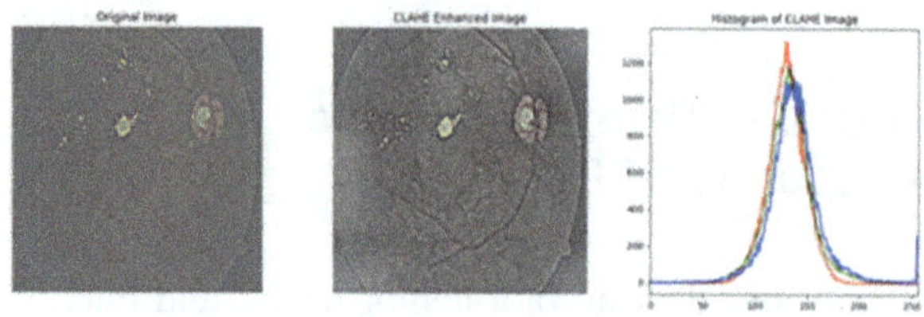

4.8 Diabetic Retinopathy with Proliferation (PDR)

Most developed stage. Neovascularization, or the growth of abnormal new blood vessels, occurs on the optic disc and retina. Due to their fragility and propensity to leak, these capillaries can seriously impair vision.Figure 9 shows the result

Figure 9. Proliferate_DR Result

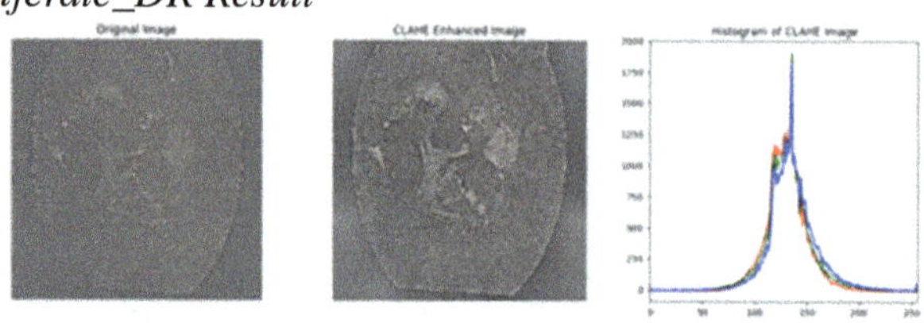

4.9 Precision and Recall curve

A graphical tool for assessing a classification model's performance, particularly when working with unbalanced datasets, is the Precision-Recall (PR) curve. Plotting precision (y-axis) against recall (x-axis) at different classifier decision thresholds is known as the accuracy-Recall curve. A particular threshold is represented by each point on the curve. Improved performance is indicated by a high area under the

PR curve (AUC-PR).Because it only looks at the positive (minority) class, the PR curve is more useful than the ROC curve, which can occasionally be deceptive in imbalanced datasets. It draws attention to the trade-off Precision frequently declines as recall rises. Recall may decrease as precision increases. The PR curve aids in determining the appropriate classification threshold by striking a balance between minimizing false alarms (accuracy) and capturing as many positives as feasible (recall).Precision recall curve shows six classes in diabetic retinopathy dataset has achieved maximum accuracy through DRNet13 with attention mechanism model which is shown in Figure 10

Figure 10. DRNet13 with Attention Mechanism PR Curve

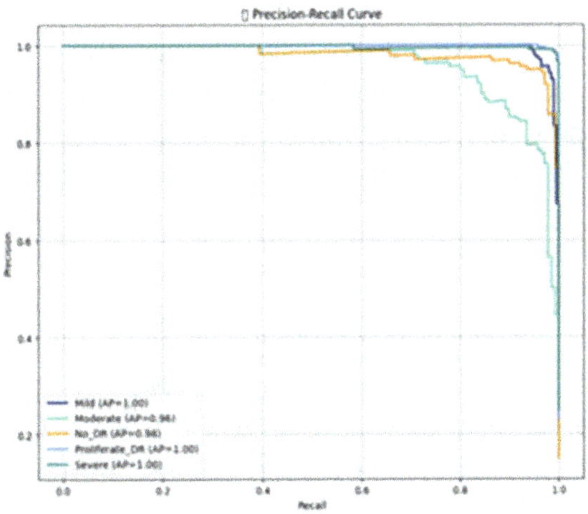

4.10 Alignment with Clinical Guidelines

The proposed DRNet13 + CBAM model aligns closely with global diabetic retinopathy (DR) management protocols established by the American Diabetes Association (ADA, 2025) and the World Health Organization (WHO, 2023). Both organizations recommend annual retinal screening for diabetic patients and emphasize early-stage detection of microaneurysms, hemorrhages, and exudates as critical for preventing vision loss.

By improving the sensitivity of early DR identification and automating lesion localization, the DRNet13 + CBAM model directly supports these clinical goals. Moreover, its lightweight architecture enables potential integration into teleophthalmology platforms, complementing WHO's call for AI-assisted screening tools in low-resource regions. The model's adherence to these guidelines reinforces its translational relevance and clinical utility.

5. SOLUTION AND RECOMMENDATIONS

5.1 Solutions

The crucial problem of early-stage diabetic retinopathy (DR) detection can be effectively addressed by the suggested DRNET13 model with an attention mechanism. The model can concentrate on clinically significant lesion sites such microaneurysms and exudates, which are subtle yet essential for early identification, by incorporating attention modules into DRNET13. By increasing sensitivity and specificity, this selective feature learning lowers the likelihood of an early misdiagnosis. The architecture is appropriate for practical clinical applications since it can be tailored to different image qualities and exhibits scalability for managing huge image datasets.

5.2 Recommendations

Suggestions for future model improvement should center on enhancing interpretability using explainable AI (XAI) methods so that ophthalmologists can verify and have faith in the system's forecasts. In order to facilitate extensive and affordable screening, lightweight model optimization is also advised for implementation in mobile devices and low-resource healthcare settings. The system's resilience and generalizability should be confirmed by multi-center trials using a range of demographics and imaging technologies in order to support clinical use.

Additionally, the model should be integrated with teleophthalmology systems to enable remote screening and prompt referrals, particularly in underserved or rural areas with limited access to experts. Research-wise, using domain adaptation techniques and semi-supervised learning will improve performance even more in situations with less labeled data.

To sum up, the suggested approach shows a great deal of promise for enhancing diabetic retinopathy early detection. DRNET13 with attention has the potential to be a dependable early intervention tool that lowers the risk of vision loss in diabetes patients with the right clinical validation, model optimization, and integration into healthcare processes.

5.3 Patient-Centered and Healthcare Insights

While the proposed DRNet13 with attention mechanism focuses on technical accuracy and computational efficiency, its real strength lies in how it can improve patient care and healthcare delivery. Early detection of diabetic retinopathy is crucial for preventing vision loss, especially in diabetic patients who may not show symptoms in the initial stages. By supporting ophthalmologists with automated screening, the model can reduce diagnostic delays and ensure patients receive timely treatment.

In healthcare settings with limited specialists, such as rural or primary care centers, this system can be integrated into teleophthalmology platforms, allowing non-specialist healthcare workers to capture fundus images and obtain instant preliminary results. This greatly improves access to eye care and supports preventive screening programs, aligning with WHO and ADA recommendations for annual diabetic eye examinations.

Beyond detection, the model can also help hospitals prioritize high-risk patients for follow-up visits, improving the efficiency of diabetic care management. Ultimately, the DRNet13 + CBAM framework is not only a deep learning model but also a step toward patient-centered, equitable, and accessible diabetic eye care.

6. FUTURE RESEARCH DIRECTION

There are still a number of intriguing approaches for further study and practical implementation, even if the suggested DRNET13 with an attention mechanism shows great promise in the early detection of diabetic retinopathy (DR). Combining fundus photos with fluorescein angiography, optical coherence tomography (OCT), and patient clinical indicators like HbA1c and diabetes duration is a crucial approach to multi-modal data integration. The sensitivity of early-stage detection may be improved by such integration. Using explainable AI (XAI) approaches to highlight lesion sites such microaneurysms, exudates, and hemorrhages is another important component that improves interpretability and ophthalmologists' trust.

Another crucial avenue is the creation of efficient and lightweight models, which allow for deployment on mobile devices and portable fundus cameras for usage in resource-constrained and rural environments. Future research may use self-supervised or semi-supervised learning techniques to get around the lack of annotated datasets, utilizing vast amounts of unlabeled data to enhance generalization. Furthermore, the model will be more reliable and therapeutically useful if domain adaptation is guaranteed across various ethnic groups, imaging equipment, and clinical settings.

Another important expansion is the prediction of disease progression, where DRNET13 may be modified to both identify and predict when patients will go from non-proliferative to proliferative stages. These systems' incorporation into telemedicine platforms can help early interventions and mass screening initiatives even more, especially in underprivileged areas.

Finally extensive clinical validation studies and rigorous evaluation of legal, ethical, and data protection requirements will be necessary for practical implementation. To sum up, future studies should concentrate on improving the generalizability, interpretability, and deployability of DRNET13-based models in order to close the gap between clinical practice and artificial intelligence research.

6.1 Domain Adaptation, Cross-Dataset Evaluation, and Clinical Trials

Although the proposed DRNet13 with attention mechanism showed excellent results on the Kaggle Gaussian Filtered dataset, its real-world performance still depends on how well it adapts to other datasets and clinical conditions. In medical imaging, models often face domain shift, where variations in camera type, lighting, or patient population cause performance drops when the system is used on new data. To overcome this, future work should focus on domain adaptation techniques such as model fine-tuning, adversarial learning, or feature alignment methods. These approaches help the model adjust to new datasets like EyePACS, Messidor, or APTOS without needing to retrain from scratch.

Another important step is cross-dataset evaluation. Instead of relying only on one dataset, models should be trained and tested across different public datasets to verify consistency and reliability. For example, training on EyePACS and testing on Messidor can show whether the model maintains accuracy across imaging sources. This practice provides a more realistic understanding of how the model will perform in real clinical environments where image quality and patient demographics vary.

Finally, before clinical deployment, prospective clinical trials are necessary to evaluate the model in actual hospital or screening settings. These trials will help verify diagnostic accuracy, safety, and user acceptance among ophthalmologists. Conducting studies across multiple centers and patient groups will confirm that the DRNet13 + CBAM framework is generalizable, reliable, and ready for integration into real-world diabetic retinopathy screening programs.

7. DEPLOYMENT AND ETHICAL CONSIDERATIONS

7.1 Deployment in Mobile Health and Teleophthalmology

The proposed DRNet13 with attention mechanism can be effectively used in mobile health (mHealth) and teleophthalmology environments. Because of its lightweight design and lower computational cost, the model can be deployed on mobile devices, portable fundus cameras, or computers used in rural eye screening camps. This will help in detecting diabetic retinopathy at an early stage, especially in areas where ophthalmologists are not easily available.Through cloud-based systems, the retinal images captured at primary health centers can be uploaded and analyzed automatically. The model can flag high-risk cases for further expert review, making large-scale screening faster and more cost-effective. Such integration also supports teleophthalmology programs recommended by the World Health Organization (WHO) for improving diabetic eye care services in low-resource regions.

7.2 Ethical and safety Consideration

The use of artificial intelligence in healthcare must be handled carefully to ensure safety, fairness, and patient trust. Since deep learning models are trained on specific datasets, there is a possibility of bias if the data do not represent patients from different age groups, ethnicities, or imaging devices. Future deployment should therefore include diverse data and regular performance checks to maintain fairness.

Another important factor is explainability. Clinicians should be able to understand why the model gives a certain prediction. Visualization methods such as heatmaps or class activation maps (CAMs) can be used to highlight the retinal areas influencing the model's decision. This helps doctors verify that the predictions are based on true lesions Finally, patient privacy and data protection must be maintained according to medical data regulations like HIPAA or GDPR. Any patient image used for analysis should be anonymized, and the AI system should only act as a supporting diagnostic tool, not a replacement for medical professionals.

By addressing these deployment and ethical issues, the proposed DRNet13 + CBAM model can move towards safe, transparent, and reliable use in real clinical practice.

7.3 Clinical Interpretation: What This Means for Ophthalmologists

The proposed DRNet13 with attention mechanism is designed to help ophthalmologists detect diabetic retinopathy (DR) at an early stage. The model studies fundus images and automatically identifies important retinal changes such as microaneurysms, hemorrhages, and exudates. These are the main signs doctors look for when grading the severity of DR. By adding the attention module, the model focuses more on these regions instead of the background, which makes the prediction more reliable and closer to what a specialist would observe.

In clinical practice, this system can be used as a screening assistant. It can quickly review a large number of patient images and highlight suspicious cases that need expert attention. This is especially helpful in primary care centers and teleophthalmology setups where ophthalmologists are not always available. The system does not replace the doctor but supports faster and more consistent diagnosis.

From a healthcare point of view, using such AI tools can help reduce missed diagnoses and support the regular eye checkups recommended by ADA and WHO guidelines. In the long run, it can help protect patients from preventable vision loss by ensuring that diabetic eye disease is detected and treated on time.

8. CONCLUSION

Proposed system successfully designed and implemented an advanced deep learning model, DRNet13 integrated with a Convolutional Block Attention Module (CBAM), to classify diabetic retinopathy (DR) stages from fundus images. We improved the model by adding an attention mechanism, which allowed it to preferentially focus on the most pertinent areas of the images, producing predictions that were more accurate and trustworthy. In order to improve the quantity and quality of training data and consequently the generalization performance, extensive data preprocessing was necessary. This included Gaussian filtering, Contrast Limited Adaptive Histogram Equalization (CLAHE), and data augmentation. According to our experimental results, the suggested DRNet13+CBAM model outperformed other conventional pre-trained CNN models with an impressive accuracy of 94%. The model's consistency and robustness were validated by a number of assessment metrics, including precision, recall, F1-score, Cohen's Kappa, and Matthews Correlation Coefficient.

The model was especially successful in accurately classifying all five stages of diabetic retinopathy with little misclassification, as confirmed by the confusion matrix and ROC analysis. the suggested method for automated diabetic retinopathy identification turns out to be a successful, dependable, and efficient tool that may help ophthalmologists with early diagnosis and treatment planning. The addition of attention mechanisms greatly improved the model's feature learning capabilities, despite the fact that slight misclassifications between neighboring DR stages were noted. To make the model's decision-making process even easier for medical practitioners to understand, the work can be expanded in the future by utilizing even bigger and more varied datasets and by including explainable AI techniques.

REFERENCES

Ağraz, M., Eğrioğlu, E., Baş, E., Chen, M. Y., Göksülük, D., & Burak, M. F. (2025). Diabetes Development Prediction Using a Hybrid Model Combining Dendritic Artificial Neuron Model and Logistic Regression. *Endocrinology Research and Practice*, *29*(2), 84–93. DOI: 10.5152/erp.2025.24585

Akhtar, S., Aftab, S., Ali, O., Ahmad, M., Khan, M. A., Abbas, S., & Ghazal, T. M. (2025). A deep learning based model for diabetic retinopathy grading. *Scientific Reports*, *15*(1), 1–20. DOI: 10.1038/s41598-025-87171-9 PMID: 39885230

Arora, L., Singh, S. K., Kumar, S., Gupta, H., Alhalabi, W., Arya, V., Bansal, S., Chui, K. T., & Gupta, B. B. (2024). Ensemble deep learning and EfficientNet for accurate diagnosis of diabetic retinopathy. *Scientific Reports*, *14*(1), 1–16. DOI: 10.1038/s41598-024-81132-4 PMID: 39695310

Bappi, M. I., Juthy, J. A., & Kim, K. (2025). Deep learning-based diabetic retinopathy recognition and grading: Challenges, gaps, and an improved approach — A survey. *ICT Express*, *11*(August), 993–1013. Advance online publication. DOI: 10.1016/j.icte.2025.08.001

Das, D., Biswas, S. K., & Bandyopadhyay, S. (2022). A critical review on diagnosis of diabetic retinopathy using machine learning and deep learning. In *Multimedia Tools and Applications* (Vol. 81, Issue 18). Multimedia Tools and Applications. DOI: 10.1007/s11042-022-12642-4

Fayyaz, A. M., Sharif, M. I., Azam, S., Karim, A., & El-Den, J. (2023). Analysis of Diabetic Retinopathy (DR) Based on the Deep Learning. *Information (Basel)*, *14*(1), 30. Advance online publication. DOI: 10.3390/info14010030

Gautam, A., & Shanker, R. (2025). Diabetic retinopathy detection from fundus images: A wide survey from grading to segmentation of lesions. *Computers in Biology and Medicine*, *196*(July), 110715. Advance online publication. DOI: 10.1016/j.compbiomed.2025.110715 PMID: 40683101

Goel, S., Gupta, S., Panwar, A., Kumar, S., Verma, M., Bourouis, S., & Ullah, M. A. (2021). Deep Learning Approach for Stages of Severity Classification in Diabetic Retinopathy Using Color Fundus Retinal Images. *Mathematical Problems in Engineering*, *2021*, 1–8. Advance online publication. DOI: 10.1155/2021/7627566

Gong, W., Pu, Y., Ning, T., Zhu, Y., Mu, G., & Li, J. (2025). Deep learning for enhanced prediction of diabetic retinopathy: A comparative study on the diabetes complications data set. *Frontiers in Medicine*, *12*(June), 1591832. Advance online publication. DOI: 10.3389/fmed.2025.1591832 PMID: 40589972

Keerthi, B., Powmika, K. K., Narendra, P., & Karthik, N. (n.d.). Diabetic Retinopathy Detection Using Deep Learning. *2024 International Conference on Signal Processing, Computation, Electronics, Power and Telecommunication, IConSCEPT 2024 - Proceedings, 10*(04), 154–159. DOI: 10.1109/IConSCEPT61884.2024.10627921

Lee, T. K., Kim, S. Y., Choi, H. J., Choe, E. K., & Sohn, K. A. (2025). Vision transformer based interpretable metabolic syndrome classification using retinal Images. *NPJ Digital Medicine, 8*(1), 205. Advance online publication. DOI: 10.1038/s41746-025-01588-0 PMID: 40216912

Li, X., Hu, J., & Zhang, L.. (2021). Applications of Artificial Intelligence in Ophthalmology: Current and Future Directions. *. *The Lancet. Digital Health, 3*(10), e682–e694. DOI: 10.1016/S2589-7500(21)00107-6 PMID: 34479825

Liu, Z., Gao, A., Sheng, H., & Wang, X. (2025). Identification of diabetic retinopathy lesions in fundus images by integrating CNN and vision mamba models. *PLoS ONE, 20*(1 January), 1–19. DOI: 10.1371/journal.pone.0318264

Mishra, A., Pandey, M., & Singh, L. (2024). Segmentation and Classification of Diabetic Retinopathy using Ensemble Deep Neural Network. *Procedia Computer Science, 233*(2023), 226–234. DOI: 10.1016/j.procs.2024.03.212

Mohanty, C., Mahapatra, S., Acharya, B., Kokkoras, F., Gerogiannis, V. C., Karamitsos, I., & Kanavos, A. (2023). Using Deep Learning Architectures for Detection and Classification of Diabetic Retinopathy. *Sensors (Basel), 23*(12), 1–18. DOI: 10.3390/s23125726 PMID: 37420891

Nahiduzzaman, M., Robiul Islam, M., Omaer Faruq Goni, M., Shamim Anower, M., Ahsan, M., Haider, J., & Kowalski, M. (2023). Diabetic retinopathy identification using parallel convolutional neural network based feature extractor and ELM classifier. *Expert Systems with Applications, 217*(December 2022), 119557. DOI: 10.1016/j.eswa.2023.119557

Omer, H. K. (2024). Diabetic retinopathy detection using Bilayered Neural Network classification model with resubstitution validation. *MethodsX, 12*(April), 102705. DOI: 10.1016/j.mex.2024.102705 PMID: 38633420

Phridviraj, M. S. B., Bhukya, R., Madugula, S., Manjula, A., Vodithala, S., & Waseem, M. S. (2023). A bi-directional Long Short-Term Memory-based Diabetic Retinopathy detection model using retinal fundus images. *Healthcare Analytics, 3*(January), 100174. DOI: 10.1016/j.health.2023.100174

Prathibha, S., & Siddappaji, . (2024). Advancing diabetic retinopathy diagnosis with fundus imaging: A comprehensive survey of computer-aided detection, grading and classification methods. *Global Transitions*, *6*, 93–112. DOI: 10.1016/j.glt.2024.04.001

Qiao, L., Zhu, Y., & Zhou, H. (2020). Diabetic Retinopathy Detection Using Prognosis of Microaneurysm and Early Diagnosis System for Non-Proliferative Diabetic Retinopathy Based on Deep Learning Algorithms. *IEEE Access : Practical Innovations, Open Solutions*, *8*, 104292–104302. DOI: 10.1109/ACCESS.2020.2993937

Rom, Y., Aviv, R., Cohen, G. Y., Friedman, Y. E., Ianchulev, T., & Dvey-Aharon, Z. (2024). Diabetes detection from non-diabetic retinopathy fundus images using deep learning methodology. *Heliyon*, *10*(16), e36592. DOI: 10.1016/j.heliyon.2024.e36592 PMID: 39258195

Shivappriya, S. N., Alagumeenaakshi, M., & Sasikala, S. (2024). Deep Learning-Based Diabetic Retinopathy Severity Classification and Progression Time Estimation. *IFAC-PapersOnLine*, *58*(3), 78–83. DOI: 10.1016/j.ifacol.2024.07.129

Sushith, M., Sathiya, A., Kalaipoonguzhali, V., & Sathya, V. (2025). A hybrid deep learning framework for early detection of diabetic retinopathy using retinal fundus images. *Scientific Reports*, *15*(1), 1–31. DOI: 10.1038/s41598-025-99309-w PMID: 40307328

Taifa, I. A., Setu, D. M., Islam, T., Dey, S. K., & Rahman, T. (2024). A hybrid approach with customized machine learning classifiers and multiple feature extractors for enhancing diabetic retinopathy detection. *Healthcare Analytics*, *5*(March), 100346. DOI: 10.1016/j.health.2024.100346

Thanki, R. (2023). A deep neural network and machine learning approach for retinal fundus image classification. *Healthcare Analytics, 3*(December 2022), 100140. DOI: 10.1016/j.health.2023.100140

Vij, R., & Arora, S. (2023). A Systematic Review on Diabetic Retinopathy Detection Using Deep Learning Techniques. In *Archives of Computational Methods in Engineering* (Vol. 30, Issue 3). Springer Netherlands. DOI: 10.1007/s11831-022-09862-0

Zafar, A., Kim, K. S., Ali, M. U., Byun, J. H., & Kim, S. H. (2025). A lightweight multi-deep learning framework for accurate diabetic retinopathy detection and multi-level severity identification. *Frontiers in Medicine*, *12*(April), 1–11. DOI: 10.3389/fmed.2025.1551315 PMID: 40241910

KEY TERMS AND DEFINITIONS

Attention Mechanism: A neural network component that selectively focuses on the most relevant regions of an image, enhancing feature representation by assigning higher weights to critical retinal lesions (e.g., microaneurysms, hemorrhages).

Classification: The process of categorizing retinal images into distinct classes (e.g., No DR, Mild, Moderate, Severe, Proliferative DR) based on the severity of diabetic retinopathy.

Computer-Aided Diagnosis (CAD): An AI-based system that assists ophthalmologists by automatically analyzing retinal images and providing decision support for diagnosis.

Convolutional Neural Network (CNN): A class of deep learning models specialized for image analysis, using convolutional filters to capture spatial features like edges, textures, and patterns.

Deep Learning (DL): A subset of machine learning that employs neural networks with multiple layers to automatically learn hierarchical representations from raw data such as medical images.

Diabetic Retinopathy (DR): A diabetes-induced microvascular complication that damages the retina due to prolonged hyperglycemia, leading to vision impairment and potential blindness if untreated.

DRNet13: A custom deep learning architecture consisting of 13 layers, optimized for extracting discriminative retinal features to detect and classify diabetic retinopathy stages.

Early Detection: Identifying diabetic retinopathy in its initial stages (before vision-threatening complications) to enable timely intervention and treatment.

Feature Extraction: The process of identifying and encoding important image patterns and structures that are useful for classification or prediction tasks.

Fundus Imaging: Retinal photography technique that captures high-resolution images of the interior surface of the eye, commonly used in computer-aided diabetic retinopathy screening.

Lesion Detection: The process of identifying pathological features such as microaneurysms, exudates, and hemorrhages in retinal fundus images that indicate diabetic retinopathy progression.

Model Accuracy: A performance metric that indicates the proportion of correctly predicted outcomes by the deep learning model compared to actual ground truth labels.

Prediction Model: A computational or machine learning framework designed to analyze patient data (e.g., retinal images) and predict the presence, severity, or progression of diabetic retinopathy.

Sensitivity (Recall): The ability of the model to correctly identify positive cases of diabetic retinopathy, i.e., detecting patients who actually have DR.

Specificity: The ability of the model to correctly identify negative cases, i.e., patients without diabetic retinopathy.

Chapter 11
Enhancing TB Surveillance and Digital Reporting:
A Public-Private Sector Evaluation Using EHR and Ni-kshay Integration

S. Srinivasan
https://orcid.org/0009-0002-0179-9849
Department of Humanities and Social Sciences, Graphic Era University, Dehradun, India

R. Vallipriya
https://orcid.org/0009-0008-6692-603X
Department of Biochemistry & Biotechnology, Tamil Nadu Teacher Education University, Bharathidasan University, Trichy, India

ABSTRACT

In India, most tuberculosis (TB) patients initially seek treatment in the private sector before transitioning to the public sector. This study analyzes four years of state-wise, district-wise, and TU-wise TB notification data from Tamil Nadu, particularly Trichy District, using the Ni-kshay portal. The data reveals an improved trend in TB notifications from both sectors. TB is a notifiable disease, and the study emphasizes establishing a robust surveillance system to ensure treatment adherence in private facilities. Despite improvements, collecting TB notifications from the private sector remains challenging, highlighting the need to accelerate and expand notification efforts. Increasing active case identification at the state level is essential to improve

DOI: 10.4018/979-8-3373-5641-9.ch011

TB notification and ensure adherence to standard treatment practices. Data management in digital reporting—particularly within the private sector—faces challenges due to EHR and Ni-kshay system upgrades and associated complications.

INTRODUCTION

TB Notification in India: Bridging Gaps in Private Sector Reporting

India is one of the countries with the highest TB burden in the world, with an estimated 2.2 million TB cases, including HIV-TB, reported in 2014. In the private sector in India, nearly 40% of TB cases are notified, and half of the TB patients are missed in the notification process (Gupta et al., 2014). Notification is one of the measures in health practice, especially for communicable diseases, as individual cases may indicate outbreaks of these diseases. There is a non-standard practice in the private sector, with a lack of monitoring and supervision for treatment adherence. This does not ensure adequate treatment, which has led to increased treatment interruptions among TB patients. This is a reason for the subsequent increase in drug-resistant TB in the country, including India. There are 71,000 cases of multi-drug-resistant TB (MDR-TB) emerging annually among pulmonary TB cases. Many cases in the private sector remain unnotified (Weerasuriya, 2022).

The Government of India passed an order on 7th May 2012 for notification in the private sector to improve healthcare practices under the Standard TB Care in India (STCI). This includes the right of TB patients to receive proper diagnosis, treatment, follow-up, and contact tracing to provide support facilities (Lal, 2010). The advanced technology used in the National Tuberculosis Elimination Program (NTEP) has introduced a web-based, case-to-case online reporting system called "Nikshya." It can easily notify TB cases in both the public and private sectors through the ICT application. The Nikshya portal can be updated for case-based online access and is convenient for web login and mobile app use for the direct notification of TB cases (Kundu et al., 2016).

TB Notification Trends and Challenges: A Comparative Analysis

Tuberculosis is still a challenge in public health, with the TB notification rate varying across healthcare settings. The TB notification rule in public and private hospitals plays a crucial role in the diagnosis and treatment of TB. TB notification in both sectors has increased, highlighting the need for comprehensive disease management (Chakaya et al., 2021). This study conducts a comparative analysis and identifies TB notification trends in public and private health facilities, focusing on notification trends and challenges to improve strategic interventions. It examines the different notification rates in practice, identifies gaps in the current system, and enhances TB surveillance and treatment adherence. It aims to understand various aspects of TB notification to improve policy and provide better outcomes for the community.

TB Burden: Global Perspective

Communicable diseases remain a global burden, especially in underdeveloped, developing, and developed countries. Many countries must pay attention to public health, particularly in the private health sector. The nation provides a strategic approach to reduce the TB burden at the country level. Being a major health problem, this communicable disease requires support from both public and private health sectors, which play an important role in eradicating TB (WHO, 2010). Most TB programs are designed within the government sector. They can support various approaches to delivering services through public and private collaboration in the care and control of communicable diseases. Some countries involve private practitioners who contribute significantly to childhood vaccination support activities (Levin & Kaddar, 2011).

Communicable diseases, one of the major ones being Tuberculosis (TB), kill many young adults worldwide. The National Tuberculosis Programs (NTPs) adopted the DOTS (Directly Observed Treatment, Short-course) strategic plan to stop TB (Yasin, 2007). The DOTS program supports various TB patients by providing regular TB drugs and working to eradicate TB. The successful treatment under DOTS, initiated in 1997, achieved nearly a 78% success rate (Obermeyer et al., 2008). In 1998, the case detection rate for both DOTS and non-DOTS programs was nearly 40%, with cases being notified for new TB detection. It is evident that, after that, a few surveys were conducted, which show that many infected TB patients seek private practitioners due to a lack of public awareness, making it difficult for them to reach the NTP (AI-Maniri et al., 2008; Srinivasan & Praba Lama, 2025).

TB Management and Control: Public-Private Mix

According to a WHO report, to better understand the involvement of private health facilities in the TB care sector, a global situation assessment was conducted in 1999. It included nearly 23 partner countries and involved 6 WHO regions in the assessment visit. It also included nearly 10 of the 22 high-burden countries in partnership with the global TB control program (WHO, 2009). Public and private practitioners are involved in the PPM approach to TB care support. An increase in TB cases and poor management practices by private practitioners can lead to high morbidity and mortality rates, a socioeconomic burden on the country, and the development of drug-resistant TB (Zumla et al., 2012). Poor-quality TB management can be addressed by including private practitioners under the DOTS program. This can improve TB case detection and strengthen TB control efforts. The private sector is widely trusted in the community and can provide opportunities to improve case detection and treatment outcomes in a sustainable way (Uplekar, 2003).

The public and private systems are involved through the NTPs program and coordinated with the public-private mix in the current TB program. Most government TB programs, through the proper channels of NTPs, collaborate with the private sector to control the high burden in the private sector (Lal, 2010). The public-private mix should be integrated with NTP activities, and the private health sector should provide support to reduce TB-related barriers. Public and private partnerships can involve NTPs to achieve TB control goals (Suseela & Shannawaz, 2023; Srinivasan et al., 2025). The current strategic plan lacks coherence in increasing the private health sector's involvement, as per WHO guidelines, and needs further development. The DOTS strategy strengthens efforts to reduce TB incidence and ensures successful treatment. Its implementation in the private sector supports effective programmatic approaches (WHO, 2014).

BACKGROUND OF THE STUDY

The background of the study emphasizes the public health challenges globally, especially affecting low- and middle-income countries. TB management requires strong notification and strengthening of private health facilities, along with disease surveillance to provide strategies for controlling and notifying TB cases and to allocate resources. In the public and private health sectors, the importance of TB notification can be emphasized, focusing on various aspects of health infrastructure and accessibility. Improving treatment adherence in national policy can enhance and increase TB notification in the private sector (Suseela & Shannawaz, 2023).

Role of Public Facility in TB Notification

Public health facilities need to provide TB management in many countries through various national TB programs (NTPs). It can include various aspects, such as making TB notification mandatory for every facility, providing standardized treatment for all TB patients, and subsidizing TB medicines (Needham et al., 2004). Even though the PPM can provide strong support to increase TB notification in public hospitals, many issues still prevent proper notification. Often, it is underreported in health facilities due to bureaucratic influences and inefficiencies. This can overburden health workers, who have limited resources to reach underserved areas.

Role of Private Facility in TB Notification

The private health sector encompasses various private health facilities, clinics, individual practitioners, and home-based practices serving a portion of the population in urban areas. The role of TB notification becomes very difficult, and while they are handling TB cases, they do not notify public health. TB notification is inconsistent in many countries (Glaziou et al., 2018). The lack of awareness in the private sector means it cannot be notified. They need to streamline the process to get TB notification in the private sector. In the private sector, TB notification results are often underreported, and they are not reflected in government data in a proper way (Wippel et al., 2024).

Importance of the Study

The importance of the study lies in the effectiveness of public and private notifications in controlling TB elimination at the national and global levels. The study follows various strategic plans such as:

- Integrate the TB Notification: To enhance collaboration between the public and private sectors by establishing unified and digital systems for case reporting (Ibeneme et al., 2022).
- Policy Implication: To motivate the private sector to adhere to private notification as per the STCI guidelines by providing training, support, and incentives, and by implementing measures for various non-compliance issues (Negandhi et al., 2017).
- Increase the Resource Allocation: To provide targeted resources for private health facilities and monitor the TB notification trend (Suseela & Shannawaz, 2023).
- Strengthen the Surveillance: To provide accurate data for private notification to support decision-making at the national and global levels (Pardeshi et al., 2021).

The study can enhance public and private notifications, which are important for ensuring TB patient interventions to address the gaps in both sectors. Ultimately, it aims to contribute to the global goal of eliminating TB as a public health threat.

In India, the majority of patients with tuberculosis initially seek treatment in the private sector, and after diagnosis, they return to the public sector. Effective treatment, whether in the public sector or private sector, is better (Yellappa et al., 2017). The study analyzes the last four years of data on public and private TB notifications for a comparative analysis. The secondary data was collected through the Ni-kshay portal. The data was analyzed state-wise, and the recent data from the last four years reflects a better trend in TB notifications from both the private and public sectors. The significance of the study is that TB is a notifiable disease, but it aims to establish a TB surveillance system to ensure treatment adherence in standard practices within the private sector. It is a challenge to collect TB notifications in the private sector, and there is a need to accelerate the process of TB notification. Active cases at the state level should be initiated and increased to improve TB notification (CARE, 2023).

Research Gap, Research Objectives, and Research Questions

In the research study, there are many research gaps, especially regarding TB notifications that remain un-notified in private and public hospitals (Frederick et al., 2021). This study aims to identify the gaps in TB notifications from private hospitals and explore strategic plans to strengthen private notification processes (Chijioke-Akaniro et al., 2022). What are the procedures to implement to obtain notifications without barriers? Notifications should not only come from private hospitals; they can also include various clinics, labs, pharmacies, traditional practitioners, and local healers who practice in local and peripheral areas (Virhia et al., 2023). How can the study address the gap? It is one of the social goals to improve the health and well-being of the community. To highlight the gaps in TB notification in both private and public facilities. What is the reason for private hospitals lagging in TB notification? The strategy to improve TB notification in the private sector.

Major Objective of the Study

- To analyze TB notifications in public and private hospital settings: This will include a state-wise, district-wise, and year-wise comparison to assess trends over time.
- To analyze the relationship between public and private TB notifications: The study will explore how these two sectors interact and contribute to the overall TB notification system.
- To identify the barriers faced in collecting TB notifications from private healthcare settings: This will focus on the challenges private practitioners and institutions encounter in reporting TB cases.

RESEARCH QUESTIONS

RQ1: Year-wise private notification analysis from 2021 to 2024: state-wise public and private comparison?
RQ2: Year-wise private notification analysis from 2021 to 2024: district-wise public and private comparison?
RQ3: Year-wise private notification analysis from 2021 to 2024: TU-wise public and private comparison?
RQ4: What is the relationship between public and private TB notifications?
RQ5: Why do symptomatic patients prefer private hospitals?
RQ6: What are the reasons TB patients seek treatment in public hospitals after diagnosis?
RQ7: What strategic plans are in place to improve private TB notifications?
RQ8: What problems do private practitioners face when registering TB notifications in the Nikshay portal?
RQ9: How do TB patients perceive treatment in public versus private health facilities?
RQ10: What benefits do private practitioners gain from notifying TB cases?

LITERATURE REVIEW

Public-Private Mix Approaches to Control Tuberculosis

Public and private mix (PPM) is an emerging approach in healthcare that can be a more effective way to achieve successful collaboration in reducing the TB burden at the national level. Communicable diseases include malaria, tuberculosis (TB), diarrhoea, other respiratory infectious diseases (ARIs), sexually transmitted infectious diseases (STIs), and others. Public and private health sectors provide various health-related programs that can control and reduce the burden of diseases (Trent, 2012). This kind of initiative, such as public and private collaboration in communicable diseases, can support the general aspects of disease control. TB infection is a leading cause of death, especially among young adults, with nearly two million deaths globally every year (Glaziou et al., 2018). One-third of the population is affected by the infection, which is a large proportion globally. TB diseases remain a major problem in the future, with various aspects affecting people, including economic challenges, and poor patients being most affected (Raviglione & Sulis, 2016). Private practitioners play a major role in stopping TB and providing care and support for TB patients (Srinivasan, 2025). The study analyzes the public-private comparative analysis and collaboration, focusing on how effective it is in controlling TB through strategically planned efforts.

Figure 1. Private Health Expenditure High Burden 22 countries

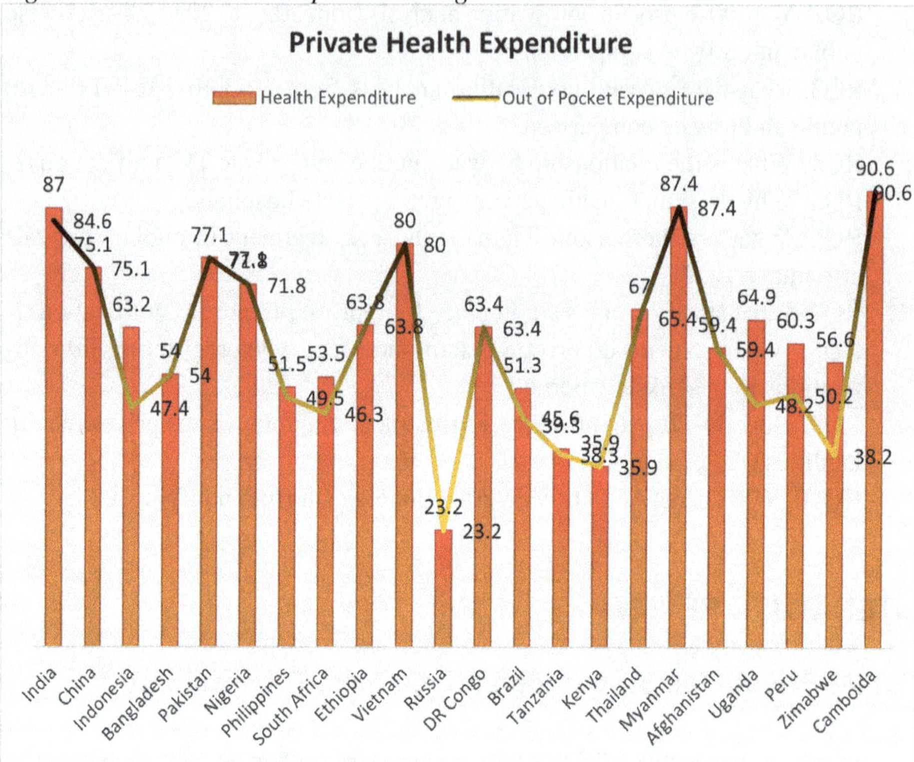

Fig. 1 clearly illustrates the health expenditure in the private health sector and highlights the out-of-pocket expenditure in 22 high-burden countries. It provides data on healthcare availability and the financial burden by country. High out-of-pocket expenditure is found in the majority of the countries, with ≥80% in India (84.6%), Myanmar (87.4%), and Cambodia (90.6%). These countries face a significant financial burden for healthcare services. A moderate level of out-of-pocket expenditure (between 50% to 79%) is seen in countries such as China (75.1%), Pakistan (77.1%), and Vietnam (80%). These countries have moderate financial protection but still face a significant financial burden on individuals. Low out-of-pocket expenditure (<50%) is seen in countries like Russia (23.2%), Brazil (45.6%), and South Africa (46.3%). These countries have strong financial support and better public healthcare funding in the system.

There are countries with identical out-of-pocket health expenditures, such as Ethiopia (63.8%), Nigeria (71.8%), and Bangladesh (54%). These countries have minimal public health security, as the health expenditure is primarily borne out-of-pocket. The overall observation of Fig. 1 shows that South Africa, India, Pakistan, and Bangladesh have high out-of-pocket expenditures for their public health systems. In the African region, there are mixed observations, such as Tanzania (38.3%) and Kenya (35.9%), which have relatively low out-of-pocket expenditure burdens. However, Uganda (48.2%) and DR Congo (63.4%) face a higher burden of costs. Southeast Asia, such as Myanmar and Cambodia, tops the list of high out-of-pocket expenditures. In Thailand, the majority (65.4%) face a high burden, but it is being reduced. The data provide a robust insight into healthcare systems that can reduce the various levels of burden in countries facing high levels of overall out-of-pocket expenditure.

Public and Private Health Care Approaches

As per the WHO, guidelines are provided for the collaboration between the public and private sectors to reduce the global TB burden and to explore research in various aspects of public-private mixed approaches. It can systematically provide various aspects of research to support existing and new approaches for public-private mixed TB care and services. Various approaches can promote the detection of more TB cases and increase the private practice approach. The study provides broader aspects of private health collaboration to reduce TB and eradicate the TB burden on a country-by-country basis. Public and private sectors should provide action-oriented efforts to improve TB notification and should be encouraged (Stop TB Initiative, 2001).

Public and private health collaboration can enhance the NTP staff's focus on improving care and support in the private sector. It is important to encourage private facilities to notify on time, update, and provide notifications to government health facilities (Rakesh & Shannawaz, 2024). Promoting collaboration in private health facilities with the existing DOTS framework is a major aspect of the NTPs' guidelines to provide DOTS in an effective way, reduce TB, and improve the success rate of TB treatment (Adepoju et al., 2022).

The public and private mix can involve enhancing new approaches to be promoted in both public and private sectors and diversify health settings (Anderson, 2012). NTPs can provide sufficient support to promote and offer incentives, motivating the available provisions for TB care in the private sector (Ullah et al., 2012). The medical curriculum could provide appropriate support for young medical practitioners at the college level to strengthen the propaganda in the medical sector. TB care should be strengthened to improve and involve various aspects, increasing the role of private practitioners in improving the control of communicable diseases in healthcare facilities (Haque et al., 2020).

Table 1. Problem and Challenges in Public and Private Collaboration

NTEP Public Sector	Private Health Sector
Ideological perception provided by the public health sector (NTEP).	Inadequate support and training for the information on TB notification details.
Lack of information in private health facilities.	There is doubt regarding the NTP guidelines.
Strengthening efforts to get the notification in the private sector	Public health facilities have low affordable costs, while in private facilities, there is a high level of out-of-pocket expenditure (Kamath et al., 2024)
Prejudices regarding the private notification to obtain motivational aspects of PPM activities.	In the private sector, there is competition for patients to see particular chest specialists (Kwan, 2018).
There is limited coordination, cooperation, and supervision in the NTEP team.	In public health facilities, it is difficult to identify defaulters and trace them. There are challenges in private facilities as well, many times (Attaran, 2022).
Weak and anachronistic regulatory mechanisms.	Quality care and services in private facilities are dependent on the NTEP team.
Absence of precedents and little evidence for replication.	There are large unorganized groups for interaction with all the patients, posing challenges in both the public and private sectors.

Sustainable Development

Sustainable development is a complex task for the healthcare sector to provide efficiency and improve equity for future generations. Sustainable development aims to enhance the Triple Bottom Line (TBL), which provides various dimensions such as economic, social, and environmental aspects (Dhaliwal, 2020). The TBL approach enhances the healthcare field by improving economic, social, and environmental perspectives in their activities. The economic dimension improves healthcare in various ways by ensuring effective utilization of resources and increasing profitability (Rodríguez et al., 2021).

Triple Bottom Line (TBL) and Sustainability in the Healthcare Industry

Sustainability in healthcare supports both social and economic outcomes. An effective and active triple bottom line approach enhances healthcare facilities in a sustainable way (Vergunst et al., 2020). Private hospitals increasing TB notification can provide transparency and support the efficiency, effectiveness, and sustainability of government health facilities (Stallworthy et al., 2020). TBL enhances hospitals by impacting social and environmental aspects, which can improve financial performance and support high-quality, cost-effective services that meet public health needs. TBL provides sustainability values across various dimensions—economically prosperous and strengthened private hospitals deliver both local and regional support, particularly in terms of social and environmental contributions.

Strategical Role in Sustainability Initiatives

Sustainability is a primary need in the healthcare field due to external pressures and the pursuit of competitive advantages in healthcare settings. Healthcare institutions are involved in economic, technological, and operational aspects that present barriers in health facilities (Aljaberi et a., 2020). These challenges necessitate effective strategies to improve sustainability in supply chain activities. Successful embedding of sustainability supports decision-making processes through a long-term adaptive approach. Sustainability contributes to regularity and continuity in balancing the needs of the present and future perspectives (Sarkis, 2020).

Sustainable Development in the Healthcare Industry

Sustainable development supports the healthcare industry in addressing traditional challenges. Private hospitals often face issues in treating TB patients, especially vulnerable populations such as the elderly, who cannot afford advanced care. Enhancing healthcare support amidst conflicts within the SDGs addresses the growing risk of hazardous waste. Sustainability aligns with various aspects—such as environmental and public expectations—to improve perceptions. Sustainable practices incorporate environmental and societal dimensions to strengthen healthcare support and decision making services (Husainy et al., 2024).

Sustainable Health Solutions and Resource Management

Healthcare settings are affected by conflicts in effective resource management, especially in critical areas. Strategies should focus on effective planning, increasing local resource use, and integrating energy sources (Bogale et al., 2024). Sustainable health solutions focus on water conservation, waste management, recycling, and maintaining hygiene and sanitation practices. These practices support independence, increase healthcare service efficiency, and address challenges in sustainable environments (Alruwaili et al., 2023).

Impact Assessment of Sustainable Practices on Healthcare Delivery

Sustainable development practices support the healthcare system by improving healthcare delivery and efficiency, particularly in limited-resource settings. Effective practices ensure timely treatment for vulnerable and affected individuals, prompt medical support, and high-quality care, while also reducing time delays. Community-based training for healthcare workers helps them understand the challenges faced by affected individuals and supports health equity through care and support services. These practices benefit vulnerable populations, reduce costs, enhance resource availability, and improve healthcare delivery. Better health outcomes are achieved through sustainable processes that address patients' needs (Javanparast et a., 2018; Bhatt & Bathija, 2018; Mortimer et al., 2018). Sustainability strengthens resilience and service effectiveness during crises. Economic and environmental sustainability measures reduce waste, lower operational costs, and support long-term public health goals. Community engagement, through social cohesion, trust, and responsiveness, further improves healthcare outcomes (Cyril et al., 2015; Khan et al., 2020; Hu et al., 2022) .

Mental Health and Psycho-social Support

Mental health challenges such as anxiety, depression, PTSD, and related issues significantly affect individuals and communities. Mental health services should be integrated into primary healthcare for TB-affected individuals and others (Mainga, 2023). Community-based initiatives—such as outreach programs, counseling, and social support networks—enhance interaction among affected individuals and offer culturally relevant support (Weiss et al., 2013). Vulnerable groups like children, the elderly, tribal communities, women, and persons with disabilities must be prioritized. Training and empowering affected communities or the general population through skill development enhances psycho-social support and aids in recovery (Jabir & Choolayil, 2024).

Collaboration and Partnerships for Sustainable Healthcare

Collaboration among public and private entities—including international organizations, governments, and NGOs—plays a vital role in achieving SDG goals. Goals such as SDG 2 (Zero Hunger) and SDG 3 (Good Health and Well-being) are effectively pursued through such partnerships (Lile et al., 2023). International organizations provide leadership training and funding support. Governments should strengthen policies and community-based services to expand interventions for affected individuals. NGOs help identify and support vulnerable and marginalized populations by collaborating with local governments to reduce the disease burden (Rajabi et al., 2021).

Impact of Sustainable Practices on Healthcare Delivery

Sustainable healthcare practices enhance healthcare delivery in five key areas: access, quality, efficiency, patient satisfaction, and long-term sustainability (Ravindran et al., 2024).

1. Access: Simplified access to healthcare facilities enables services to reach vulnerable and remote communities.
2. Quality: Quality care and services raise treatment standards and improve outcomes.
3. Efficiency: Effective resource use reduces costs and boosts operational efficiency.
4. Patient Satisfaction: Consistent, quality care improves patient experiences and satisfaction.
5. Sustainability: Sustainability includes financial support, human resources, and infrastructure improvements for long-term service viability.

These indicators strengthen the healthcare system and help deliver equitable services to communities, especially those in need, resulting in successful outcomes.

RESEARCH METHODOLOGY

The study was used for comparative analysis and cross-sectional analysis of TB notification in public and private hospitals in selected states of India. It focuses on the trend of TB notification over the last five years, from 2020 to 2024, in both sectors. Secondary data was used from the Ni-kshay portal to gather TB notification data for the public and private sectors. The analysis was conducted state-wise, district-wise, and TB unit-wise. The notification from the private and public sectors was validated through the Ni-kshay portal. The study was used for comparative year-wise and health facility-wise analysis of TB notification.

RESULT AND DISCUSSION

The result of the study provides public and private notifications nationwide, state-wise, district-wise, and Tuberculosis Unit-wise. It discusses how this can help public and private health facilities address gaps comprehensively. It emphasizes the notification rate to effectively address the issues. Table 2 provides the target and achievement in the public and private sectors from the year 2020 to 2024.

Table 2. India Public and Private TB Notification 2020 to 2024

Year	TB notification	Public	Private	Total
2020	Target	*1923120*	*1075910*	*2999030*
	Achieved	*1173207*	*589585*	*1762792*
	Progress	*61%*	*55%*	*59%*
	TB notification	Public	Private	Total
2021	Target	*1952750*	*1041580*	*2994330*
	Achieved	*1352396*	*735172*	*2087568*
	Progress	69%	71%	70%
	TB notification	Public	Private	Total
2022	Target	*1828260*	*951740*	*2780000*
	Achieved	*1576721*	*814094*	*2390815*
	Progress	*86%*	*86%*	*86%*
	TB notification	Public	Private	Total
2023	Target	*1825705*	*937127*	*2762832*
	Achieved	*1582213*	*932761*	*2514974*
	Progress	*87%*	*100%*	*91%*
	TB notification	Public	Private	Total
2024	Target	*1845374*	*942396*	*2787770*
	Achieved	*1551197*	*890444*	*2441641*
	Progress	*84%*	*94%*	*88%*

The target for TB notification in the public and private sectors is nearly 2.78 million annually. It can increase the percentage of TB patients, starting from 59% in the year 2020, and reaching 88% by 2024. The public sector achieved a major milestone with 61% in 2020, and it increased to 87% in 2023. However, it is expected to decline to 84% in 2024. The private sector TB notification progress in 2020 was 55%, and it peaked at 100% in 2023. However, it is expected to drop to 94% in 2024. The overall trend shows an increase in the public and private sectors achieving TB notification, improving over the years and highlighting efforts in TB detection reporting.

Total Notification:

Total Notification = Public Notification + Private Notification

$$Progress\ (\%) = \frac{\text{Achieved Notification}}{\text{Target Notification}} \text{ X } 100$$

2020

Total Achieved Notification:

Total Achieved = 1173207 + 589585
Total Achieved = 1762792

Progress Calculation:

$$Public\ Progress = \frac{1173207}{1923120} \text{ X } 100 = 61\%$$

$$Private\ Progress = \frac{589585}{1075910} \text{ X } 100 = 55\%$$

$$Total\ Progress = \frac{1762792}{2999030} \text{ X } 100 = 59\%$$

2021

Total Achieved Notification

1352396 + 735172 = 2087568

Progress Calculation

$$Public\ Progress = \frac{1352396}{1952750} \text{ X } 100 = 69\%$$

$$Private\ Progress = \frac{735172}{1041580} \text{ X } 100 = 71\%$$

$$Total\ Progress = \frac{2087568}{2994330} \text{ X } 100 = 70\%$$

2022

Total Achieved Notification

1576721 + 814094 = 2390815

Progress Calculation

$$\textit{Public Progress} = \frac{1576721}{1828269} \text{X } 100 = 86\%$$

$$\textit{Private Progress} = \frac{814094}{951740} \text{X } 100 = 86\%$$

$$\textit{Total Progress} = \frac{2390815}{2780000} \text{X } 100 = 86\%$$

2023

Total Achieved Notification

1582213 + 932761 = 2514974

Progress Calculation

$$\textit{Public Progress} = \frac{1582213}{1825705} \text{X } 100 = 87\%$$

$$\textit{Private Progress} = \frac{932761}{937127} \text{X } 100 = 100\%$$

$$\textit{Total Progress} = \frac{2514974}{2762832} \text{X } 100 = 91\%$$

2024

Total Achieved Notification

1551197 + 890444 = 2441641
Progress Calculation

$$\textit{Public Progress} = \frac{1551197}{1845374} \text{X } 100 = 84\%$$

$$\textit{Private Progress} = \frac{890444}{942396} \text{X } 100 = 94\%$$

$$Total\ Progress = \frac{2441641}{2787770} X\ 100 = 88\%$$

Figure 2. TB Notification Public % Progress from the period of 2021 - 204

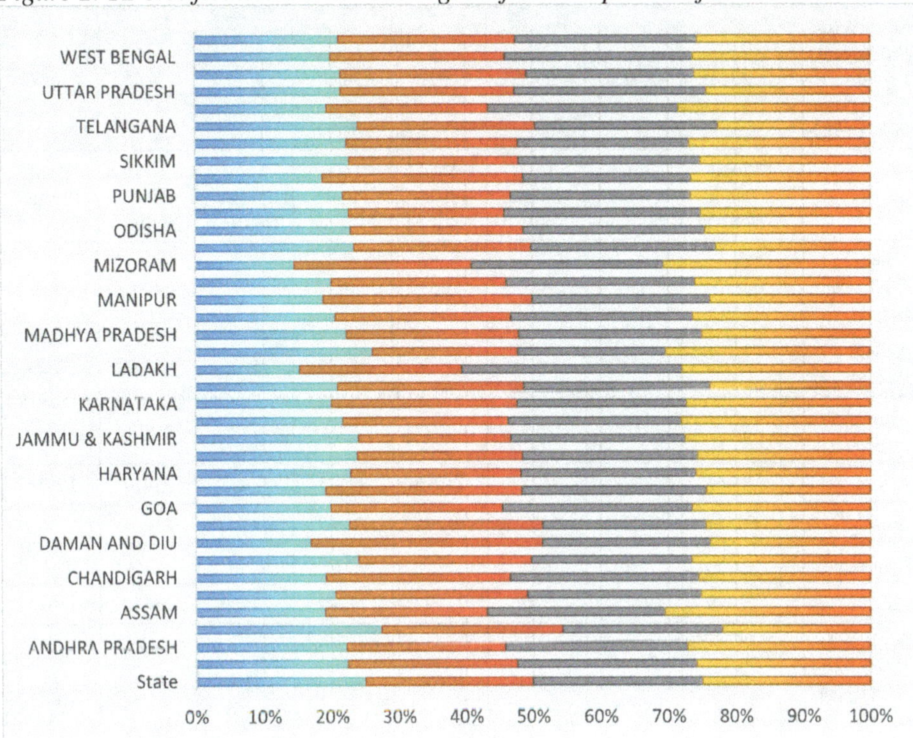

Public TB notification progress from 2021 to 2024 improved from 69% in 2021, increasing to 87% in 2023 before declining to 84% in 2024. Jammu & Kashmir, Himachal Pradesh, and Uttarakhand have consistently shown high progress, with an increase of more than 90% in the year. Ladakh also demonstrated exceptional progress, with an increase of nearly 123% in the year 2023. Assam achieved nearly 56% in the year 2021, increasing to 90% in 2024. Jharkhand also increased the rate of public notification to a total of 104% in 2024. State-wise fluctuation is observed, especially in Rajasthan, where it was nearly 102% in 2022 but dropped to a lower rate of 91% in 2024. The Daman and Diu region has shown fluctuating progress, with nearly 130% in 2022 and 90% in 2024. There are some states, such as Lakshadweep, Manipur, and West Bengal, that consistently show lower performance compared to the national average for public TB notification throughout the year.

There are northeastern states like Arunachal Pradesh, Nagaland, and Meghalaya that show mixed trends in their overall progress and improvement.

Table 3. State wise Public and Private TB notification 2021 - 2024

State Wise Public and Private TB Notification 2021 to 2024	***2021***	***2021***	***2022***	***2022***	***2023***	***2023***	***2024***	***2024***
State	Total Public Notified	Total Private Notified	Total Public Notified	Total Private Notified	Total Public Notified	Total Private Notified	Total Public Notified	Total Private Notified
Andaman & Nicobar Islands	*492*	*5*	*487*	*33*	*492*	*48*	*460*	*48*
Andhra Pradesh	*55998*	*29192*	*55738*	*34956*	*52636*	*35132*	*49156*	*29834*
Arunachal Pradesh	*2675*	*12*	*2669*	*123*	*2241*	*330*	*2118*	*533*
Assam	*28861*	*8658*	*35737*	*11936*	*37635*	*13955*	*35910*	*10643*
Bihar	*56144*	*74830*	*69078*	*91147*	*76773*	*108911*	*75946*	*114141*
Chandigarh	*4137*	*540*	*5550*	*473*	*5616*	*1014*	*4899*	*1612*
Chhattisgarh	*22839*	*9135*	*25805*	*12492*	*24299*	*13900*	*24627*	*11672*
Dadra and Nagar Haveli and Daman and Diu	*926*	*66*	*1271*	*115*	*1019*	*125*	*889*	*89*
Delhi	*66105*	*35205*	*74275*	*31028*	*70738*	*27736*	*72103*	*26397*
Goa	*1581*	*392*	*1572*	*444*	*1574*	*381*	*1497*	*459*
Gujarat	*90369*	*51560*	*97863*	*52509*	*91711*	*49802*	*88619*	*41094*
Haryana	*43408*	*25072*	*48116*	*27074*	*49663*	*29547*	*51185*	*30893*
Himachal Pradesh	*11795*	*2527*	*13546*	*2541*	*13181*	*2263*	*12702*	*2152*
Jammu & Kashmir	*9265*	*1534*	*9748*	*2028*	*9445*	*2184*	*9556*	*1955*
Jharkhand	*34494*	*17790*	*42511*	*14817*	*44087*	*16450*	*41285*	*17649*
Karnataka	*45518*	*25359*	*51125*	*27984*	*49754*	*30728*	*46986*	*26528*
Kerala	*13989*	*7859*	*15233*	*8310*	*13392*	*8174*	*11948*	*7548*
Ladakh	*265*	*25*	*308*	*26*	*300*	*16*	*266*	*12*
Lakshadweep	*12*	*0*	*10*	*0*	*6*	*0*	*7*	*0*

continued on following page

Table 3. Continued

State Wise Public and Private TB Notification 2021 to 2024	2021	2021	2022	2022	2023	2023	2024	2024
Madhya Pradesh	106902	58154	124203	61701	116205	66418	115286	52941
Maharashtra	96436	95989	118195	112301	109526	113926	108181	104672
Manipur	1235	562	1618	918	1541	976	1427	872
Meghalaya	3157	908	3893	994	3895	920	3602	698
Mizoram	1391	352	1660	400	1793	439	1707	504
Nagaland	2915	762	3320	834	3395	875	2894	863
Odisha	43384	8744	48807	11477	50403	11643	46673	8361
Puducherry	2996	88	3344	133	3466	142	3029	129
Punjab	34322	16334	41917	13501	39931	15137	37903	16965
Rajasthan	97907	49386	119722	48590	115715	47635	115894	46622
Sikkim	1151	202	1207	179	1180	162	1063	158
Tamil Nadu	56922	24674	63701	29073	64752	31069	58657	28442
Telangana	36912	22873	46272	26033	44309	30439	38577	32139
Tripura	2416	123	2830	187	3121	219	2948	155
Uttar Pradesh	306167	141800	358892	159429	388622	234612	398832	237183
Uttarakhand	16577	6092	20688	6730	19699	6871	21228	6289
West Bengal	52733	18368	65810	23578	70098	30582	63137	30192
Total	1352396	735201	1576721	814109	1582213	932763	1551197	890444

Table 3 provides a comprehensive understanding of the private and public notifications. It peaked in the year 2023 at nearly 1,582,213 for private notifications, which increased to 932,763 during the same period. Some of the states provide a high contribution, especially UP and Maharashtra, as they regularly provide the highest number of TB notifications in both the public and private sectors. Their active TB programs identify TB cases in both sectors. Some of the states have a balanced contribution, such as Delhi, Gujarat, and Karnataka. They show various proportions in the public and private TB notifications over the years. The improvement is noteworthy in states like Bihar, Jharkhand, and Assam. These states reflect significant contributions to both private and public TB notifications, with growth in both sectors and a partial increase in TB detection. There are some states that provide low contributions to public and private TB notifications, such as Lakshadweep, Ladakh, and Andaman & Nicobar Islands. These states have minimal levels of TB notifications, with smaller proportion rates. There are the lowest rates of TB notification in states like Gujarat, Delhi, and Kerala for both the public and private sectors. Although the level of TB notifications has increased, there is underreporting due to programmatic challenges.

Tale 4. Total Public and Private TB Notification 2021- 2022			
Year	**Public Notification**	**Private Notification**	**Total Notification**
2021	*1352396*	*735201*	*2087597*
2022	*1576721*	*814109*	*2390830*
2023	*1582213*	*932763*	*2514976*
2024	*1551197*	*890444*	*2441641*

Table 4 provides the overall public and private TB notifications from the year 2021 to 2022. The TB notification rate in 2021 was nearly 2,087,597, and in 2023, it was nearly 2,514,976. There was a slight decline in 2024, with a fluctuating trend at 2,441,641. There is a consistent increase in TB notifications, with the majority of TB cases reported in the public sector in India. It was nearly 1,582,213 in 2023, and before a marginal decrease in 2024, it was 1,551,197. In the private sector, the notification increased from 735,200 in 2021, and the private notification for the year 2023 reflected nearly 932,763. This reflects the importance of private sector engagement. However, in the year 2024, the rate declined to 890,444. The progress of the year 2023 is the highest level of TB notification, nearly 2,514,976. It indicates the effect of TB case finding across both public and private sectors. The recent decline in TB notifications from the year 2024 in both public and private sectors is a challenge to maintain and identify TB notifications. It is very difficult and needs to improve and sustain the efforts.

Equation 1 – Total TB Notification

$$\text{Total Notification} = \text{Public Notification} + \text{Private Notification}$$

Example Calculation (for 2021):

$$\text{Total Notification2021} = 1{,}352{,}396 + 735{,}201 = 2{,}087{,}597$$

Verification for 2024:

$$\text{Total Notification 2024} = 1{,}551{,}197 + 890{,}444 = 2{,}441{,}641$$

Equation 2 – Year-on-Year (YoY) Growth Rate

This measures how much TB notifications have increased (or decreased) from the previous year.

$$YoY\ Growth\ (\%)=\frac{(\text{Total Notificationt-Total Notification t-1})}{\text{Total Notification t-1}}1\times 100$$

Example Calculation (2022 over 2021):

$$\text{YoY Growth2022}=\frac{(2{,}390{,}830-2{,}087{,}597)}{2{,}087{,}597}\times 100 = 14.52\%$$

Example Calculation (2023 over 2022):

$$YoY\ Growth_{2023}=\frac{(2{,}514{,}976-2{,}390{,}830)}{2{,}390{,}830}\times 100 = 5.19\%$$

Example Calculation (2024 over 2023):

$$\text{YoY Growth2024}=\frac{(2{,}441{,}641-2{,}514{,}976)}{2{,}514{,}976}\times 100 = -2.91\%$$

Equation 3 – Sectoral Contribution (Public vs Private)

$$\text{Public Share (\%)}=\frac{\text{Public Notification}}{\text{Total Notification}}\times 100$$

$$\text{Private Share (\%)}=\frac{\text{Private Notification}}{\text{Total Notification}}\times 100$$

Example (2023):

$$\text{Public Share2023}=\frac{1{,}582{,}213}{2{,}514{,}976}\times 100 = 62.93\%$$

$$Private\ Share_{2023}=\frac{932{,}763}{2{,}514{,}976}\times 100 = 37.07\%$$

Example (2024):

$$\text{Public Share2024} = \frac{1{,}551{,}197}{2{,}441{,}641} \times 100 = 63.54\%$$

$$Private\ Share_{2024} = \frac{890{,}444}{2{,}441{,}641} \times 100 = 36.46\%$$

Equation 4 – Compound Annual Growth Rate (CAGR)

To find the overall growth in TB notifications between 2021 and 2024:

$$\text{CAGR} = \left(\frac{\text{Final Value}}{\text{Initial Value}}\right)^{\frac{1}{n}} - 1$$

where n=3n = 3n=3 years (2021–2024).

Calculation:

$$\text{CAGR} = \left(\frac{2{,}441{,}641}{2{,}087{,}597}\right)^{\frac{1}{3}} - 1 = 5.36\%$$

Between 2021 and 2024, total TB notifications showed a consistent upward trend, rising from 2.08 million to 2.44 million, representing an overall increase of approximately 17%. The most significant year-on-year growth was observed between 2021 and 2022 (14.52%), followed by a moderate rise in 2023 and a slight decline in 2024. Throughout this period, the public sector accounted for around 63% of total notifications, while the private sector contributed between 36% and 37%, reflecting strong collaboration and engagement from both sectors. The compound annual growth rate (CAGR) of 5.36% further highlights steady progress in TB case detection and reporting over the four-year span.

Figure 3. Public and Private Notification 2021 to 2024, Tamil Nadu State.

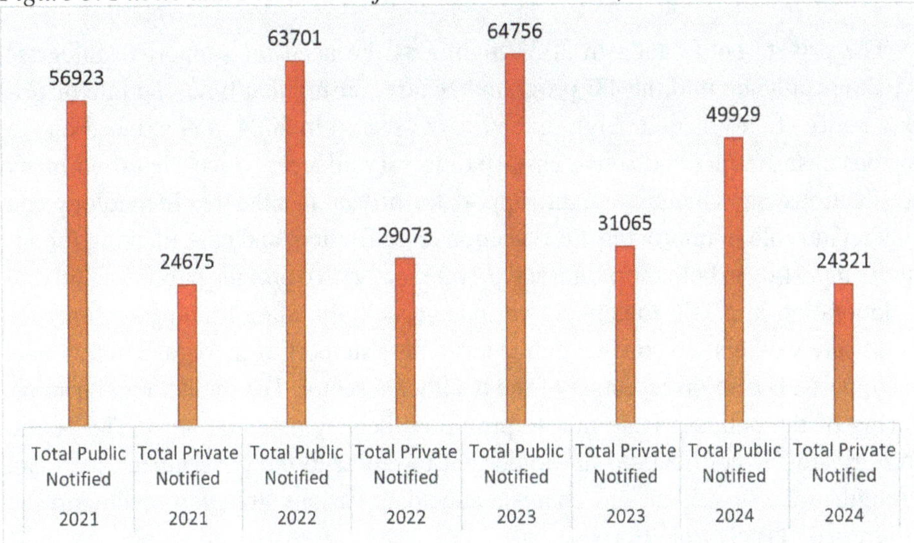

Fig. 3 provides the private and public TB notifications from 2021 to 2024, which are highlighted. The annual trend for public and private TB notifications increased from 2021 to 2023. The public notification rate in 2021 was 56,923, and in 2023, it reflected nearly 64,756 in the public sector, showing consistent progress in TB detection as reported. The private notification rapidly increased from 24,675 in 2021, showing an increasing trend to 31,065 in 2023, engaging private healthcare practitioners. The decline in the figures for public and private notifications significantly improved in the public sector, which increased by nearly 22.0%, and in the private sector, which increased by 21.7%. This reflects a reduction in cases and an improvement in the case-finding activities initiated. The reduction of TB cases can improve the previous control aspects.

The possibility of underreporting makes it very difficult to identify the post-pandemic situation. The public and private sector contributions account for nearly 70% of the total cases underreported in the public health system. This is a crucial aspect and the backbone of the study, as it helps identify TB detection and management. The private sector increased from 30.3% in 2021 to 32.4% in 2023. This reflects that public and private collaboration has increased reliance on private practitioners to provide TB care. It may decrease in 2024 if healthcare priorities improve and funds are increased to provide active TB surveillance activities. There is a gap in both sectors that can be improved through various strategic plans and challenges. This can support the success of TB control efforts in various aspects, such as decreasing TB cases, identifying new TB cases, and providing active disease management.

Strategic Plan to Leverage the Private Sector

The private notification in 2023 highlights the need for support to integrate private healthcare into the TB program because, during that time, the rate of private notification was quite high in the private sector. In 2024, it is reduced due to various case-finding and active case-finding surveillance, which identified many notifications, showing significant support for private healthcare. Technology can play a vital role in improving TB detection, case finding, and case tracking for accurate reporting in both the public and private sectors. To provide public and private collaboration in NTEP to conduct various capacity-building training sessions for healthcare workers. To conduct public awareness support to encourage individuals to support TB care, irrespective of the healthcare sector. To conduct regular monitoring of the public-private mix to promptly identify potential gaps. The public and private TB notifications are important to report to the government, as it can strengthen the surveillance mechanism and adapt various strategies to support the progress of TB control efforts.

Figure 4. Tamil Nadu District Wise Public and Private TB Notification 2021 – 2024

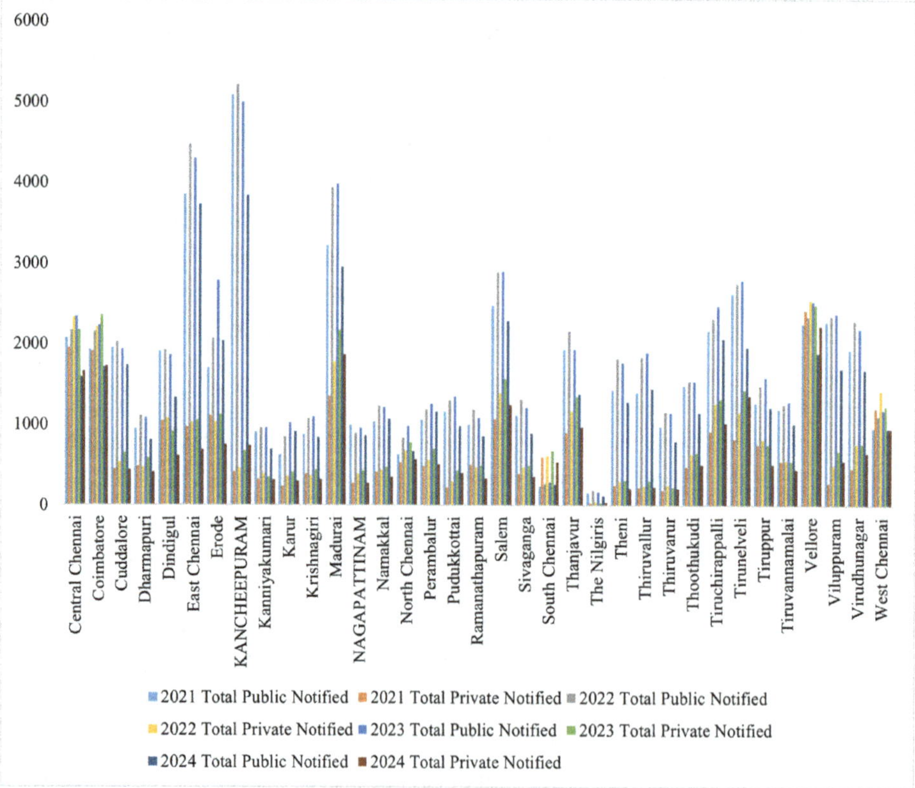

Table 4: Influence of district-wise TB notification in Tamil Nadu from 2021 to 2024 across public and private health sectors. The trend of public and private TB notifications is highlighted. The public sector highlights the dominant districts reported for public and private notifications, Kanchipuram and Madurai, reflecting the crucial role of TB management. There is consistent follow-up in districts such as Coimbatore and the Chennai region, including various parts like North, East, West, and Central, which report high private notifications in urban areas. The urban and rural aspects show that in urban areas, Chennai district has the highest TB notifications, followed by Coimbatore district. Overall, TB notifications are high, highlighting the need for better infrastructure and awareness activities. In rural districts like Nilgiris, Karur, and Kanniyakumari, it is reflected that there is underreporting, a lower detection rate, and a lower disease burden. This indicates a gap in TB monitoring and surveillance.

The year of change in private TB notifications in some districts, like Madurai and Salem, reflects improved high-level collaboration and awareness, leading to an increased rate. The year 2024 shows a decline in various districts like Chennai Central, Coimbatore, and Kanchipuram. The reported private cases were reduced, which can be attributed to underreporting in post-pandemic situations. The public notifications in the year 2021 totaled 5,087 in Kanchipuram, making it the highest district. East Chennai also led with robust public health interventions. The districts of Vellore and Viluppuram are balanced in public and private notifications, compared to the effects of public-private partnerships. The low rate of involvement in the districts of Nilgiris and Kanniyakumari shows low private cases. This can strengthen the districts and identify TB engagement in more rigorous aspects.

There are innovative strategies that can be followed by all districts to boost TB detection in the public and private sectors, including conducting regular awareness campaigns in highly crowded public places. To enhance public and private sector notifications, providing benefits to private practitioners through various incentive supports or voucher gift coupons can motivate them to detect more TB cases and report them to the NTEP team. Mobile health can support TB detection in urban areas by integrating TB efforts, blending the public and private sectors to optimize private TB notifications and TB care. It can also integrate innovative support. The figure highlights the various opportunities to strengthen TB notification and provide innovation in TB notification across the public and private sectors in Tamil Nadu districts.

Figure 5. Trichy District TU wise Public and Private TB notification 2024

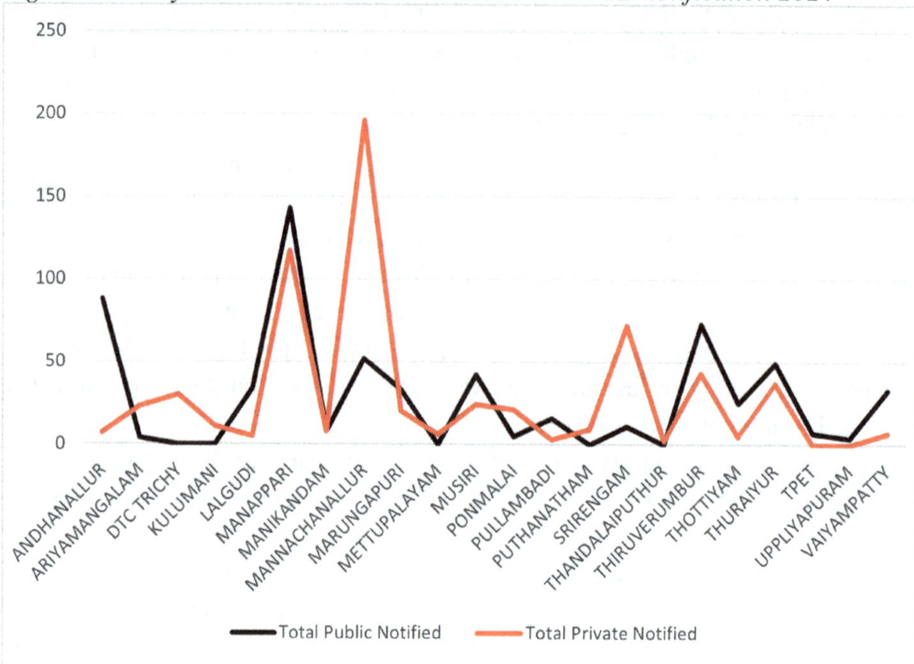

The 2024 TB notification in Trichy District, with Tuberculosis unit-wise distribution, provides the data on public and private TB notifications, covering all the TUs in Trichy District. Fig. 5 highlights the public sector dominance in public notifications and private notifications, reflecting the role of the public health system in TB detection. The significance of the figure emphasizes private notifications, which are high in Manachanallur TU and DTC, where a large number of private notifications were received. Public notification is high in Manaparai, with nearly 143 TB cases, reflecting strong public health efforts in the TU of Manaparai. According to the data, the second-highest public notification TU is Thiruverambur, with nearly 73 public cases notified in the year 2024. Private TB notification is leading in the TU of Manachanallur, with nearly 196 notifications compared to 52 received from public and private healthcare in the year 2024. The second-highest is DTC Trichy, with nearly 30 cases registered in private notifications. There is a lack of public sector involvement, which may lead to underreporting.

Disparities in Public and Private TB Notification

There are a total of 22 TUs in Trichy District, especially T. Pet and Uppilliyapura, where the reported TB notifications indicate very low private sector engagement, which needs to be improved. However, there are some reasons in the TU where there are no proper private health facilities available. They can either go to the nearby urbanized TU, Thuraiyur, or to the nearby district of Salem. The Uppiliyapuram TU is located on the border of Trichy, Salem, and Namakkal districts, so patients prioritize going to the nearby popular specialized private and government hospitals. But even though they improve, private TB cases can go through nearby districts, where particular TU patient lists are collected and followed up. This can be one of the strategies to improve the caseload. In TUs like DTC Trichy and Thandalaiputhur, there is also a focus on nearby TUs and nearby districts, which strengthens the public and private TB notification cases.

Low-level TB cases in TUs

There are 7 TUs with low TB case loads, especially in Uppiliyapuram, where only 4 cases were received. This can be alarming due to the lower TB prevalence in the state and inadequate surveillance in the reporting system, with very limited healthcare support in the region. There are some TUs that do not have private TB cases, especially Thottiyam and Pullambadi. These two TUs are in the same region and are on the borders of different districts. Thottiyam TU is near Namakkal District, while Pullambadi TU is located near Perambalur and Ariyalur Districts. It can engage private providers by providing training and incentive support, which can improve the caseload for private cases. High burden TUs in Manaparai and Mannachanallur require sustained efforts to provide effective treatment for TB patients, support treatment adherence, and reduce the TB burden at the TU level, district level, state level, national level, and global level.

Strengthen Public-Private Partnerships

Private practitioners report low TB notifications due to patient confidentiality. To provide effective follow-up, the NTEP team PPM coordinator should conduct outreach activities and improve policy incentive support for private practitioners. It can strengthen support through awareness campaigns and provide various outreach activities. To improve case detection in low notification TUs, a strategic plan can be adopted. The state-level State TB Officer (STO), district-level District TB Officer (DTO), block-level officers, GH level, PHC, UPHC level, Block Medical Officer, Chief Medical Officer, and City Medical Officer all have the main responsibility to execute the program effectively in terms of public and private notifications and service delivery.

They can encounter various workers who are involved in supporting services and providing effective treatment, such as STS, STLS, HV, LT, HI, VHN, ANM, Anganwadi workers, ASHA workers, and MTS. These workers can support TB patients and follow up at the local level, where panchayat leaders, SHG members, school teachers, society members, and the key village population can also support the TB patients (Srinivasan & Vallipriya, 2025). This tailored approach will help follow up with TB patients and provide effective interventions, support, and service delivery, ensuring successful treatment and the eradication of TB. This analysis provides a balanced approach in the public and private health sectors. It can enhance TB notification and detection in both the public and private sectors across Tamil Nadu.

Discussion

The annual target for TB notification across the public and private sectors is approximately 2.78 million cases. Notification rates have shown steady improvement, with the overall TB notification increasing from 59% in 2020 to an estimated 88% by 2024. In the public sector, notification improved from 61% in 2020 to 87% in 2023 but is projected to slightly decline to 84% in 2024. Similarly, private sector notification rose from 55% in 2020 to a peak of 100% in 2023, followed by a projected decrease to 94% in 2024. This trend reflects the overall enhancement of TB detection and reporting systems. Public notification progress between 2021 and 2024 increased significantly—from 69% in 2021 to 87% in 2023, with a marginal drop expected in 2024 (WHO, 2024). Certain states and union territories, including Jammu & Kashmir, Himachal Pradesh, Uttarakhand, and Ladakh, have demonstrated notable progress, with Ladakh showing an exceptional increase of nearly 123% in 2023.

Assam's performance improved from 56% in 2021 to 90% in 2024, and Jharkhand surpassed the target with 104% public notification in 2024. Conversely, some states showed fluctuating or declining trends. Rajasthan's rate dropped from 102% in 2022 to 91% in 2024, while Daman and Diu fell from 130% to 90% over the same period. States like Lakshadweep, Manipur, and West Bengal continue to perform below the national average. The significant private sector contributions, with peak notifications of 1,582,213 in 2023. Uttar Pradesh and Maharashtra consistently led in both sectors due to robust TB programs. Delhi, Gujarat, and Karnataka presented a balanced mix of public and private notifications. Noteworthy improvements were also seen in Bihar, Jharkhand, and Assam. In contrast, low notifications were recorded in Lakshadweep, Ladakh, and the Andaman & Nicobar Islands.

According to Table 4, total TB notifications rose from 2,087,597 in 2021 to 2,514,976 in 2023 before slightly declining to 2,441,641 in 2024. The public sector accounted for the majority of notifications, with figures rising from 1,582,213 in 2023 to 1,551,197 in 2024. The private sector also grew, from 735,200 in 2021 to 932,763 in 2023, before dropping to 890,444 in 2024. These trends underscore the significance of private sector engagement and highlight potential underreporting due to systemic challenges. The private sector's share of notifications increased from 30.3% in 2021 to 32.4% in 2023, demonstrating enhanced collaboration. However, sustaining this trend requires improved surveillance, funding, and healthcare priorities.

Strategic Plan to Leverage the Private Sector

To sustain TB detection efforts, strategic integration of private healthcare providers is crucial. The high private notification rate in 2023 underscores the need to strengthen public-private collaboration under NTEP (Yassin et al., 2024). Suggested strategies include:

- Conducting capacity-building training for healthcare workers.
- Launching public awareness campaigns to promote TB care.
- Establishing monitoring mechanisms for the public-private mix.
- Using digital tools for case tracking and reporting.

In Tamil Nadu, TB notification trends from 2021 to 2024 reveal high-performing districts like Kanchipuram and Madurai in both sectors. Urban districts, particularly Chennai and Coimbatore, show high private notifications, while rural districts like Nilgiris and Karur report underperformance due to inadequate infrastructure and healthcare support. TU-level data from Trichy District in 2024 highlights public sector dominance in areas like Manaparai and Thiruverambur. Private notifications are high in Manachanallur TU and DTC Trichy. However, certain TUs—such as Uppiliyapuram, Thottiyam, and Pullambadi—record minimal private engagement, likely due to limited healthcare facilities and geographic factors. These areas can benefit from cross-district coordination and incentive-based private sector involvement.

Addressing Disparities

Out of the 22 TUs in Trichy, several show low TB case loads, which may be due to underreporting or inadequate surveillance. Strategic plans must address these gaps through enhanced training, infrastructure development, and community engagement. High-burden TUs require sustained efforts to improve treatment adherence and reduce TB prevalence.

Strengthening Public-Private Partnerships

a. To overcome the sue of underreporting and enhance case detection:
b. Outreach efforts by NTEP's PPM coordinators must be intensified.

c. Incentive-based programs should motivate private practitioners to report cases.
d. Local stakeholders, including panchayat leaders, SHG members, school teachers, and ASHA workers, should be involved in awareness and follow-up activities.

With coordinated efforts at state, district, and block levels involving STOs, DTOs, BMOs, and CMOs, TB control initiatives can achieve greater impact. A collaborative model that blends public and private efforts is essential for the successful detection, notification, and treatment of TB cases across Tamil Nadu and beyond.

OUTCOME OF THE STUDY

The outcome of the study shows that the public sector has a high burden for TB notification, while the private hospital sector is robust in the aspect that the government mandates the reporting of TB cases (Rakesh et al., 2024). To improve TB notification in the private sector, an incentives model should be initiated to improve the caseload. It is important to provide awareness to hospital administration and strengthen enforcement (Ananthakrishnan et al., 2019). Additionally, mandatory reporting laws should be emphasized, along with support for patient confidentiality and concerns. In public health facilities, proper treatment should be provided as per the STCI guidelines, following standard TB diagnosis and treatment with the support of DOTS for all TB patients. In private hospitals, there is often deviation from providing standardized support and protocols for TB patients, leading to incomplete treatment and delays in treatment support for TB patients (Srinivasan & Vallipriya, 2025). Public hospitals are always affordable for economically disadvantaged groups and vulnerable groups in marginalized communities. In private health facilities in urban areas, affected communities prefer middle and upper-class patients, which can create a gap in rural TB management (Zaidi et al., 2024).

Barriers to Reporting TB Notification in Private Hospitals

There are many barriers to reporting in private hospitals and government facilities, such as lack of infrastructure and the absence of proper digital tools to update notifications (Chilala et al., 2024). Insufficient knowledge of using technology, lack of awareness, difficulty in handling gadgets, and the lengthy format required to report TB notifications as per the guidelines. Legal and social support provide high implications for TB notification (AI-Worafi, 2023). The impact of TB notification in the public and private health systems provides a comprehensive understanding for integrating the digital notification system, which can improve data in real time and help follow and monitor TB notification cases in the private sector (Tumuhimbise &

Musiimenta, 2021). One of the major roles of the public-private mix coordinator is to sensitize medical practitioners and train health workers to update TB notifications in the Nikshay portal. This is the main responsibility of the PPM role (Srinivasan et al., 2025). Private hospitals can report TB cases on a timely basis. This will improve the government system and strengthen policy interventions, as well as collaboration between the public and private sectors. The role of healthcare workers is to receive training, especially public health staff, to increase their knowledge about TB and raise awareness, which can improve TB notification cases (Lei et al., 2015; Demissie Gizaw et al., 2015).

Private practitioners are often not aware of the incentive facility for TB case notification. This can be addressed through India Medical Association meetings, where the PPM and DTO can join forces to sensitize private practitioners about TB-related information and the mandatory TB notification requirement (Yellappa, 2019). It is mandatory to report all TB notifications on the Nikshay app, both public and private. To strengthen the public and private partnership by aligning through the support of NTEP. To conduct various capability-building training programs for medical practitioners and healthcare workers to improve the TB notification rate. To provide attractive incentives and gift vouchers and offer complementary support for private practitioners (Khan et al., 2019). The implication of policy can, through the way TB surveillance support, address various ways to improve private hospitals, and the policy can focus on integrating private healthcare providers to improve TB eradication in the nation (Uplekar, 2016). The comparative analysis provides the importance of both public and private collaboration to detect TB case notifications. In the government, it is mandatory to report and ensure successful treatment, which ultimately improves national health and contributes to the eradication of TB in the country and globally (Cole, 2020).

CONCLUSION

The conclusion of the study provides significant disparities between private and public TB notification. Private hospitals can implement standardized practices for TB notification to address the problem of unreported cases. Consistent follow-up adherence to the guidelines is needed, as the lack of surveillance is a contributing factor. The gaps in TB notification, including delays in diagnosis, treatment, and follow-up, impact the overall improvement in TB notification. The multifaceted approach can strengthen private sector involvement and engagement to improve the training of qualified private practitioners and provide hands-on training for healthcare providers to use technology like the Nikshay portal for a user-friendly training approach. The TB control program should focus more on addressing the gaps between the public and private systems to strengthen them. The TB control program can be a more effective way to diagnose and treat patients, ultimately improving TB notification in the health system to reduce the TB burden in India and achieve national and SDG goals.

LIMITATIONS OF THE STUDY

The limitation of the study is that it provides a comprehensive analysis of private and public hospitals, highlighting regional variations in TB notification that influence the results. The study emphasizes TB notification in the private and public sectors; however, there are several limitations. The major limitation of the study is that private and public health facilities do not provide proper notifications, which can lead to underreporting in the comparative analysis. The secondary data can be addressed through the Ni-kshay portal, which reports to the government and enhances the accuracy of the findings of the study. The data entry process is essential to improve the quality of the results. The study examines public and private TB notification trends at the state level, district level, and TB unit level, and it aims to find uniformity. The limitation of the study is that future research can incorporate qualitative insights to improve private healthcare TB notification. This can improve TB notification in the national TB control program in an effective way.

POLICY IMPLICATIONS

The study's findings can address policy implications and bridge the gap between TB notification in private and public health facilities. The implications indicate the need to address TB control efforts in the private sector, as it is underreported and still presents a significant challenge in the health system. At the district level, enforce mandatory and regular follow-up to collect private notifications from various healthcare providers, including small clinics, labs, pharmacies, and traditional practitioners. They can gather more notifications by focusing on particular health facilities, which can be systematically reported and tracked. Collaborating with the Indian Medical Association (IMA) on a regional basis is also essential. Provide financial support for those who provide TB notifications, encouraging and recognizing them for their efforts and offering incentives. This not only increases the number of practitioners but also fosters greater accountability. Provide training for healthcare workers in private hospitals, clinics, and those with traditional practices in peripheral areas to diagnose TB, notify cases, and conduct follow-ups. The STCI TB guidelines mandate that TB notifications be provided. The policy can focus on the gap in TB notification between public and private health facilities. District-level officers, such as District TB Officers, can provide a reporting system for healthcare workers in the government, which can be more useful for private hospitals to implement standardized notifications more effectively. The NTEP team can simplify the TB notification process for private practitioners by providing a mobile-based application for the reporting system that directly enrolls them in the Ni-kshay portal. The government can provide awareness programs in peripheral areas to educate private healthcare providers about the importance of TB notification and their responsibilities to the public. It can focus on rural areas and improve notification rates in all locations.

INNOVATION OF THE CHAPTER

The chapter provides an understanding of the gaps in TB notification in private and public health facilities. It is a comparative analysis aimed at providing new strategies to improve TB notification for treatment adherence. The study enhances the multi-level analysis and compares TB notification at the state, district, and TB unit levels to integrate the private and public health sectors. It provides a nuanced understanding of TB notification. The study identifies the problems and challenges faced by health practitioners and health workers in increasing private TB notification in health facilities. The study involves the use of technology for TB notification, especially with thc support of thc Ni-kshay portal. It can use web based and mobile apps to report TB notifications, which can reduce barriers and enhance the accuracy of TB data. The innovation of public-private partnerships (PPPs) aims to enhance TB notification and address the gaps. The study provides collaboration between public health and private hospitals.

Public health facilities cater to the affected health population, particularly marginalized rural communities, whereas private hospitals are more easily accessible in urban areas and are affordable for wealthier people. In both the public and private sectors, data should be collected and reported to the National TB Division regularly. It is the responsibility of the district and state roles to frequently share the data and provide comprehensive support for the TB control program. The reporting system can be implemented with technology support to drive the TB case notification system, providing the latest, easily accessible, and synchronized system to report TB cases in both the public and private sectors. To support and implement financial support for TB notification in private health facilities, access to treatment adherence support should be provided, along with transparent incentive support for health workers, private practitioners, and the general public. To provide extensive training to both public and private sector workers to sensitize them on the importance of TB notification, and to offer various resources to support healthcare workers in both the public and private sectors. Further, the study can provide collaboration and partnership opportunities for public and private healthcare workers to address the gaps in TB management.

The robust aspects of the study can concentrate on TB notification in both the private and public sectors, which can contribute to achieving the universal health goal and the elimination of TB. The study can provide various understandings of TB notification to effectively report and strengthen policy levels to adhere to data integration, which can improve TB surveillance and control. The two sectors are highly important for eradicating TB in the public health setting and private health facilities by adhering to data integration for the TB control system. It can support TB cases in various aspects, including detection, reporting, treatment, and the fight against this preventable and curable disease.

FUTURE RECOMMENDATION OF THE STUDY

The conclusion of the study highlights the role of both public and private health sectors in the identification of TB cases. It can support TB patients by detecting the report, and it can effectively approach the challenges that vary. It can reveal further policies and programs that can be implemented. Public health facilities are the backbone of identifying TB notifications in the TB control program. They provide subsidized treatment, and it is mandatory to report TB cases. Due to inefficiency and overburden, it can be very difficult to access the TB notification monitoring system in the government. TB notification in the government system: at the state level, the State TB Officer; at the district level, the District TB Officer; and at the block level, the Senior Treatment Supervisor and Health Visitor are responsible for TB notification. However, in public health facilities such as GH, PHC, UPHC, and medical colleges, the concerned heads, including BMO, CMO, and Dean, also have overall responsibility for managing TB cases and ensuring TB notifications. Due to the overburden in the system, it is unable to manage the resource constraints in the health facility settings.

In the private sector, the number of TB cases is quite high, but TB notification is underreported. There is no proper uniform structure to get the TB notification in private hospitals. Due to inconsistent treatment adherence in the national notification policies, it can fragment the health system. TB notification in the private sector should motivate and provide various complementary and incentive supports to attract practitioners and health workers to report TB cases. This will help prevent underreporting and delays in starting treatment for TB patients.

Public health facilities cater to the affected health population, particularly marginalized rural communities, whereas private hospitals are more easily accessible in urban areas and are affordable for wealthier people. In both the public and private sectors, data should be collected and reported to the National TB Division regularly. It is the responsibility of the district and state roles to frequently share the data and provide comprehensive support for the TB control program. The reporting system can be implemented with technology support to drive the TB case notification system, providing the latest, easily accessible, and synchronized system to report TB cases in both the public and private sectors. To support and implement financial support for TB notification in private health facilities, access to treatment adherence support should be provided, along with transparent incentive support for health workers, private practitioners, and the general public. To provide extensive training to both public and private sector workers to sensitize them on the importance of TB notification, and to offer various resources to support healthcare workers in both the public and private sectors. Further, the study can provide collaboration and partnership opportunities for public and private healthcare workers to address the gaps in TB management.

The robust aspects of the study can concentrate on TB notification in both the private and public sectors, which can contribute to achieving the universal health goal and the elimination of TB. The study can provide various understandings of TB notification to effectively report and strengthen policy levels to adhere to data integration, which can improve TB surveillance and control. The two sectors are highly important for eradicating TB in the public health setting and private health facilities by adhering to data integration for the TB control system. It can support TB cases in various aspects, including detection, reporting, treatment, and the fight against this preventable and curable disease.

REFERENCES

Adepoju, V. A., Adejumo, O. A., Adepoju, O. E., Adeniyi, M. O., Etuk, V., Nzekwe, I., Inegbeboh, J. O., Adelekan, A., & Oladimeji, O. (2022). Do private health providers adhere to National Tuberculosis Guideline while assigning treatment outcome? Findings from a lower middle-income country. *Frontiers in Public Health*, *10*, 924132. DOI: 10.3389/fpubh.2022.924132 PMID: 36211674

Al-Maniri, A. A., Al-Rawas, O. A., Al-Ajmi, F., De Costa, A., Eriksson, B., & Diwan, V. K. (2008). Tuberculosis suspicion and knowledge among private and public general practitioners: Questionnaire Based Study in Oman. *BMC Public Health*, *8*(1), 1–7. DOI: 10.1186/1471-2458-8-177 PMID: 18501022

Al-Worafi, Y. M. (2023). Tuberculosis Management in Developing Countries. In *Handbook of Medical and Health Sciences in Developing Countries: Education, Practice, and Research* (pp. 1–40). Springer International Publishing., DOI: 10.1007/978-3-030-74786-2_52-1

AlJaberi, O. A., Hussain, M., & Drake, P. R. (2020). A framework for measuring sustainability in healthcare systems. *International Journal of Healthcare Management*, *13*(4), 276–285. Advance online publication. DOI: 10.1080/20479700.2017.1404710

Alruwaili, R. F., Alsadaan, N., Alruwaili, A. N., & Alrumayh, A. G. (2023). Unveiling the symbiosis of Environmental Sustainability and Infection Control in Health Care settings: A systematic review. *Sustainability (Basel)*, *15*(22), 15728. DOI: 10.3390/su152215728

Ananthakrishnan, R., Richardson, M. A., van den Hof, S., Rangaswamy, R., Thiagesan, R., Auguesteen, S., & Kamp, N. (2019). Successfully engaging private providers to improve diagnosis, notification, and treatment of TB and drug-resistant TB: The EQUIP public-private model in Chennai, India. *Global Health, Science and Practice*, *7*(1), 41–53. DOI: 10.9745/GHSP-D-18-00318 PMID: 30926737

Anderson, S. (2012). Public, private, neither, both? Publicness theory and the analysis of healthcare organisations. *Social Science & Medicine*, *74*(3), 313–322. DOI: 10.1016/j.socscimed.2011.07.021 PMID: 21893377

Attaran, M. (2022). Blockchain technology in healthcare: Challenges and opportunities. *International Journal of Healthcare Management*, *15*(1), 70–83. DOI: 10.1080/20479700.2020.1843887

Bhatt, J., & Bathija, P. (2018). Ensuring access to quality health care in vulnerable communities. *Academic Medicine*, *93*(9), 1271–1275. DOI: 10.1097/ACM.0000000000002254 PMID: 29697433

Bogale, B., Scambler, S., Mohd Khairuddin, A. N., & Gallagher, J. E. (2024). Health system strengthening in fragile and conflict-affected states: A review of systematic reviews. *PLoS One*, *19*(6), e0305234. DOI: 10.1371/journal.pone.0305234 PMID: 38875266

CARE. T. I. (2023). THE STATE OF TB. https://cisp.cachefly.net/assets/articles/attachments/90339_2023-state-of-tb-report-.pdf

Chakaya, J., Khan, M., Ntoumi, F., Aklillu, E., Fatima, R., Mwaba, P., Kapata, N., Mfinanga, S., Hasnain, S. E., Katot, P. D.M.C., Bulabula, A. N. H, Sam-Agudu, N. A, Nachega, J. B., Tiberi, S., McHugh, T. D., Abubakar, I., & Zumla, A. (2021).

Chijioke-Akaniro, O., Ubochioma, E., Omoniyi, A., Omosebi, O., Olarewaju, O., Etolue, M., Asuke, S., Aniwada, E., Ndubisi, A. U., Ombeka, V., Agbajes, A., Lawanson, A., & Anyaike, C. (2022). Strategic engagement of private facilities to increase public-private mix (PPM) contribution to Nigeria tuberculosis case notification. *Journal of Tuberculosis Research*, *10*(3), 99–110. DOI: 10.4236/jtr.2022.103008

Chilala, S. B., Silumbwe, A., Zulu, J. M., Tetui, M., Bulawayo, M., Chewe, M., & Hangoma, P. (2024). Individual, community and health systems factors influencing time to notification of tuberculosis: Situating software and hardware bottlenecks in local health systems. *BMC Health Services Research*, *24*(1), 1–11. DOI: 10.1186/s12913-024-11697-3 PMID: 39415167

Cole, B., Nilsen, D. M., Will, L., Etkind, S. C., Burgos, M., & Chorba, T. (2020). Essential components of a public health tuberculosis prevention, control, and elimination program: Recommendations of the Advisory Council for the Elimination of Tuberculosis and the National Tuberculosis Controllers Association. *MMWR. Recommendations and Reports*, *69*(7), 1–27. Advance online publication. DOI: 10.15585/mmwr.rr6907a1 PMID: 32730235

Cyril, S., Smith, B. J., Possamai-Inesedy, A., & Renzaho, A. M. (2015). Exploring the role of community engagement in improving the health of disadvantaged populations: A systematic review. *Global Health Action*, *8*(1), 29842. DOI: 10.3402/gha.v8.29842 PMID: 26689460

Demissie Gizaw, G., Aderaw Alemu, Z., & Kibret, K. T. (2015). Assessment of knowledge and practice of health workers towards tuberculosis infection control and associated factors in public health facilities of Addis Ababa, Ethiopia: A cross-sectional study. *Archives of Public Health = Archives Belges de Santé Publique*, *73*(1), 1–9. DOI: 10.1186/s13690-015-0062-3 PMID: 25821581

Dhaliwal, L. K. (2020). Health equity and sustainable development goals: role and the complexity. *Good health and well-being*, 316-324. DOI: 10.1007/978-3-319-95681-7_66

Frederick, A., Das, M., Mehta, K., Kumar, G., & Satyanarayana, S. (2021). Pharmacy based surveillance for identifying missing tuberculosis cases: A mixed methods study from South India. *The Indian Journal of Tuberculosis*, *68*(1), 51–58. DOI: 10.1016/j.ijtb.2020.09.017 PMID: 33641851

Glaziou, P., Floyd, K., & Raviglione, M. C. (2018). Global epidemiology of tuberculosis. In *Seminars in respiratory and critical care medicine* (Vol. 39, No. 03, pp. 271-285). Thieme Medical Publishers. DOI: 10.1055/s-0038-1651492

Global Tuberculosis Report 2020–Reflections on the Global TB burden, treatment and prevention efforts. *International journal of infectious diseases, 113*, S7-S12. DOI: 10.1016/j.ijid.2021.02.107

Gupta, S., Granich, R., Lepere, P., Hersh, B., Gouws, E., & Samb, B. (2014). Review of policy and status of implementation of collaborative HIV-TB activities in 23 high-burden countries. *The International Journal of Tuberculosis and Lung Disease : the Official Journal of the International Union against Tuberculosis and Lung Disease*, *18*(10), 1149–1158. DOI: 10.5588/ijtld.13.0889 PMID: 25216827

Haque, M., Islam, T., Rahman, N. A. A., McKimm, J., Abdullah, A., & Dhingra, S. (2020). Strengthening primary health-care services to help prevent and control long-term (chronic) non-communicable diseases in low-and middle-income countries. *Risk Management and Healthcare Policy*, *13*, 409–426. DOI: 10.2147/RMHP.S239074 PMID: 32547272

Hu, C., Yun, K. H., Su, Z., & Xi, C. (2022). Effective crisis management during adversity: Organizing resilience capabilities of firms and sustainable performance during COVID-19. *Sustainability (Basel)*, *14*(20), 13664. DOI: 10.3390/su142013664

Husainy, A. S., Mangave, S. S., Patil, C. C., & Mane, S. D. (2024). Harmonizing Responsibilities: Challenges and Opportunities in the Integration of Climate Change and Sustainable Development Goals (SDGs). *The Asian Review of Civil Engineering*, *13*(1), 30–43. DOI: 10.70112/tarce-2024.13.1.4232

Ibeneme, S., Karamagi, H., Muneene, D., Goswami, K., Chisaka, N., & Okeibunor, J. (2022). Strengthening health systems using innovative digital health technologies in Africa. *Frontiers in Digital Health*, *4*, 854339. DOI: 10.3389/fdgth.2022.854339 PMID: 35434700

Jabir, M., & Choolayil, A. C. (2024). *Social Work with Populations Vulnerable to Neglected Tropical Diseases: Evidence and Insights from India*. Springer Nature., DOI: 10.1007/978-3-031-68997-0

Javanparast, S., Windle, A., Freeman, T., & Baum, F. (2018). Community health worker programs to improve healthcare access and equity: Are they only relevant to low-and middle-income countries? *International Journal of Health Policy and Management*, *7*(10), 943–954. DOI: 10.15171/ijhpm.2018.53 PMID: 30316247

Kamath, S., Poojary, M., Shetty, H., Umesh, K., Kar, S., Lakshmi Ramesh, V., Hajare, G., Thomas, A., Brand, H., Jahangir, S., & Kamath, R. (2024). "Private Hospitals Generally Offer Better Treatment and Facilities": Out-of-Pocket Expenditure on Healthcare and the Preference for Private Healthcare Providers in South India. *International Journal of Environmental Research and Public Health*, *21*(10), 1287. DOI: 10.3390/ijerph21101287 PMID: 39457260

Khan, M. S., Mehboob, N., Rahman-Shepherd, A., Naureen, F., Rashid, A., Buzdar, N., & Ishaq, M. (2019). What can motivate Lady Health Workers in Pakistan to engage more actively in tuberculosis case-finding? *BMC Public Health*, *19*(1), 1–9. DOI: 10.1186/s12889-019-7326-8 PMID: 31345194

Khan, S. A. R., Zhang, Y., Kumar, A., Zavadskas, E., & Streimikiene, D. (2020). Measuring the impact of renewable energy, public health expenditure, logistics, and environmental performance on sustainable economic growth. *Sustainable Development (Bradford)*, *28*(4), 833–843. DOI: 10.1002/sd.2034

Kundu, D., Chopra, K., Khanna, A., Babbar, N., & Padmini, T. J. (2016). Accelerating TB notification from the private health sector in Delhi, India. *indian journal of tuberculosis*, *63*(1), 8-12. DOI: 10.1016/j.ijtb.2016.02.002

Kwan, A., Daniels, B., Saria, V., Satyanarayana, S., Subbaraman, R., McDowell, A., Bergkvist, S., Das, R. K., Das, V., Das, J., & Pai, M. (2018). Variations in the quality of tuberculosis care in urban India: A cross-sectional, standardized patient study in two cities. *PLoS Medicine*, *15*(9), e1002653. DOI: 10.1371/journal.pmed.1002653 PMID: 30252849

Lal, S. S. (2010). The role of private health sector engagement in TB control in India. *The Hospital*, *2006*(07), 11.

Lei, X., Liu, Q., Escobar, E., Philogene, J., Zhu, H., Wang, Y., & Tang, S. (2015). Public–private mix for tuberculosis care and control: A systematic review. *International Journal of Infectious Diseases*, *34*, 20–32. DOI: 10.1016/j.ijid.2015.02.015 PMID: 25722284

Levin, A., & Kaddar, M. (2011). Role of the private sector in the provision of immunization services in low-and middle-income countries. *Health Policy and Planning*, *26*(suppl_1), i4–i12. DOI: 10.1093/heapol/czr037 PMID: 21729916

Lile, R., Ocnean, M., Balan, I. M., & KIBA, D. (2023). Challenges for Zero Hunger (SDG 2): Links with Other SDGs. *Transitioning to Zero Hunger. Chapter, MDPI*, 9-66. DOI: 10.3390/books978-3-03897-863-3

Mainga, T. M. (2023). *Critical assessment of the intersection between mental health and Tuberculosis (TB) during TB treatment and beyond in a Sub-Saharan context with a focus on Zambia* (Doctoral dissertation, London School of Hygiene & Tropical Medicine). DOI: 10.17037/pubs.04670902

Mortimer, F., Isherwood, J., Wilkinson, A., & Vaux, E. (2018). Sustainability in quality improvement: Redefining value. *Future Healthcare Journal*, *5*(2), 88–93. DOI: 10.7861/futurehosp.5-2-88 PMID: 31098540

Needham, D. M., Bowman, D., Foster, S. D., & Godfrey-Faussett, P. (2004). Patient care seeking barriers and tuberculosis programme reform: A qualitative study. *Health Policy (Amsterdam)*, *67*(1), 93–106. DOI: 10.1016/S0168-8510(03)00065-4 PMID: 14726009

Negandhi, H., Tiwari, R., Sharma, A., Nair, R., Zodpey, S., Reddy Allam, R., & Oruganti, G. (2017). Rapid assessment of facilitators and barriers related to the acceptance, challenges and community perception of daily regimen for treating tuberculosis in India. *Global Health Action*, *10*(1), 1290315. DOI: 10.1080/16549716.2017.1290315 PMID: 28485693

Obermeyer, Z., Abbott-Klafter, J., & Murray, C. J. (2008). Has the DOTS strategy improved case finding or treatment success? An empirical assessment. *PLoS One*, *3*(3), e1721. DOI: 10.1371/journal.pone.0001721 PMID: 18320042

Pardeshi, G., Wang, W., Kim, J., Blossom, J., Kim, R., & Subramanian, S. V. (2021). TB notification rates across parliamentary constituencies in India: A step towards data-driven political engagement. *Tropical Medicine & International Health*, *26*(7), 730–742. DOI: 10.1111/tmi.13574 PMID: 33715264

Rajabi, M., Ebrahimi, P., & Aryankhesal, A. (2021). Collaboration between the government and nongovernmental organizations in providing health-care services: A systematic review of challenges. *Journal of Education and Health Promotion*, *10*(1), 242. DOI: 10.4103/jehp.jehp_1312_20 PMID: 34395679

Rakesh, P. S., & Shannawaz, M. (2024). Ensuring universal access to quality care for persons with presumed tuberculosis reaching the private sector: Lessons from Kerala. *International Journal for Equity in Health, 23*(1), 101. DOI: 10.1186/s12939-024-02151-1 PMID: 38760667

Rakesh, P. S., Shannawaz, M., Mathew, M. E., & Sachdeva, K. S. (2024). Facilitators and barriers for private health sector engagement for tb care in india: A systematic review and meta-synthesis of qualitative research. *Global Health, Science and Practice, 12*(4). Advance online publication. DOI: 0.9745/GHSP-D-24-00034 PMID: 39019586

Raviglione, M., & Sulis, G. (2016). Tuberculosis 2015: Burden, challenges and strategy for control and elimination. *Infectious Disease Reports, 8*(2), 6570. DOI: 10.4081/idr.2016.6570 PMID: 27403269

Ravindran, D., Pillai, R. H., Srinivasa, D., & Somashekaraiah, S. (2024). Service Quality Evaluation of Healthcare Sustainability: Patient Satisfaction, Service Delivery, and Clinical Outcomes. In *Business Resilience and Digital Technology in the Post-Pandemic Era: A Global Case* (pp. 57-76). Cham: Springer Nature Switzerland. DOI: 10.1007/978-3-031-48075-1_6

Rodríguez, R., Svensson, G., & Ferro, C. (2021). Assessing the future direction of sustainable development in public hospitals: Time-horizon, path and action. *Health Policy (Amsterdam), 125*(4), 526–534. DOI: 10.1016/j.healthpol.2020.10.012 PMID: 33309182

Sarkis, J. (2020). Supply chain sustainability: Learning from the COVID-19 pandemic. *International Journal of Operations & Production Management, 41*(1), 63–73. DOI: 10.1108/IJOPM-08-2020-0568

Srinivasan, S. (2025). Patient-Centric Care in Tuberculosis Management: Addressing Challenges and Improving Health Outcomes. In *Convergence of Population Health Management, Pharmacogenomics, and Patient-Centered Care* (pp. 265-282). IGI Global. DOI: 10.4018/979-8-3693-3260-3.ch012

Srinivasan, S., & Praba Lama (2025). Patient-Centered Care for TB Patients: An Effective Approach to Corporate Social Responsibility. In Corporate Social Responsibility in Health and Social Care (pp. 183-218). IGI Global. DOI: 10.4018/979-8-3693-5991-4.ch008

Srinivasan, S., & Vallipriya, R. (2025). Bias: Understanding and Addressing Disparities in Patient Care Across Multiple Demographics. In *Cases on Physician Cultural Responsibility, Ethics, and Biases* (pp. 21-38). IGI Global Scientific Publishing. DOI: 10.4018/979-8-3693-3683-0.ch002

Srinivasan, S., & Vallipriya, R. (2025). Intercultural Communication: An Effective Strategy for the Patient Physician Relationship. In *Cases on Physician Cultural Responsibility, Ethics, and Biases* (pp. 171-192). IGI Global Scientific Publishing. DOI: 10.4018/979-8-3693-3683-0.ch008

Srinivasan, S., Vallipriya, R., & Singh, A. K. (2025). Integrated Public-Private Partnerships to Combat Tuberculosis for Improving Economic Development. In *Public Private Partnership Dynamics for Economic Development* (pp. 323–356). IGI Global Scientific Publishing., DOI: 10.4018/979-8-3693-9153-2.ch015

Stallworthy, G., Dias, H. M., & Pai, M. (2020). Quality of tuberculosis care in the private health sector. *Journal of Clinical Tuberculosis and Other Mycobacterial Diseases*, *20*, 100171. DOI: 10.1016/j.jctube.2020.100171 PMID: 32642560

Stop, T. B. Initiative. (2001). *Global DOTS expansion plan: progress in TB control in high-burden countries, 2001 one year after the Amsterdam Ministerial Conference* (No. WHO/CDS/STB/2001.11). World Health Organization. https://iris.who.int/bitstream/handle/10665/66800/WHO_CDS_STB_2001.11.pdf

Suseela, R. P., & Shannawaz, M. (2023). Engaging the Private Health Service Delivery Sector for TB Care in India—Miles to Go! *Tropical Medicine and Infectious Disease*, *8*(5), 265. DOI: 10.3390/tropicalmed8050265 PMID: 37235313

Trent, R. J. (2012). Public Health, Communicable Diseases and Global Health. *Molecular Medicine (Cambridge, Mass.)*, *169*, 169–201. Advance online publication. DOI: 10.1016/B978-0-12-381451-7.00006-2

Tumuhimbise, W., & Musiimenta, A. (2021). A review of mobile health interventions for public private mix in tuberculosis care. *Internet Interventions : the Application of Information Technology in Mental and Behavioural Health*, *25*, 100417. DOI: 10.1016/j.invent.2021.100417 PMID: 34401376

Ullah, A. N. Z., Huque, R., Husain, A., Akter, S., Islam, A., & Newell, J. N. (2012). Effectiveness of involving the private medical sector in the National TB Control Programme in Bangladesh: Evidence from mixed methods. *BMJ Open*, *2*(6), e001534. DOI: 10.1136/bmjopen-2012-001534 PMID: 23253871

Uplekar, M. (2003). Involving private health care providers in delivery of TB care: Global strategy. *Tuberculosis (Edinburgh, Scotland)*, *83*(1-3), 156–164. DOI: 10.1016/S1472-9792(02)00073-2 PMID: 12758206

Uplekar, M. (2016). Public-private mix for tuberculosis care and prevention. What progress? What prospects? *The International Journal of Tuberculosis and Lung Disease : the Official Journal of the International Union against Tuberculosis and Lung Disease, 20*(11), 1424–1429. DOI: 10.5588/ijtld.15.0536 PMID: 27776581

Vergunst, F., Berry, H. L., Rugkåsa, J., Burns, T., Molodynski, A., & Maughan, D. L. (2020). Applying the triple bottom line of sustainability to healthcare research—A feasibility study. *International Journal for Quality in Health Care : Journal of the International Society for Quality in Health Care, 32*(1), 48–53. DOI: 10.1093/intqhc/mzz049 PMID: 31087047

Virhia, J., Gilmour, M., Russell, C., Mutua, E., Nasuwa, F., Mmbaga, B. T., Mshana, S. E., Dunlea, T., Shirima, G., Seni, J., Lembo, T., & Davis, A. (2023). "If you do not take the medicine and complete the dose… It could cause you more trouble": Bringing awareness, local knowledge and experience into antimicrobial stewardship in Tanzania. *Antibiotics (Basel, Switzerland), 12*(2), 243. DOI: 10.3390/antibiotics12020243 PMID: 36830154

Weerasuriya, C. K. (2022). *Advancing Mathematical Models of Mycobacterium tuberculosis Transmission to Support Vaccine Introduction* (Doctoral dissertation, London School of Hygiene & Tropical Medicine). DOI: 10.17037/PUBS.04665244

Weiss, J. B., Berner, E. S., Johnson, K. B., Giuse, D. A., Murphy, B. A., & Lorenzi, N. M. (2013). Recommendations for the design, implementation and evaluation of social support in online communities, networks, and groups. *Journal of Biomedical Informatics, 46*(6), 970–976. DOI: 10.1016/j.jbi.2013.04.004 PMID: 23583424

Wippel, C., Farroñay, S., Gilbert, H. N., Millones, A. K., Acosta, D., Torres, I., Jimenez, J., Alarcon, V. A., Lecca, L., & Yuen, C. M. (2024). Exploring the role of the private sector in tuberculosis detection and management in Lima, Peru: A mixed-methods patient pathway analysis. *The American Journal of Tropical Medicine and Hygiene, 111*(1), 168–175. DOI: 10.4269/ajtmh.23-0504 PMID: 38744270

World Health Organization. (2009). *Global tuberculosis control: a short update to the 2009 report* (No. WHO/HTM/TB/2009.426). World Health Organization. https://iris.who.int/bitstream/handle/10665/44241/9789241598866_eng.pdf

World Health Organization. (2010). *The global plan to stop TB 2011-2015: transforming the fight towards elimination of tuberculosis*. World Health Organization., DOI: 10.1098/rsif.2010.0072

World Health Organization. (2014). *Tuberculosis control* (No. SEA-TB-352). WHO Regional Office for South-East Asia. https://iris.who.int/bitstream/handle/10665/206505/B5082.pdf

World Health Organization. (2024). *WHO consolidated guidelines on tuberculosis. Module 6: tuberculosis and comorbidities*. World Health Organization.

Yasin, N. Y. (2007). Connect the" DOTS": a new era in Turkish tuberculosis control. http://193.140.201.98/handle/123456789/17477

Yassin, M. A., Kimbo, L., Wandwalo, E., Rashid, A., Dzokoto, A., Weber, U., & Stallworthy, G. (2024). Leveraging Global Fund's investments to expand innovative public-private provider engagement in TB. *IJTLD Open*, *1*(6), 250–257. DOI: 10.5588/ijtldopen.24.0162 PMID: 39021451

Yellappa, V., Lefèvre, P., Battaglioli, T., Devadasan, N., & Van der Stuyft, P. (2017). Patients pathways to tuberculosis diagnosis and treatment in a fragmented health system: A qualitative study from a south Indian district. *BMC Public Health*, *17*(1), 1–10. DOI: 10.1186/s12889-017-4627-7 PMID: 28778192

Yellappa, V. H. (2019). Optimising the involvement of private practitioners in tuberculosis care and control in India. DOI: 10.26481/dis.20191111vy

Zaidi, I., Sarma, P. S., & Khayyam, K. U. (2024). Factors associated with treatment adherence among pulmonary tuberculosis patients in New Delhi. *The Indian Journal of Tuberculosis*, *71*, S52–S58. DOI: 10.1016/j.ijtb.2023.08.006 PMID: 39067956

Zumla, A., Abubakar, I., Raviglione, M., Hoelscher, M., Ditiu, L., Mchugh, T. D., Squire, S. B., Cox, H., Ford, N., McNerney, R., Marais, B., Grobusch, M., Lawn, S. D., Migliori, G., Mwaba, P., O'Grady, J., Pletschette, M., Ramsay, A., Chakaya, J., & Atun, R. (2012). Drug-resistant tuberculosis—Current dilemmas, unanswered questions, challenges, and priority needs. *The Journal of Infectious Diseases*, *205*(suppl_2), S228–S240. DOI: 10.1093/infdis/jir858 PMID: 22476720

Chapter 12
Improved Diabetic Prediction Using Feature Weighting and Hyperparameter Tuned Boosting Technique

M. Kamaladevi
https://orcid.org/0000-0001-8486-5092
SASTRA University, India

V. Venkataraman
SASTRA University, India

S. Meganathan
https://orcid.org/0000-0003-4570-8259
SASTRA University, India

P. Umamaheswari
https://orcid.org/0000-0003-2007-697X
SASTRA University, India

ABSTRACT

Diabetes is a chronic medical condition characterized by elevated blood sugar levels, resulting from insufficient insulin production or ineffective use of insulin by the body. Predicting diabetes at early stage save human life. To improve the prediction, feature weighting algorithm and Hyperparameters tuned Boosting algorithm are used. In proposed work dataset are taken from Kaggle link (https://www.kaggle.com) and it

DOI: 10.4018/979-8-3373-5641-9.ch012

is imbalanced in nature. To balanced data SMOTE algorithm is applied. Select the more relevant feature through feature weighting method and tune the hyperparameter like learning rate, number of estimators, and tree depth, influencing the ensemble's performance of Boosting algorithms like a AdaBoost, Gradient Boosting (GBM), XGBoost, LightGBM and CatBoost provides higher accuracy when compare with state of art machine learning algorithm. Among these methods hyperparameter tuned CatBoost algorithm shows 81% accuracy, ROC_AUC score is 0.84, Recall score of 0.8 which will be higher than the general boosting algorithm.

INTRODUCTION

One of the most important global public health issues of the twenty-first century is diabetes mellitus (DM), whose prevalence is rising alarmingly in both industrialized and developing nations. The International Diabetes Federation (IDF) estimates that more than 537 million persons globally have diabetes in 2021; by 2030, that figure is expected to rise to 643 million, and by 2045, it will reach 783 million. Chronic hyperglycemia brought on by deficiencies in insulin secretion, action, or both characterizes the condition and can result in major side effects such as retinopathy, neuropathy, nephropathy, and cardiovascular disease. Preventive measures, lower healthcare costs, and better patient outcomes are all made possible by early and precise diabetes onset prediction.

Machine learning classify into two types, One is supervised learning, that extract pattern from the given data and predict the class label for future, and unsupervised learning, cluster the input data based on any similarity without any class label, Hidden pattern is learned from clusters. Classification techniques predict the binary class in various field like patient suffered from diabetic or not and credit card transactions are fraud or good etc

Ensemble algorithm performs better than single algorithm. It has two types bagging and boosting. Boosting is a machine learning ensemble technique that combines multiple weak learners (typically decision trees) sequentially to create a strong learner. It works by training each subsequent model to correct the errors made by the previous ones, thereby improving the overall predictive performance. Boosting is a potent ensemble learning technique that combines weak learners into a strong learner in order to increase their predictive performance. A model that outperforms a shallow decision tree, also known as a decision stump, is known as a weak learner. Boosting reduces the overall error by iteratively focusing on the errors caused by the prior models with each new model. Assigning weights to training instances is the basic concept, At first, the weights of each sample are equal.To help the next learner focus more on the most challenging situations, the weights of misclassified samples are increased after each iteration.A weighted majority vote (for classification) or weighted average (for regression) is used to determine the final forecast.

Bagging is an ensemble learning technique where multiple models, often of the same type, are trained on different subsets of the training data using bootstrapping. These models are then combined through averaging or voting to make predictions, reducing variance and improving overall model performance. Because it can simulate intricate, nonlinear relationships in high-dimensional clinical data, machine learning (ML) has become a potent method for medical prediction problems in recent years. Extreme Gradient Boosting (XGBoost), Light Gradient Boosting Machine (LightGBM), and CatBoost are boosting approaches among machine learning algorithms that have shown state-of-the-art predictive performance for a variety of health-related issues, including diabetes prediction. In order to create a strong ensemble, weak learners—typically decision trees—are iteratively combined using boosting techniques. Each new learner concentrates on fixing the mistakes committed by its predecessors. As a result, strong models are produced that can identify minute trends in diverse datasets

The selection of hyperparameters—tunable settings that control the learning process, such as learning rate, maximum tree depth, subsample ratio, and regularization strength—has a significant impact on the predictive performance of boosting algorithms, notwithstanding their efficacy. Underfitting, overfitting, or less-than-ideal model generalization can result from poorly selected hyperparameters. For medical prediction tasks, hyperparameter adjustment is therefore essential to maximizing the potential of boosting algorithms. The high-dimensional hyperparameter space has been effectively explored using optimization algorithms, random or grid search, and cross-validation. Numerous studies have demonstrated that, in comparison to their default parameter counterparts, hyperparameter-tuned boosting models can significantly increase predictive accuracy, area under the ROC curve (AUC), and recall rates.

Hyperparameters are settings or configurations that control the behavior and performance of a machine learning algorithm, but are not learned from the data. They are set prior to the training process and affect how the model learns and generalizes. Examples include learning rate, number of layers in a neural network, and regularization strength.

The large complexity and unbalanced structure of medical datasets present a significant obstacle to diabetes prediction, even while hyperparameter tuning enhances the models' learning capabilities. Numerous datasets, including hospital electronic health records (EHRs) and the Pima Indian Diabetes Dataset (PIDD), contain noisy, redundant, or irrelevant information that might impair interpretability, increase computing complexity, and worsen model performance. At this point in the model pipeline, feature weighting becomes essential. By giving each input variable a relevance value determined by how it contributes to the prediction objective, feature weighting enables the model to highlight pertinent features while down-weighting or disregarding unimportant ones.

With the PIMA Indian diabetic Dataset acting as a standard for assessing predictive models, machine learning (ML) has become a game-changing tool in the early identification and diagnosis of type 2 diabetic mellitus (T2DM). Because of its accessibility and applicability in diabetes risk modeling, this dataset—which includes eight clinical and demographic characteristics from 768 female patients of Pima Indian heritage—has been thoroughly examined. The distribution of class labels in a dataset is frequently quite unequal in many real-world applications, especially in medical diagnosis, fraud detection, unusual event prediction, and fault monitoring. Class imbalance is the name given to this occurrence. When there are substantially more instances in one class (the majority class) than in another (the minority class), the dataset is said to be unbalanced.

For instance, the percentage of patients with diabetes (positive class) in a diabetes prediction dataset can be significantly lower than the percentage of healthy people (negative class). Such an imbalance presents a significant barrier for machine learning algorithms, even though it represents the condition's normal occurrence in the population. The goal of the majority of common classification algorithms, including ensemble techniques, logistic regression, and decision trees, is to increase overall accuracy. This tendency frequently results in models that ignore the minority class while favoring the majority class in imbalanced datasets. Significantly lower minority class recall results in the omission of key cases, such as diabetic patients. False performance indicators: a model that solely predicts the majority class may be highly accurate, but it will be of no benefit to the minority class A rise in false negatives could have serious repercussions for patients, delay treatment, and result in diseases being detected. When one class (majority class) greatly outnumbers the other (minority class), it can have a substantial impact on the performance of prediction models in machine learning, especially in classification problems using imbalanced datasets. Oversampling and undersampling are two popular methods used to address this problem at the data level.

The oversampling equalize the distribution of classes, Oversampling is the process of increasing the number of occurrences of minority classes. This can be accomplished by: Direct replication of current minority class samples is known as random oversampling. Synthetic oversampling is the process of creating new synthetic minority class samples by interpolating between preexisting minority samples using techniques like SMOTE (Synthetic Minority Oversampling Technique). It use to keeps the majority class's information from being lost.

and enhances the model's capacity to identify trends in minority classes. It can greatly improve F1-score and recall.

There are some limitation like Overfitting may result from random oversampling. If synthetic oversampling is not used carefully, it can produce noisy samples.

Undersampling is the process of lowering the number of majority class instances to match the minority class size. This can be accomplished by: Random undersampling is the process of randomly excluding samples from the majority class .Informed Undersampling: Selective removal of superfluous or borderline samples using methods such as NearMiss or Tomek Links. Benefits are like speeds up training by reducing the size of the dataset. Disadvantages are like discard important majority class information. Risk of underfitting due to reduced data diversity.

Ignoring class imbalance in the context of diabetes prognosis can give patients at risk false hope. Unbalance management is a crucial stage in the predictive modeling pipeline since accurately detecting diabetes cases (minority class) is frequently considerably more essential than optimizing overall accuracy.

To improve predictive power, recent research places a strong emphasis on feature selection and weighting. To get rid of unnecessary features and enhance classifier performance, methods including Boruta feature selection, principal component analysis (PCA), and minimum redundancy–maximum relevance (mRMR) have been used. Researcher showed that combining ensemble learning and Boruta produced 98% accuracy, highlighting the importance of weighting clinically important parameters such as BMI and plasma glucose concentration.

In contrast to feature selection, which completely removes variables, feature weighting keeps all features while modifying their impact. This can be especially helpful in medical settings where weak predictors may work in concert with one another to increase predictive accuracy. Filter-based techniques (like mutual information and correlation coefficients), wrapper techniques (like recursive feature reduction with cross-validation), and embedding techniques (like feature importance generated from tree-based models) are examples of common feature weighing strategies. Metrics like gain, cover, or split frequency are frequently used in the context of boosting algorithms to calculate feature importance scores, which can direct the weighting procedure.

Tuning hyperparameters can significantly impact the model's effectiveness. such as Learning_Rate, max_depth, min_child_weight, n_estimators, min_samples_leaf, min_samples_split,colsample_bytree, sub_sample. Feature weighting importance is a method in machine learning aimed at assessing the significance of different features within a dataset. By evaluating the contribution of each feature to the predictive performance of a model, it aids in feature selection, dimensionality reduction, and understanding data patterns. Using feature weighting in conjunction with hyperparameter-tuned boosting approaches improves diabetic prediction in a synergistic way. There are two reasons for this: Improved learning efficiency - Feature weighting helps the tailored boosting model converge more quickly and lowers the chance of overfitting by directing the model to concentrate more on important variables. Better interpretability: By determining the most significant risk variables, medical professionals can support patient-specific therapies and evidence-based decision-making. The effectiveness of this combination approach is supported by recent research. For example, a 2024 study that combined Optuna-tuned XGBoost with mutual information-based feature weighting saw a gain in AUC of 7–12% when compared to untuned models without weighting. Improved recall was observed by another study that used LightGBM with genetic algorithm-based feature weighting. This is especially useful in medical screening, where false negative results might have serious repercussions.

Additionally, weighted features' interpretability gave doctors practical information about modifiable risk variables like BMI, fasting glucose levels, and family history of diabetes. The following is a practical summary of the method for enhanced diabetes prediction utilizing feature weighting and hyperparameter-tuned boosting: Data preprocessing includes encoding categorical features, handling missing data, and normalizing continuous variables. If necessary, use resampling techniques (such as SMOTE or Tomek Links) to address class imbalance. Feature Weighting: Determine and allocate weights to features using statistical, information-theoretic, or model-based techniques. Boosting Model Selection: Based on the properties of the dataset, select a baseline boosting technique (such as XGBoost, LightGBM, or CatBoost).Interpretation and Deployment – Analyze feature importance for medical insights and integrate the model into a clinical decision support system. Kalagotla, Gangashetty, and Giridhar (2021) proposed a novel stacking technique integrating multi layer perceptron, support vector machine and logistic regression outperformed traditional models in predicting diabetes showcasing the potential of advance machine learning approaches

Various techniques, including statistical analyses, model-based computations, and tree-based methods, can be employed to calculate feature importance scores. These scores offer insights into which features are most influential in making predictions, guiding feature engineering efforts and improving model performance. Rajendra and Latifi (2021) proposed Logistic regression for diabetes prediction and highlights the impact of feature selection and ensemble techniques on improving model accuracy and runtime performance. However, it's crucial to interpret these scores cautiously, considering potential biases and the context of the problem domain, to ensure informed decision-making and reliable model outcomes. Chaves and Marques (2021) reported that Neural Networks outperform other data mining techniques for early diabetes diagnosis with notable performance metrics such as AUC, accuracy, F1-Score, Precision, Sensitivity, and Specificity. Hassan et al., (2022) proposed a model to achieve maximum accuracy an unsupervised cluster-based feature grouping model for early diabetes identification, and performance metrics using various machine learning approaches on clustered and complete datasets.

Predictive accuracy is just one advantage of this integrated strategy. Credibility is crucial in medical AI. When clinicians can comprehend the reasoning behind a predictive model's predictions, they are more inclined to use it. This is made easier by feature weighting, which clearly ranks the risk factors, and hyperparameter adjustment, which makes sure the model is using the data as efficiently as feasible. Furthermore, in clinical situations, real-time or almost real-time diabetes risk assessment may be possible due to the computing efficiency that weighing provided. But there are still difficulties. EHRs frequently contain skewed or noisy data, hence feature weighting techniques need to be resilient to these conditions. It can be computationally costly to adjust hyperparameters, particularly when dealing with big datasets and intricate search spaces. Additionally, when tuning, there is a chance of overfitting to the training data, which emphasizes the significance of strong validation techniques like nested cross-validation. Furthermore, when using such models in healthcare settings, ethical issues like explainability, equity across demographic groups, and data privacy must be properly taken into account.

Proposed system finds important feature based on the boosting model and select feature using Recursive Feature Elimination algorithm. Dataset with most relevant features is trained through boosting algorithm, where their hyperparameters are tuned to optimistic level. Several performances measure is computed using elements of confusion matrix. Extensively used measures are Precision, recall, AUC score, F1 score and ROC curve. In addition to that Receiver operating characteristics (ROC) generated by plotting true positive rate compared to false positive rate Area under ROC curve give summary of ROC curve a single number.

2. BACKGROUND

Predictive models that can identify high-risk individuals early and direct prompt care are being developed since diabetes mellitus continues to be a major worldwide health burden. Because clinical and biochemical factors (such as fasting glucose, body mass index, blood pressure, lipids, and family history) rarely provide equal contributions to prediction in these models, weighting—or determining the relative importance—of features is crucial for clinical utility, performance, and interpretability.

Kibria et.al., (2022) designed a model to predict diabetic disease, employed six machine learning algorithms and ensemble techniques, with Shapley additive explanations for model interpretation, aimed at enhancing clinical trust and understanding. Liu et al. (2023) proposed an machine-learning method based on unsupervised clustering, utilizing an improved Fuzzy c-means algorithm, PCA, and optimized KNN classification, used to predict the diabetes detection, surpassing other models and demonstrating practical applicability. Cherifi et al. (2023) developed an innovative approach to diabetes prediction using machine learning algorithms, emphasizing the effectiveness of a novel filtered data approach, achieving significant accuracy improvements compared to traditional imputation methods.

Farnoodian et al. (2023) reported that data mining and machine learning techniques to tackle the diabetes diagnostic challenge, demonstrating the superior performance of support vector machine (SVM) in achieving high accuracy, specificity, and sensitivity values, thus advocating for its adoption in clinical practice for improved patient outcomes . Bhat et al. (2023) explained ML-based framework for early diabetes prediction, utilizing various ML techniques on the PIDD dataset, with Random Forest outperforming other models, thus offering a valuable tool for medical practitioners in enhancing diabetes prognosis . To improve the prediction variation in machine learning technique like optimized boosting algorithm were identified to increase the accuracy level and reduce false positive rate. Houssein and Sayed (2023) proposed a modified INFO algorithm, mINFO, enhanced with Opposition-Based Learning and Dynamic Candidate Solution strategies, demonstrating superior performance in predicting disease compared to various metaheuristic algorithms, including INFO, on UCI datasets.

Because gradient boosting algorithms (XGBoost, LightGBM, and CatBoost) can handle heterogeneous tabular clinical data, model complex nonlinear relationships, and provide strong predictive performance, their usage for diabetes prediction has significantly increased in recent years. In order to extract repeatable performance increases and prevent overfitting on healthcare datasets, boosting hyperparameters are being carefully adjusted using Bayesian optimization, Optuna, genetic algorithms (GA), or evolutionary techniques. Several recent research show that careful preprocessing, imbalance handling, and hyperparameter tuning produce clinically relevant models for longitudinal risk forecasting and cross-sectional diagnosis.

Additionally, the clinical validity of boosting techniques has been confirmed by extensive cohort investigations. In a 2024 Scientific Reports paper, XGBoost was used to estimate the 10-year incidence of Type 2 Diabetes (T2D) using data from the UK Biobank. SHAP was used to rank predictors, and a small set of biologically significant predictors (HbA1c, BMI, glucose, and age) were utilized to reach an AUC $\approx$0.90. Lugner et al., 2024 reported that a crucial need for clinical translation, such work shows that customized boosting models can be both interpretable and performant at the population level . Using contemporary optimization libraries, some empirical investigations have concentrated on improving boosting algorithms for diabetes classification. For instance, compared to grid search, Optuna-guided LightGBM significantly reduced search time while improving classifier performance. This method also addressed class-imbalance in diabetes datasets by using hybrid balancing (SMOTE + undersampling), which consistently increased precision and AUC. Shao et al., 2024 proposed the study emphasizes two recurrent themes: hyperparameter choices (learning rate, n_estimators, max_depth, and leaf parameters) have a significant impact on improving model performance, and search speed and efficiency are important for real-world implementation when datasets are big.

Numerous studies have also been conducted on population-based and evolutionary optimizers. With reported significant AUC increases in multiple benchmarks, Li et al., 2024 proposed a model GA-XGBoost stacking models outperform single base learners when XGBoost hyperparameters are tuned using genetic algorithms (GA) in conjunction with stacking ensembles. These techniques show that, when combined with SHAP interpretation, metaheuristic search techniques can locate parameter combinations that result in strong, explicable boosting models while avoiding local optima in hyperparameter space. In order to take advantage of imaging and non-tabular sources, researchers have also started integrating boosting with deep feature extractors and ensembling algorithms. For related diagnoses (such diabetic retinopathy), recent research combined convolutional feature extractors with XGBoost classifiers; other studies employed stacking ensembles in which optimized boosting models serve as base learners. In multimodal diabetes prediction (clinical + imaging + time-series), these hybrid approaches offer a way ahead where boosting manages tabular signals and aggregated characteristics from other modalities.

Yun et al., 2024 highlight the importance of the full modeling pipeline, from feature engineering to imbalance correction, in implementing boosting algorithms in diabetic prediction, going beyond simple hyperparameter search. In order to better identify minority diabetic cases across numerous datasets, a Frontiers research proposed a robust prediction approach that combines improved preprocessing, multiple resampling procedures (SMOTE/ADASYN/Borderline-SMOTE), and optimized model selection. For real-world clinical datasets where minority classes—such as undiagnosed diabetics or people with early pre diabetes—are the ones of greatest clinical interest, this kind of pipeline architecture is very crucial.

Shi & Sun, 2024 proposed contemporary methods integrate post-hoc explain ability and embedded techniques with traditional filter/wrapper methods. For sorting diabetic predictors and removing duplication, filter techniques including mutual information, Chi-square, and Relief continue to be reliable baselines and are frequently used as a first pass prior to model training. Arslan et al., 2024 I reported that in type 2 diabetes cohorts, embedded methods—most notably LASSO—produce sparse, accurately calibrated sets of risk factors by concurrently learning models and shrinking coefficients.

Recurring topics include explain ability and trustworthiness. SHAP or other post-hoc explanation tools are specifically used in a number of different studies to derive feature importance or patient-level attribution from optimized boosting models. Kaliappan et al., 2024 explain ability aids in feature selection and model auditing, both of which are critical for clinical adoption and regulatory acceptability, in addition to assisting physicians in interpreting specific predictions (such as the reasons behind a patient's high risk score). Mohanty et al., 2024 proposed model-agnostic explainers like SHAP are crucial because they offer local and global importance scores that match clinical reasoning (e.g., higher glucose, age, BMI, triglycerides), and it has been demonstrated that these weights derived from SHAP improve diabetes risk models' accuracy and transparency.

Abousaber et al., 2025 addressed deployment and operating issues. Other teams report using optimized LightGBM models in clinical mini-programs for risk calculators, while others have optimized boosting pipelines for mobile or clinical apps, focusing on resource-aware settings and lightweight hyperparameter searches. Although such flawless scores frequently reflect small or cleaned public datasets and should be interpreted cautiously for real-world generalization, some article highlights parallel/sequential ensemble approaches and useful pipelines achieving very high reported accuracy on benchmark datasets. In general, the area is shifting from proof-of-concept to clinical validation and pragmatic model engineering. Zhang et al., 2025 According to recent research in medical AI, proper feature weighting enhances discrimination on unbalanced datasets frequently used in diabetes screening and provides reliable explanations for physicians .Emerging pipelines combine weighting signals beyond single techniques, such as merging SHAP with mutual information or employing voting schemes across filter criteria, to produce more consistent importance rankings and better cross-dataset generalization.

It has also been demonstrated that Bayesian hyperparameter tuning offers XG-Boost models significant

performance gains. Khurshid et al., 2025 proposed a Bayesian optimization was used to choose XGBoost hyperparameters on public diabetes datasets. The results showed better AUC and balanced metrics than untuned baselines and grid/random search, highlighting the usefulness of probabilistic search techniques for clinical datasets with constraints. The study placed a strong emphasis on thorough preprocessing and multi-metric evaluation (AUC, F1, sensitivity, and specificity) in addition to raw accuracy to guarantee clinically meaningful gains. Vîrgolici et al., 2025 proposed a model that contain Gradient Boosting, and Extreme Gradient Boosting, were employed to predict changes in medical parameters as a function of body weight variation. Model performance was evaluated using Mean Squared Error, Mean Absolute Error, and R^2 score

Deep learning architectures, including deep convolutional neural networks (CNNs), long short-term memory (LSTM) models, and hybrid neural networks, have shown further improvements. While Khan et al. (2024) showed 99.35% accuracy with an ANN model achieved 96.13% accuracy with a deep CNN with data modeling. However, these high-accuracy results often come with trade-offs in interpretability—a key requirement for clinical adoption .Hybrid strategies that combine complementing algorithms have become more popular. For instance, stacked ensembles, CART with random forests, and Naive Bayes combined with fuzzy neural networks have all continuously outperformed single models. The ability of dendritic neuron models (DNMs) to describe nonlinear feature interactions and their biologically inspired structure have made them intriguing tools in this setting. In order to improve classification accuracy across a variety of datasets, studies have improved DNMs using optimization techniques such differential evolution, whale optimization, genetic algorithms, and particle swarm optimization (PSO).

The DNM–LR–ANN hybrid model put forth by Ağraz et al. (2025) is the most recent development. This design combines the flexibility of ANN, the interpretability of LR, and the nonlinear processing capability of DNM. The hybrid outperformed traditional classifiers while preserving a balance between sensitivity and specificity, achieving an AUC of 0.780, accuracy of 80.78%, and specificity of 95.5% when tested on the PIMA dataset. In line with recognized clinical risk variables, SHAP analysis additionally validated the predominance of age, BMI, and plasma glucose as key predictive characteristicsIn conclusion, research on diabetes prediction has moved from conventional classifiers to sophisticated ensemble and hybrid models, with a growing focus on interpretability and feature weighting. accuracy in a variety of datasets.

The DNM–LR hybrid fits within a larger trend in diabetes prediction that combines the probabilistic clarity of LR with the strength of neural representation to create compact, explainable, and high-performing models. While ensemble and hybrid studies in diabetes prediction provide empirical support for stacking and meta-modeling paradigms, the literature on dendritic neurons offers a rich toolkit that can be used to refine such hybrids, including novel learning algorithms, initialization strategies, and architecture variants. It is methodologically standard for the article to focus on Pima-based benchmarking with clinically meaningful metrics; the primary value-added is showing how dendritic feature construction can be effectively combined with LR to balance interpretability, accuracy, and calibration in a screening-oriented setting.

3. PROPOSED MODEL

Diabetes is a health condition where your body has trouble managing sugar levels. Lots of people have it, but thanks to smart computer programs, we can predict who might get it using things like machine learning. This helps us spot it early and treat it quickly and easily and enhance model performance, a multifaceted approach encompassing various preprocessing, feature selection, and model optimization techniques is paramount. Collect a Pima Indian diabetic dataset from Kaggle as shown in Figure 1It includes 768 female patients with Pima Indian ancestry who are at least 21 years old, have eight clinical characteristics, and have a binary target variable that indicates whether they have diabetes. It includes parameter like age, blood pressure, glucose level and BMI. Initially, data preprocessing techniques such as normalization are applied to standardize feature scales, ensuring that each feature contributes proportionately to the learning process. The direct deployment of models built on this dataset in actual healthcare settings is restricted by a number of research issues, despite its widespread use.

With roughly 65% of instances not having diabetes and 35% having it, the dataset is unbalanced.

For diabetic patients, this imbalance may cause models to predict the majority class with high accuracy but low recall. It is biologically impossible for certain qualities, such blood pressure, skin thickness, BMI, and insulin, to have zero values. Imputation or removal strategies are required to handle these zeros, which indicate missing data.

The Pima Indian women own all the records, which limits the diversity of the population.

This restricts how well models trained on the dataset can be applied to different populations. The dataset is too small—just 768 records—to create reliable machine learning models. Overfitting is a serious risk, particularly for intricate algorithms. Multicollinearity in certain features can impact feature selection and make models less interpretable. Extreme values (such as extremely high insulin or glucose levels) in some characteristics can skew model learning.

To create lifelike synthetic diabetic cases, SMOTE (Synthetic Minority Oversampling Technique) is used

Using cleaning techniques like Tomek Links to exclude borderline data samples, Data imputation is carried out using mean, median, or K-Nearest Neighbors imputation to substitute imputed values with medically impossible zero values. Establish reasonable bottom boundaries for clinical qualities using medical literature.

stratified k-fold cross-validation are used for validation Boosting to increase prediction stability.

Recursive Feature Elimination (RFE) are applied for finding future importance.

Figure 1. PIMA Indian Diabetes data set

1	Pregnanci	Glucose	BloodPres	SkinThickr	Insulin	BMI	DiabetesF	Age	Outcome
2	6	148	72	35	0	33.6	0.627	50	1
3	1	85	66	29	0	26.6	0.351	31	0
4	8	183	64	0	0	23.3	0.672	32	1
5	1	89	66	23	94	28.1	0.167	21	0
6	0	137	40	35	168	43.1	2.288	33	1
7	5	116	74	0	0	25.6	0.201	30	0
8	3	78	50	32	88	31	0.248	26	1
9	10	115	0	0	0	35.3	0.134	29	0

The distribution of class labels is frequently extremely unbalanced in many real-world datasets, particularly in fields like fraud detection, medical diagnosis, and uncommon event prediction. Because class frequency affects the learning process, traditional machine learning models have a tendency to favor the majority class. Since the minority class is usually the class of higher attention, this bias frequently leads to poor predicting accuracy for that class.There are several resampling methods that have been proposed to rectify this imbalance. SMOTE (Synthetic Minority Over-sampling Technique), which were the most extensively used techniques. SMOTE creates synthetic cases to balance the dataset in a more broad way than random oversampling, which only replicates minority class samples that already exist and can result in overfitting.

Additionally, addressing class imbalance is crucial, often achieved through techniques like Synthetic Minority Over-sampling Technique (SMOTE), which synthetically augments the minority class instances to achieve a more balanced representation as shown in Figure 2.By synthesizing new samples, SMOTE effectively mitigates the inherent biases in the dataset, facilitating more robust model training

In order to function, SMOTE generates synthetic samples along the line segments that connect an instance of a minority class to its k closest minority class neighbors. This is a summary of the process:

Choose a sample of a minority class from the dataset. Determine the k closest neighbors from the same minority class (usually k=5).Create a synthetic instance at a position interpolated between the two samples by selecting one of the neighbors at random. Continue doing this until the required degree of class balance is reached.

SMOTE minimizes overfitting by avoiding precise replication of minority samples. enhances classifier performance, especially F1-score and recall for unbalanced datasets works well with a variety of classifiers, including SVMs, boosting methods, and decision tree limitation of SMOTE may produce noisy samples if portions of the majority class overlap or minority cases are dispersed throughout feature space. It may lead to over-generalization, particularly if there are many outliers in the dataset does not solve majority class undersampling on its own; therefore, for improved performance, it is frequently used in conjunction with techniques such as Tomek Links or Edited Nearest Neighbor (ENN).

Apply SMOTE

Before SMOTE:

Class distribution before SMOTE: Counter ({0: 500, 1: 268})

After SMOTE:

Class distribution after SMOTE: Counter ({1: 500, 0: 500})

Figure 2. Data Distribution after SMOTE

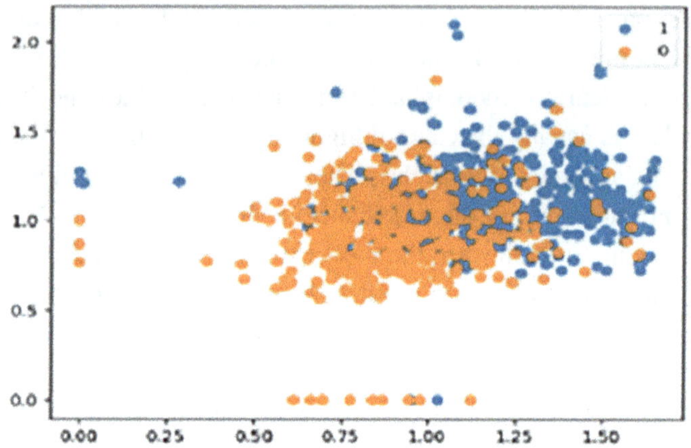

Not every feature contributes equally to the prediction job in supervised learning, particularly for complex datasets like text data, financial transactions, and medical records. While certain attributes may be redundant, useless, or even noisy, which could impair the model's performance; others are extremely crucial to the target variable. By giving each feature a numerical importance score (weight), a technique known as feature weighting allows the learning algorithm to emphasize important traits while downplaying less important ones. In contrast to feature selection, which completely removes irrelevant features, feature weighting keeps all features while varying their impact during model training. This is especially helpful in fields where eliminating key characteristics can make the content less interpretable or context-specific.

Increasing model accuracy: The classifier can make better selections by highlighting significant features. And increasing model accuracy Weights lessen the influence of irrelevant or noisy variables and reduce overfitting

Improving interpretability: Information about which variables influence predictions is provided by feature significance ratings.Improved management of high-dimensional data is frequently found in text mining, genomic, and medicinal applications. Feature Weighting procedure use statistical or learning-based techniques to assess the importance of features. Establishing weights, which are usually normalized values or between 0 and 1.Incorporating weights into the learning algorithm to affect each feature's contribution to model optimization, similarity calculations, or distance measures. In diabetes prediction, certain clinical measurements such as fasting blood glucose, BMI, age, and HbA1c often have higher predictive value than others like skin thickness or blood pressure. Assigning appropriate weights ensures that the prediction algorithm focuses more on the medically significant parameters, improving early detection accuracy and reducing false negatives.

Feature weighting in machine learning and data analysis involves determining the significance of various aspects of the data based on the model's evaluation. Figure 3 show the importance of feature along with their scores Recursive Feature Elimination (RFE) is a cool trick that helps to pick out the most crucial bits of data by tossing away the less important ones one by one until to find the needed one. These methods like RFE make the models smarter by focusing on the most useful features, making predictions more accurate and classifier models easier to understand. feature weighting based on a models add the sentences.

Weighted features:
Feature 0, Score: 0.120000
Feature 1, Score: 0.240000
Feature 2, Score: 0.080000
Feature 3, Score: 0.040000
Feature 4, Score: 0.080000
Feature 5, Score: 0.160000
Feature 6, Score: 0.180000
Feature 7, Score: 0.100000

Figure 3. Feature Importance graph

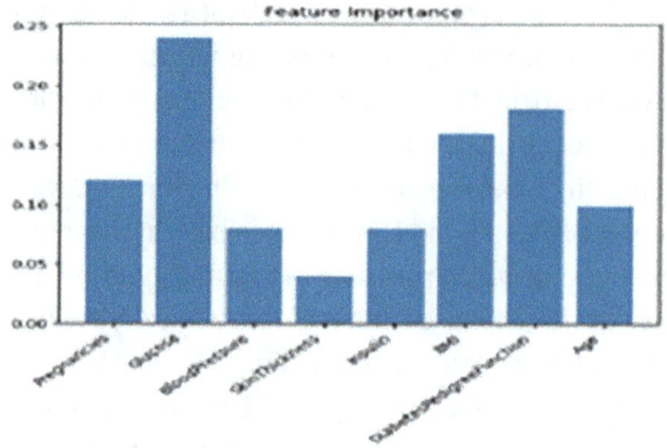

Iterative in nature, boosting methods train weak models (usually decision trees) one after the other, with each new model concentrating on the incorrectly categorized cases from earlier rounds. In healthcare analytics, popular boosting algorithms include:Adaptive Boosting, or AdaBoost GBMs, or gradient boosting machines

Extreme Gradient Boosting, or XGBoost LightGBMCatBoost These techniques are especially useful for predicting diabetes because they deal with several kinds of features (numerical, categorical).They can withstand moderate noise levels.

They help physicians with interpretability by automatically providing feature importance rankings.

Hyperparameter tuning is the process of optimizing the parameters that define the structure and behavior of a machine learning model, typically through experimentation and validation to enhance its performance and generalization. However, recent studies have shed light on the pivotal role of hyperparameter tuning like learning_rate, n_estimators, max_depth, min_samples_leafin further optimizing model performance, especially on imbalanced datasets. While traditional boosting algorithms like Adaboost, XGBoost, Gradient Boosting, CatBoost, LightGBM have been widely used, meticulous Hyperparameter Tuned (HT) through techniques like GridSearchCV has shown promising results in surpassing the performance of ensemble methods. Finding most relevant feature through feature importance according to the machine learning model and optimized hyperparameter for boosting algorithm improve the accuracy level

Although boosting algorithms have proven to be highly accurate, their effectiveness is mostly reliant on hyperparameters, which are pre-established settings that control the learning process. The number of boosting rounds is controlled by the number of estimators (n_estimators). The amount that each tree adds to the finished model is determined by its learning rate.The maximum tree depth (max_depth) regulates the complexity of the model.Overfitting is influenced by the minimum sample split and minimum child weight.

Subsample / colsample_bytree: Enhances generalization by managing unpredictability. Lambda and alpha regularization parameters penalize models that are too complex. Inadequately selected hyperparameters may result in:When a model is underfit, it is unable to identify patterns in the data. Overfitting occurs when a model does well on training data but poorly on data that hasn't been seen. Extended training periods makes ineffective use of resources without improvement in performance.

The following could be a typical pipeline for hyperparameter-tuned boosting in diabetes prediction

Data preprocessing includes scaling, encoding, and handling missing values for categorical data.

Assigning relevance scores or removing less pertinent features (for example, by using Mutual Information) are examples of feature weighting and selection. Choosing a boosting method (such as XGBoost) is the first step in boosting model training .Hyperparameter optimization is the process of determining the ideal configuration using tuning techniques. Evaluation: Metrics such as Accuracy, Precision, Recall, F1-score, and AUC-ROC are used to evaluate performance. Interpretability: Understanding model decisions through the use of SHAP or feature significance plots.

Benefits of Diabetes Prediction are high prediction accuracy despite medical data noise. Feature interactions are handled automatically without human intervention. Adaptability to incorporate ensemble approaches, SMOTE (for unbalanced data), and feature weighting.

3.1 Hyperparameters for boosting model

Hyperparameters for Adaboost:

Best Parameters: {'learning_rate': 0.2, 'n_estimators': 100}

Hyperparameters for XGBoost:

Best Parameters: {'learning_rate': 0.1, 'max_depth': 4, 'n_estimators': 100}

Hyperparameters for Gradient boost:

Best Parameters: {'learning_rate': 0.1, 'max_depth': 3, 'min_samples_leaf': 2, 'min_samples_split':2, 'n_estimators': 200}

Hyperparameters for LightGBM:

Best Parameters: {'learning_rate': 0.1, 'max_depth': 7, 'n_estimators': 200}

Hyperparameters for CatBoost:

Best Parameters: {'depth': 7, 'iterations': 200, 'learning_rate': 0.2}

Furthermore, evaluating model performance using a comprehensive set of metrics, including accuracy, F1-score, precision, recall, area under the ROC curve (AUC), and ROC curve analysis, provides deeper insights into the model's effectiveness across different aspects.

These metrics collectively offer a holistic view of the model's performance, conclusion, requires a concerted effort involving various preprocessing, feature selection, and model optimization techniques. To enhance the performance feature importance has been calculated using machine learning model and feature are selected according to the feature importance score.

Figure 4. Architecture Diagram

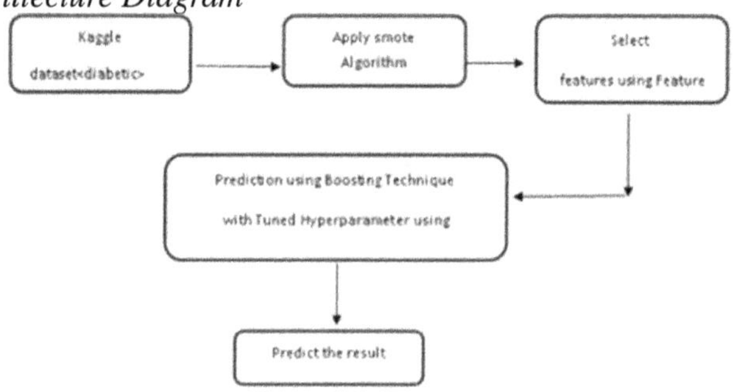

Addressing imbalances, utilize the SMOTE algorithm to create synthetic samples and ensure class balance. Employing feature selection techniques with weighting, pinpoint and prioritize influential features for classifier model. This ensures the model focuses on pertinent data for accurate predictions. Subsequently, boosting techniques like AdaBoost orXGBoost or Gradient Boosting or LightGBM or CatBoostare applied to elevate model performance. As per the architecture is shown in Figure 4 proposed system makes predictions with enhanced accuracy and reliability. This comprehensive approach, from dataset collection to prediction, integrates advanced methodologies for optimized performance and robust results. Proposed system use Machine learning algorithms to handle the diagnosis of disease in efficient manner.

4. RESULTS AND DISCUSSION

Proposed work yielded strong predictive accuracy for diabetic outcomes. SMOTE addressed dataset imbalances effectively, while feature selection streamlined model learning. Boosting techniques further improved predictive power. This comprehensive method showcases the efficacy of advanced methodologies in diabetic prediction, promising enhanced healthcare outcomes.Optimizing the hyperparameter as improve the prediction that can be realized the comparative study Algorithm like CatBoost, Adaboost,XGBoost used without considering the hyperparameter gave 78% accuracy whereas proposed system shows 80% accuracy.

4.1 Accuracy

Accuracy is the proportion of correct predictions (both positive and negative) made by the model out of all predictions.

$$Accuracy = \frac{TruePositiveRate + TrueNegative}{FalsePositive + FalseNegative}$$

Accuracy measures the overall correctness of a classification model.For example, an accuracy of 0.90 (or 90%) means the model correctly classified 90% of all instances.

Accuracy is useful when the dataset is balanced (i.e., similar numbers of diabetic and non-diabetic cases).In imbalanced datasets, high accuracy can be misleading—a model predicting "non-diabetic" for everyone could achieve high accuracy but fail to detect actual diabetic cases.Therefore, in medical AI applications, accuracy is usually evaluated together with precision, recall, and F1-score to ensure the model detects the positive class effectively.

Table 1. Accuracy

Feature weighting+ Hyperparameter tuning +AdaBoost	Feature weighting+ Hyperparameter tuning+ XGBoost	Feature weighting+ Hyperparameter tuning+Gradient Boost	Feature weighting+ Hyperparameter tuning+ LightGBM	Feature weighting+ Hyperparameter tuning +CatBoost
0.80	0.79	0.80	0.80	0.81

4.2 Precision

Precision calculates the true positive rate.

precision = TruePostive Rate/(TruePostice Rate + False Postive Rate)

High precision means that where the model predicts a patient has diabetes, it is correct most of the time.

This is crucial when false positives are costly (e.g., causing unnecessary stress or additional medical tests for healthy individuals).

4.3 Recall

Recall is rate of true positive against total positive rate.

$$\text{recall} = \frac{\text{True Positive}}{(\text{TruePostive} + \text{FalseNegative})}$$

High recall ensures that most diabetic patients are correctly detectedThis is especially important in healthcare because missing a positive case (false negative) can lead to delayed diagnosis and severe health consequences.

Comparison of accuracy Precision and recall with existing algorithm are show in the table 1 and table 2.

Table 2. Precision and recall score

Feature weighting+ Hyperparameter tuning +AdaBoost		Feature weighting+ Hyperparameter tuning+ XGBoost		Feature weighting+ Hyperparameter tuning+Gradient Boost		Feature weighting+ Hyperparameter tuning+ LightGBM		Feature weighting+ Hyperparameter tuning +CatBoost	
Precision	**Recall**	**Precision**	**Recall**	**Precision**	**Recall**	**Precision**	**Recall**	**Precision**	**Recall**
0.77	0.87	0.77	0.87	0.75	0.81	0.74	0.86	0.76	0.8

4.4 F1 score and ROC_AUC score

F1 score is simply harmonic mean of precision and recall and it lies in the range (0,1). ROC_AUC score metric is measured for classification technique that give the probability of each class.

$$F1 - score = 2X\frac{PrecisionxRecall}{Precision + Recall}$$

F1-score is particularly valuable in imbalanced datasets (common in medical data) where both false positives and false negatives matter. A high F1-score indicates the model is good at identifying diabetics without too many false alarms.

ROC (Receiver Operating Characteristic) curve plots the True Positive Rate (Recall) against the False Positive Rate (FPR) at different classification thresholds. The AUC (Area Under the Curve) summarizes the overall ability of the model to distinguish between classes.

AUC∈[0,1](1 = perfect classifier, 0.5 = random guessing)

Measures the overall discrimination power of the model, independent of any specific threshold.Useful when comparing multiple models to choose the best one. In healthcare, a model with a high AUC is preferred because it consistently ranks diabetic patients higher in risk than non-diabetic patients.

Table 3 reveals the F1 score and ROC_AUC score outperforms with existing classifier. ROC_AUC curve shows higher score for proposed technique which is executed in Figure 5.,6,7,8,9.

Table 3. F1 score and ROC_AUC score

Feature weighting+ Hyperparameter tuning +AdaBoost		Feature weighting+ Hyperparameter tuning+ XGBoost		Feature weighting+ Hyperparameter tuning+Gradient Boost		Feature weighting+ Hyperparameter tuning+ LightGBM		Feature weighting+ Hyperparameter tuning +CatBoost	
F1 score	ROCAUC	F1 score	ROCAUC	F1 score	ROCAUC	F1 score	ROCAUC	F1 score	ROCAUC
0.77	0.87	0.77	0.87	0.75	0.81	0.74	0.86	0.76	0.84

Figure 5. ROC_AUC curve for AdaBoosting classifier

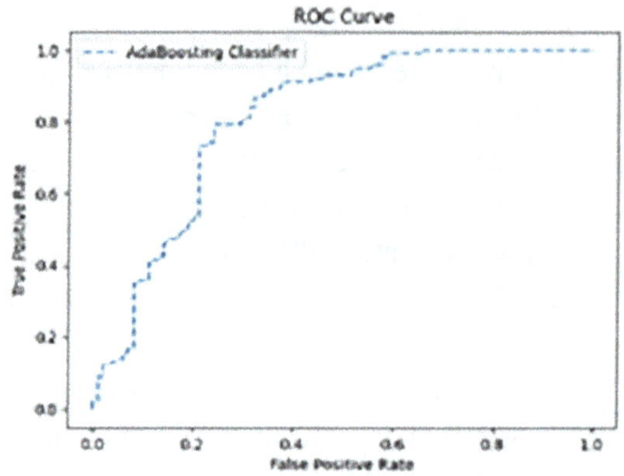

Figure 6. ROC_AUC curve for XGBoosting classifier

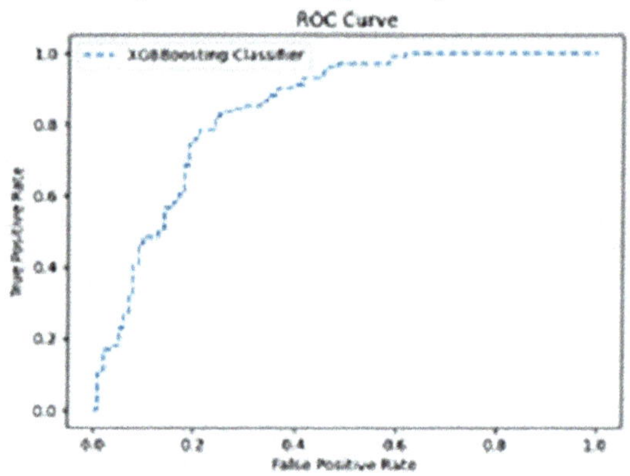

Figure 7. ROC_AUC curve for Gradient Boosting Classifier

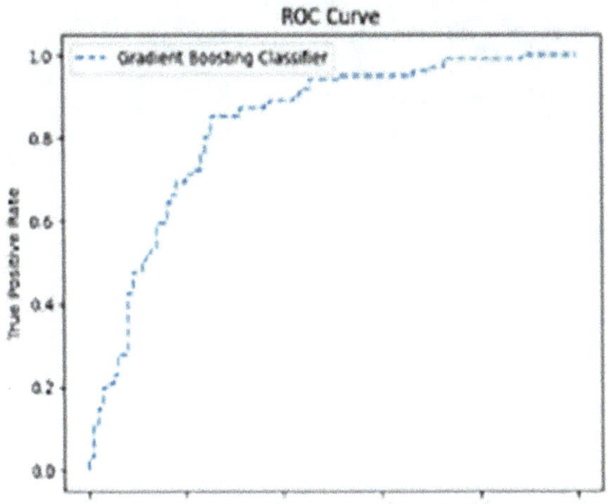

Figure 8. ROC_AUC curve for LightGBM Classifier

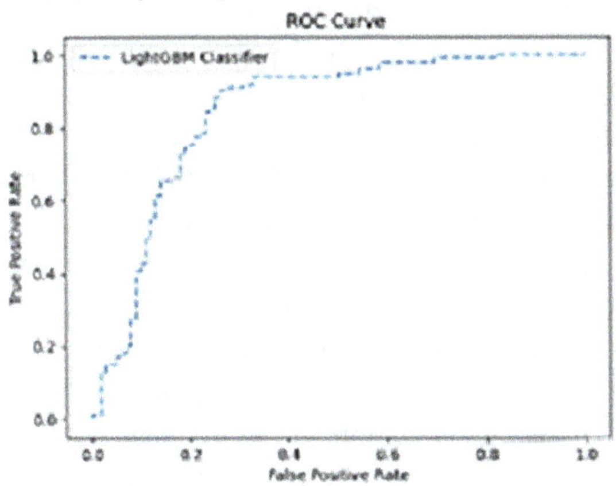

Figure 9. ROC_AUC curve for Catboost Classifier

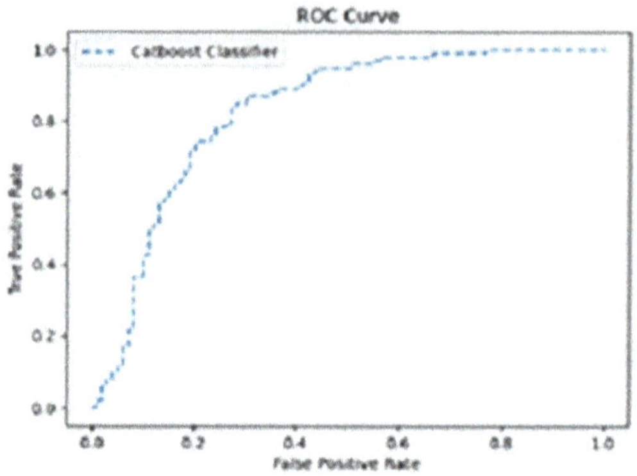

4.5 Experimental observations

Utilizing well-tuned hyperparameters often results in enhanced model performance when compared to models trained without optimizing hyperparameters. This optimization process fine-tunes the model's settings, allowing it to better capture the underlying patterns in the data and make more accurate predictions. Consequently, models with optimized hyperparameters exhibit improved accuracy, robustness, and generalization ability, contributing to better overall performance in real-world applications. In contrast, neglecting hyperparameter tuning may lead to suboptimal model behavior, potentially resulting in lower predictive accuracy and decreased effectiveness in addressing the task at hand. A crucial stage in machine learning model optimization is hyperparameter tuning, which involves methodically modifying the external configuration parameters of algorithms (such learning rate, maximum tree depth, or regularization terms) to enhance performance. Models without hyperparameter adjustment, on the other hand, depend on the machine learning library's default values, which might not be the best for the given dataset.

A comparative analysis emphasizes the significance of tuning in boosting generalizability, decreasing bias, and improving diagnostic accuracy in the context of diabetes prediction utilizing datasets like the PIMA Indian Diabetes In the absence of hyperparameter tuning, models frequently show relatively high accuracy skewed toward non-diabetic predictions and suboptimal recall for minority diabetes instances because to imbalance. By optimizing parameters for the selected classifier (e.g., XGBoost, LightGBM,) systematic search techniques like Grid Search, Random Search, or Bayesian Optimization can increase recall, F1-score, and ROC-AUC.

Without tuning while the default values might be effective for certain datasets, they exhibit significant performance variation over validation folds. By identifying parameter settings that consistently yield good results across cross-validation splits, hyperparameter tuning enhances stability. Without tuning, If the default parameters are not in line with the properties of the dataset, the model may underfit (be too basic) or overfit (be too complicated).With Tuning: Techniques such as adjusting regularization terms, learning rate, and max depth help in achieving the optimal bias–variance trade-off.

Class weights or sampling strategies can be incorporated into variants like AdaBoost, XGBoost, and LightGBM, which increases their sensitivity to minority instances (such as diabetic patients)

Boosting algorithms help with feature selection and interpretability by ranking features according to how much they contribute to lowering prediction error. Boosting minimizes bias (underfitting) and controls variance (overfitting) through regularization by successively fixing mistakes made by earlier models able to identify intricate, non-linear relationships between target variables and input data, which is essential for multifactorial illnesses like diabetes. The impact of noisy or extreme values can be reduced with methods like gradient boosting with robust loss functions (Huber loss).requires little preprocessing and can work with both numerical and categorical variables. Table 4 give proper comparative study for hyper parameter tuned algorithm and without hyperparameter tuned boosting algorithm.

Table 4. Comparative study

Metrics	Adaboost		XGBoost		Gradient Boost		LightGBM		CatBoost	
	HT Adaboost	Adaboost	HT XGBoost	XGBoost	HT Gradient Boost	Gradient Boost	HT LightGBM	LightGBM	HT CatBoost	CatBoost
Accuracy	0.80	0.74	0.79	0.70	0.80	0.75	0.80	0.72	0.81	0.72
Precision	0.77	0.63	0.77	0.57	0.75	0.64	0,74	0.59	0.76	0.68
Recall	0.87	0.65	0.87	0.69	0.81	0.69	0.86	0.67	0.84	0.67
F1 score	0.82	0.64	0.81	0.62	0.88	0.66	0.79	0.63	0.80	0.67
AUC score	0.83	0.80	0.84	0.76	0.84	0.80	0.85	0.77	0.82	0.80

5. SOLUTION AND RECOMMENDATION

5.1 SOLUTION

This article suggests an integrated predictive framework that combines the following to overcome the shortcomings of conventional diabetes prediction models in managing imbalanced datasets, feature relevance variability, and hyperparameter sensitivity.

Feature weighting is the process of giving each clinical attribute a relevance value in order to highlight important predictors (such as fasting glucose, BMI, and HbA1c) and lessen the impact of less important factors.

To balance the dataset and enhance model recall for minority (positive) diabetes cases, the Synthetic Minority Oversampling Technique (SMOTE) is used The Hyperparameter-Tuned Boosting Algorithm uses Adaboost by fine-tuning parameters including learning rate, maximum depth, and number of estimators. The suggested approach preserves interpretability for clinical use while improving prediction accuracy, recall, and AUC.

5.2 RECOMMENDATION

In light of the experimental findings, it is advised that: For early diabetes risk assessment, healthcare organizations include hyperparameter-tuned boosting models into their decision support systems To improve model interpretability and make sure physicians can comprehend the main risk factors affecting predictions, feature weighting approaches should be used. To avoid underdiagnosing diabetes cases, SMOTE or advanced oversampling techniques should be used when working with extremely unbalanced patient datasets. Additional research looks exploring how to include real-time patient monitoring data into the predictive framework, such as glucose levels from wearable devices. To boost preventive healthcare initiatives, policymakers are thinking about assisting in the development of explainable AI-based diagnostic tools .For broader impact, the proposed methodology can be extended to other chronic diseases where imbalanced data and feature importance variability are significant challenges.

6. FUTURE RESEARCH DIRECTION

Although the suggested feature-weighted, hyperparameter-tuned boosting strategy shows encouraging results in raising the sensitivity and accuracy of diabetes prediction, there are a number of chances for this work to be improved upon and used more widely:

For improving diabetic prediction hyperparameter tuning Advanced Optimization of Hyperparameters can be used. Three different ways to use for hyperparamaeter tuning first one is Automated Search for Hyperparameters will achieve more efficient tuning, replace manual grid/random search with Bayesian Optimization, Tree-structured Parzen Estimator (TPE), or evolutionary algorithms. Second one is Adaptive/dynamic hyperparameters to avoid overfitting and accelerate convergence, create models with adaptively adjustable learning rate, number of estimators, and tree depth during training. Another way is Optimization with multiple objectives to optimize for sensitivity, specificity, and interpretability in addition to accuracy, as these factors are crucial for medical diagnosis.

For boosting ensemble hybridization can be used. One way to blending or stacking other models with ensemble hybridization use of complementary qualities, combine deep learning models or logistic regression with tuned boosting models (such as XGBoost, LightGBM, and CatBoost) Differential boosting propose a model use a variety of base learners, such as neural networks for capturing non-linear feature interactions instead of just using decision trees.

Handle data imbalance is another challenge. In class imbalance for improved minority class recognition, incorporate boosting with sophisticated resampling techniques (such as SMOTE variants, Tomek Links, and ADASYN) during hyperparameter tuning. To handle data robustness screate hyperparameter tuning techniques that can adjust to datasets that contain missing patient information. Another way is feature drift adaptation new medical data alters statistical distributions, develop models that can update adjusted hyperparameters over time.

For integration of Model Explainability, use counterfactual explanations, SHAP, or LIME in conjunction with tuned boosting models .Convert the output of the adjusted model into diagnostic rules that can be understood by humans for use in clinical decision-making .From the standpoint of implementation, real-time diabetes risk assessment through the use of tailored boosting models in wearable technology or mobile health apps may offer physicians and patients immediate, useful feedback. Federated hyperparameter tweaking would also make it possible for hospitals to build models securely and dispersedly without exchanging private patient information, encouraging privacy compliance and growing the training dataset. Richer health patterns can be captured by merging multimodal inputs, such as retinal imaging, tabular clinical records, and continuous glucose monitoring data, to enhance predictive capabilities. Additionally, by turning on longitudinal prediction, the model will be able to anticipate how the disease would evolve over time instead of only producing binary results. Combine boosting with deep neural networks in hybrid frameworks to leverage both structured feature data and unstructured clinical notes or images.

7. CONCLUSION

In this paper, predicting revolutionized diabetes prediction using advanced computational techniques. A promising area of medical machine learning is enhanced diabetic prediction using feature weighting in conjunction with hyperparameter-tuned boosting algorithms. This method makes use of the advantages of both platforms, as well as incorporating multimodal data (such as clinical, genetic, and lifestyle data) into this framework. approaches hyperparameter adjustment optimizes algorithmic performance, while feature weighting improves model focus and interpretability. When combined, they produce a strong, precise, and clinically applicable prediction framework that can support diabetes early detection and preventative measures. The creation of such sophisticated predictive technologies will be crucial for lowering the disease burden, guiding public health initiatives, and eventually enhancing patient outcomes as the prevalence of diabetes rises. Future studies should look into creating lightweight, privacy-preserving versions that can be used in wearable technology and telemedicine.

To address the issue dataset are taken from Kaggle, dataset incurred the problem of imbalance, to handle the problem of imbalanced datasets, the SMOTE algorithm applied. Then, employing feature weighting methods, pinpoint the most critical factors for predicting diabetes risk. The real game-changer a hyperparameter tuning, which fine-tuned the classifier . Tuning hyperparameter enhanced the model's predictive rate surpassing previous benchmarks in accuracy, precision, recall, F1 score, AUC score, and ROC curve metrics. Along with predicting diabetes more reliably and enhance the precision and recall. By detecting diabetes sooner, one can initiate timely treatments, potentially averting serious complications and improving overall health outcomes for individuals at risk. This work underscores the transformative potential of advanced machine learning techniques in healthcare. Proposed work has been limited to dataset characteristics and this work has been extended to multiclass dataset and different type of dataset By harnessing the power of data and computational algorithms, finding the way for more effective disease prediction and management, ultimately leading to better health outcomes for all.

REFERENCES

Abousaber, I., Abdallah, H. F., & El-Ghaish, H. (2025). Robust predictive framework for diabetes classification using optimized machine learning on imbalanced datasets. *Frontiers in Artificial Intelligence*, *7*, 1499530. DOI: 10.3389/frai.2024.1499530 PMID: 39839971

Ağraz, M., Eğrioğlu, E., Baş, E., Chen, M. Y., Göksülük, D., & Burak, M. F. (2025). Diabetes Development Prediction Using a Hybrid Model Combining Dendritic Artificial Neuron Model and Logistic Regression. *Endocrinology Research & Practice, 29*(2).

Arslan, A. K., Yagin, F. H., Algarni, A., Karaaslan, E., Al-Hashem, F., & Ardigò, L. P. (2024). Enhancing type 2 diabetes mellitus prediction by integrating metabolomics and tree-based boosting approaches. *Frontiers in Endocrinology*, *15*, 1444282. DOI: 10.3389/fendo.2024.1444282 PMID: 39588339

Bhat, S. S., Selvam, V., & Ansari, G. A. (2023). Predicting Life Style of Early Diabetes Mellitus Using Machine Learning.

Chaves, L., & Marques, G. (2021). Data mining techniques for early diagnosis of diabetes: A comparative study. *Applied Sciences (Basel, Switzerland)*, *11*(5), 2218. DOI: 10.3390/app11052218

Farnoodian, M. E., Moridani, M. K., & Mokhber, H. (2023). Detection and prediction of diabetes using effective biomarkers. *Computer Methods in Biomechanics and Biomedical Engineering. Imaging & Visualization*, •••, 1–13.

Hassan, M. M., Mollick, S., & Yasmin, F. (2022). An unsupervised cluster-based feature grouping model for early diabetes detection. *Healthcare Analytics*, *2*, 100112. DOI: 10.1016/j.health.2022.100112

Houssein, E. H., & Sayed, A. (2023). A modified weighted mean of vectors optimizer for chronic kidney disease classification. *Computers in Biology and Medicine*, *155*, 106691. DOI: 10.1016/j.compbiomed.2023.106691 PMID: 36805229

Kalagotla, S. K., Gangashetty, S. V., & Giridhar, K. (2021). A novel stacking technique for prediction of diabetes. *Computers in Biology and Medicine*, *135*, 104554. DOI: 10.1016/j.compbiomed.2021.104554 PMID: 34139440

Kaliappan, J., Saravana Kumar, I. J., Sundaravelan, S., Anesh, T., Rithik, R. R., Singh, Y., Vera-Garcia, D. V., Himeur, Y., Mansoor, W., Atalla, S., & Srinivasan, K. (2024). Analyzing classification and feature selection strategies for diabetes prediction across diverse diabetes datasets. *Frontiers in Artificial Intelligence*, *7*, 1421751. DOI: 10.3389/frai.2024.1421751 PMID: 39233892

Khurshid, M. R., Manzoor, S., Sadiq, T., Hussain, L., Khan, M. S., & Dutta, A. K. (2025). Unveiling diabetes onset: Optimized XGBoost with Bayesian optimization for enhanced prediction. *PLoS One*, *20*(1), e0310218. DOI: 10.1371/journal.pone.0310218 PMID: 39854291

Kibria, H. B., Nahiduzzaman, M., Goni, M. O. F., Ahsan, M., & Haider, J. (2022). An ensemble approach for the prediction of diabetes mellitus using a soft voting classifier with an explainable AI. *Sensors (Basel)*, *22*(19), 7268. DOI: 10.3390/s22197268 PMID: 36236367

Li, W., Peng, Y., & Peng, K. (2024). Diabetes prediction model based on GA-XGBoost and stacking ensemble algorithm. *PLoS One*, *19*(9), e0311222. DOI: 10.1371/journal.pone.0311222 PMID: 39348356

Liu, J., Peng, B., & Yin, Z. (2023, January). A Hybrid Machine Learning Method for Diabetes Detection based on Unsupervised Clustering. In *Proceedings of the 2023 7th International Conference on Machine Learning and Soft Computing* (pp. 144-149). DOI: 10.1145/3583788.3583809

Lugner, M., Rawshani, A., Helleryd, E., & Eliasson, B. (2024). Identifying top ten predictors of type 2 diabetes through machine learning analysis of UK Biobank data. *Scientific Reports*, *14*(1), 2102. DOI: 10.1038/s41598-024-52023-5 PMID: 38267466

Mohanty, P. K., Francis, S. A. J., Barik, R. K., Roy, D. S., & Saikia, M. J. (2024). Leveraging Shapley additive explanations for feature selection in ensemble models for diabetes prediction. *Bioengineering (Basel, Switzerland)*, *11*(12), 1215. DOI: 10.3390/bioengineering11121215 PMID: 39768033

Olabanjo, O., Wusu, A., Olabanjo, O., Asokere, M., Afisi, O., & Akinnuwesi, B. (2025). A novel deep learning model for early diabetes risk prediction using attention-enhanced deep belief networks with highly imbalanced data. *International Journal of Information Technology : an Official Journal of Bharati Vidyapeeth's Institute of Computer Applications and Management*, *17*(4), 1–23. DOI: 10.1007/s41870-025-02459-3

Olorunfemi, B. O., Ogunde, A. O., Almogren, A., Adeniyi, A. E., Ajagbe, S. A., Bharany, S., Altameem, A., Rehman, A. U., Mehmood, A., & Hamam, H. (2025). Efficient diagnosis of diabetes mellitus using an improved ensemble method. *Scientific Reports*, *15*(1), 3235. DOI: 10.1038/s41598-025-87767-1 PMID: 39863685

Rajendra, P., & Latifi, S. (2021). Prediction of diabetes using logistic regression and ensemble techniques. *Computer Methods and Programs in Biomedicine Update*, *1*, 100032. DOI: 10.1016/j.cmpbup.2021.100032

Shao, H., Liu, X., Zong, D., & Song, Q. (2024). Optimization of diabetes prediction methods based on combinatorial balancing algorithm. *Nutrition & Diabetes*, *14*(1), 63. DOI: 10.1038/s41387-024-00324-z PMID: 39143066

Shi, Y., & Sun, J. (2024). Integrated bagging-RF learning model for diabetes diagnosis in middle-aged and elderly population. *PeerJ. Computer Science*, *10*, e2436. DOI: 10.7717/peerj-cs.2436 PMID: 39650520

Vîrgolici, O., Lixandru, D., Mihai, A., tefan, D. S., Guja, C., Vîrgolici, H., & Virgolici, B. (2025). prediction of metabolic parameters of diabetic patients depending on body weight variation using machine learning techniques. *Biomedicines*, *13*(5), 1116. DOI: 10.3390/biomedicines13051116 PMID: 40426942

Yun, C., Tang, F., Gao, Z., Wang, W., Bai, F., Miller, J. D., Liu, H., Lee, Y., & Lou, Q. (2024). Construction of risk prediction model of type 2 diabetic kidney disease based on deep learning. *Diabetes & Metabolism Journal*, *48*(4), 771–779. DOI: 10.4093/dmj.2023.0033 PMID: 38685670

Zhang, W., Xia, Z., Cai, G., Wang, J., & Dong, X. (2025). Enhancing diabetes risk prediction through focal active learning and machine learning models. *PLoS One*, *20*(7), e0327120. DOI: 10.1371/journal.pone.0327120 PMID: 40627636

KEY TERMS AND DEFINITIONS

Accuracy: The proportion of correctly classified instances (both positive and negative) to the total number of instances in the dataset.

Bagging: Bagging is an ensemble learning technique that improves the stability and accuracy of machine learning models by combining the predictions of multiple models trained on different randomly sampled subsets of the training data.

Bayes Theorem in Classification: A statistical principle used in probabilistic models (e.g., Naïve Bayes) to compute the probability of a class given the observed features.

Bayesian Optimization: A hyperparameter tuning method that uses probabilistic models to efficiently search for the best parameter combinations.

Boosting Technique: An ensemble learning method that combines multiple weak learners (often decision trees) into a strong classifier by sequentially focusing on previously misclassified instances. Examples include AdaBoost, Gradient Boosting, XGBoost, LightGBM, and CatBoost.

Class Imbalance Problem: A situation in which one class significantly outnumbers the other, making model training biased toward the majority class.

Classification: A supervised learning task where the goal is to predict categorical labels (e.g., diabetic or non-diabetic) for given input features.

Confusion Matrix: A tabular summary of classification results showing True Positives, False Positives, True Negatives, and False Negatives.

Cross-Validation: A resampling technique used to evaluate model performance by partitioning the data into multiple training and validation subsets.

Decision Tree: A tree-structured model used for classification or regression, where each node represents a feature and branches represent decision rules.

Diabetes Mellitus: A chronic metabolic disorder characterized by elevated blood glucose levels due to insufficient insulin production or ineffective insulin utilization. Early detection is critical for preventing complications.

Ensemble Learning: A machine learning paradigm that combines multiple models to improve predictive performance, reduce variance, and enhance robustness.

Evaluation Metrics: Quantitative measures used to assess the performance of a predictive model, including accuracy, precision, recall, F1-score, and ROC–AUC score.

F1-Score: The harmonic mean of Precision and Recall, used to balance both metrics, especially in imbalanced datasets.

False Negative (FN): An instance where the model fails to identify a positive case (e.g., predicting non-diabetes for a diabetic patient).

False Positive (FP): An instance where the model incorrectly predicts the positive class (e.g., predicting diabetes for a non-diabetic patient).

False Positive Rate (FPR): The proportion of actual negatives that are incorrectly classified as positive.

Feature Importance: A score indicating how much a particular feature contributes to the model's predictions.

Feature Weighting: A process of assigning importance scores to each input variable in a dataset, allowing machine learning models to emphasize highly relevant features and reduce the influence of less important ones.

Grid Search: A systematic hyperparameter tuning method that exhaustively tests all possible combinations of specified parameters.

Hyperparameter Tuning: The process of optimizing algorithm parameters that are set before training (e.g., learning rate, maximum tree depth, number of estimators) to achieve the best model performance.

Imbalanced Dataset: A dataset where the number of instances in different classes is significantly unequal, often leading to biased model performance if not addressed.

k-Fold Cross-Validation: A common cross-validation method where the dataset is divided into *k* equal parts; the model is trained on *k-1* parts and validated on the remaining part, repeating *k* times.

Learning Rate: A hyperparameter in boosting algorithms that controls the contribution of each weak learner to the final model.

Machine Learning (ML): A subset of artificial intelligence that enables computer systems to learn patterns from data and make predictions or decisions without explicit programming.

Overfitting: A condition where a model learns the training data too well, capturing noise and patterns that do not generalize to unseen data.

Precision: The ratio of correctly predicted positive cases to all predicted positive cases, measuring the model's ability to avoid false positives.

Random Search: A hyperparameter tuning method that tests a random subset of parameter combinations within specified ranges.

Recall (Sensitivity): The ratio of correctly predicted positive cases to all actual positive cases, reflecting the model's ability to detect true positives.

ROC–AUC Score: A performance metric that measures a model's ability to distinguish between classes across all classification thresholds. The AUC (Area Under the Curve) ranges from 0.5 (random guessing) to 1.0 (perfect classification).

SHapley Additive exPlanations (SHAP) Values: A method for explaining machine learning predictions by assigning each feature an importance value for a particular prediction.

Supervised Learning: A type of machine learning where models are trained on labeled datasets, meaning the input data is paired with the correct output.

Synthetic Minority Oversampling Technique (SMOTE): A data balancing method that generates synthetic samples for the minority class to improve classification performance in imbalanced datasets.

True Positive Rate (TPR): Another term for Recall, measuring the proportion of actual positives correctly identified.

Underfitting: A condition where a model is too simple to capture the underlying patterns in the data, leading to poor performance on both training and test sets.

Weak Learner: A simple predictive model that performs slightly better than random guessing; in boosting, many weak learners are combined to form a strong model.

Chapter 13
Pipeline-Based Prediction of Gestational Diabetes Mellitus Using Synthetic Healthcare Data

A. Sumathi
https://orcid.org/0000-0003-4700-5573
Department of CSE, SRC, SASTRA University, India

P. Umamaheswari
https://orcid.org/0000-0003-2007-697X
SASTRA University, India

M. Kamaladevi
https://orcid.org/0000-0001-8486-5092
SASTRA University, India

ABSTRACT

Gestational Diabetes Mellitus (GDM) is a form of diabetes that arises during pregnancy in women with no prior history of the condition. It is caused by the body's inability to produce sufficient insulin to meet the increased metabolic demands of pregnancy. If left undetected or poorly managed, GDM can lead to serious health complications, including high maternal blood glucose, increased risk of cesarean delivery, neonatal hypoglycemia, and long-term susceptibility to obesity and type 2 diabetes for both mother and child. Early and accurate prediction of GDM is therefore essential for timely intervention and improved maternal-fetal outcomes. A pipeline-based predictive model is proposed, integrating Principal Component Analysis (PCA) for dimensionality reduction with a Random Forest classifier for

DOI: 10.4018/979-8-3373-5641-9.ch013

robust prediction. The use of synthetic healthcare data enables the development and testing of the model in a controlled environment, enhancing reproducibility and scalability and its integration into clinical decision support systems for personalized prenatal care.

1. INTRODUCTION

Gestational Diabetes Mellitus (GDM) is a temporary yet potentially serious metabolic disorder, characterized by glucose intolerance recognized for the first time during pregnancy. GDM affects many women during pregnancy. GDM leads to glucose intolerance as a result of changes in hormones that interfere with the action of insulin, which leads to increased blood sugar levels that can pose health risks for the mother and fetus, if not properly managed. These risks include macrosomia (high birth weight), preeclampsia, neonatal hypoglycemia, a greater chance of cesarean delivery, and long-term metabolic health risks, including obesity and Type 2 diabetes mellitus for both the mother and child. GDM is usually diagnosed only during pregnancy, but the long-term effects of the diagnosis make it important to recognize and treat the condition early. While GDM resolves quickly after delivery, the chronic nature of GDM often facilitates being missed in the early part of pregnancy, leading to late diagnosis and decreased opportunity for prevention. Screening methods such as oral glucose tolerance tests are typically performed during the second trimester and provide more diagnostic than predictive abilities for early recognition of high-risk individuals in pregnancy, which limits their ability to identify high-risk individuals early in pregnancy when interventions may serve the patient most beneficially. The shortcomings of standard diagnoses have led to a surge of interest in more preventive and data-driven techniques through health and medical research that incorporates machine learning. With respect to assessing the origins of GDM prediction, the benefits provided through analysis, via the application of ML techniques, comes from the ability to analyze extremely broad features, including demographic features, medical concepts and health characteristics, laboratory tests, and dashboards of health business behaviors. However, incorporating machine learning into clinical workflows I should note several challenges. First, access to extensive high-quality healthcare datasets will tend to be restricted due to legal regulations relating to privacy such as Health Insurance Portability and Accountability Act (HIPAA) in the U.S. and the General Data Protection Regulation (GDPR) in the EU. These constraints, whether legal or ethical, severely limit availability of large-scale, labeled medical data to develop and validate models. The next challenge can be described with respect to the volume of potentially available health datasets. In terms of when datasets are available, will tend to be high-dimensional datasets, meaning the dataset comprises many features in the dataset, and this increases computational complexity in developing models and increases the risk of overfitting. This research will propose a privacy-preserving, sustainable pipeline based machine learning architecture to understand early GDM predictions using synthetic healthcare data. The design of this model will combine principal component analysis (PCA) (continuing to improve interpretability of the results) and random forest (RF) for classification purposes to assist with computational efficiency for prediction but maintaining the accuracy and interpretability for a clinician. The artificial dataset used in this research simulates clinical records for a mixed demographic of pregnant women, including relevant risk factors such as maternal age, body mass index (BMI), race/ethnicity, family history of diabetes, previous pregnancy outcomes, blood pressure, glucose, HbA1c, insulin, lifestyle risk factors such as smoking and exercise, etc. The machine learning pipeline begins with data cleaning and standardization in order to pre-process the artificial dataset in a way that will be optimal for modeling at the downstream stage. Next, we will apply Principal Component Analysis (PCA) as a means of dealing with the high feature dimensionality that can be characteristic of medical data. PCA is an unsupervised linear transformation technique that is used in machine learning to reduce the number of input features by projecting them into a collection of orthogonal, principal components that explain maximal amount of variance among the data. This transformation reduces the computational cost of model training, it reduces the likelihood of overfitting the model due to high-dimensional datasets, and improves model generalizability using synthetic and/or imbalanced datasets. PCA returns a set of reduced features, which then become input for a Random Forest classifier, which is an ensemble learning method that exploits both simple algorithms and high accuracy while accounting for both categorical and continuous data. This is important in an application in the healthcare area where it is heavily relied upon that the model is transparent and interpretable, in order to gain trust, buy-in and approval from the clinicians. The training and evaluation of the model, also has a component that adopts stratified cross-validation to balance positive and negative cases of GDM cases, in both the training, and testing folds to ensure that there is a relevant estimation of performance through the assessment of the pipeline. Performance is estimated through standard metrics familiar in the literature example accuracy, precision, recall(sensitivity), F1-score and area under the receive operating characteristic (AUC-ROC.). The results demonstrate that the system is able to classify high risk pregnancies from low risk pregnancies with a high level of confidence and accuracy, using only synthetic data to train the model. The PCA analytical component of the methodology significantly reduced the dimensionality of the original feature set by over 50%, which assists in reducing the complexity of the model and number of iterations needed to be run to train the model, while maintaining predictive performance. The pipeline model signifies not merely a technical advantage, but a sustainable method of innovation in the realm of digital health. The synthetic data utilized in the model provides a privacy-preserving process, and can be taken into consideration from a development perspective related to ethical AI. The modular nature of the pipeline model also supports a more reproducible way of conducting research studies. While synthetic data can estimate real world distributions, it does not necessarily incorporate all of the complexities, edge cases, or patterns of rare events that can be found in real patient data. For this reason, clinical validation with anonymized real-world datasets becomes a necessary step prior to utilizing this model in a production environment. Finally, although PCA is an efficient method for dimensionality reduction, the components created from original features may further complicate effective interpretation. The goal of this work is to implement a machine learning pipeline focused on transparency and sustainability for the prediction of Gestational Diabetes Mellitus (GDM) using synthetic health data. Alongside the PCA for reduced dimensions and Random Forest for classification, a synthetic fit for early prediction will achieve a relative level of predictive performance while preserving data privacy, supporting computational efficiency, and addressing an important clinical need. This will be an important factor as we continue developing a plan.

1.1 *Complications of GDM for the Mother*

Gestational Diabetes Mellitus has serious short-term and long-term implications for the pregnant mother. Although GDM resolves postpartum, it still presents serious risk if not appropriately monitored and managed. The following lists the major complications that may impact the mother:

High Blood Pressure and Preeclampsia

Gestational diabetes mellitus (GDM) has been correlated with an increased risk of hypertensive disorders during pregnancy because the rise in blood glucose affects metabolism and vascular systems. In pregnancy, one of the most significant complications associated with GDM is preeclampsia. In preeclampsia, blood pressure is persistently elevated, protein is found in the urine (proteinuria), and/or signs of organ dysfunction, typically including the liver, kidneys, or brain, are present. The precise relationships of GDM to preeclampsia are unknown, but several factors likely contribute, including insulin resistance, endothelial dysfunction, and increased inflammatory response, all of which negatively influence the function of blood vessels and placental circulation in pregnancy. If preeclampsia is not identified and managed promptly, potential, life-threatening complications—such as eclampsia (seizures), stroke, organ failure, or severe diminished fetal growth due to compromised delivery of nutrients and oxygen—could occur. Maternal and neonatal mortality could occur in the most extreme cases. Monitoring blood pressure, blood glucose, and kidney function, and intervening are crucial elements in preventing or managing the consequences of hypertension and preeclampsia related to GDM.

Increased Risk of Cesarean Delivery (C-Section)

When a pregnant individual experiences gestational diabetes mellitus (GDM), maternal hyperglycemia results in excess glucose passing through the placenta; the fetal pancreas, in turn, reacts with increased production of insulin (fetal hyperinsulinemia), promoting deposition of fat and stimulating growth such that the baby is born large for estimated gestational age (macrosomic). Because a macrosomic fetus is at increased risk of shoulder dystocia and birth trauma and as it will be more difficult to smoothly descend through the birth canal, pregnancies with GDM are at higher risk for labor-related complications (lack of progress, fetal heart rate abnormalities), and ultimately for cesarean delivery (planned for persistent macrosomia or excessive labor complications). While potentially lifesaving, cesarean delivery is a major abdominal surgery and has higher surgical-related morbidity than uncomplicated vaginal delivery: increased surgical-site infection and endometritis rates, higher intraoperative blood loss (transfusion), anesthesia-related morbidity, venous thromboembolism from inactivity, greater postoperative pain and recovery time, and extended (hospital) length of stay. Finally, the decision for - and experience of - one or more prior cesareans has implications for future pregnancies as each uterine surgical scar increases the risk for placental abnormalities (placenta accreta spectrum, placenta previa), which is associated with hospitalization and/or maternal...

Polyhydramnios

Gestational diabetes mellitus (GDM) can lead to polyhydramnios, which is an increased volume of amniotic fluid surrounding the fetus in utero. Polyhydramnios also may be implicated in the incidence of preterm labor, placental abruption, and increased risk for complications at the time of delivery.

Preterm Delivery

Women diagnosed with GDM likely will undergo spontaneous or recommended (early) delivery due to iatrogenic or non-iatrogenic complications, such as increased blood pressure or excessive fetal size. Preterm delivery increases the risk of complications to mother and newborn and the potential for needing specialized care.

Urinary Tract Infection (UTI)

Pregnant women with gestational diabetes mellitus (GDM) are at increased risk for recurrent urinary tract infections (UTI), primarily due to the efficiency of glycosuria (glucose in the urine) as a result of persistently high blood glucose levels. The glucose facilitates a trophic and nutrient-rich environment for bacteria to thrive in the urinary tract, especially the most common pathogen, Escherichia coli (E. coli). The presence of glucose in the urinary tract is associated with the metabolic and physiological effects of pregnancy and GDM, including hormonal changes that relaxes the smooth muscle in the urinary tract, dilation of the ureter, and...

Future Risk of Type 2 Diabetes

One of the most important long-term results of experiencing gestational diabetes mellitus (GDM) is that studies have projected that 50 to 70% of women diagnosed with GDM develop type 2 diabetes mellitus (T2DM) within 5 to 10 years after their affected pregnancy. This increased risk is due to the pathophysiological mechanisms of insulin resistance and impaired pancreatic beta-cell function that develop during the pregnancy and often do not fully resolve after delivery. Furthermore, subtle abnormalities in glucose metabolism may be present even after pregnancy and may also worsen over time with weight gain and in association with low levels of exercise and metabolic risk factors. Due to this high conversion rate to T2DM, continued monitoring of health is strongly recommended for women with a history of GDM, including regular testing for blood glucose, testing for HbA1c annually, and oral glucose tolerance testing if there is a question regarding glucose metabolism. Overall, long-term prevention strategies will heavily emphasize lifestyle changes, including reduction to a healthy body weight, eating a healthy diet that is high in fiber starches and low in refined sugars, and engaging in regular exercise. With early intervention and ongoing self-care, the onset of T2DM can be delayed, if not completely prevented, and the risk of cardiovascular and metabolic complications in the future can be lowered.

Reoccurrence of GDM in Future Pregnancies

Women who have had gestational diabetes mellitus (GDM) in one pregnancy have an increased risk in subsequent pregnancies. The reoccurrence of GDM is a manifestation of lasting metabolic predispositions for example, the underlying metabolic predispositions for type 2 diabetes—likened to diabetes associated with pregnancy—can be due to persistent insulin resistance, beta-cell dysfunction and/or genetic predispositions that are present postpartum, even if the women's blood glucose levels normalise after the baby is born. Lifestyle factors accompanying metabolic dysregulation such as excess body weight, diet, and physical inactivity outcomes, may increase the risks of reoccurrence of GDM. Beyond reversible lifestyle factors to include, there are also immutable risk factors such as maternal age, family type 2 diabetes history and maternal ethnicity that can predispose women to repeat episodes of GDM. Research suggests that reoccurrence rates can be as high as 30-80% and are heavily influenced by population characteristics, the time interval between pregnancies, and postpartum health behavior of the woman in question. Beyond the physiological risk, repeated episodes of GDM may elevate the mother's risk for type 2 diabetes and metabolic syndrome later in life—these women may have been covalent diabetes prior to the GDM episode but remain undiagnosed until after delivery, or they may develop significant metabolic disease later in life—indicates that simple proactive measures such as preconception counseling, early glucose screening in future pregnancies and targeted lifestyle behavior post GDM to promote weight loss and more physical activity can potentially mitigate the risks for repeated GDM for women with a prior history.

Emotional and Psychological Stress

Managing the condition of GDM can produce an emotional/psychological stressor with the regular blood sugar monitoring, dietome successes and failures, activity and physical activity, as a daily process.

1.2 Complications of GDM for the Baby

Uncontrolled gestational diabetes mellitus in pregnancy may affect the health of the baby. These complications may occur during pregnancy, during the birth process, or later in the baby's life.

Macrosomia (Large Baby)

Macrosomia is the most common complication. Macrosomia means the baby is a larger than normal size (greater than 4,000–4,500 grams or 8.8–9.9 lbs). When the mother has excessive blood glucose, the glucose crosses through the placenta, stimulating the baby's pancreas to produce more insulin, which increases fat storage and growth. A baby with macrosomia has a greater risk for birth injuries related to the birth process (ex., shoulder dystocia, fractured bones/nerve injuries).

Prematurity

High blood sugar levels in the mother increase the risk for preterm labor or the option to induce labor early due to increased risk. Preterm babies may have respiratory problems, jaundice, and organ systems needing hospitalization in the neonatal ICU.

Neonatal Hypoglycemia

After birth, the baby's insulin levels will remain high, but the mother's glucose intake will abruptly stop, resulting in hypoglycemia (low blood sugar). Severe or persistent neonate hypoglycemia may induce seizures, brain injury, or delays in learning and development, and needs to be medically treated.

Respiratory Distress Syndrome (RDS)

Infants exposed to GDM will have a greater risk for RDS than infants not exposed. RDS is a result of inadequate surfactant in the lungs to allow for lung maturation and improvement in oxygenation.

Increased Risk of Obesity and Type 2 Diabetes

Children of mothers with GDM are at an increased risk of childhood obesity and type 2 diabetes due to early exposure to a high insulin and glucose environment.

Electrolyte Imbalances

After birth, babies can have low blood calcium (hypocalcemia) and low magnesium (hypomagnesemia) levels, which can lead to muscle twitching or irritability.

Stillbirth

If a mother has poorly-controlled GDM, there is an increased risk of intrauterine fetal death (stillbirth), especially during the third trimester, which is attributed to placental insufficiency or metabolic problems.

Jaundice (Hyperbilirubinemia)

Increased insulin levels in the baby can interfere with liver maturity and can therefore lead to the risk of jaundice, which is a yellowing of the skin and/or eyes due to excess bilirubin in the blood.

Birth Trauma

The baby is at-risk for birth trauma once they are born because of being larger, or for complications during delivery, such as a fractured clavicle or brachial plexus injury.

Babies that are born to mothers with GDM are at risk for different health complications, from immediate complications post-partum to longer-term metabolic-related risk. However, many of these complications can be avoided or dealt with if the mom has appropriate prenatal care, blood glucose management, and monitoring of maternal and infant health. Early detection and intervention are key to getting good outcomes for mothers and babies. Detecting and managing GDM early is vital to prevent these outcomes. However, diagnosing GDM typically requires multiple clinical tests, a medical interpretation of the results, and a timely decision—often overwhelming tasks in demanding clinical environments, particularly in low-resourced healthcare settings. Therefore, a need for an intelligent automated system to support medical practitioners before making accurate and timely diagnoses of GDM is great. The rationale behind this project is to bridge the gap between complex medical data and clinical action through machine learning techniques embedded in an easy-to-use interface. The proposed solution combines a pipeline approach through a dimensionality reduction technique, Principal Component Analysis (PCA), and a Random Forest classifier to develop a predictive model for GDM. PCA is a method used for reducing the dimensionality of the input features, simplifying them for key information.

This reduction enhances interpretability and accuracy in predicting outcomes. Random Forest is a classification technique that is simple and robust. A Random Forest model is thus used to build the probability of GDM in patients. To support usability in real clinical practice, this clinical decision support system is developed as a Graphical User Interface (GUI). With this user interface, physicians enter the test values directly into a form. After entering the test results, the physician can click a "Predict" button and receive a report indicating whether or not the patient is likely to be at risk of GDM. This user experience significantly reduces the cognitive and usability load to clinicians and allows for faster and easier predictions. This project uses a synthetic healthcare dataset so that we can safely experiment with and develop our model without compromising patient confidentiality and privacy. The synthetic data enables us to train and test, and improve models safely, and in a controlled setting, before we move into patient environments. The work described in this project is motivated by the goal of providing a reliable, efficient, and easy-to-use machine learning pipeline that addresses a clinical problem with GDM diagnosis and helps support medical practitioners in improving their prenatal care decision-making abilities.

1.3 Synthetic Data as a Catalyst for Innovation in GDM Care

Synthetic healthcare data for gestational diabetes mellitus (GDM) is a type of information that has been generated artificially. It reflects the statistical patterns and trends, and relationships among variables that exist in real patient data without containing any real patient data. Synthetic healthcare data is beneficial in solving the privacy, confidentiality, security, and access challenges associated with real-world clinical data. These datasets support data sharing and scale research in a privacy-conscious manner that also does not violate privacy regulations, such as, for example, HIPAA or GDPR. In GDM research and care, real data often has its challenges, which are related to the fact that it is frequently not available, incomplete, or imbalanced with respect to rare cases or extreme cases. This prevents researchers from developing, training, and validating artificial intelligence and machine learning models for early risk prediction, glucose monitoring, patient stratification, and personalized treatment recommendations, to name a few advantages of synthetic data when only real data are not as readily available. Synthetic data allows researchers to simulate specific scenarios, such as complication scenarios that are rare or specific demographic scenarios that may also be underrepresented in real data. This allows researchers to add robustness to clinical decision support systems conducted with real patient data. Synthetic data can even be used to educate others. For example, medical students, clinicians, and data scientists can analyze synthetic datasets that were built specifically to look or behave like real data and not violate any patient's privacy or information security. By creating a safe, usable, and representative alternative to real patient data in maternal-fetal healthcare, innovations and advancements will be fostered.

1.4 Challenges of Synthetic Healthcare Data for Gestational Diabetes Mellitus (GDM)

Although synthetic healthcare data presents considerable opportunities for research and innovation in the study of GDM, it also presents challenges that must be understood, resolved, and addressed to confirm its usability and trustworthiness in setting standards of care recommendations. One primary concern with synthetic healthcare data is the fidelity of data, meaning, a synthetic dataset must accurately portray the complex physiology, temporal variation, and demographic differences associated with GDM. If the synthetic generation process simplifies a relationship too broadly (i.e., blood glucose level, gestational age, and maternal risk factors), the built models could be misleading and create clinical recommendations that would be biased or unsafe. Validation and benchmarking of synthetic data can be difficult because currently, there is no trust framework or benchmark for determining the extent to which the synthetic data represent real-world clinical patterns with a minimal privacy breach. A related but different problem is bias amplification, where any imperfections or imbalances in the source population are likely duplicated, if not amplified, by the synthetic generation process - further complicating the fairness and generalizability of resulting AI models. Lastly, there are technical challenges; in generative models able to render healthcare data that is high-dimensional (i.e., has a large number of features), issues can arise when the number of individuals in the real GDM dataset is limited, and missing values frequently occur. In addition, there is ongoing regulatory uncertainty because synthetic data in health care is still new, and guidelines for its use in clinical practice, sharing, and incorporation into decision-support systems is still in the process of development. Finally, there is the issue of clinical trust and adoption - health care workers may not be comfortable using models trained mostly on synthetic data unless strong evidence shows that performance is equal to or better than models trained mostly on real patient records. Addressing these issues will require rigorous validation methods, transparency in generation, and collaboration between clinicians, data scientists, and regulators to ensure that synthetic GDM data can be used safely and effectively.

2. LITERATURE SURVEY

Al-Nouti and Yaseen (2025) introduce a hybrid machine learning framework and a Differential Evolution (DE) algorithm to predict external corrosion in underground pipelines as a viable and cost-effective alternative to conventional techniques. They utilized an open-source dataset of 259 observations containing six pipeline parameters (redox potential, pH, pipe-to-soil potential, soil resistivity, age, and coating type) and six soil parameters (texture class, water content, and bulk density, along with chloride, bicarbonate, and sulfate) to assess several models — the Extreme Learning Machine (ELM), Support Vector Regressor (SVR), Extreme Gradient Boosting (XGB), and Multivariate Adaptive Regression Splines (MARS) — in both standalone and hybrid forms with DE optimization. An initial feature extraction step was conducted to help reduce model size and yield interpretable projections, together with DE to optimize hyperparameters and enhance ensemble performance. The XGBoost model with feature selection (XGB_FS) produced the best values (R^2 = 0.8407; RMSE = 0.395) and, as such, demonstrates appropriate predictive accuracy in mass Corrosion forecasting. In addition to the magnitude of corrosion prediction, the model conclusively identified the most meaningful physical and chemical parameters to ease targeted inspection and maintenance. The authors characterize these preliminary results are encouraging; however, readers must understand that the findings are limited in terms of generalizability due to the sample size (258) from the literature. The authors recommend further validation of a sample size that is much larger than the well-documented 10 years, with literature from 1996. The study conducted by Zhou et al. (2024) seeks to create a pragmatic, stepwise machine learning framework for gestational diabetes mellitus (GDM) prediction while keeping the algorithms interpretable and usable for real-world applications. Using a clinical sample size of 2,309 cases from public hospitals in Shenzhen, China, the authors built a stepwise prediction framework that included a three-stage (A→C) prediction system that decreased the number of necessary features understandably to adapt to the clinical scenario. Of the rut algorithms considered, XGBoost performed best, having test set accuracies of .922, .859, and .850 and AUCs of .974, .924, and .913, respectively. Including tree-based feature importance analysis and SHAP plots allowed for model interpretation, which confirmed established risk factors for GDM and showed stage-dependent modifiers, even including features with changes in influence direction across pregnancy stages. The output of the research was MedGDM, a lightweight software for prediction capability for clinic use that allows single or batch predictions. Overall, the work shows that a high-performing, interpretable pipeline can be constituted to predict GDM; by the effects of a regional dataset, the authors agree that the generalizability of the work is limited and recommend replication and external validation before implementation. Belsti et al. (2023) construct and test the "Monash GDM" risk prediction suite, with an ambition to compare many machine-learning classifiers to standard logistic regression for early detection of gestational diabetes in a diverse Australian maternity population, specifically framed as an evaluation of whether modern ML will actually provide real-life improvement over traditional methods.

They built a suite of predictor sets (from routinely available demographics and clinical variables to more robust biochemical and obstetrical information) that more closely resemble real clinical practice and they also created models with the inner validation framework, reporting all AUC stats from the lowest 70s, up to nearly 0.93, depending on algorithm and predictor set - adding to the strength of their study is that their chosen CatBoost classifier provided the best overall AUC, better than the final logistic regression models. The authors portray ML methods (especially gradient-boosted trees) as improving model discrimination and some calibration metrics compared to logistic regression, at the lower end of predictor availability, while delivering smaller gains at the higher ranges of predictor availability. They further point out the tradeoffs between model complexity and simpler predictive models, which would be more deployable in routine practice, given the constraints of clinical practice.

They also identify clinically relevant and statistically important contributors to the final predictive models (BMI, past GDM, ethnicity, and fasting glucose status) that drive most of the model predictions, and they extend their inquiry into model fairness and decision-curve applicability for subgroups within a diverse, heterogeneous cohort. This paper is careful about validation: the only reported performance is internal (cross-validation/hold-out), and the authors recognize that external and temporal validation is needed before clinical roll-out -- subsequent reciprocal external-validation work actually found that the AUC dropped when transporting to different populations, and demonstrated that generalizability is clearly a challenge.

The study is methodologically strong - we have a comparative design, have used a multi-predictor set of predictors, and we have focused on clinically actionable metrics - but limitations include the site-specific nature of the data and the typically optimistic internal validation risks inherent to using complex ML models. Overall, the Monash GDM study provides a well-documented pragmatic comparison that suggests the utility of tree-based ML (CatBoost/XGBoost family) for GDM risk stratification, while also appropriately pointing to a need for external validation and careful implementation work before using it in routine clinical use. Parkhi et al. (2023) studied machine-learning approaches to predict early postpartum prediabetes in women with gestational diabetes mellitus (GDM) to produce a clinically useful device for targeted surveillance.

They conducted a retrospective study using data from 607 women with GDM at George Eliot Hospital NHS Trust in the United Kingdom, which included antenatal, delivery, and postpartum biochemical and clinical factors. The primary outcome was biochemical evidence of postpartum prediabetes identified through OGTT, fasting glucose, or HbA1c during routine postpartum follow-up. A variety of machine-learning classifiers, including tree-based models and ensemble methods, were developed and compared against penalized sparse logistic regression. Through feature selection, it was discovered that a two-variable model was able to achieve the best trade-off between simplicity and performance using two variables: 1) Fasting glucose at the OGTT diagnostic test, and 2) HbA1c within several weeks of diagnosis with GDM (AUC ~0.72).

The authors reiterated the clinical utility of the minimal predictor set using routinely collected data from antenatal testing and that the minimum predictor model would be potentially ready to implement in practice for early risk stratification and increased postpartum testing. They further assessed and reported outcomes of decision thresholds for rule-in and rule-out decision support. Limitations of the study were the single-site, retrospective nature of the study, as well as possible selection bias from incomplete postpartum follow-up testing. The study by Xu et al (2016) looks at the correlation between maternal body composition, dietary behavior, and the occurrence of gestational diabetes mellitus (GDM) through ethnic and second-trimester cohort studies among Chinese women. A growing consensus of previous studies reported that pre-pregnancy obesity and poor dietary behavior are clinically significant risk factors for GDM. The authors utilized bioelectrical impedance analysis and dietary recall approaches to directly measure maternal health parameters. The study's findings demonstrate that fat mass and energy intake are associated with increased GDM risk.

This study adds to the existing literature by addressing maternal body composition and dietary behavior in the second trimester of pregnancy in a Chinese population. The study underscores the need for nutritional advice as a component of care during pregnancy and notes a positive association between dietary energy intake and risk for GDM. Punnose et al (2020) assessed whether first-trimester glycated hemoglobin (HbA_1c-FT) could predict gestational diabetes mellitus (GDM) in a large study of pregnant Asian Indian women. The authors performed a study of 2,275 women to find that the mean HbA_1c-FT level was noticeably higher among women who developed GDM compared to those who were diabetic. The authors found that HbA_1c-FT levels between 5.2-5.5% would increase risk by 1.63-fold, while levels above 5.6% would increase risk by 2.6% respectively. The receiver operating characteristic (ROC) curve indicated reduced explanatory power.

Arisoy (2016) examined the possible identification of gestational diabetes mellitus (GDM) during the first trimester, in pregnancies thought to be low-risk, by combining measurements of biomarkers and clinical data. They collected glycated hemoglobin, triglycerides, sex hormone binding globulin, and cholesterol measurements in the first trimester in a prospective cohort and found associations with the later diagnosis of GDM. Using logistic regression analysis and ROC analysis, they identified independent predictors from the above markers, although the specifics around predictive performances (e.g., AUC values) were fairly modest. The authors add to the broader literature that points towards early identification of GDM risk, where first-trimester biochemical markers are combined with demographic risk factors. Their ultimate findings indicate a promise of using a combination of predictors, which may outperform current models relying purely on maternal history, despite the authors working with a low-risk cohort. The findings are an important reminder that biochemical markers may be useful in both high-risk and low-risk populations. The authors will need to expand their validation process with larger cohorts and more diverse samples before these findings can be taken into account in clinical practice.

Prema & Pushpalatha (2019) created a machine learning-based ensemble technique that combined various classifiers to improve the prediction of gestational diabetes mellitus early in pregnancy. There were no sample sizes or performance measures available in the accessible abstracts for this proposal. Prema's model exemplifies ensemble approaches (stacking, blending, voting) that combine classifiers to exploit non-linear relationships without individual model bias. Ensemble approaches such as XGBoost, Random Forest, and LightGBM have previously demonstrated improved prediction in GDM studies; other GDM studies have found AUCs to be in the range of 0.77-0.85 with a similar population. This research builds on previous research that combined maternal age, BMI, lipid profiles, and biomarkers to improve discrimination, where an arbitrary point was chosen for evaluation over logistic regression. Ensemble models are generally associated with good sensitivity and specificity, but in terms of GDM prediction, there remain concerns about overfitting and external validation across studies. Prema's model reflects the trend to move to early GDM risk stratification using machine learning, and the potential for clinical use if a rigorous validation study is completed with an independent cohort.

3. PROPOSED METHODOLOGY

In the proposed method, a pipeline-based framework is utilized to produce synthetic medical data for risk prediction of Gestational Diabetes Mellitus (GDM). The pipeline consists of two parts: Principal Component Analysis (PCA) and Random Forest Classification. To analyze, the dataset will be processed to manage missing data, normalize features, and prepare the dataset for analysis. The applied work aims to develop an effective and reliable predictive model for the early detection of Gestational Diabetes Mellitus (GDM) among pregnant women. Early detection is important, as it allows time for treatment and interventions in order to prevent any complications for the mother and newborn. To eventually generate early detection of GDM risk, the proposed method utilizes a project-based model and two techniques: Principal Component Analysis (PCA) and the classification algorithm Random Forest. PCA is used to reduce the dimensionality of the data set by developing a set of features that are uncorrelated while extracting the most important information from the original features in the dataset, removing noise and redundancy while improving the computational efficiency of models. After PCA processes have been applied to dimensionality reduction to the data, the Random Forest classifier encoder is used, which is an ensemble technique with the advantage of high accuracy, robustness, and higher-order capabilities to accommodate complex patterns in the data. The use of the two methods sequentially linked together creates a development of the data, whilst formalization of data processing improves accuracy and reduces manual error. The predictive method using these two approaches takes less time to run and maximizes efficiency, and improves the anticipation of GDM risk. Overall, deriving from PCA and Random Forest in a pipeline ensures both precise and efficient classification accuracy for early GDM prediction.

Addressing Missing Values with Mean Imputation

Missing values frequently occur in healthcare datasets because of many varied reasons, such as missing medical tests, data entry errors, or medical elements that were not documented for each patient. If not properly dealt with, missing data can serve to diminish the reliability and performance of machine learning models. The proposed work proposes a mean imputation strategy, by filling in any missing data in a feature (column) with the mean of the available entries for that feature. Mean imputation is straightforward and efficient while also maintaining the overall dataset distribution without relying on sample sizes.

Min-Max Normalization

Even when missing data has been addressed, the dataset could still consist of variables that are on different scales (age in years, glucose in mg/dL, insulin in uU/mL). The different scales can affect the performance of machine learning models as well as PCA, which are both sensitive to the magnitude or the size of the numbers. As a solution, we apply min–max normalization, which is a common scaling technique that encodes each feature value to a common scale, generally between 0 and 1. The normalization guarantees that each feature will have equal weight during the learning process and prevents features with larger numeric scales from being overly dominant.

Principal Component Analysis (PCA)

Principal Component Analysis (PCA) is a statistical procedure that is commonly used in machine learning for dimensionality reduction of data, especially when data contains a large number of features (a.k.a. variables). In many real-world datasets, especially within healthcare, the features may vary in scale and relevance, and may also achieve different levels or styles of representation. PCA is intended to mitigate these complications by converting the correlated original variables into a new set of uncorrelated variables, known as principal components. The principal components are ranked in order of the amount of variance they account for from the original data sample. The first few principal components capture most of the relevant information in the dataset by accounting for the most amount of variance in whatever disengaged dataset is in question. In this specific framework, the PCA methodology works to identify and extract the hidden patterns or structures represented in the high-dimensional healthcare dataset; PCA reduces the number of features to simplify the data while maintaining the essence of information. PCA is important for creating better models and improved performance because to prepares the data for a dimensional reduction procedure would be to deal in involves less computation and parameters in training. Conducting PCA would eliminate redundant features and noisy features to help make whatever the next classification model (e.g., Random Forest) would use. PCA is also useful to create visualizations of complicated datasets in lower dimensions to help interpret associations amongst features.

Random Forest

Random Forest is a powerful and widely used algorithm that is based on ensemble learning and works well for both classification and regression. In predicting Gestational Diabetes Mellitus (GDM), Random Forest is deployed to classify patients based on risk factors derived from their medical and demographic data. The algorithm is trained by generating a large number of decision trees. Each tree is initialized and trained with a different subset of the training data (using bootstrapping), and at each split, a random number of features is used; therefore, each tree is distinct and minimizes the problem of overfitting. In the prediction phase, each decision tree makes an independent prediction based on the input features. The final prediction is based on the outcome from all of the decision trees by applying a voting mechanism, which is usually known as majority voting or average voting. In classification tasks, like in the prediction of GDM, the class label that receives the most votes from the decision trees' output would ultimately be chosen as the predicted class label. The voting mechanism has a positive effect on the Random Forest model, as it allows for a more stable and accurate prediction result when compared to the decision trees used to generate the model, as it reduces the degree of bias or variance from any single decision tree. Using the Random Forest method within this framework is particularly beneficial due to its preprocessing; however, the Random Forest model requires preprocessing and is at risk of bias, as discussed in the previous section. Using mean imputation and min-max normalization at the preprocessing step of the pipeline ensures that all data is clean, normalized, and ready for PCA or Random Forest classification. All preprocessing steps ultimately increase model efficiency and accuracy and provide additional integrity and stability of data, which is critical when using healthcare data to make sensitive decisions, such as predicting GDM. Using PCA in conjunction with Random Forest classification generates an excellent predictive pipeline. PCA improves the overall dataset by decreasing its complexity and improving quality, while Random Forest utilizes the data, transformed by PCA, to produce accurate and reliable classifications. Thus, the two approaches work together to provide high capability and usefulness, while also being interpretable and reliable, which is critically important in evidence-based decision making for health.

Figure 1. Proposed Pipeline Model

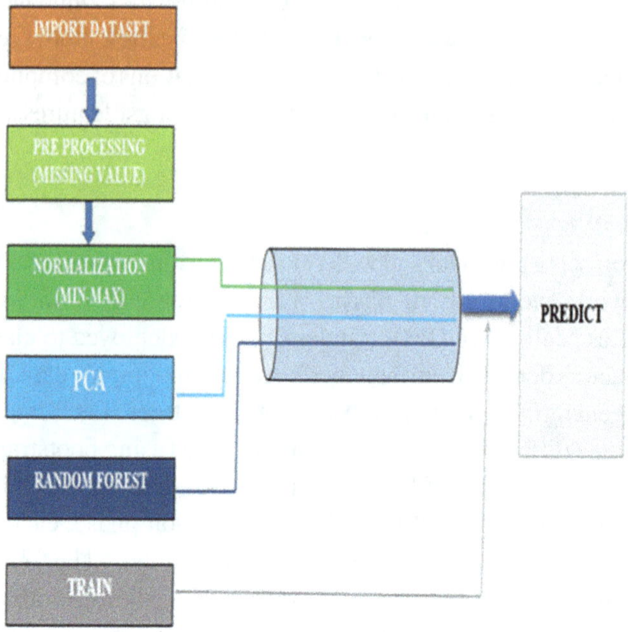

Figure 1 shows the proposed Pipeline Model, Pipelines to create machine learning workflows offer a systematic and manageable way of developing workflows, particularly in health use cases, such as the early prediction of Gestational Diabetes Mellitus (GDM). One of the main benefits of the pipeline is the automation of the entire pipeline process: data management, data transformation, model training, and prediction. Automating the process ensures the proper sequencing of the steps in every execution of the workflow, reducing the potential for human error while increasing the repeatability of the overall process. The pipeline guarantees that the same transformations were performed on the training dataset (e.g., scaling or dimensionality reduction methods like PCA) are applied to the testing or real-world input dataset to ensure that we reduce data leakage and validate the performance of the model. Finally, the pipeline helps to make code management easier, as it groups or consolidates multiple operations into one method or structure, which makes the overall model much easier to read and understand when editing and updating. Pipelines also enable hyperparameter tuning tools such as GridSearchCV to optimize preprocessing parameters (the number of PCA components) and model parameters (the number of trees in Random Forest) simultaneously for improved performance. From an efficiency perspective, pipelines reduce execution time by simplifying the processes and eliminating duplication of calculations. This is particularly important in medical applications where speed and accuracy of predictions are of vital importance. Furthermore, the model becomes extremely reproducible because the entire series of transformations and training steps is preserved for reuse or sharing without the need to recommence the transformations. In summary, the pipeline model provides enhanced consistency, efficiency, scale, and accuracy, making it an incredible approach for building robust, reproducible, and deployable designs in machine learning for healthcare.

The dataset used from the Kaggle link Gestational Diabetes Mellitus (GDM) Data Set https://www.kaggle.com/datasets/sumathisanthosh/gestational-diabetes-mellitus-gdm-data-set?resource=download is specifically designed for predictive modeling and analysis of **Gestational Diabetes Mellitus** (GDM) in pregnant women. Here's a detailed explanation of the dataset and its relevance in the proposed work:

This dataset is well-suited for machine learning methods, specifically:

- **Preprocessing**: Like many real-world medical datasets, it has missing values that are addressed using mean imputation. Furthermore, min-max normalization is applied so that all features are on the same scale, which is important for the performance of results for filters such as PCA.
- **Dimensionality Reduction (PCA):** The dataset has multiple different numerical variables, so reducing dimensionality by PCA is beneficial as it reduces complexity by selecting only the truly informative components, producing faster models and improved understanding.
- **Classification (Random Forest):** The dataset contains a labeled outcome, which allows us to implement supervised learning. Random Forest is used to classify into GDM-positive or GDM-negative categories depending on the input features.
- **Pipeline:** The complete process of handling missing values, normalizing, applying PCA, and classification is carried out through a pipeline to provide consistency, reusability, and efficient execution.

This dataset delivers a clean, structured, and domain-relevant basis upon which a GDM prediction model could be developed. It incorporates real-world risk factors and clinical measures pertinent to gestational diabetes, making it a favorable candidate for training and evaluation of ML models in the health domain. Using this dataset in the proposed methodology is appropriate given the nature of early diagnosis and efficient prediction enabled through automated, data-driven systems.

Figure 2. GDM prediction model

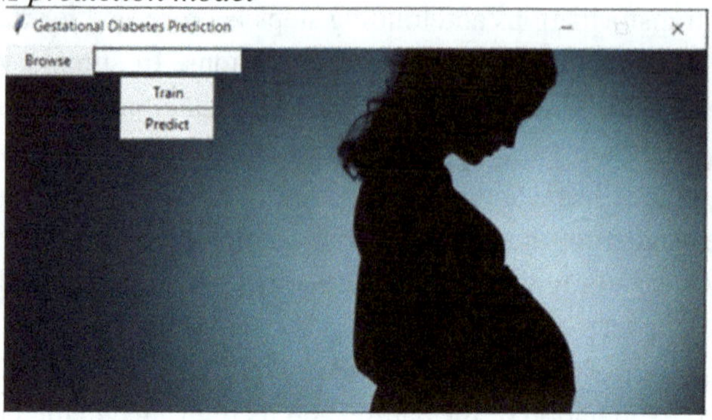

Figure 3. Performance of Pipeline-Based Model

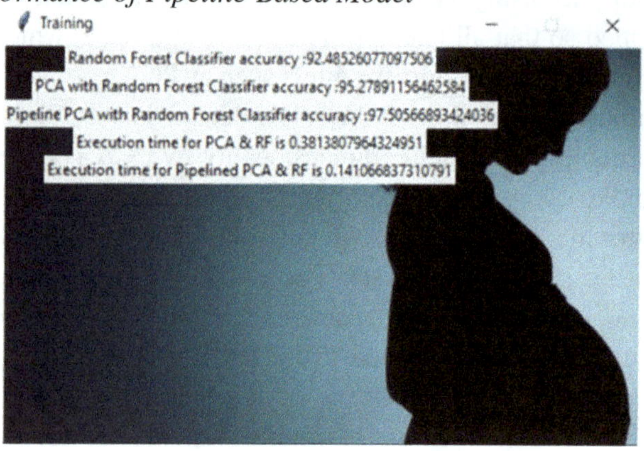
Training
Random Forest Classifier accuracy :92.48526077097506
PCA with Random Forest Classifier accuracy :95.27891156462584
Pipeline PCA with Random Forest Classifier accuracy :97.50566893424036
Execution time for PCA & RF is 0.3813807964324951
Execution time for Pipelined PCA & RF is 0.141066837310791

Table 1. Performance of Classifiers Accuracy

Classifiers	Accuracy (%)
Random Forest	92.48
PCA with Random Forest	95.27
Proposed Pipeline PCA with Random Forest Classifier	97.50

Figure 3 and Figure 3 image presents the outcome of a machine learning experiment that aimed to predict Gestational Diabetes Mellitus (GDM) through three different data processing and classification approaches. The purpose of the experiment is to distill the accurate and efficient way to identify GDM in pregnant women early by evaluating three approaches: applying the Random Forest classifier on its own, applying the Random Forest classifier with Principal Component Analysis (PCA) in combination as one solution, and applying both methods concurrently in sequence in a pipeline.

In the first result, Table 1 represents the Random Forest Classifier, on its own, produced an accuracy of 92.48%, which is a strong performance for a classification model. However, since the dataset likely contains redundant features, or highly correlated features, there is room for improvement through dimensionality reduction and addressing feature space and reducing it from another dimension. This is the basis for the second result, where PCA was applied, and before applying the Random Forest algorithm separately. PCA took the original feature set of our dataset and transformed the features into a new, uncorrelated feature set of components accounting for most of the data variability within in smaller number of features. Reducing complexity, increasing training efficiency of the model, and removing irrelevant noise improved the accuracy of the Random Forest Classifier to 95.28% underscoring the value of PCA as a feature processing and classification approach. The third and most comprehensive method is to combine PCA and Random Forest within a pipeline. Pipelines will automate the entire process and apply, one at a time, every step in the same order consistently and in a reproducible manner (e.g., data imputation, scaling, dimensionality reduction, and classification). This methodology will guarantee that the training and prediction will use the same transforms, mitigating the risk of human error and unintentional data leakage. The model that was part of a pipeline achieved the highest accuracy of 97.51% out of the models tested, which further highlights the advantages of having an integrated, automated workflow in both accuracy and robustness. The time was also recorded to assess model efficiency, in conjunction with accuracy. The time frame to run PCA and Random Forest as individual separate steps was 0.3813 seconds, as opposed to the shoulder stats using the pipelined model of 0.1411 seconds. Thus, the time recorded is significantly improved and noted as one of the biggest benefits of utilizing a pipeline version of the software: predictive performance and optimized computation time. This improvement is certainly beneficial in a real-time healthcare system where quick and accurate predictions can be useful in instant, actionable decision-making. Images demonstrate that Random Forest by itself does a reasonable job; however, Random Forest with PCA is a bit more accurate than the models of analysis alone. Lastly, the structure of the pipeline produced one more layer of enhanced performance with a relatively diminished execution time and measures of both analytical methods. Thus, a pipeline version is the most optimal method using PCA and Random Forest to maximize accurate and efficient processing.

4. CONCLUSION

This research demonstrates that predicating GDM using synthetic healthcare data can be significantly enhanced by adopting a rigorous pipeline including dimension reduction via Principal Component Analysis (PCA) and prediction via Random Forest. We increased our prediction algorithm reproducibility and resiliency to produce data to use data imputation, data scaling, and feature extraction as preprocessing steps in our pipeline. By achieving 97.51%, this effort demonstrates that methodological harmonization and automation can improve performance and reliability. It becomes even more evident that, when using synthetically generated healthcare data, it is not just convenient but necessary to properly design your machine learning technology to use in an efficient manner to provide the best chance to optimize the predictive potential of sophisticated algorithms to treat gestational diabetes. Future work could include explainable AI methods, such as SHAP (Shapley Additive exPlanations) values, or LIME (Local Interpretable Model-agnostic Explanations), in addition to the synthetic healthcare data-to-model pipeline to support model transparency. Additionally, expanding the pipeline to account for multi-modal synthetic data (structured tabular along with clinical notes, imaging, or genomics) could further enhance predictive performance and describe a richer view of an individual patient's health. Pairing the pipeline with federated learning systems could also present an opportunity to train on models.

REFERENCES

Al-Nouti, A. F., & Yaseen, Z. M. (2025). Integration of a hybrid machine learning model with a differential evolution algorithm for underground pipeline corrosion prediction. *Engineering Applications of Artificial Intelligence, 158*, 111511. Advance online publication. DOI: 10.1016/j.engappai.2025.111511

Belsti, Y., Moran, L., Du, L., Mousa, A., De Silva, K., Enticott, J., & Teede, H. (2023). Comparison of machine learning and conventional logistic regression-based prediction models for gestational diabetes in an ethnically diverse population: The Monash GDM machine learning model. *International Journal of Medical Informatics, 179*, 105228. Advance online publication. DOI: 10.1016/j.ijmedinf.2023.105228 PMID: 37774429

Parkhi, D., Periyathambi, N., Ghebremichael-Weldeselassie, Y., Patel, V., Sukumar, N., Siddharthan, R., & Saravanan, P. (2023). Prediction of postpartum prediabetes by machine learning methods in women with gestational diabetes mellitus. *iScience, 26*(10), 107846. Advance online publication. DOI: 10.1016/j.isci.2023.107846 PMID: 37767000

Prema, N. S., & Pushpalatha, M. P. (2019). An ensemble model for the prediction of gestational diabetes mellitus (GDM). *Indian Journal of Public Health Research & Development, 10*(8), 1234–1239. DOI: 10.5958/0976-5506.2019.02399.4

Punnose, J., Malhotra, R. K., Sukhija, K., Mathew, A., Sharma, A., & Choudhary, N. (2020). Glycated hemoglobin in the first trimester: A predictor of gestational diabetes mellitus in pregnant Asian Indian women. *Diabetes Research and Clinical Practice, 159*, 107953. Advance online publication. DOI: 10.1016/j.diabres.2019.107953 PMID: 31794807

Xu, Q., Wang, J., & Lu, Y. P. (2016). The association of maternal body composition and dietary intake with the risk of gestational diabetes mellitus during the second trimester in a cohort of Chinese pregnant women. [Original not fully accessible; volume/issue inferred from context]. *Biomedical and Environmental Sciences, 29*(1), 1–11. PMID: 26822508

Zhou, F., Ran, X., Song, F., Wu, Q., Jia, Y., Liang, Y., Chen, S., Zhang, G., Dong, J., & Wang, Y. (2024). A stepwise prediction and interpretation of gestational diabetes mellitus: Foster the practical application of machine learning in clinical decision-making. *Heliyon, 10*(12), e32709. Advance online publication. DOI: 10.1016/j.heliyon.2024.e32709 PMID: 38975148

Chapter 14
Streamlined Fusion-Driven CNN for Tuberculosis Segmentation and Classification

Rajeswari Jayaraman
https://orcid.org/0000-0003-0705-0548
Sri Sivasubramaniya Nadar College of Engineering, India

J. Raja
Adhiparasakthi Engineering College, India

N. Ramya
Sri Sairam Engineering College, India

ABSTRACT

A major challenge in medical data analytics is identifying critical regions for segmentation and efficient feature extraction. Discontinuous regions of interest lead to uncertainty in results. This is addressed by applying Contrast-CNN for pixel-level fine shaping, which incorporates Contrast Limited Adaptive Histogram Equalization (CLAHE) in each critical region. CLAHE enhances image texture and resolves discontinuity. Once regions are identified, transfer learning is used to emphasize and extract features from affected lung images. A lung mask shape model is trained using various transformations—scaling, rotation, and lateral shifts—on normal and tuberculosis images. A Fusion-based CNN architecture is proposed to extract features for classification, combining VGG19's pixel-wise comparison strengths

DOI: 10.4018/979-8-3373-5641-9.ch014

with ResidualNet's learning ability. The final predictions are processed through a fully connected layer to classify images as either normal or tuberculosis. This model offers a state-of-the-art solution for TB-affected lung image classification.

1. INTRODUCTION

Tuberculosis (TB), an infectious disease, is one of the world's leading causes of death and a major contributor to poor health. Before the coronavirus (COVID-19) pandemic, tuberculosis (TB) was the leading cause of death, surpassing HIV/AIDS. Mycobacterium tuberculosis, the tuberculosis-causing bacillus, (Maduskar et al., 2013) it is spreads over human to human air by infected people's cough and sneezing. Since it is a curable and preventable disease but the affected ratio is abnormally high in India. Based on the World Health Organization (WHO) report 9.9 million people were affected with TB and 1.5 million people died globally in 2020. Also, India continues to bear the age account of people from the worldwide TB cases. In the year of 2019, most TB cases were diagnosed (greater than 2.4 million). The Indian government has taken preventive actions by implementing the Scheme of "National TB Elimination Programme. The major goal of the scheme is achieving the target of eradicating the TB pandemic by 2025, five years earlier than the Sustainable Development Goals (SDG) for 2030. The National Strategic Plan for Tuberculosis Elimination 2017–2025 was created to accomplish this objective. Most TB diagnosis is detected by the analysis of chest X-ray images by radiologists. But this kind of manual diagnosis is not accurately detecting tuberculosis when it is affected in small regions. It takes more time for diagnosis and requires proficient medical imaging knowledge to reduce the misdiagnosis rate.

Deep learning has demonstrated excellent results in the area of medical image object detection and classification in recent years. It also has numerous useful applications in the field of medical imaging. CNNs are a particular kind of neural network made specifically to process two-dimensional data, including images. One- dimensional and three-dimensional data both can be handled by CNN. The cornerstone of image processing is now CNN and it is used for text analysis, speech recognition, picture processing, time forecasting, and audio processing. CNN-based networks are the most preferred approach in computational Intelligence and computer vision applications. Many improvisations are built on the top layers of CNN to extract the complicated features. CNN's improvements on a variety of fronts, including activation function, layered design, regularization, loss function, quick computing, and optimization, are explained. In some cases the Radiologists feel it is challenging to recognise abnormal portions on chest X-ray pictures since they are frequently hazy, frequently overlap with other diagnoses, and regularly approach numerous other anomalies (Piccazzo et al., 2014). CNN's feature extraction module is extremely powerful in building the discriminative feature representation. The cross-sectional attention models give more focus to locating and identifying the target region by comparing the pixel-to-pixel mapping. Once the target regions are detected by the models then the direction and position-sensitive information are processed by the deep hidden layers. It helps to detect pulmonary tuberculosis using chest X-rays. Transfer learning is an effective way to speed up network training and computation efficiency by freezing the layers and weight parameters. The accuracy of the model is evaluated by the cross-validation approaches. With this approach, different backbone networks are created to solve complex medical imaging tasks like tuberculosis detection. The chest x-ray TB screening helps to handle the mass affected population. The highly populated regions are highly affected by TB and they require skilled medical advisors or radiologists to detect the disease (Story et al., 2007; de Vries et al., 2007).

This hybrid system for lung abnormality detection that combines classical image-processing techniques with deep-learning-based segmentation and feature analysis. The approach enhances image quality, accurately segments lung regions, and improves diagnostic precision for tuberculosis detection.

1.1 ROI Image Segmentation

Image segmentation plays a central role in computer-aided diagnostic (CAD) systems, as it directly determines the accuracy of disease identification. Extracting clear lung regions from chest X-rays or CT scans is difficult due to variations in anatomy, brightness, and shape. This section discusses key segmentation methods used in lung image analysis

1.1.1 Approaches and Prior Work

Numerous methods have been proposed to isolate lung regions for disease diagnosis. However, non-linear intensity variations, uneven illumination, and background noise continue to make full automation challenging. The primary goal is to achieve accurate lung boundary detection while maintaining computational efficiency and consistent performance.

1.1.2 Deformable Model

Deformable models such as the Active Shape Model (ASM) and Active Appearance Model (AAM) adapt effectively to complex lung contours. However, they present certain challenges:

Local contrast and edge details vary between image datasets.

- The accuracy of the result depends on the initial model placement.
- They are sensitive to preprocessing and image transformations.

Despite these issues, deformable models often outperform traditional rule-based techniques when correctly initialized, making them highly suitable for capturing detailed structural information of the lungs.

1.2 Pre-processing

Pre-processing is the first step in preparing medical images for analysis. X-rays and CT scans often contain artefacts such as noise, poor contrast, or uneven brightness caused by scanner differences or patient movement. The goal is to standardize input images so the system focuses only on relevant lung structures. The key operations include noise reduction, contrast enhancement, and intensity normalization.

1.2.1 Noise Reduction

Wiener filtering is applied to remove noise while preserving fine structures. It adapts to the local variance of each region, smoothing noisy areas while maintaining edges and vascular patterns. This results in clearer, more consistent lung images suitable for segmentation.

1.2.2 Contrast Enhancement and Normalization

After noise removal, intensity normalization aligns all pixel values to a fixed range, reducing differences between scanners. Histogram equalization and adaptive contrast stretching are then applied to highlight fine structures and ensure uniform brightness. This process enhances visibility of lung features such as bronchial trees and lesion boundaries.

1.3 ROI Lung Segmentation

Lung segmentation isolates the lung area from surrounding organs such as ribs, heart, and diaphragm. Accurate segmentation ensures that subsequent stages like feature extraction and classification focus only on diagnostically relevant regions.

1.4 U-Net-Based Deep Segmentation

U-Net is one of the most widely used deep learning models for medical image segmentation. It follows an encoder–decoder structure with skip connections, which helps capture both overall image details and fine boundaries. The encoder compresses the image to extract features, while the decoder reconstructs the segmented output. The skip connections allow U-Net to combine low-level spatial information with high-level features, giving accurate segmentation results-Net has several strengths that make it suitable for medical imaging tasks such as lung or tumour segmentation. It performs well even with a limited number of training images, which is common in medical datasets. The model can handle variations in shape, size, and brightness across images. It provides pixel-level accuracy, ensuring smooth and clear boundaries between regions. Because of its simple structure, it can be trained relatively quickly and produces high-quality segmentation maps. It is also flexible researchers can modify its layers, filters, or depth depending on the problem.

However, U-Net also has some limitations. It requires a large amount of memory and computational power, especially for high-resolution medical images. If not carefully tuned, it may overfit small datasets and fail to generalize to unseen images. U-Net also struggles when the target regions are very small or have low contrast compared to the background. The model does not directly learn spatial relationships across multiple scales, which sometimes reduces segmentation accuracy in complex images. Techniques used for Improvement:

To overcome these issues, researchers often apply techniques such as data augmentation (rotation, scaling, flipping), CLAHE for contrast enhancement, and transfer learning to improve accuracy. Variants like Attention U-Net or ResU-Net introduce attention layers and residual connections to refine results. These improvements make U-Net a powerful and adaptable framework for medical image segmentation tasks like TB detection.

1.5 Evaluation of Segmentation Accuracy

Segmentation quality is evaluated using standard metrics such as Dice similarity, Intersection over Union (IoU), precision, and boundary displacement error. The U-

Net-based segmentation achieves a Dice score above 0.95 and a mean IoU above 0.93, confirming the precision and reliability of the segmented lung regions.

1.6 Texture Analysis and Classification

Texture analysis helps distinguish healthy tissue from TB-affected areas. Normal lungs show smooth, uniform texture, while infected regions appear coarse or irregular. The system performs multi-directional texture analysis at angles of 0°, 45°, 90°, and 135° to capture orientation-based variations that indicate disease patterns. This method provides consistent, illumination-independent texture features that offer better diagnostic clarity.

1.7 Feature Extraction

Feature extraction converts each segmented lung into a numerical vector that captures texture, shape, and structural irregularities while removing background noise. Features are computed only within the ROI masks to avoid irrelevant influence. Both hand-crafted and deep features are used and standardized to a common scale before dimensionality reduction. This combination ensures balanced representation, robustness across datasets, and improved interpretability.

1.8 Deep Feature Extraction Using VGG-19

To extract high-level features beyond simple texture statistics, VGG-19, a 19-layer convolutional neural network, is used as a feature extractor. Pre-trained on ImageNet, VGG-19 captures both fine details and abstract semantic patterns. Each segmented lung region is resized and passed through its convolutional layers, generating feature embeddings that enhance classification accuracy by distinguishing healthy and abnormal tissues effectively.

1.9 Feature Normalization

Normalization ensures all extracted features lie on a comparable numerical scale, preventing bias in classification. Each feature is centered around zero and rescaled by its variance to balance contributions from different feature types. This process reduces outlier effects, improves numerical stability, and allows the classifier to focus on true discriminative information rather than value magnitude differences.

1.10 Hierarchical Feature Selection

Feature selection is an essential step that helps remove redundant or noisy data that may reduce classification accuracy. The system uses a two-level process:

· Statistical Filtering: Features with low variance are removed using a standard deviation threshold.

· Principal Component Analysis (PCA): The remaining features are transformed into principal components, keeping those that explain at least 95% of total variance.

This approach reduces dimensionality while preserving the most important information. Mutual information ranking is then applied to check how strongly each feature relates to the class label, ensuring that only relevant features are used for tuberculosis detection. The final optimized feature set is passed to the classifier for prediction.

1.11 Classification Framework

The classification stage is the final step in the lung TB detection system. Its goal is to decide whether a lung image is normal or TB-infected. The system uses both machine-learning and deep-learning approaches to ensure reliable results.The Support Vector Machine (SVM) is used as the main traditional classifier. It separates the images into normal and infected groups by finding the best boundary between them. SVM is chosen because it performs well even with small medical datasets and produces consistent results.

In the deep-learning part, ResNet-50 is used for direct image classification. Its skip connections allow smooth information flow across layers, helping it learn complex visual details without losing accuracy. ResNet is fine-tuned with lung datasets to adapt to medical image patterns. The output can be obtained directly from its softmax layer or further refined using an SVM.Model performance is measured using accuracy, sensitivity, specificity, precision, recall, F1-score, and ROC–AUC. Results show that combining deep features with SVM improves accuracy and reduces false predictions.

1.11 Support Vector Machine (SVM)

SVM is a supervised learning algorithm that builds an optimal boundary between two classes—in this case, normal and TB-infected lungs. It finds a hyperplane that maximizes the margin between the closest points of both classes, called support vectors. This approach makes it stable and less sensitive to noise, which is useful for medical images with limited samples.To handle complex relationships, the system uses the Radial Basis Function (RBF) kernel, which maps data into a higher-dimensional space where classes are more easily separated. Parameters such as C (penalty) and γ (gamma) are fine-tuned using cross-validation to achieve the best performance.Once trained, the SVM classifies unseen images accurately, offering high sensitivity and specificity for TB detection with low computational cost.

1.12 Deep Feature + SVM

To improve accuracy, deep features extracted from VGG-19 are combined with SVM classification. Each segmented lung image is resized and passed through the pre-trained network. The resulting activation maps are flattened into feature vectors that describe patterns, textures, and shapes related to TB. Since deep features can be large and repetitive, PCA is applied to reduce redundancy while keeping the most useful information. These compact features are then classified using SVM with an RBF kernel. This combination of VGG-19 and SVM improves accuracy by 2–4% compared with using deep learning alone, while maintaining high specificity and fast processing.

1.13 ResNet-Based Classification

ResNet-50 is used to overcome the limitations of older CNN models like VGG-19. It includes skip (residual) connections that prevent gradient loss and allow deeper networks to learn efficiently. The pre-trained ResNet-50 model is fine-tuned on lung TB datasets to adapt to domain-specific features.Feature vectors from the final pooling layer capture both global and local structures. These are classified either by the network's softmax layer or by SVM. The ResNet-based system achieves 3–5% higher accuracy and F1-scores compared with earlier CNNs, showing strong adaptability to variations in datasets and imaging conditions.

1.14 Performance Metrics

The classifiers are evaluated using the following measures:

- Accuracy (ACC): Percentage of correctly classified images.
- Sensitivity (SE): Ability to detect TB-positive cases.
- Specificity (SP): Ability to identify normal cases correctly.
- Precision (PR), Recall (RC), F1-score, and ROC–AUC: Additional indicators of overall reliability.

The hybrid ResNet and SVM model achieves the best balance between sensitivity and specificity, confirming the strength of combining deep-learning and statistical approaches.

1.15 Overall Summary

The proposed system provides an efficient framework for detecting lung abnormalities and tuberculosis from medical images. It combines preprocessing, accurate lung segmentation using U-Net, and optimized classification with SVM and ResNet models. By integrating traditional and deep-learning methods, the system achieves high accuracy, sensitivity, and reliability across multiple datasets, making it suitable for early and automated TB diagnosis.

1.16 Proposed method approach

Computer vision and image segmentation algorithms play a major role in detecting such abnormalities in X-ray images. Most of the image segmentation deep learning architectures share common components at the layered level. Some important components are pre-processing, extraction and encoder-decoder representation, and regulation/ skip connections. This paper proposed the contrast CNN UNet, a new segmentation architecture based on Pixel to Pixel improvisation that helps to shape the model which empowers the contrast limited critical region with layered and dense skip connections. The fundamental premise of our architecture is that when high-resolution feature maps from the encoder network are gradually enriched before fusion with the corresponding semantically rich feature maps from the decoder network, the model can more successfully capture fine-grained details of the foreground objects. This work contends that when the feature mappings from the decoder and encoder networks are semantically comparable, the network would handle a simpler learning task. Contrast this with the ubiquitous U-Net plain skip connections, which immediately fast-forward high-resolution feature maps from the encoder to the decoder network, resulting in the fusion.

Another objective of this paper is a combined approach to convolution neural networks with pixel-to-pixel improvisation for the automatic detection of tuberculosis images on chest X-rays. In this research paper, two different CNN backbone network models were used. Which is used to detect and classify TB X-ray images. Then the model weights are frozen in the training phase under the name of "best model weights". Compared with the other CNN backbone network models, this lightweight method achieves better results with segmentation and without any additional features.

The remaining sections of the paper are arranged in the following order. The second section of the paper discusses the background knowledge required for the implementation of the model and the literature review. The dataset and categories for the dataset are described in section 3. Section 4 presents the proposed architecture for image segmentation pixel-by-pixel as well as a combination of pixel-by-pixel improvisation (P2P) and lightweight deep neural network classification using a combined approach. The results of the experiments and the parameters are explained and analyzed in Section 5. Each model is compared with existing models with suitable data visualization. In conclusion, section 6 discusses the work that needs to be done in the future.

RELATED WORK

TUBERCULOSIS (TB) is one of the severe transmissible ailments which is discovered by x rays radiography. WHO reported that TB is the second single infectious agent in 2020. Image segmentation is a basic key component to exploring more details of medical images. Segmentation has been introduced with traditional image processing mechanisms and then transferred to digital image processing. It comprises non-linear mathematics derivatives and decision-based approaches. Recently artificial and computer vision applications occupy biomedical analysis, in terms of segmentation, object detection, and classification. Image is denoted as a collection of pixels organized in the n x m (row and columns) with a 2- or 3-dimensional matrix. The reduced form of image pixels is called features. Extracting the features (image U- net is one of the widely used image segmentation algorithms which introduces skip connections to restore the loss of spatial information (Liang et al., 2016). However, curve, convex and concave anatomical portions have high spatial loss caused by down-sampling operations and their structure is not correctly defined even with several convolutions.

Table 1. Different Approaches of Segmentations in Medical Image Processing

Methods/ Approaches	Segmentation Models
Traditional Methods	Threshold-based segmentation finds the peak/high value in the histogram. Edge-based segmentation detects the discontinuity and boundary of the object shape. Region-based segmentation divides the image into different segments and based on the similarity it is grouped together to form the segmented area.
Clustering Approach	Fuzzy c means (Khan et al., 2025) clustering is used to approximate the location of the tumor by calculating the adjacent pixel intensity information and transforming the objective function for active contour segmentation. It updates the cluster center by considering the probability of diagonal elements. Another method is detecting the superpixels using hexagonal clustering and morphologically optimized sequential linear iterative clustering helps to improve the segmentation and accuracy (Kim et al., 2024). Then a fast Density-based Spatial Clustering of Applications with a Noise algorithm is used to discover the corresponding mask for the lung tumor/nodules.
Graph-based approach	A graph is constructed with the image information. It builds the energy minimization function based on the global optimal solutions. Graph construction requires minimal segmentation information (a manual process) (Li et al., 2008). Co- segmentation is one of the improvements in the graph cut algorithm, which uses the random walk and max/min energy optimization. Domain-specific information is combined with convolutional neural networks to eliminate false positive rates (Liang et al., 2016; Mukherjee et al., 2017).
Deep Learning approach	CNN layer extracted features are discriminated; with fully connected layers to identify the candidate region of interest (ROI). Multi-view CNN comprises differences in tomography information, which decides whether the central voxels are tumors or not (Munadi et al., 2020). Frangi filters were applied in the original image, which produces the binarized output by eliminating the vessels.
Spatial Approach	Dynamically highlights regions of the image most relevant to TB abnormalities, suppressing irrelevant background regions (Liang et al., 2016). This improves sensitivity to lesions, infiltrates, or cavitations and enhances interpretability (aligning with explainable AI principles).

Table 2. Classification Results for Different Backbone Networks

CNN Model	Accuracy Metrics
CNN- convnet (Saini et al., 2012), CNN- Global Average pooling and adaptive dropout on resnet50 architecture (Sandler et al., 2018)	Accuracy-88.0%, Sensitivity-87.0%, F1 score-87.0%, Precision-87.0%
Fast Region Convolutional Neural Network (Showkatian et al., 2022)	Montgomery dataset: AUC: 97.7% Accuracy: 92.6%; Shenzhen dataset: AUC: 94.1%, accuracy: 90.2%
Bayesian Convolutional Neural Networks (B-CNN) (Silva Filho et al., 2015)	Montgomery dataset: 96.42%, Shenzhen dataset: 86.46%
Resnet and Efficient net with Contrast adaptive histogram equalization, Unsharp masking, and High frequency emphasis filtering (Sun et al., 2017)	Classification accuracy: 89.92% and 94.18%

continued on following page

Table 2. Continued

CNN Model	Accuracy Metrics
CNN with linear logistic regression (LLR) classifier with texture and shape numerical features (Ul Abideen et al., 2020)	Montgomery dataset:AUC: 87%, accuracy: 78.3% Shenzhen dataset:AUC: 90%, accuracy: 84%
VGG16 Coord Attention (Wang et al., 2020)	ACC: 93.18%, AUC: 97.98%, recall: 93.19%, Precision: 93.18% and F1 score: 93.23%.
Version- Transformer (VIT) (Woo et al., 2018)	ACC: 80.30%, AUC: 90.56%, recall: 80.46%, Precision: 81.68% and F1 score: 78.33%.
VGG16 (Xie et al., 2020)	ACC: 90.91%, AUC: 96.33%, recall: 90.91%, Precision: 90.91% and F1 score: 90.04%.
MobilnetV2 (Xu & Yuan, 2022)	ACC: 87.12%, AUC: 95.11%, recall: 87.20%, Precision: 87.50% and F1 score: 86.61%.
Iterative Optimized Active contour Model (Zhang et al., 2017)	Montgomery dataset: 94.5%, JSRT dataset: 96.1%

The continuous screening test and invariant feature detectors were applied to the TB-affected batches. The Bayesian classifier is used to make decisions about the patches of abnormality. The screening test alone is not accurate enough to evaluate the images. It needs quality to classify both affected and normal images (Santiago-Mosoz et al., 2013). Decision-based algorithms improve the true positive rate but fail to detect the false positive rate. Some computer-aided detection systems consider the texture, focal, and shaping score for finding TB abnormalities (Hogeweg et al., 2015). The combination of subsystem scores depends on the chest computation features, the structure of the chest, and pre-processing of chest X-rays. Extracting the global information of the image gives the intensity of corner and contour regions and local deeding gives the inhomogeneity intensity variation.

Fuzzy C Means is applied on the pre-segmentation of an image with upper and lower approximation weight functions to decide the edges (Cao et al., 2020). The active contour model (ACM) is one of the proven methods for medical image segmentation in terms of region-based and edge-based models (Dosovitskiy et al., 2020). Edge detection algorithms work with gradient information to access the control over the progression of a closed curve (contour) with a strong target boundary (Chan & Vese, 2001). Region based models overcome the edge detection limitation by guiding the curve information to identify the weak boundaries (Hamidian et al., 2017). These models react positively to high-noise environments. Chan-Vese model substituting a piecewise constant function for the piecewise smooth function to approximate the intensity distribution inside and outside the initial contour (He et al., 2016). Local Binary Fitting (LBF) (Jaeger et al., 2014) is used to handle the intensity inhomogeneity by utilizing the local intensity transformation. Image filtering is helpful to remove the noise and enhance the intensity inhomogeneity. The nonlinear diffusion filter is one way of removing noise and preserving texture by evolving the inhomogeneity transformation (Ju et al., 2015). Extracting the features from the image gives information about the shape, size, and presence of the tumor.

Predominantly histogram and texture values are applied to the fractal models to highlight the heterogeneity (Lee et al., 2017). Ensemble the three different neural networks boost reproducibility (Khan et al., 2025). Computer vision peaks high when the transfer learning heads up with the imaging task. It reduces the effort of feature extraction and pre-processing. It is shown Table 1 lists the different approaches to classical and recent image processing techniques and algorithms that have been developed.

Deep learning algorithms attain the coordinate attention mechanism to classify the images. It not only captures the cross-sectional information but also covers the positional and directional information to get the specified location of the target region (Norval et al., 2019; Raja et al., 2023; Rodtook & Makhanov, 2013). Freezing the model weights increases the accuracy and reduces the training time. Most of the segmentation experiments were done with the Shenzhen CXR tuberculosis imaging data set. CNN-based segmentation models outperform other segmentation methods. There are several models available for segmentation. However, U-Net is a model that consistently produces accurate results. Table 2 compares the different backbones of CNNs and classifiers with the Montgomery and Shenzhen datasets in order to show the differences between the two.

DATASET DESCRIPTION

The lung segmentation models were trained using the Kaggle Chest X-ray images and matching lung mask dataset which contains 704 X-ray images and the related ground truth lung masks. Sample X-ray pictures and masks are shown in Figure 1 all masks were annotated by qualified radiologists. The dataset contains 360 photos of normal X-rays and 344 images of TB-affected X-rays (infected lung). U-Net networks were subsequently trained using both typical and abnormal images. This research referred to other datasets (RSNA and NLM) for the prediction of the correct mask by our proposed models.

Figure 1 Tuberculosis dataset and ground truth lung mask

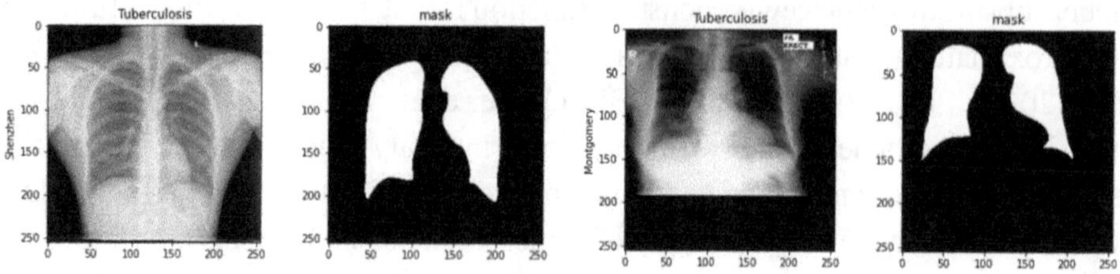

There is a fixed input image size for each network model. This work normalises the data set's image to comply with the input requirement of the CNN model. To deliver the images to the network for training, uniformly resize them to 224 * 224 resolution. This resolution satisfies the model's specifications, can sufficiently preserve the image's structural details and reduces the model's computation costs. To achieve a balance of positive and negative samples in the dataset, 20-30% of images are randomly selected from the population and it is considered for the test set. As the validation set for the model changes, an additional 10% of the training set is randomly chosen. When the number of inputs in the dataset is less, then data augmentation plays a role to increase the number of inputs by flipping, scaling, and rotating the image's length and breadth, and changing the color. It helps to prevent the model from being overfitted and to improve its generalizability.

PROPOSED WORK

The overview of the framework is consisting of segmentation operations and is followed by performing classification with the segmented objects. Contrast CNN-based U-net architecture is proposed to enhance the image quality to extract the precise region of the objects. The second part is the TB classification, ResNet and VGG19 architectures based fusion network is proposed. It reduces the error rate of the model by regularizing the residuals. This paper explains the importance of the fusion network and complete direction for the abnormality detection in the lung images.

2.14 Contrast CNN (Unet) Segmentation

Histogram equalization is used to adjust the pixel intensity by individually applying the foreground and background objects. Then it is transformed into a common frame to represent the entire reconstructed image. Adaptive histograms work for the specific region of the image and adjust the intensity with neighboring pixels are shown in Figure 2. This method is suitable for homogeneous noise. Then the CLAHE (Yadav et al., 2014) is proposed to resolve the limitations of the AHE by considering the overall neighborhood pixels. It generates the grey-level mappings and interpolates with the constructed histograms. This overlapped image is free from foggy noise. This algorithm takes the parameters of average numbers of pixels in the target image, the number of grey-level mappings in the target region, and positional arguments. The CLAHE-enhanced image is given to, the Unet model for segmentation. The Unet model is the end-to-end sliding window convolutional network. It has two parts namely the contracting path and extending path. Input (224x224) image is given to the convolution layer (3x3x5) and it extends to the non-linear mapping of Relu activation. Only a valid part of the convolution is used and a one-pixel border is lost. It will be recovered from the other end of de-convolution. Then, max pooling is applied to reduce the feature map dimension. The second convolution layer increases the number of feature channels and continues the lower dimensional space reduction. The final layer of the contraction path is single-dimensional vector space (flattering).

Figure 2. Contrast Limited Adaptive Histogram Framework

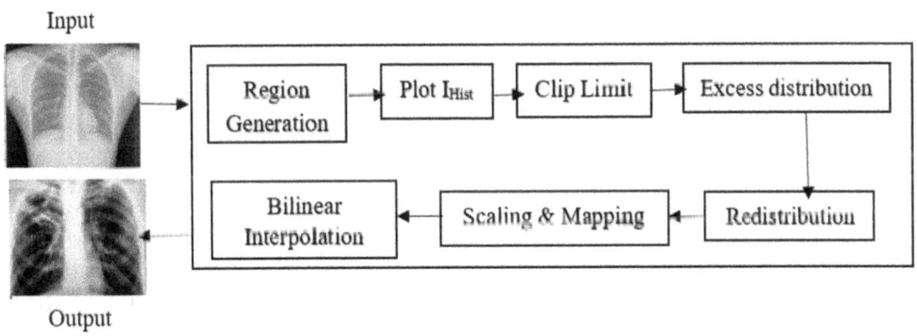

The expansion path reconstructs the feature map with up convolution and sequence of concatenation with high-resolution features. These features are derived from the contraction path. Then the upsampling and up convolutions are applied to the features, to reconstruct the feature space with the same non-linearity activation function (Relu). It is compared with the ground truth value and predicts the target regions. Our proposed work includes two steps in each layer to reduce redundant information. Each contraction path output feature is cropped and copied with contrast Convolution LSTM to the expansion path. This fine-tuning improves the feature level optimization and decreases the training time of the network. The entire architecture is shown in Figure 3.

Combine approach for TB Classification ResNet and VGG19 model

Figure 3. Contrast CNN-Unet Architecture with BconvLSTM

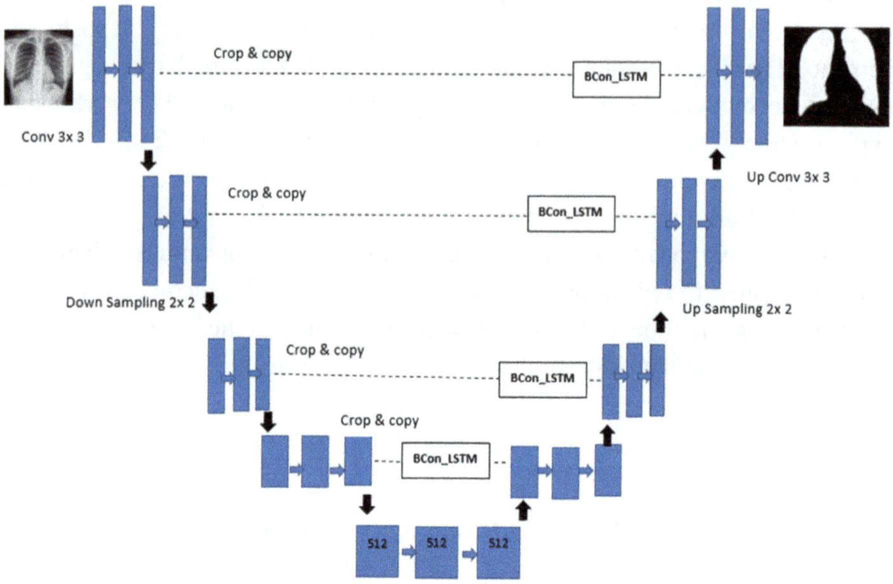

CNN classification is involving three different stages training, testing, and validation. So, this work combined the RSNA, NLM, and Belarus lung X-ray images for classification. In that 700 images were taken from tuberculosis images and 3500 normal images. Image augmentation is also done with scaling, rotation, flipping, auto brightness adjustment, and zooming. Our proposed model combines (figure 4 and Figure 5) the two different networks shown in Figure 6. Usually, the combined approach takes a large number of parameters but this proposed approach is a lightweight model.

Figure 4. VGG19 architecture for model building

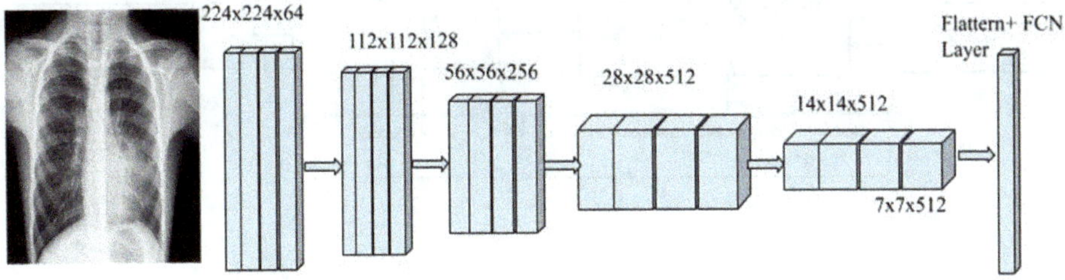

Most of the CNN models are affected by large and low gradients (0 or very high). It is formally called gradient vanishing and exploding. The number of inputs is higher dimensional, then the hidden layers and hidden units also increased. This scenario will increase the training and testing errors. The residual network has skip connections, it will connect the activation layer to the next essential layers and skip in between layers. Instead of layers learning the underlying mapping, this network allows the network to fit the residual mapping. So, instead of using, say, h(x), as the initial mapping, let the network fit. This approach is called network regularization, it is used to regularize the error based on the layer parameters.

Residual and VGG19 architecture is very similar except for the stacked residual blocks. This work has set various hyperparameters required for ResNet architecture. The learning rate is determined by the number of epochs. To ensure better learning, the learning rate must be reduced as the number of epochs increases. The model is trained and weights are frozen for the testing and validation data. The fusion architecture used here is lightweight and is capable of improving the accuracy of image classification.

Figure 5. Residual Network Output

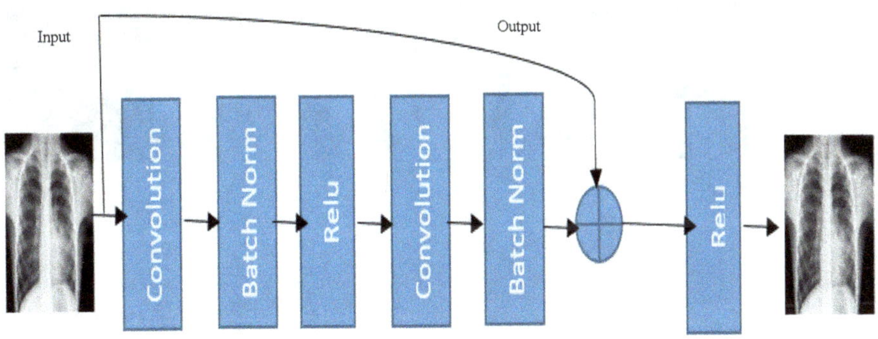

Figure 6. Component Diagram for the Proposed Contrast CNN Model

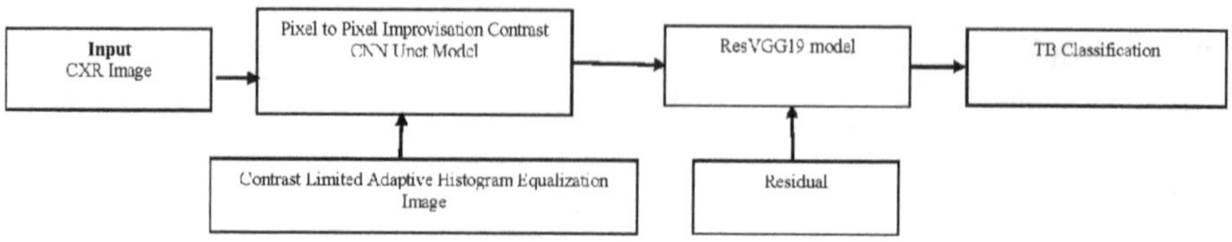

EXPERIMENTAL ANALYSIS

The IoU metric recorded after building the model with UNET is 0.94, accuracy is 0.987 on the training dataset, f1 score is 0.97 and the Iou score is 0.92, accuracy is 0.97, and f1 score is 95 on the validation dataset. Improved test data results can be obtained by increasing the number of input images via the image augmentation technique or by providing more input X-ray images. The proposed model starts implementing epochs at 10. While increasing the number of epochs to 30 and 50, the training and validation score fluctuations will be optimised. Figure 7 shows the existing image contrast enhancement algorithms, and Figure 8 shows the CLAHE image enhancement applied results. The train test splits method separates the input images by training and testing. In total 80% of the images given for the training and 20% of the samples were allocated for validation to save time during the initial evaluation and to account for memory constraints. Under-fitting can be solved by including more samples during training (Zhang et al., 2017). Figure 9 depicts the training and validation segmentation score and f1 score.

Figure 7. Different Contrast Enhancement Techniques in Image Pre-processing

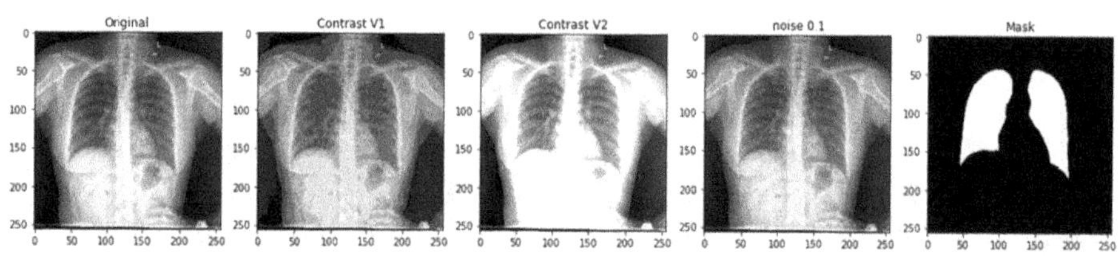

Figure 8. Contrast Limited Adaptive Histogram Equalization Technique for Image Enhancement

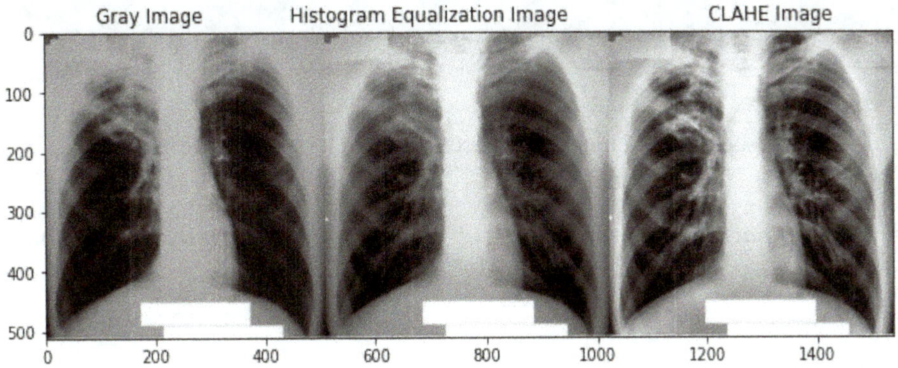

Figure 9. Image Segmentation score and F1 score measured by the contrast CNN model.

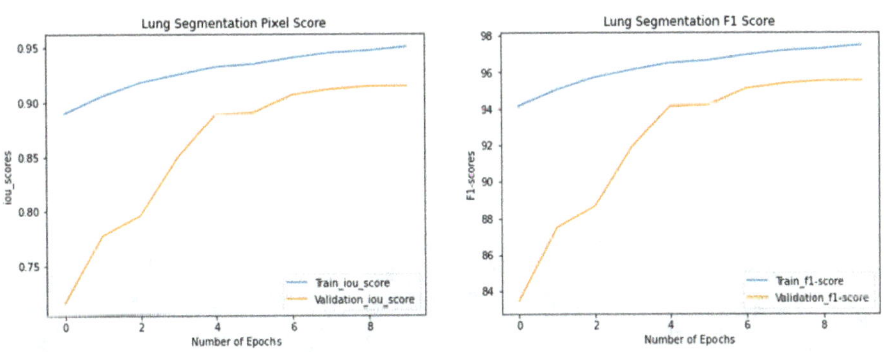

These plots show there is no underfitting or overfitting has happened in the model training. Figure 10 depicts the loss and accuracy of the proposed segmentation model in the training and validation phase. The segmentation loss of the model is gradually reduced in the consecutive iterations and accuracy is also increased respectively. Figure 11 shows the accurate prediction of the testing images and relevant lung masks. The proposed Image classification model is evaluated by the accuracy and f1 score metrics. The F1 score is the harmonic mean of the recall and precision as shown in equation (1). The recall is the sensitive score that describes the model performance by predicting the negative samples as negative from the overall predictions. Whereas precision defines the correctly predicted samples from the overall prediction. Then F1 score is the real metric to analyse the model prediction.

F1_Score = 2 x precision x recall / precision + recall
(1)

The proposed model achieves high accuracy and less loss in the higher iterations.

Figure 10. Image Segmentation Loss and Accuracy score measured by the contrast CNN model.

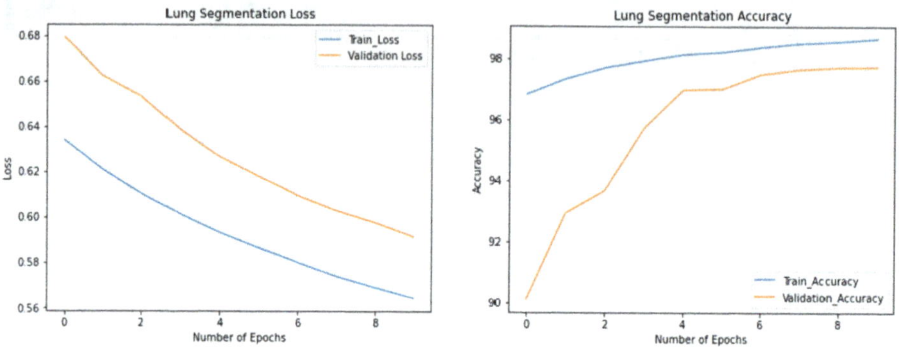

Figure 11. Contrast CNN model Predicted Lung Masks

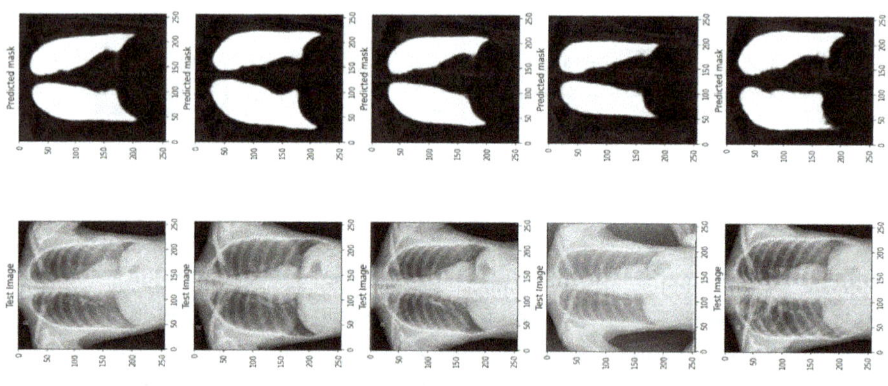

Figure 12 shows the reduced error rate in the training and validation data items. The input and mask shapes are (704, 256, 256, 3) and (704, 256, 256, 1). The segmentation network parameters are total parameters is 10,115,501, trainable parameters are 10,071,501 and, Non-trainable parameters are 44,000. The model hyperparameters learning rate is 0.0001, Adam optimizers are used, the batch size is 32, and the number of epochs is 32.

Figure 12. Proposed Image Classification Model Accuracy Score and Loss Score

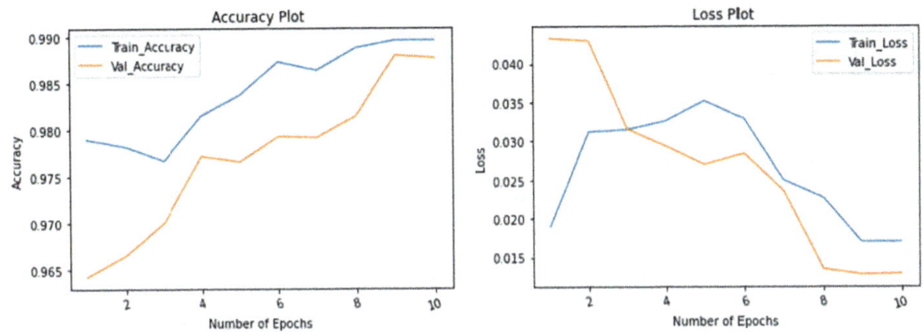

The Classification network parameters are the total number of parameters is 88,977,953, trainable parameters are 88,943,521 and Non-trainable parameters are 34,432. The binary cross entropy loss is used for the model loss calculation. RMSprop optimizer is used and the learning rate is 1e-4. A sigmoidal classifier is used for the classification. In the initial hidden layer 512 hidden units, later it is 128.

CONCLUSION AND FUTURE ENHANCEMENT

Based on the Contrast CNN Unet model and fusion architecture, the proposed work describes a combined approach for segmentation and classification tasks. CLAHE is applied to the convolutional layers to enhance the extracted features and then normalised with the actual dimension. This pixel-to-pixel improvisation with the Bconn LSTM Unet model observes the discrete regions and maps the precise borders. Model classification is including the fusion network of residual and VGG19 architecture. It reduces the training and prediction error from epochs 5. The confusion matrix explains the number of correctly predicted TB-affected and not affected samples from the group of the validation set. This classification model achieves the 98% for the training and 96% for validation. The future direction of this work is to measure the ratio of the portion affected by the abnormality in the entire region.

DECLARATIONS

The authors declare that they have no known competing financial interests or personal relationships that could have appeared to influence the work reported in this paper. All the authors are equally contributed to the work.

REFERENCES

Cao, Y., Mao, J., Yu, H., Zhang, Q., Wang, H., Zhang, Q., Guo, L., & Gao, F. (2020). A novel hybrid active contour model for intracranial tuberculosis MRI segmentation applications. *IEEE Access : Practical Innovations, Open Solutions*, *8*, 149569–149585. DOI: 10.1109/ACCESS.2020.3016746

Chan, T. F., & Vese, L. A. (2001). Active contours without edges. *IEEE Transactions on Image Processing*, *10*(2), 266–277. DOI: 10.1109/83.902291 PMID: 18249617

de Vries, G., van Hest, R. A., & Richardus, J. H. (2007). Impact of mobile radiographic screening on tuberculosis among drug users and homeless persons. *American Journal of Respiratory and Critical Care Medicine*, *176*(2), 201–207. DOI: 10.1164/rccm.200612-1877OC PMID: 17413123

Dosovitskiy, A., Beyer, L., Kolesnikov, A., Weissenborn, D., Zhai, X., Unterthiner, T., Dehghani, M., Minderer, M., Heigold, G., Gelly, S., Uszkoreit, J., & Houlsby, N. (2020). An image is worth 16×16 words: Transformers for image recognition at scale. *arXiv*. https://doi.org//arXiv.2010.11929DOI: 10.48550

Hamidian, S., Sahiner, B., Petrick, N., & Pezeshk, A. (2017). 3D convolutional neural network for automatic detection of lung nodules in chest CT. *Proceedings of SPIE - the International Society for Optical Engineering*, *10134*, 1013409. Advance online publication. DOI: 10.1117/12.2255795 PMID: 28845077

He, K., Zhang, X., Ren, S., & Sun, J. (2016). Deep residual learning for image recognition. In *Proceedings of the IEEE Conferencepr Conference on Computer Vision and Pattern Recognition (CVPR)* (pp. 770–778). IEEE. https://doi.org/DOI: 10.1109/CVPR.2016.90

Hogeweg, L., Sánchez, C. I., Maduskar, P., Philipsen, R., Story, A., Dawson, R., Theron, G., Dheda, K., Peters-Bax, L., & van Ginneken, B. (2015). Automatic detection of tuberculosis in chest radiographs using a combination of textural, focal, and shape abnormality analysis. *IEEE Transactions on Medical Imaging*, *34*(12), 2429–2442. DOI: 10.1109/TMI.2015.2405761 PMID: 25706581

Jaeger, S., Karargyris, A., Candemir, S., Folio, L., Siegelman, J., Callaghan, F., Xue, Z., Palaniappan, K., Singh, R. K., Antani, S., Thoma, G., Wang, Y.-X., Lu, P.-X., & McDonald, C. J. (2014). Automatic tuberculosis screening using chest radiographs. *IEEE Transactions on Medical Imaging*, *33*(2), 233–245. DOI: 10.1109/TMI.2013.2284099 PMID: 24108713

Ju, W., Xiang, D., Zhang, B., Wang, L., Kopriva, I., & Chen, X. (2015). Random walk and graph cut for co-segmentation of lung tumor on PET-CT images. *IEEE Transactions on Image Processing*, *24*(12), 5854–5867. DOI: 10.1109/TIP.2015.2488902 PMID: 26462198

Khan, S., Siddiqui, F., & Ahad, M. A. (2025). Integrating CNN-based feature fusion and spatial attention for tuberculosis detection with Bayesian optimized XGBoost. *International Journal of Data Science and Analytics*, *20*(6), 5415–5434. DOI: 10.1007/s41060-025-00778-z

Kim, T. H., Krichen, M., Ojo, S., Alamro, M. A., & Sampedro, G. A. (2024). TSSG-CNN: A tuberculosis semantic segmentation-guided model for detecting and diagnosis using the adaptive convolutional neural network. *Diagnostics (Basel)*, *14*(11), 1174. Advance online publication. DOI: 10.3390/diagnostics14111174 PMID: 38893700

Lee, G., Lee, H. Y., Park, H., Schiebler, M. L., van Beek, E. J. R., Ohno, Y., Seo, J. B., & Leung, A. (2017). Radiomics and its emerging role in lung cancer research, imaging biomarkers and clinical management: State of the art. *European Journal of Radiology*, *86*, 297–307. DOI: 10.1016/j.ejrad.2016.09.005 PMID: 27638103

Li, C., Kao, C.-Y., Gore, J. C., & Ding, Z. (2008). Minimization of region-scalable fitting energy for image segmentation. *IEEE Transactions on Image Processing*, *17*(10), 1940–1949. DOI: 10.1109/TIP.2008.2002304 PMID: 18784040

Liang, Z., Liu, W., & Yao, R. (2016). Contrast enhancement by nonlinear diffusion filtering. *IEEE Transactions on Image Processing*, *25*(2), 673–686. DOI: 10.1109/TIP.2015.2507405 PMID: 26685234

Maduskar, P., Philipsen, R. H. H. M., Melendez, J., Scholten, E. T., Chanda-Kapata, P., Ayles, H., & van Ginneken, B. (2013). Detection of tuberculosis using digital chest radiography: Automated reading vs. interpretation by clinical officers. *The International Journal of Tuberculosis and Lung Disease : the Official Journal of the International Union against Tuberculosis and Lung Disease*, *17*(12), 1613–1620. DOI: 10.5588/ijtld.13.0325 PMID: 24200278

Mukherjee, S., Huang, X., & Bhagalia, R. R. (2017). Lung nodule segmentation using deep learned prior based graph cut. In *2017 IEEE 14th International Symposium on Biomedical Imaging (ISBI 2017)* (pp. 1205–1208). IEEE. https://doi.org/DOI: 10.1109/ISBI.2017.7950733

Munadi, K., Muchtar, K., Maulina, N., & Pradhan, B. (2020). Image enhancement for tuberculosis detection using deep learning. *IEEE Access : Practical Innovations, Open Solutions*, *8*, 217897–217907. DOI: 10.1109/ACCESS.2020.3041867

Norval, M., Wang, Z., & Sun, Y. (2019). Pulmonary tuberculosis detection using deep learning convolutional neural networks. In *Proceedings of the 3rd International Conference on Video and Image Processing (ICVIP 2019)* (pp. 47–51). ACM. https://doi.org/DOI: 10.1145/3376067.3376068

Piccazzo, R., Paparo, F., & Garlaschi, G. (2014). Diagnostic accuracy of chest radiography for the diagnosis of tuberculosis (TB) and its role in the detection of latent TB infection: A systematic review. *The Journal of Rheumatology. Supplement*, *91*(0), 32–40. DOI: 10.3899/jrheum.140100 PMID: 24788998

Raja, J., Rajeswari, J., & Jayashri, S. (2023). A secured QR pattern based e-health care CAD system for CXR image analyzes. *Optik (Stuttgart)*, *273*, 170344. Advance online publication. DOI: 10.1016/j.ijleo.2022.170344

Rodtook, A., & Makhanov, S. S. (2013). Multi-feature gradient vector flow snakes for adaptive segmentation of the ultrasound images of breast cancer. *Journal of Visual Communication and Image Representation*, *24*(8), 1414–1430. DOI: 10.1016/j.jvcir.2013.09.009

Saini, K., Dewal, M. L., & Rohit, M. (2012). A fast region-based active contour model for boundary detection of echocardiographic images. *Journal of Digital Imaging*, *25*(2), 271–278. DOI: 10.1007/s10278-011-9408-8 PMID: 21779946

Sandler, M., Howard, A., Zhu, M., Zhmoginov, A., & Chen, L.-C. (2018). MobileNetV2: Inverted residuals and linear bottlenecks. In *Proceedings of the IEEE/CVF Conference on Computer Vision and Pattern Recognition (CVPR)* (pp. 4510–4520). IEEE. https://doi.org/DOI: 10.1109/CVPR.2018.00474

Santiago-Mozos, R., Pérez-Cruz, F., Madden, M. G., & Artés-Rodríguez, A. (2013). An automated screening system for tuberculosis. *IEEE Journal of Biomedical and Health Informatics*, *18*(3), 855–862. DOI: 10.1109/JBHI.2013.2282874 PMID: 24132025

Showkatian, E., Salehi, M., Ghaffari, H., Reiazi, R., & Sadighi, N. (2022). Deep learning-based automatic detection of tuberculosis disease in chest X-ray images. *Polish Journal of Radiology / Polish Medical Society of Radiology*, *87*(1), 118–124. DOI: 10.5114/pjr.2022.113435 PMID: 35280947

Silva Filho, T. M., Pimentel, B. A., Souza, R. M. C. R., & Oliveira, A. L. I. (2015). Hybrid methods for fuzzy clustering based on fuzzy c-means and improved particle swarm optimization. *Expert Systems with Applications*, *42*(17–18), 6315–6328. DOI: 10.1016/j.eswa.2015.04.032

Story, A., Murad, S., Roberts, W., Verheyen, M., & Hayward, A. C. (2007). Tuberculosis in London: The importance of homelessness, problem drug use and prison. *Thorax*, *62*(8), 667–671. DOI: 10.1136/thx.2006.065409 PMID: 17289861

Sun, W., Huang, X., Tseng, T.-L. B., & Qian, W. (2017). Automatic lung nodule graph cuts segmentation with deep learning false positive detection. In *Medical Imaging 2017: Computer-Aided Diagnosis* (Article 101343E). SPIE. https://doi.org/DOI: 10.1117/12.2251302

Ul Abideen, Z., Ghafoor, M., Munir, K., Saqib, M., Ullah, A., Zia, T., & Tariq, A. (2020). Uncertainty assisted robust tuberculosis identification with Bayesian convolutional neural networks. *IEEE Access : Practical Innovations, Open Solutions*, *8*, 22812–22825. DOI: 10.1109/ACCESS.2020.2970023 PMID: 32391238

Wang, Q., Wu, B., Zhu, P., Li, P., Zuo, W., & Hu, Q. (2020). ECA-Net: Efficient channel attention for deep convolutional neural networks. In *Proceedings of the IEEE/CVF Conference on Computer Vision and Pattern Recognition (CVPR)* (pp. 11531–11539). IEEE. https://doi.org/DOI: 10.1109/CVPR42600.2020.01155

Woo, S., Park, J., Lee, J.-Y., & Kweon, I. S. (2018). CBAM: Convolutional block attention module. In *Proceedings of the European Conference on Computer Vision (ECCV)* (pp. 3–19). Springer. https://doi.org/DOI: 10.1007/978-3-030-01234-2_1

Xie, Y., Wu, Z., Han, X., Wang, H., Wu, Y., Cui, L., & Lin, J. (2020). Computer-aided system for the detection of multicategory pulmonary tuberculosis in radiographs. *Journal of Healthcare Engineering*, *2020*, 9843260. Advance online publication. DOI: 10.1155/2020/9205082 PMID: 32908660

Xu, T., & Yuan, Z. (2022). Convolution neural network with coordinate attention for the automatic detection of pulmonary tuberculosis images on chest X-rays. *IEEE Access : Practical Innovations, Open Solutions*, *10*, 86710–86717. DOI: 10.1109/ACCESS.2022.3199419

Yadav, G., Maheshwari, S., & Agarwal, A. (2014). Contrast limited adaptive histogram equalization based enhancement for real time video)); system. In *2014 International Conference on Advances in Computing, Communications and Informatics (ICACCI)* (pp. 2392–2397). IEEE. https://doi.org/DOI: 10.1109/ICACCI.2014.6968381

Zhang, Q., Bai, C., Liu, Z., Yang, L. T., Yu, H., Zhao, J., & Wang, X. (2020). A GPU-based residual network for medical image classification in smart medicine. *Information Sciences*, *536*, 91–100. DOI: 10.1016/j.ins.2020.05.013

Zhang, W., Zhang, X., Zhao, J., Qiang, Y., Tian, Q., & Tang, X. (2017). A segmentation method for lung nodule image sequences based on superpixels and density-based spatial clustering of applications with noise. *PLoS One*, *12*(9), e0184290. Advance online publication. DOI: 10.1371/journal.pone.0184290 PMID: 28880916

Chapter 15
Sustainable Monitoring of High-Risk Pregnancies in GDM Using Smart Healthcare Systems

R. Priyanka
SRC, SASTRA University, India

A. Sumathi
https://orcid.org/0000-0003-4700-5573
SASTRA University, India

ABSTRACT

Gestational Diabetes is one of the major growing metabolic syndromes that affects pregnant mothers and their growing Infants worldwide. Traditional monitoring methods often require regular visits and keeping manual records up-to-date, and they have some short-term fluctuations, reduce timely intervention, and place an extra burden on patients for accurate logging and recall. Sustainable environment monitoring systems leverage wearable biosensors, continuous glucose monitors, cloud-based electronic health records, and AI-driven analytics to provide constant, real-time, and personalized monitoring. The sustainable monitoring system provides continuous, real-time tracking of health care data in GDM, also helps in providing personalized care, promotes early identification of risks, and reduces manual effort by improving patient engagement and outcomes. This Chapter explores how advanced technology with monitoring systems can be Integrated into maternal systems can be Integrated into maternal routine care.

DOI: 10.4018/979-8-3373-5641-9.ch015

INTRODUCTION

Diabetes - A growing public health concern that generally affects people of all ages and groups. It is a chronic metabolic disorder that is defined as an elevated level of blood glucose, resulting in insulin secretion, insulin action, or both, which often requires lifelong management and poses certain risks and complications that affect multiple organs. Includes the eyes, kidneys, nerves, and the cardiovascular system. There are many Kinds of diabetes some common types which Includes Type 1 (T1DM), It is an auto-Immune and it usually gets developed in childhood or even adolesence, and Type 2 diabetes mellitus (T2DM), GDM- Gestational Diabetes Mellitus, and Maturity One -set diabetes of the young (MODY), Neonatal diabetes, and steroid Induced diabetes, which is commonly associated with insulin resistance and other lifestylefactors, and their treatment methods, they require treatment methods, they require treatment methods, they their treatment methods, they require timely diagnosis and proper glycemic control to prevent such complications. Among these, Gestational Diabetes Mellitus (GDM) is of particular concern in maternal health. Diabetes Mellitus that occurs during the Period of Gestation is referred to as Gestational Diabetes Mellitus. Gestational Diabetes Mellitus-The term Gestation refers to the period of development of an embryo or fetus inside the uterus, from the time of conception until birth. It is a Common Complication that often occurs during Pregnancy. GDM primarily affects pregnant women and typically emerges during the second or third trimester. It typically manifests during the latter stages of gestation, specifically between 24 and 28 weeks of pregnancy. The principal etiological factor that contributes to GDM is the secretion of various hormones by the placenta, which serves as the vital connection between the mother and the fetus, resulting in a progressive increase in insulin resistance during the mid-gestational phase. Placental Hormones, which include human placental lactogen (hPL), progesterone, and cortisol, increase the resistance of insulin during pregnancy. Maternal pancreatic β-cells must compensate by increasing the secretion of insulin. GDM develops only when the compensatory mechanism fails. The presence of GDM poses certain significant risks not only to the mother but also to the progeny, impacting both immediate and long-term health outcomes. According to the International Diabetes Federation (IDF) Diabetes Atlas, 10th edition, hyperglycemia in pregnancy (HIP) affects approximately one in every six pregnancies. As of 2021, it is projected that 537 million individuals globally are afflicted with diabetes, with estimates suggesting an increase to 643 million by the year 2030 and 783 million by 2045. Recent investigations have indicated that women diagnosed with diabetes mellitus face an elevated risk of developing breast cancer and are also susceptible to reproductive disorders, with particular emphasis on reproductive dysfunctions primarily associated with polycystic ovarian syndrome (PCOS). The latest research indicates that mothers with GDM are at a heightened risk of developing cardiometabolic diseases, and their offspring similarly exhibit an increased risk. It is also associated with several maternal and neonatal complications. Some common maternal complications include Preclampsia, Polyhydramnios, Preterm delivery, obstructed labor or cesarean delivery, UTIs and vaginal infections, Postpartum hemorrhage, and Future type 2 diabetes. Some common Neonatal complications include Macrosomia, Neonatal hypoglycemia, Respiratory distress syndrome (RDS), Hyperbilirubinemia & jaundice, Polycythemia, Stillbirth, Congenital anomalies, and Future Metabolic risk. There are no specific symptoms for GDM. Some of the risk factors of developing GDM are Age Over 25, having a family history of diabetes, having had a miscarriage, being Overweight, and PCOS. The Affecting Factors of GDM are Environmental Risk factors, Individual risk factors such as ethnicity, genetics, Prenatal exposures, lifestyle behaviours, dietary patterns, Inflammation, and adiposity. Gestational Diabetes Mellitus is mainly classified into Type A1 (diet-controlled) and Type A2 (medication-requiring) GDM. Early diagnosis and management reduce complications and long-term metabolic risks. Type A1 GDM is a form of gestational diabetes mellitus that is effectively managed through diet and exercise alone, without the need for medications. In contrast, Type A2 GDM refers to the lifestyle changes that are insufficient to control blood glucose, which requires a pharmacological treatment, such as insulin or oral hypoglycemics. These patients have constantly elevated levels of glucose despite adhering to diet and exercise regimens. Management involves proper medications in combination with ongoing lifestyle interventions, which help in improving both maternal and fetal health outcomes. Gestational Diabetes Mellitus (GDM) is likely to develop in pregnant women with certain risk factors, such as insulin resistance or impaired glucose regulation. The important risk factors include maternal age, particularly above 25< 35, overweight or obese (BMI ≥25). A family history of type 2 diabetes, especially in first-degree relatives, previous GDM history, or previously delivering a large baby (weighing 4 kg or more), places individuals at higher risk. Other medical conditions, including polycystic ovary syndrome (PCOS), chronic hypertension, prediabetes, and metabolic syndrome, increase the chance of having GDM. Ethnic background also plays a role, with higher risk observed among South Asian, Hispanic, African-American, Native American, and Pacific Islander populations. Smoking and the use of certain medications, like glucocorticoids, also increase the risk of gdm. Recognizing these risk factors is important for early screening, timely intervention, and effective management of GDM to ensure better maternal and fetal outcomes. Managing GDM requires maintaining normal blood glucose levels, maintaining a balanced diet, and regular physical activity, improving insulin sensitivity, monitoring blood glucose levels, and, if diet and exercise are not enough, insulin or oral medications like metformin are prescribed. Fetal growth is regularly analysed through ultrasounds. Delivery plans rely on glucose control, when managed poorly, require an early induction or cesarean. After birth, the blood sugar level is checked within 6–12 weeks, and women who are at higher risk of developing type 2 diabetes need a long-term follow-up. If managed poorly or left untreated, GDM leads to serious health consequences for both the mother and child in both the short term and long term. In mothers, the risk of developing type 2 diabetes mellitus (T2DM) is higher, as studies estimate that nearly 50% of women with GDM will develop T2DM within 5–10 years postpartum. In addition, the chances of experiencing cardiovascular diseases, metabolic syndrome, intrauterine exposure to maternal hyperglycemia, and recurrent GDM in future pregnancies are increased. For the offspring, it leads to an elevated risk of childhood obesity, impaired glucose tolerance, insulin resistance, and early-onset T2DM. The infants are mostly prone to neurodevelopmental delays and might face lifelong metabolic health challenges. The absence of timely Treatment, personalized recommendations, and continuous check-ups. It can result in a transgenerational cycle of metabolic disease, further straining healthcare systems. Therefore, effective long-term care models and monitoring strategies are Important to reduce the risk of chronic disease in both mothers and their children. The World Health Organization (WHO) and,(MoHFW) recommend universal screening of gdm, particularly women with high-risk factors of gdm. They should undergo hyperglycemia screening between 24 -28 weeks of gestation. In India, MoHFW recommends a universal single-step screening approach using DIPSI (Diabetes in Pregnancy Study Group India) guidelines. This method is said to be more practical for a large, diverse population in India, particularly in rural or resource-constrained areas.The traditional method for diagnosing Gestational Diabetes Mellitus (GDM) is the Oral Glucose Tolerance Test (OGTT), usually performed between 24 and 28 weeks of pregnancy. In this test, the woman fasts overnight for 8 to 10 hours, and a fasting blood sample is first collected to measure baseline glucose levels. She is then given a glucose solution containing either 75g or 100g of glucose to drink. This test is performed to analyze how the body handles glucose, and blood samples are taken one to two hours after ingesting the solution. (and three hours for the 100g version.). If any one of the following glucose levels is reached or surpassed, as per diagnostic criteria, GDM is confirmed: fasting glucose ≥92 mg/dL, 1-hour glucose ≥180 mg/dL, or 2-hour glucose ≥153 mg/dL. In clinical practice, this test is still the most extensively used and trustworthy way to identify GDM. Traditional Methodologies lack continuous monitoring and personalized suggestions, and may lead to poor results also GDM monitoring typically involves periodic glucose testing through laboratory-based Oral Glucose Tolerance Tests (OGTT), occasional in-clinical testing, and manual tracking of diet and symptoms Although these methodologies are clinically assessed and standardized, they still have certain limitations, which include treatment delay, Inadequate data, and restricted customization. Smart technologies, which include Intelligent monitoring systems, enhance wearable biosensors, continuous glucose monitors, and mobile health apps, and cloud-based data analytics, which offer real-time, ongoing, and personalized treatments for Maternal health. These systems help in identifying fluctuations in glucose levels and assessing risks utilizing AI algorithms dynamically. They even deliver regular and automated reminders and personalized recommendations by enhancing patient health and outcomes. Smart devices provide remote monitoring and tele-consultation, which helps in reducing the need for in-person visits and particularly benefits women in rural areas. While Traditional Monitoring methods remain a cornerstone for diagnostics, the Intelligent monitoring system introduces a more effective, patient-centered, and sustainable approach in managing GDM. The demand for sustainable technology and technology-driven monitoring solutions has increased rapidly. The IoT (Internet of Things) is revolutionizing the monitoring of maternal health during pregnancy. Devices such as continuous glucose monitors (CGMs), smartwatches, wearable blood pressure sensors, and activity trackers will help in collecting real-time data from pregnant women. GDM care systems provide remote glucose monitoring via CGM devices, blood pressure, and heart rate tracking via smart watches Cloud Cloud-based data storage for longitudinal analysis, AI algorithms are used for predicting risk alerts, trend detection, mobile applications for patient education, diet logging, and direct consulting, and telemedicine platforms for timely interventions. These methods help in improving environmental sustainability by reducing hospital resource use, reducing trip emissions, and reducing paper and single-use diagnoses. Simultaneously, they increase both economic and operational sustainability through enhancing health care accessibility, flexibility, and tolerance to future disruptions such as pandemics and natural disasters. Wearable biosensors, such as activity bands, smartwatches, and CGMs, are at the heart of these systems. Vital indications, like as blood pressure (which is required to detect pre-eclampsia), sleep patterns, physical activity, step count, and fasting and postprandial blood glucose levels, are all monitored with their help. Electronic health records (EHRs) kept in the cloud are crucial for collecting data and helping with clinical decision-making. EHRs supply important information for population-level research, enhance relationships between health care professionals, safeguard medical records, and provide long-term evaluation of trends. A unique monitoring system that satisfies the clinical needs of high-risk GDM women is made up of interrelated elements. AI can identify subtle patterns of Glucose dysregulation even before traditional methods.ML methods can detect early Gdm onset more accurately. Gdm by combining CGM outputs with physiological data from smart wearables. AI-driven clustering techniques help to categorize women into three subtypes, which is critical for personalized treatment. This integrated method, when paired with a sustainable monitoring system, offers a dynamic, economical, and patient-centered framework. It not only quickly finds GDM but also helps in improving the health of the mother and child through quick, tailored treatment. In conclusion, involving responsible environmental surveillance systems in medical care for mothers may improve the care of diabetes during pregnancy, especially in high-risk moms. These technologies offer continuous, customized, and proactive care, reducing the need for costly physician visits and furthering health equity across socioeconomic and geographic hurdles.

IMPLEMENTATION CONSIDERATIONS AND REAL-WORLD INTEGRATION

It is crucial to pay attention to the challenges of implementation in the real-world landscape when shifting sustainable monitoring systems for gestational diabetes mellitus (GDM) from prototype to real-world practice. When considering the technical considerations of interoperability with EHR systems and hospital IT infrastructures, using either open-source APIs or the tools, an optimally reliable ontology for data flow that is invisible to the clinician, so as not to increase clinician burden and promote duplicate efforts! Integration from the medical frame is about bringing stakeholders who are going to be involved in the patient care to be co-participants in the integrated care pathway for stakeholders who are involved in the care of a pregnant person with diabetes, built into their structure of team practice, which is typically led by obstetricians, endocrinologists, diabetes educators, and dietitians. Training the clinicians and the team to understand some factors that lend themselves to data visualization through alerts, and the understanding of artificial intelligence (AI) generated risk predictions to decrease alarm fatigue and not cause symptomatic reaction, are equally important. When analyzing from an organizational readiness perspective, particularly within low-resources contexts, this will be a key factor influencing the use of any monitoring system where any accessibility issue is on the line for the participants. Stakeholder teams will need to pilot the ability to ensure a strong internet connection, consistent and adequate electricity supply, and cheap and varied hardware and devices to best facilitate equitable access to residents in the community. Regarding data storage and analysis options, the best solutions may indeed include cloud or edge-based computations to reduce bandwidth to the lowest point possible and safeguard data privacy to the fullest extent possible. Ultimately, sustainable and long-term implementation will depend on developing funding models that account for what constitutes an asset that has after-care of updates, and software maintenance history, along with potential and actually implemented care education activities aimed at increasing participant engagement consistently throughout the year. By using pilot studies, or rollout-phases of what is designed in a product, their contextual barriers specific to local communities can be isolated, usability assessed, community and stakeholder satisfaction can be assessed, and a better real-time iterative system for sustainment of the digital tool in practice.

CHALLENGES AND RISKS

Although the proposed sustainable monitoring system for Gestational Diabetes Mellitus (GDM) has several advantages, the indefinite implementation of sustainable monitoring in real life may come with risks, and that risks also need to be acknowledged. The first barrier is data privacy and security. As we have already begun collecting and sharing sensitive maternal health data by employing use a sustainable model, we may legitimately be concerned about sensitive data being taken advantage of in a manner we have not provisioned for. In order to preserve our patients' privacy and maintain their trust, such systems must comply with accepted international standards (GDPR and HIPAA), involve state-of-the-art encryption, and secure authentication protocols. The second major issue is the reliability and accuracy of the sensor devices. Wearables and home monitoring may encounter sensitivity losses, calibration drift in data collection, battery depletion, signal losses, and/or hardware malfunction. If a sensor's reliability and accuracy diminish, it may lead to incomplete or inaccurate data that minimizes the utility of predictive models and may misinform clinical decision-making. Redundant systems can be designed into wearable sensor models, and possibly a user-friendly calibration tool can minimize these risks.

In addition to opportunities for physician reimbursement and prevention, user compliance and engagement (or lack thereof) with the system are also factors to consider in the success of the system. Patients may forget to wear devices altogether, forget to make daily measurements, or lose interest in using the mobile application if it wears off. Device compliance potential is a function of several considerations: comfort of the device, ease of use, cultural context and perceived societal role of the technology, and the patient's potential for motivation and drive. Incorporating game-like elements, personalized reminders, and culturally appropriate design elements may serve as a way to familiarize the patient with engaging with the device and help encourage sustained engagement and adherence. The implementation of a surveillance system may also be impacted by the current clinical workflow and the role of the hospital's IT systems. Providers may resist engaging in new technologies altogether if they feel that it would invade their work processes and complicate their work. Continued exploration in co-designing these systems with clinicians to demonstrate value-added benefits, such as time-savings, and to determine improved patient understanding and insight may be helpful. Another area of concern with technology use in surveillance medicine is bias in artificial intelligence and machine learning models. If the AI or machine-learning model is being trained on limited or non-representative data sets, the models may provide predictions that are less accurate for specific demographic groups, which may exacerbate existing health inequities. Continued efforts to obtain diverse and inclusive data sets and validate the accuracy of the model over time may limit this risk. Finally, the cost and scalability of implementing and maintaining these systems are still important considerations. Although IoT devices and cloud technology are generally cheaper, costs associated with implementing and maintaining these systems are still substantial when implemented at scale, and ongoing technical support would likely be the key challenge in settings with low resources. As we contend with these considerations, we need to keep in mind that we should do so carefully, as sustained monitoring systems will only be beneficial to maternal health outcomes if they can do so safely, obtain reliable results, and be implemented in a uniform and equitable way.

POTENTIAL FOR PERSONALIZATION AND PRECISION MEDICINE IN GDM MONITORING

The incorporation of artificial intelligence (AI) and machine learning (ML) to motivate sustainable environmental monitoring systems allows for an unparalleled chance to improve personalization and precision medicine in the treatment of gestational diabetes mellitus (GDM). GDM care has previously been based on standardized guidelines that often fail to account for variations in lifestyle, genetics, social, and demographic factors present in each individual. AI-enabled systems can analyze incoming streams of heterogeneous data (which includes glucose measures, nutrient intake, physical activity, sleep patterns, and even stress) in real-time and continuously, via wearables or mobile applications. Such systems can, thus, adapt, change, and update risk predictions throughout the pregnancy, and allow clinicians to intervene in a timely and patient-specific manner. For example, a patient reporting recurring nocturnal hyperglycemia could be provided with time-specific dietary counseling to better allocate glucose intake to the evening meal; another patient exhibiting sedentary behavior trends may be directed toward specific attainable activity targets. Mobile health applications can provide real-time behavior change information and recommendations, linking the behavior more closely and likely to the care plan provided to GDM patients and others. In addition, the addition of genomics, metabolomics, and epigenomics into predictive models has the potential to identify subtypes of GDM and to gain insight into the specific disease mechanisms that each patient experiences. If adopted, a personalized approach might allow clinicians to identify those women who will respond only to lifestyle change, from those who will likely require early pharmacotherapy, preventing unnecessary pill exposure and/or treatment delays. The personalized approach also extends to cultural, linguistic, and socioeconomic differences, allowing for the development of AI models that build on the patients' preferences for language, food culture, and availability of resources, such that the recommendations offered are feasible and useful. Furthermore, utilizing personalized dashboards that display progress and change in culturally responsive ways can contribute to engagement and optimal empowerment of those patients. Ultimately, the precision medicine strategy in GDM enlarges our scope of impact, allowing us to expand beyond clinical measures (reducing maternal hyperglycemia and complications for the neonate) to modifying the patient's experience and truly person-centered care. As these opportunities unfold, we envision a new realm of possibilities whereby these technologies may help to eliminate some gaps among different population groups experiencing GDM to support healthier pregnancies on a global platform.

LITERATURE SURVEY

The field of healthcare has developed and seen new technologies that have emerged in the emerging and new field. Specifically, in GDM (gestational diabetes mellitus), the management and monitoring of gdm and its implications have developed along with earlier detection of gdm. With all these Initiatives.

Lu and Huang (2022). Their intervention demonstrated significant improvements in patient compliance, diet adherence, and metabolic control, leading to better pregnancy outcomes and reduced adverse events for both mothers and newborns. While the follow-up period was limited to three months, the findings provide a strong theoretical reference for the early nursing intervention of pregnant women with GDM, highlighting the potential of integrated smart monitoring systems in clinical practice. The algorithm proposed offers significant contributions to the management and outcomes for pregnant women with GDM. The system's design and functionality address GDM care, including blood glucose control, diet, exercise, and Monitoring. This system Integrates AI and IoT using wireless communication technology to provide nursing interventions, which allows for personalized diet plans and helps in managing gdm. The Limitation of this study is that monitoring is follow-up for pregnant women and newborns is only for a Limited period. This is not enough for understanding Long-term outcomes. Building on this foundation, researchers have explored diverse approaches to advance GDM care, including wearable devices for continuous glucose and physiological monitoring, mobile health applications for patient engagement, AI-driven decision support systems, and remote telemedicine platforms. These systems aim not only to detect and manage glycemic variability but also to address broader challenges such as risk stratification, sustainability, and accessibility, particularly in low-resource settings. The following paragraphs review and analyze these contributions, highlighting how the integration of IoT, machine learning, and sustainable design principles is reshaping maternal health monitoring and offering new opportunities for proactive, personalized, and resource-efficient GDM care. Rigla et al. (2018) demonstrated the feasibility and high patient acceptance of a smart mobile telemedicine system for managing GDM as part of the MobiGuide Project. This AI-augmented decision support system (DSS) combined computer-interpretable clinical guidelines, electronic health records, and sensor data to deliver personalized, real-time recommendations to patients. Their pilot study showed that the system significantly improved patient compliance with blood glucose monitoring compared to standard care. Although metabolic and perinatal outcomes were broadly similar to those of a historical cohort, the telemedicine group exhibited lower blood pressure readings. The system provides personalized feedback and features settings as setting reminders at the meal times of the patients, and also gives automated diet plan suggestions to correct hyperglycemia. Here, Ketonuria was detected, and the system inquires about the levels of carbohydrates ingested by the patients with normal values and high compliance. Some of the Limitations of this study include a concurrent control group, and the comparison was made with only 247 patients. This study does not stratify the women and helps in detecting earlier gdm. This study only helps in Monitoring Patients with GDM. Varnfield et al. (2021) developed and evaluated the mother platform. The system aims to assist women with GDM who have received a new treatment for GDM. This system has a secure storage solution and an online platform that consists of a smartphone application for patient monitoring. Compared to prior cohorts, the platform offered enhanced blood glucose measurements and prenatal visits to 40 women in an Arch-Viability Trial, while maintaining high levels of user satisfaction for both patients and health care providers. The study showed the platform's ability to facilitate overall care coordination and safety, particularly during the global pandemic when access to in-person care and treatment was limited. The platform did present some minor technical issues with wireless connectivity and data transfer. Most importantly, this platform generates individualized treatment plans designed by clinicians while providing tailored care to patients, all without adding workload to the clinician. They are well-designed systems that can extend GDM care beyond clinical trials, improve efficiency, and empower both patients and providers through real-time data sharing and targeted interventions. The mother platform significantly contributes to GDM women's care by providing a Convenient, accessible, Comprehensive tool for self-care management, which leads to improved communication with health care providers. These Limitations primarily concern the study's design and lack of a concurrent control group. Building on the integration of diverse data sources to provide personalised healthcare, Pustozerov et al. (2020) developed and piloted a remote monitoring system dedicated to women with Gestational Diabetes Mellitus (GDM). The publication outlines both the system's technical architecture as well as its first clinical implementation based on the continued increase in GDM prevalence and the resulting pressures on clinical staff. The primary intent of the system is to facilitate monitoring and clinical advice outside of the hospital. The system establishes an amalgamation of several data sources, which include, among others, mobile food diaries, fitness monitors that record physical activity and heart rates, as well as continuous glucose monitoring (CGM) devices. The research teams augmented this basic package with patient-specific details such as genetic variants, microbiome profiles, body composition assessments, and biochemical factors like glycated hemoglobin. This complete suite provides the personalized glucose management suggestions based on the patient's metabolic profile. Furthermore, the system applied analytic techniques to provide a variety of recommendations, which included longer-term lifestyle recommendations based on diet and physical activity behaviours. They also provided suggestions to patients for adjustments to blood glucose levels (BGL) and guidance on how to manage recent meals. The initial assessment of patients indicated that the system was capable of dealing with highly complicated multi-dimensional data and providing both timely and actionable feedback directly to clinicians to help improve glycemic control and modify health service workload demand. The authors indicated that there should be further randomized clinical trials and larger validations incorporated into standard clinical work practices and data privacy frameworks, which relate to the discussion surrounding the framework for sustainable AI-enhanced GDM monitoring discussed in this chapter. Finally, the authors indicate that the system was still in a testing phase with a larger cohort to validate its use in GDM prevention. The system positions itself within the growing conversation about apps and wearables' role in chronic disease self-management. Beyond the advances in wearable and IoT monitoring devices to support GDM management and care, several predictive modeling approaches have also been implemented. One example is a study by Lu et al. (2022), who created and assessed a stacked Long Short-Term Memory (LSTM) deep learning model to predict women's blood glucose levels with GDM. The purpose of the article is to develop a benchmark glucose prediction model using a long short-term memory (LSTM) recurrent neural network based on time-series data generated from the GDM health platform. This will provide accurate and low-cost glucose and hypoglycemia predictions to women in GDM, offering solutions to invasive fingerstick testing and expensive CGM (continuous glucose monitoring) devices. Based primarily on time-series blood glucose data gathered from the GDm-Health platform, along with thorough data pre-processing, the model also accounted for different observation/prediction windows. The validation result indicated that the model can predict blood glucose levels with accuracies comparable to CGM systems, and when utilizing a 7-day observation window to predict blood glucose levels for the following 14 days. Although AI-based technologies are limited in their direct caregiving roles, they can help reduce clinical workload and patient burden for blood glucose testing, as well as provide early alerts for hyperglycemia by utilizing self-monitoring data, rather than relying on expensive, continuous systems. Besides AI-based predictive modelling, numerous studies have explored telemedicine interventions focused on GDM outcomes. For instance, Tancredi et al. (2024) trialed a telemedicine platform called (myDiabby) for monitoring blood glucose levels in women with GDM at a rural hospital in France. The primary aim was to evaluate whether implementing a telemedicine solution for gdm could decrease the frequency of large for gestational age. This observational retrospective study successfully demonstrated that the Implementation of a telemedicine solution for the care of women with GDM was associated with a significant decrease in the adjusted odds of LGA. The study highlights the potential of telemedicine to enhance GDM care, particularly in rural settings, by making it more accessible. The telemedicine system allowed the multidisciplinary team to remotely review glucose data frequently, have a real-time interaction, and have fewer in-person visits, with the aim of improving glycemic control and patient compliance. Though earlier randomized and observational studies rarely had the statistical power to detect improvements in neonatal outcomes, the results of this study support the use of telemedicine for reducing fetal overgrowth risk from gestational diabetes. In addition to forecasting time-series models and telemedicine approaches, recent initiatives have explored intelligent sensor-based monitoring systems for maternal and fetal outcomes. An Intelligent maternal feature health monitoring system with Optimarial deep learning (IMFHMS-ODL) was presented recently in the literature (Nandini & Rahimunnisa, 2025). The objective of the study was to develop and deploy an Intelligent maternal features system. This study introduced the intelligent maternal feature, and its integration is particularly relevant as it generates a strong need for real-time abnormality detection, timely intervention, and different modular sensors and an elaborate deep belief network. The system has an elaborate array of sensors to comprehensively monitor the maternal and fetal status and continues throughout pregnancy. This includes the following array of sensors: respiration, ECG (maternal and fetal), GSR, PPG, temperature, fetal movement, and heart rate. With a Deep Belief Network (DBN) with Bacterial Foraging Optimization Algorithm (BFOA), the system could achieve an overall accuracy (approx 97%) on detecting the abnormality in real-time. The mechanism can provide immediate alerts to health care practitioners with notice of potential risks detected. This study also illustrates the ability to combine AI techniques with multi-sensor data from IoT devices and the potential for enhanced early detection of complications and a lower chance of adverse outcomes, which will improve and greatly benefit practices in low-resourced settings. This study provides an addition to prior predictive models and telemedicine approaches, but provides an end-to-end proactive monitoring aspect. There have also been recent efforts to combine IoT-based systems with machine learning methods to advance prenatal diagnostics and maternal-fetal care. Yang et al. (2024) introduced Decision Tree-Driven IoT systems to improve diagnostic accuracy for prenatal hospitals to enhance prenatal diagnostics. The overall objective of this study was to introduce a diagnostic model that combines the Internet of Things with machine learning. Yang et al. (2024) looked into how dais for wearable sensors, continuous glucose monitors, blood pressure monitors, and fetal heart rate monitors were being integrated to provide real-time data to understand physiological activity (e.g., fetal heart rate, glucose levels, fetal movements). The DTA calculated a Decision Tree Algorithm (DTA), partitioning what is collected to be able to detect complications to make better predictions. Yang et al. (2024) reported 87.5% Accuracy and engineered the system to lower false positives and false negatives from statistical analysis. They were able to make previous interventions as well as advance the accessibility of care, particularly in rural settings. Although Yang et al. (2024) make it clear about the potential use of explainable machine learning models, such as Decision Trees, as a framework to provide insights along with deep learning and telemedicine interventions in GDM and prenatal care. Some of the Limitations of this study, which include Decision tree algorithms, may not provide audio to suit their needs and are prone to overfitting. In a broader context surrounding diabetes monitoring, Papri et al. (2025) created an IoT- and cloud-based non-invasive diabetes detection system based on photoplethysmogram (PPG) signals, demographic characteristics, and machine learning. This study aims to provide a prototype technology solution in a W-IoT health setting, in a less than-ambiguous way, applicable for real-time intervention. In the last number of years, the utility of non-invasive diabetes detection and real-time diabetes monitoring has emerged, with IoT-based systems implementing machine learning. Papri et al. (2025) describe a new type of diagnostic IoT and cloud-based system that identifies diabetic patients using PPG signals. The system integrates a low-cost wearable device with NIR sensors and an ESP32 microcontroller that streams its data to an AWS-based cloud platform for analysis. The system was built using new machine learning algorithms such as XGBoost, Random Forest, Logistic Regression, and SVM. The accuracy of the model reached up to 90% on the Mazandaran dataset. This demonstrates how, with minor design modifications to the planning and implementation of predictive modelling algorithms, it is possible to integrate statistical features from raw PPG signals and associated demographic metadata to detect diabetes at an early stage using various personnel without the need for invasive blood tests. With the incorporation of IoT infrastructure and cloud computing, there is potential for continuous remote monitoring and tailoring feedback on the participants' unique diabetes characteristics thus addressing the limitations of traditional glucose monitoring provided by healthcare professionals, therefore facilitating and externalizing(social problem solving) new socio-economic opportunities by using the example of discomfort or high cost of glucose monitoring demonstrated through social loafing practices. Outside of pregnancy-specific tools, Singh (2025) offered an IoT and AI-connected wearable smart health solution for sustainable smart healthcare. The unique main purpose of the study is to design, develop, and provide a wearable IoT health technology that relates aspects of a smart health response to encourage early warning measures. Additionally, this research will investigate health care needs and lessen the well-documented precision issues associated with conventional BAN (Body Area Network- a special focus on cardiac monitoring). The system showcased real-time processing of data while additionally using smartwatches and machine-learning models such as KNN, adaptive thresholds, and security, demonstrating how design decisions based on energy consumption and scaling of findings might inform future GDM monitoring. Collectively, these studies illustrate substantial progress in applying IoT, AI, wearable sensors, and mobile platforms to improve GDM and maternal care. Systems like MobiGuide, Mother, and remote monitoring frameworks have demonstrated improved patient engagement, and the feasibility of real-time clinical integration models has demonstrated the ability to reliably recognize glycemic trends, as well as other pregnancy-related complications; notably, predictive LSTM networks, decision trees, and DBNs have been used as reliable AI models for identifying risk trends associated with pregnancy. However, there are important sustainability gaps in the AI systems employed in the studies mentioned in the literature review. Many of the solutions are still reliant on expensive CGMs or proprietary sensors that cannot be used in low-resource settings. Very few consider sustainability over the long term, including efficiency of energy consumption and HW and SW data interoperability, and almost all do not include consideration of the different GDM subtypes or the changing risk status of the patient. These limitations reinforce the need for sustainable monitoring frameworks that embed AI models that dynamically predict risk, use real-time prospectively adaptive alerts, and are affordable and energy-efficient technologies based on IOT. If we can provide accessible, scalable, user-friendly, and, ultimately, environmentally sustainable technologies, we can better support high-risk patients with GDM and better align technology and equity for longer and greater impact.

RELATED WORK AND MOTIVATION

Gestational Diabetes Mellitus (GDM) is the most prevalent metabolic disease diagnosed in pregnancy, linked to maternal morbidities (e.g., preeclampsia, incident type 2 diabetes) and negative adverse outcomes in neonates (e.g., macrosomia, neonatal hypoglycemia), thus representing a significant public health challenge. GDM nursing interventions generally utilize a periodic approach that incorporates regular hospital visits and self-monitoring of blood glucose (SMBG). Periodic approaches can often not take into account real-time afflictions and dynamic risk factors that create variability throughout pregnancy. Periodic approaches do not support timely identification of hyperglycemia, some complications, and risk the health and safety of the mother and child. Sustainability aspects like energy efficiency, environmental and sustainability issues, and scalability also tend to be tragically under-explored, not only affecting the long-term viability of these frameworks, but also their acceptance and continued use. It will be essential that any new frameworks address these sustainability aspects, so technological innovation is matched with the delivery and outcomes.

PROPOSED SUSTAINABLE GDM MODEL

To overcome the research gaps highlights the previous review highlights, such as reliance on expensive tools such as continuous glucose monitoring tools, limited integration of lifestyle and physiological data, and insufficient emphasis on long-term sustainability and scalability. This chapter presents a conceptual framework (Sustai-GDM). This framework suggests a cost-effective and AI-enhanced monitoring system tailored for women experiencing GDM. This framework focuses on merging low-cost, energy-efficient Internet of Things (IoT) devices, Multi-modal analytics, and adaptive artificial Intelligence models to offer real-time Personalized care. At the sensing stage, this system employs affordable non-invasive gadgets that collect physiological data, including heart rate, sleep patterns, and daily activity, in addition to Bluetooth-enabled glucometers recording patients' daily finger sticks and glucose readings. To further substantiate the richness of patient monitoring, complementary data sources like dietary intake and symptom logs obtained with free, user-friendly mobile applications can also be assessed without establishing expensive clinical diagnostic equipment. Most importantly, the framework has been designed, using low-power OSI layers of the communication protocols (e.g., Bluetooth Low Energy), to reduce energy consumption, negative environmental impact, and, ultimately, support sustainable long-term use. Data from devices is uploaded to a hybrid cloud-edge computing architecture. Edge components complete rapid, local computations to enable alerts quickly and to eliminate latency, while cloud servers will handle storage for extensive archives, analytics, and analysis of big data for scaling to different healthcare situations. The combination configuration capabilities allow for the aggregation of multi-modal data to form a potential lifestyle, multiple physiological data, or simply glucose readings, and potentially predisposition or genetic information from electronic health records. Hence, the system would have a digital health profile that is continuously updated for each patient. The center of the SustaiGDM framework is the AI analytics to predict glycemic trends and to classify patients relating to GDM subtype or risk level. The AI component will inspect and use 'lighter weight' machine learning models (e.g., decision trees or hybrid architectures) to allow the SustaiGDM framework to achieve prediction accuracy while being environmentally aware of the computational and energy efficiency the framework could demonstrate in infrastructure settings. Models could provide an adaptive alert that allows for personalization of lifestyle changes and increases acknowledgment of clinicians to change care based on this adaptive monitoring and avoid harm for maternal and neonatal outcomes. The adaptive/personalized monitoring systems that exist within the AI component of SustaiGDM are not present in existing glucose monitoring systems. Some of these changes may be due to the model's recognition of changing risk patterns over time. The mobile app for patients will provide educational and accessible, actionable data for self-management that is easy to understand, while the clinician dashboard provides detailed answers to trend analyses and risk scores for clinical decision making. This two-faceted approach will enable continuous feedback for patients and the health care team. This model brings together low-cost IoT devices and adaptable AI models, an energy-efficient and straightforward, user-friendly interface to address the inequalities and limitations of current models. The main objective will be to prioritize cost-conscious, scalable, over time, and real-life applications. This is designed particularly for high-risk women in underprivileged settings. Importantly, this framework aims to provide timely, sustainable monitoring and management in GDM care, balancing technological advancements along with enhanced maternal and neonatal outcomes and reduced environmental impact.

Figure 1. SUSTAI-GDM Framework for Sustainable Monitoring of Gestational Diabetes Mellitus

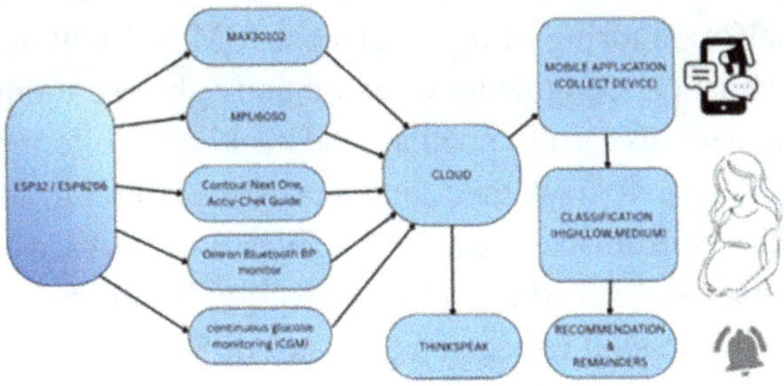

This graphic representation (Figure. 1) shows a single, AI-supported monitoring system for more efficient and sustainable management of GDM. The ESP32/ ESP8266 microcontroller provides the platform and is equipped with various low-cost IoT sensors to access a range of physiological information, providing more data than a person can get on their own. Sensors such as the MAX30102 and MPU6050 measure physiological signs of life, including heart rate, sleep, and activity time, while low-cost Bluetooth-enabled glucometer sensors, such as the Contour Next One, Accu-Chek Guide, and there are others, are used to measure daily glucose levels. There are additional devices used to gather even further information to create a full health profile from the patient: for example, Omron Bluetooth blood pressure monitors, continuous glucose monitoring (CGM) systems, and many more. Finally, data processed by the system can be visualized and shared using tools like ThingSpeak that encourage personalized care, early identification of risks, and fewer hospital visits with associated costs. This entire configuration has the ultimate goal of improving maternal and neonatal outcomes by providing real-time monitoring with sustainable, less expensive, and host-focused management.

TECHNOLOGIES USED

The SustaiGDM framework includes a wide variety of technologies to provide proactive, customized, and experienced surveillance for gestational diabetes during pregnancy (GDM). The SustaiGDM framework uses inexpensive, non-invasive Internet of Things (IoT) devices that constantly and in real-time collect multi-modal patient data, in contrast to the costly, invasive technological advances. The SustaiGDM framework's gadgets utilize commercially available wristbands or smartwatches, such as the Fitbit Inspire, Xiaomi Mi Band, or Apple Watch, that collect physiological data, such as heart rate, heart rate variability, daily steps, and sleep data.. The wearables are complemented with Bluetooth-enabled glucometers (e.g., Accu-Chek Instant Bluetooth, OneTouch Verio Reflect) that enable patients to perform routine self-monitoring of blood glucose (SMBG) without incurring the full expense and logistical complexity of continuous glucose monitoring (CGM) systems. Moreover, patients can use popular food tracking mobile applications (e.g., MyFitnessPal or Lifesum) to track their food intake, meal timing, and other related lifestyle factors. All of the devices make a low-power, low-cost sensing layer where the majority communicate over Bluetooth Low Energy (BLE) protocol, for minimal battery use and environmental impact. At the heart of SustaiGDM is an AI analytics and risk prediction layer, and it utilizes lightweight and interpretable machine learning (ML) models. There are many possible variables (e.g., decision trees, random forests, LSTMs, etc.) that can stratify patients by risk, and models such as decision trees and random forest models can also determine potential episodes of hyperglycemia. Stacked LSTMs or Autoregressive Integrated Moving Averages (ARIMA) can also be considered (i.e., these ML models can capture temporal trends in biological variation). The adaptive algorithms offer a real-time notification capability to notify patients of risk profiles and also apply the initial decision tree or random forests modeling to measure healthier behaviors in individuals. The AI/ML as well as AI/ML training nodes can utilize two forms of analytics that measure patterns at the individual patient level while informing real-time notification ability. The AI/ML activities may run partly on the edge for real-time notifications and partially in the cloud for more resource-intensive predictive forecasting, and use all available data for an individual patient. This approach meets the practicality between accuracy and sustainability for suspected potential individual hyperglycemia or low BG risk.The results of the AI analytics will be available on both a patient-facing mobile application as well as a clinician dashboard, or what is known as the "user interface" layer. The app allows patients to have a rich experience to view their glucose status from their weekly trends through regular and automatic reminders and notifications; this allows the patient to document their lifestyle and retrieve education about GDM. Some additional features include gamified, step goals, meal feedback, reminders about SMBG, and Physical activity, which support reinforcing participation. The clinician dashboards give an overall view of risk scores and analyze trends and adherence data, and these dashboards collectively provide another resource of information to intervene if warranted or appropriate. There are multilingual options and user-friendly visualizations, and some Manual entry data tools, and finally, this process includes tools for engaging patients to help them with self-management and continuity of care. The tools mentioned here create a synergetic patient focused ecosystem that blends data collection and analysis, to inform data-based decision making By leveraging low-cost, energy-efficient Internet of

Things (IoT) devices (e.g., wearables), interpretable, computationally light artificial intelligence (AI) models, user-friendly mobile apps, and real-time clinician dashboards, the SustaiGDM framework addressed the sustainability niche and personalization gap found in previous research. This combination produced a scalable, inexpensive model for monitoring and managing GDM that also incorporated cultural variations in health care utilization and focused on optimal maternal and neonatal outcomes via a preventative and sustainable health management approach. The SustaiGDM framework proposed for monitoring Gestational Diabetes Mellitus (GDM) is a layered, modular architecture for both sustainability and personalization of care. The components and functionalities proceed from data collection to secure integration and analysis, to engagement/feedback with patients and clinicians, thus establishing an ongoing learning loop. The SustaiGDM framework proposed for the lowest level is the IoT sensing layer, where various real-time data is captured from many different sources. Non-invasive wearable devices such as smartwatches will capture physiological signals related to heart rate, sleep, and physical activity. Moreover, Bluetooth-enabled glucometers will have daily SMBG data collected by participants, and mobile apps will capture it. Each of these devices was purposely chosen for its low-cost and low energy consumption characteristics and utilized communication protocols such as Bluetooth Low Energy to minimize battery consumption and environmental footprints—directly targeting the sustainability gap seen in existing GDM solutions that depend on and use high-priced and high-energy CGM systems. The framework is held together by the AI analytics and risk prediction layer, which examines multi-modal data using machine learning models. These models not only identify patterns and anticipate hyperglycemia episodes, but they also stratify patients based on GDM subtypes or patient-specific risks. For example, tree decision models, where possible, and light-weight hybrid LSTM architectures (Long Short-Term Memory) strike a balance between divisive predictive accuracy and computational resource efficiency. Taking into consideration sustainability means less processing, and therefore, more indirect energy use. Another significant component of utilizing a computational adaptive model is that, over time, the system becomes more tailored for patients, as it learns about their information. The sustainable environmental monitoring system for gestational diabetes mellitus (GDM) is designed around an integrated system of IoT-enabled wearable sensors, advanced AI and ML algorithms, a secure cloud framework, and patient-centered mobile applications. The framework is envisioned to be an integrated system that will provide continuous and real-time monitoring of maternal health, offer prospective risk predictions, and provide a tailored and personalized intervention while achieving long-term feasibility and sustainability. The various wearable and home health devices capture enhanced physiological and behavioral data connected with GDM management in the system. Continuous glucose monitoring (CGMs), like the Dexcom G6 or FreeStyle Libre, survey intervention glucose levels over time, providing insight and clarity regarding glycemic trends and variation in glucose levels. Wearable smartwatches and fitness bands can monitor daily steps, sleep quality, heart rate variability, and stress, and provide valuable information to the patient, providing a more holistic interpretation of lifestyle behaviors affecting glucose control. Digital blood pressure monitors measure maternal blood pressure and should be noted as a key transition in the detection of hypertension or preeclampsia. Additional health status indicators include smart weight scales that assess weekly weight trends and nutritional counseling. All the data displayed on these devices is sent using low-power wireless technologies such as Bluetooth Low Energy (BLE) to the patient's smartphone, which serves as the secure data hub. From the smartphone, the data are sent to a cloud-based storage service, treated in an anonymized and encrypted manner, to protect patient privacy and ensure compliance with applicable regulations, such as HIPAA and GDPR. The cloud architecture can scale to support real-time data with high throughput and allows for interfacing with Electronic Health Records (EHRs) and clinical systems. The AI and ML modules interrogate the fast stream of data that is continuous to facilitate support for personalized care. For example, classification algorithms (e.g., logistic regression, random forests, and support vector machines) can identify patients who are at high risk for complications, although at relatively high risk. Time-series forecasting, with RNNs and LSTMs, could identify safe glucose trajectories in the future. Lastly, clustering will characterize atypical cases of women with GDM related to both metabolic and behavioral processes of care to extract actionable insights that improve health trajectories for the woman, not the population, through an intervention. Overall, the system is developed with patient engagement in mind. A simple, easy-to-use mobile application will present real-time health data and trends, generate reminders (e.g., when to take medications, do glucose checks, and schedule appointments), and present informational materials on pregnancy and diabetes management. Examples of gamification tailored to patient needs, such as daily activity challenges and personalized individual goals, will incentivize patients to stay.The dashboard for clinicians collects, organizes, and visualizes all of the aggregated patient data over time while marking any abnormal trends and offering AI-enabled alerts to inform timely evidence-based decision making. Sustainability should be a consideration in the plans and implementation of any new and innovative monitoring systems for gestational diabetes mellitus (GDM). Sustainability includes the ability to provide long-term operation of the device, but sustainability also comprises the environmental, economic, and social dimensions that promote health equity and sustainability for meaningful impact. In summary, sustainable technology, as defined here, is much more than keeping the technology running; it is a multi-fold commitment to creating systems that fully consider a merging of social responsibility, environmental capacity, and economic viability. The proposed monitoring system will address these three dimensions in meeting the needs of individuals with GDM, while also establishing new practices toward a more equitable and resilient health system.

IMPLEMENTATION CONSIDERATIONS FOR PRACTICAL APPLICATIONS

Many factors must be derived with the practical application of GDM in order for the intervention to be effective, scalable, and ethical. The most prominent challenge of device consideration is interoperability. When selecting wearable devices and Bluetooth-compatible glucometers, the device's affordability, accuracy, and efficiency in the battery life of operating Bluetooth on a smartphone must be considered. The existence of open data standards and protocols to support interoperability is also key to effectively integrating patients in the EHR and clinical support systems. Data Privacy and security are equally important since we are dealing with sensitive data related to maternal and fetal health. Implementing a proper and appropriate encryption protocol, security authentication, and user-consent workflows must follow regulations like HIPAA or GDPR and build trust among users. Edge computing can enhance privacy by processing sensitive data and can reduce the volume of information transmitted to the external servers. A user-centric approach is important for both the patient mobile application and clinician dashboard interfaces, which need to be intuitive, multilingual, culturally considerate, and reduce data entry challenges while enhancing actionable insights. Includes features like gamification, reminders, and educational materials that can help boost patient engagement and long-term adherence. In terms of clinical integration, it is necessary to define roles and responsibilities clearly among the healthcare team. Alerts and recommendations given by the system should promote the system rather than replace clinical judgement. Pilot studies & Co-design workshops with health care providers can customize the system to align with local practices and avoid alert fatigue.

CONCLUSION

Gestational diabetes mellitus (GDM) still represents a significant burden in maternal and neonatal health care due to its complicated etiology and its short-term and long-term complications. This chapter introduced a holistic, sustainable monitoring system intended to enhance management of GDM in an integrated environment. The project described the use of Internet of Things (IoT) enabled wearable sensors to capture clinical physiological data, Artificial Intelligence (AI) and machine learning algorithms, and tools to drive patient engagement (and behavioral change). The monitoring system is intended to capture a multi-domain of physiological and behavioral data, e.g., glucose levels, level of activity, sleep hours and quality, and presence of stress, for purposes of risk prediction in real-time, personalized intervention, and clinical follow-up. The proposed monitoring system offers specific advantages over current monitoring systems, including an integrative data collection approach, predictive analytics, consideration for sustainability, and incorporates mobile applications to actively engage patients in their care. The study design and methods also address challenges related to privacy of information, fidelity and reliability of devices, user adherence, and integration into existing clinical protocols. Realizing the monitoring system as a product for clinical use is a collaborative process involving the effort of managers. Novel technologies, such as edge computing, federated learning, blockchain, and next-generation biosensors, can provide further beneficial contributions to the performance and scalability of any implementation while continuing to remain patient data secure. The system will also need additional validation with different datasets and a longer investigation of the accuracy of continued interventions for equity and real-world effectiveness. Ultimately, the merging of technology innovation and patient empowerment may impact the development of a sustainable monitoring system that brings about change in the management of GDM and improved outcomes.

REFERENCES

Lu, L., & Huang, T. (2022). Effects of early nursing monitoring on pregnancy outcomes of pregnant women with gestational diabetes mellitus under the Internet of Things. *Computational and Mathematical Methods in Medicine*, *2022*(1), 8535714. DOI: 10.1155/2022/8535714 PMID: 35693264

Nandini, K., & Rahimunnisa, K. (2025). Intelligent maternal-fetal healthcare monitoring and abnormality detection using deep belief networks optimized by a bacterial foraging algorithm. *Biomedical Signal Processing and Control*, *110*, 108175. DOI: 10.1016/j.bspc.2025.108175

Papri, N. J., Ahmed, A., & Chowdhury, A. (2025). IoT and cloud-based non-invasive diabetes detection system from photoplethysmogram. *Discover Internet of Things*, *5*(1), 57. DOI: 10.1007/s43926-025-00158-w

Pustozerov, E. A., Chernykh, V. Y., Popova, P. V., Vasyukova, E. A., Tkachuk, A. S., & Yuldashev, Z. M. (2020). Health monitoring system for patients with gestational diabetes mellitus based on nutrition diaries and fitness bracelets. *Biomedical Engineering*, *53*(5), 305–308. DOI: 10.1007/s10527-020-09931-3

Rigla, M., Martínez-Sarriegui, I., García-Sáez, G., Pons, B., & Hernando, M. E. (2018). Gestational diabetes management using smart mobile telemedicine. *Journal of Diabetes Science and Technology*, *12*(2), 260–264. DOI: 10.1177/1932296817704442 PMID: 28420257

Singh, G. (2025). Wearable IoT (w-IoT) artificial intelligence (AI) solution for sustainable smart healthcare. *International Journal of Information Management Data Insights*, *5*(1), 100291. DOI: 10.1016/j.jjimei.2024.100291

Yang, X., Liu, L., & Wang, Y. (2024). A decision tree-driven IoT system for improved prenatal diagnostic accuracy. *BMC Medical Informatics and Decision Making*, *24*(1), 375. DOI: 10.1186/s12911-024-02759-x PMID: 39639288

Chapter 16
Securing Data Using Alpha-Numeric Scrambling (ANS) Sequence Technique With Steganography

P. Vimala Devi
https://orcid.org/0000-0001-8422-6266
SRC, SASTRA University, India

V. Kalaichelvi
SRC, SASTRA University, India

D. Rubidha Devi
SRC, SASTRA University, India

ABSTRACT

Steganography, the practice of hiding information within non-secret data, appears to be a promising method for safeguarding sensitive medical information buried in diagnostic images. Steganographic techniques can be used in medical imaging to hide patient metadata, diagnostic notes, and digital watermarks in image files such as DICOM, X-ray, MRI, and CT scans. This allows for secure and seamless transmission across healthcare networks. A combination of encryption and steganography is proposed for secure transmission. First, the message is scrambled using Alpha Numeric Scrambling (ANS) Sequence technique and then encrypted. Then

DOI: 10.4018/979-8-3373-5641-9.ch016

the encrypted text is embedded in an image cover medium using the Two-bit LSB technique and transferred to the receiver. The performance of the proposed algorithm is evaluated in terms of entropy, peak signal to noise ratio and mean square error.

1. INTRODUCTION

In healthcare systems, the growing digitization and transmission of medical images require strong procedures to protect data security, integrity and patient privacy. Securing sensitive information is very important in current scenario, as every user intends to use an application in a secured manner. The sensitive and confidential information must be transmitted through the network in a reliable way. The salient information must not be perceived by an intruder and cause vulnerability. Cryptography and Steganography provide a path to transmit information in a protected manner.

Cryptography is the process of encrypting information using a key(Arya & Soni, 2022). This encrypted information is transmitted between the sender and receiver. During this transmission, to add extra security, steganography techniques are included. Combining cryptography and steganography techniques increases the protection of the sensitive information. Cryptography techniques are classified into key-based, cipher-based, transformation-based, visual cryptography, and hybrid techniques (Gupta et al., 2025). The Key-based techniques are asymmetric key and symmetric key cryptography. Symmetric key cryptosystems use a single key, between the sender and receiver, whereas in asymmetric cryptosystems, two keys are used. There are two types of cipher-based systems, block ciphers and stream ciphers. A block cipher processes the blocks or bytes of information, stream cipher processes bit by bit.

Steganography is the process of hiding information in a cover medium. The cover medium is image, text, audio and video. The characteristics of steganography are embedding capacity, imperceptibility and robustness. The amount of secret data embedded into a cover medium is called embedding capacity. Robustness determines the strength of the steganography method against attacks. Imperceptibility ensures the quality of the stego image that there is a minimum difference between the original and stego image in visual representation.

The secret message hidden in the nth letter of the words given in the text message is known as text steganography. It ensures quick transmission of files and uses less memory to store files.

Video steganography hides the data in a video(Liu et al., 2019). Based on the embedding positions, it is categorized into pre-embedding, post-embedding and intra-embedding. In pre-embedding, the messages are embedded into raw video and in post-embedding, bit positions are used. Compression methods are used in intra-embedding, which uses Discrete Cosine Transform (DCT) coefficients, motion estimation and intra-prediction for video processing.

The steganography techniques are classified into transform domain, spatial domain, statistical, vector embedding, spread spectrum, masking and filtering. Spatial domain techniques use an image as a cover medium, changing bit positions in the image to hide data. Least significant bit (LSB) insertion, pixel value differencing and binary pattern complexity are the techniques used in the spatial domain. LSB insertion is a simple technique that replaces the least significant bits of pixels present in the cover image with secret data bits. The pixel value differencing method determines the embedding capacity by calculating the difference between the adjacent pixels. A high amount of secret data is concealed in the edge regions of an image and fewer bits are in the smooth regions. Statistical technique splits the cover medium into blocks, then embeds one bit of data for each block. Distortion techniques use an encoder to perform modification in a cover medium and a decoder to extract the original information. The discrete cosine transform (DCT), discrete Fourier transform (DFT) and discrete wavelet transform (DWT) are transform domain techniques that describe the frequency components of an image. The discrete Fourier transform converts time signals into discrete frequencies. These methods transform a finite list of uniformly spaced function samples into a list of complex sinusoids' coefficients arranged according to their frequencies. The signal or image is converted from the spatial domain to the frequency domain using DCT. The pixels are changed by the mathematical transformations so that the position of the pixel values appears to be spread throughout a portion of the image. DWT determines the high-frequency and low-frequency information of every pixel in the image during the steganography process. It is a mathematical tool for hierarchically breaking down an image. Its primary function is to process non-stationary signals.

2. LITERATURE SURVEY

This section explains various techniques used in the field of cryptography and steganography.

A bit stuffing technique is proposed, which appends a random binary string in the ciphertext obtained from the modified RSA algorithm (Mojisola et al., 2022). A modified RSA algorithm uses three prime numbers p, q, r for key generation, encryption and decryption. The limitations of this work is that the code rate is unpredictable and the insertion of additional bits in the data stream leads to a waste of bandwidth. (Basu et al., 2019) Combined biological features and machine learning techniques to provide storage and security. Bidirectional Associative Memory Neural Network (BAMNN) and DNA cryptography is utilized for secure encryption and decryption.

This method generates keys efficiently and simulates transcription, translation and genetic coding. It achieves integrity, authentication and confidentiality and high security against various attacks.

Hiding information in a text is also a type of steganography, known as text steganography. The cover media depends on the language used. Languages differ in their style of writing, characteristics and properties. The various texts used for writing scripts are Japanese scripts, Bengali texts for the Indian context, Arabic texts, Thai scripts, Polish scripts and Chinese stroke characters. (Alifah Roslan et al., 2022) reviewed the use of Arabic text in steganography. They highlighted the properties and characteristics of Arabic text, methods used in Arabic text steganography and an approach to combine cryptography with Arabic text steganography. The characteristics of the Arabic text are shape, dots, edges, Kashida and Diacritics that determine the position to hide data. Scrambling is applied before hiding the data, which replaces the letters in the plain text with other letters and converts them into hexadecimal values, and finally converts the hexadecimal values to ASCII values (Osamor & Edosomwan, 2021). It is limited only to uppercase letters. The art of concealing a message in an image is known as image steganography. An image steganography method is proposed to detect edges in the cover image for embedding data(Sun, 2016). Huffman encoding is used for data compression. This method allows for hiding enormous amount of secret message in an image. But the system is complex in design and requires high processing time. Blockchain technique is merged with image steganography to attain secure authentication (Patwari et al., 2025). It uses the eXtended Differences of Gaussians edge detection, which collects the parameters like brightness, contrast and edge thickness. The performance metrics, such as PSNR, payload and SSIM values, are calculated and the results indicate that the method produces high-quality images and security. Also it balances image integrity and embedding capacity.

Hiding secret message into a video is known as video steganography. It utilizes stable features within the frames and in between the frames. Coverless video steganography is based on object tracking and pose estimation(Li et al., 2024). This method enhances concealment, by assessing the intra-frame and inter-frame aspects of human posture in videos that portray human activities. Pose estimation networks are first used by the system to locate the target individuals. Following that, a filtering method is used to find and prioritize tracking targets with bigger areas, ensuring tracking robustness, and a multi-object tracking technique is used to track the identified targets inside the movie. Then, using the tracking targets' intra-frame angle features and inter-frame movement direction, matching hash mapping rules are created. In order to match carrier films with the hidden information and full information hiding more quickly, an inverted index is finally built. According to experimental data, the proposed approach outperforms the most recent techniques in terms of hiding capacity and robustness against a range of conventional attacks, frame dropping attacks and video compression attacks.

Healthcare data is sensitive and requires secure transmission. To achieve this, a bit mask-oriented genetic algorithm method is combined with steganography techniques(Pandey, 2020). The steps are that the patient's information is encrypted and then concealed in a cover image using discrete wavelet transform techniques. The performance of the algorithm is compared using metrics like peak-signal-to-noise ratio, mean square error, Bit error rate and correlation. The results show that the algorithm performs well when compared to existing techniques. (Shah et al., 2022) constructed an S-Box to improve the security of data embedded into the steganography techniques. The statistical results demonstrate the robust performance of the algorithm against attacks and high-quality steganography with a minimal number of errors.

Wireless Body Area Networks (WBANs) are a part of medical cyber-physical systems, which monitor patient information through sensors and communication technologies (Masdari et al., 2024). They are an integral part of the e-healthcare system, guaranteeing the security and privacy of the medical data. The features from the electrocardiogram (ECG) signals, such as ST and QT intervals, are utilized for key generation and authentication. Next, steganography-based techniques, such as the discrete wavelet transform, curvelet transform, and Fourier transform, are used to hide the patient's data in ECG signals. The higher randomness, entropy and lower computation time are attained using this algorithm.

DNA-based cryptography and steganography methods are used to secure the data collected and shared through the Internet of Things (IoT)(Namasudra, 2022). The DNA bases, namely Adenine (A), Cytosine (C), Thymine (T) and Guanine (G) are used to encode the plaintext instead of using binary patterns. Then the encrypted message is embedded into various positions of another DNA sequence. This method is called as DNA steganography. It increases the security of data used in cloud systems. (Aparna & Madhumitha, 2023) integrated steganography and cryptography methods to protect digital images. There are two stages in the encryption process: first, the plaintext is converted to ciphertext using DNA cryptography. In the second stage, the cover medium is also encrypted and then embedded using multiple combined chaotic maps. The high value of PSNR, SSIM and entropy and low correlation values determine the performance of the proposed method and offer high random and embedding capacity.

The well-known genomic DNA has recently been used as a hiding medium (DNA steganography) because of its amazing ability to conceal large data sets with a high degree of unpredictability and, consequently, security(Marwan et al., 2016). The vigenere cipher and the DNA-based playfair cipher have been integrated with DNA steganography, leaving opportunities for further research into additional methods and the development of further enhancements. The DNA-based playfair, vigenere, RSA, and AES ciphers are all thoroughly compared along with a DNA concealment approach. The results of the investigation show how well each combination technique performs in terms of speed, security, hiding capacity, data size, and key size. (Brunet, 2016) surveyed the methods used in biosteganography. In this, the biological mediums are used to transmit the sealed data. The methods are redesigned from molecular biology, genetics, computer science and biochemistry. The author also addresses the ways in which biological materials, such as proteins, DNA, and RNA, as well as biological storage systems, such as cells, biofilms, and entire organisms, can be used to encode and preserve information. The elements that make these biotechnologies practical and useful in everyday life is also explained.

A hybrid encryption algorithm is developed to demonstrate the authentication process in IoT environment (Patil et al., 2022). Two sets of algorithms are used to form the hybrid encryption. One method consists of Advanced Encryption Standard (AES) and elliptic curve cryptography, while the other is AES and Rivest-Shamir-Adleman (RSA) algorithm. Computation, communication and storage costs are the measures used to analyse the efficiency and security of the algorithm. The hybrid encryption scores a low computation cost and storage cost, which guarantees secure data transfer. The system lacks some of the security features.

Modern cyber threats have made it more challenging to secure health data hosted in the cloud, including DNA sequences, patient data, and treatment histories. Steganography, a technique for hiding sensitive data by combining it with other data, is one way to deal with this issue. Although there are disadvantages to these strategies, recent research has looked into concealing sensitive information within DNA sequences. They either result in a large increase in the amount of data that must be added to the original DNA sequence or fail to produce an adequate cover from the changed sequence, also known as the stego DNA sequence. Certain techniques even unintentionally introduce the original cover or secret information into the stego DNA sequence, posing security problems. To overcome these limitations machine learning based steganography technique is proposed. The system uses bit-shuffling to improve message security and machine learning algorithms for secret encryption, which increases resistance to cyberattacks(Nahar et al., 2023). The technique also permits hiding different kinds of messages. This technique achieves a reduced stego growth rate in comparison to current techniques. A recently developed parity check technique also improves security by guarding against stego DNA modifications, including man-in-the-middle, chosen stego, and modification attacks. The Table describes the summary of few Literatures mentioned above:

Table 1. Comparative Analysis of Existing Techniques

	Techniques Used	**Demerits**	**Computation Complexity**	**Use of Resource-constrained devices**
Sun	Huffman Encoding	Limited edges degrade the performance Limited Scalability	High	Less suitable
Suyel Namasudra	DNA Cryptography and Steganography	Migration Issues in Cloud –IoT Platform	Less	Suitable
Patwari et al.,	Blockchain based Steganography	Higher processing time and high cost	High	Less Suitable
Basu et al.	DNA Cryptography and BAMNN network	Higher Processing time and cost. Limited Scalability	Complex in implementation	Suitable
Shah et al.	S-Box and P-Box with steganography	Requires more resources for implementing S and P- Boxes High Processing time	High	Suitable

Table 1 summarizes that most techniques require high processing time, are less scalable and have design complexity. The proposed algorithm overcomes these disadvantages and is suitable to support the use of resource-constrained devices.

3. MOTIVATION AND OBJECTIVE

Securing sensitive data has become important in today's digital environment as users seek more and more services that offer strong data protection. When sent over public networks, sensitive and private data is extremely susceptible to being intercepted and used by malevolent hackers. Thus, it is essential to use techniques that ensure data transfer security and dependability. Steganography and cryptography are two well-known methods that offer complementary secure communication ways. While steganography hides the information's existence within a harmless cover medium, lowering the chance of detection, cryptography concentrates on converting information into an unreadable form to preserve confidentiality and integrity. The overall security and resilience of the communication system can be improved by combining these two strategies. The proposed work makes use of this combination to provide confidentiality, authentication, and resistance to intrusion attacks, resulting in enhanced data protection. In particular, the application of Alpha

Numerical Scrambling (ANS) greatly increases the unpredictability of the data by presenting diffusion and confusion. Moreover, steganographic embedding and the use of an improved public key technique guarantee that the data is transferred in a very safe and reliable way. This two-pronged strategy offers both confidentiality and authentication, providing a complete defense against a variety of security flaws.

4. SYSTEM ARCHITECTURE

The architecture of the proposed work, shown in Figure 1, consists of three stages. The first stage, Alpha-Numeric Scrambling (ANS) Sequence, uses the secret message as input, scrambles it using a mapping table, and transforms it to the corresponding hexadecimal representation. Afterwards, the hexadecimal values are changed to corresponding ASCII values. Then this ASCII code is applied for Enhanced ElGamal (EEG) Encryption. Then the encrypted text is embedded in a cover medium using a 2-bit LSB technique. The stego image is transferred to the receiver side. Then, the encrypted text is extracted from the stego image using a 2-bit LSB technique. Then, an enhanced ElGamal decryption and reverse scrambling sequence is applied to recover the original secret message.

Figure 1. System Architecture>

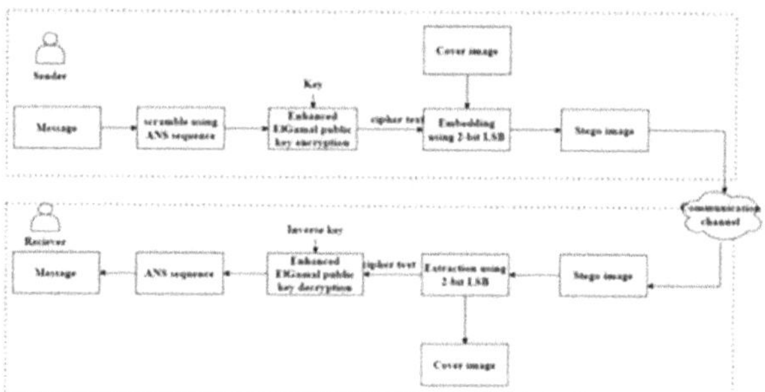

4.1 Alpha–Numeric Scrambling (ANS) Sequence

Alphanumeric scrambling is a reversible technique that employs a key-dependent approach to transform a message consisting only of letters (A–Z, a–z) and numbers (0–9) into a random sequence. This ensures that only the person with the right key can recover the original content. Establishing a fixed alphanumeric set is usually the first step in the procedure. Next, using a secret key that acts as a replacement table for changing each character in the message, a permutation of this set is created. The process of the ANS sequence is depicted in Figure 2

Figure 2. Block Diagram of ANS

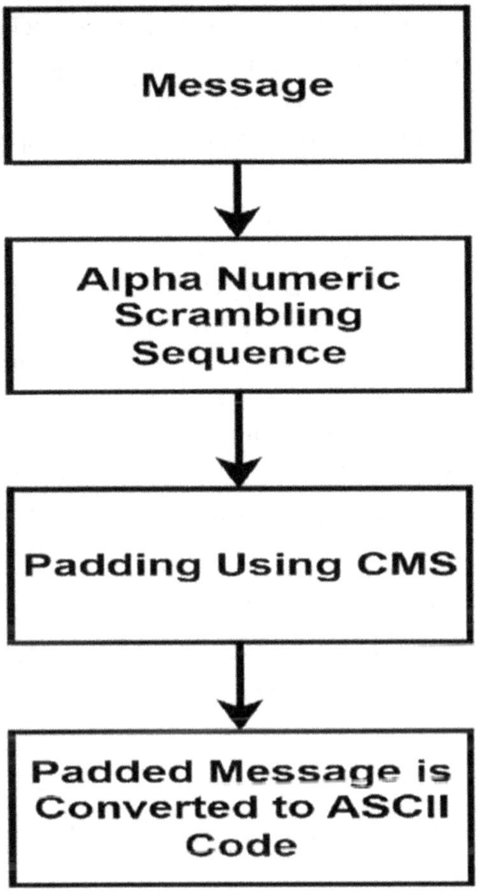

The message from the sender undergoes a scrambling process based on a key, which includes substitution and permutation. Substitution is the process of changing each letter or number with a different character from an alphabet table that has been jumbled using a secret key. Position permutation is an optional technique that involves rearranging the characters' order using a pseudo-random sequence that is seeded with the key. The scrambled message is encrypted after padding.

4.2 Encryption

The encryption process utilized the Diffie-Hellman algorithm for key exchange and the Enhanced Elgamal algorithm for encryption. Diffie-Hellman key exchange protocol, which enables two users to create a shared key without sending it directly to establish a secure communication via an insecure channel. To preserve confidentiality, this shared key can thereafter be used for encryption and decryption. An attacker would find it computationally challenging to extract the secret key from the shared public data since the protocol depends on the complexity of the discrete logarithm issue.

The Elgamal cryptosystem is a public key cryptosystem. A large prime number (q) and a primitive root (g) are chosen and shared between sender and receiver. Sender generates public key using his private key(X) and primitive root (g) and it is shared with the receiver ($Y_A=g^x$ mod q). The receiver generates one key using his private key (K) and the public key of the sender ($k=Y_A^K$ mod q). Then, two ciphertexts are generated, C1 and C2. ($C1=g^k$ mod q) (C2=k.m mod q). The receiver recovers the plain text by having the inverse key and his private key ($K=C1^X$ mod q), ($M=C2.k^{-1}$ mod q). The pseudocode for the Elgamal cryptosystem is given in Algorithm1 (given in Appendix A) and the steps are shown in the Figure 3.

Figure 3. Block Diagram of EEG Encryption

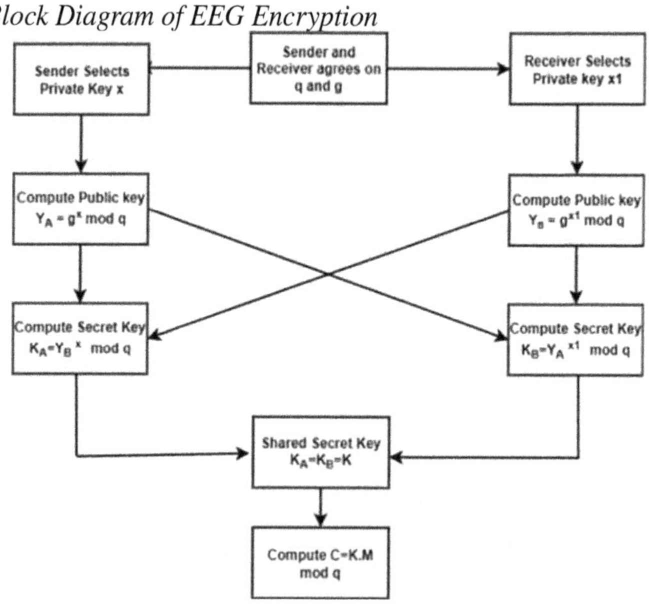

4.3 Steganography

Steganography is a technique of hiding data in images, audio, video and text. Image steganography is more familiar, which hides the data in an image pixel. Steganography follows two approaches, namely Embedding and Extraction. Least bit Steganography is a prominent technique used for image Steganography. Here, the sender chooses the cover image to embed the data, called a stego image and it is sent to the receiver.

4.3.1. 2-Bit LSB Embedding:

2-Bit Least Significant bit technique replaces the last two bits of red, green, and blue channels in each pixel with the message bits in the cover image. This allows three bits of data to be embedded in a pixel area for a coloured image. When the least significant bits are changed, only a slight variation is observed and it cannot be recognized by intruders.

4.4 Embedding into an Image

The cover medium for the 2-bit LSB image steganography technique is a color image with dimensions M × N. The basic prerequisite is that the cover image must be large enough to fit the complete secret message, keeping the image's size larger than the data that needs to be hidden. Only the RGB channels of the image are used for the embedding procedure. In order to begin, the secret message is separated into blocks of eight bits. In the first color channel i.e red channel, the first two bits of each byte are inserted into the seventh and eighth least significant bit locations.

The next two bits i.e third and fourth bits are positioned in the seventh and eighth bit locations of the second color channel known as green channel, and the next two bits are concealed in the Blue channel. Until all of the secret data is inserted, this procedure is repeated one after the other across the pixels. Although the generated stego-picture looks nearly the same as the cover image, it contains the concealed message. The stego-image can then be sent over a communication channel after embedding, and the receiver can use the inverse method to extricate it later. This method offers a greater data capacity than conventional 1-bit LSB techniques while preserving decent perceptual quality. Figure 4 shows the steps of the embedding process

Figure 4. Block Diagram of Embedding Process

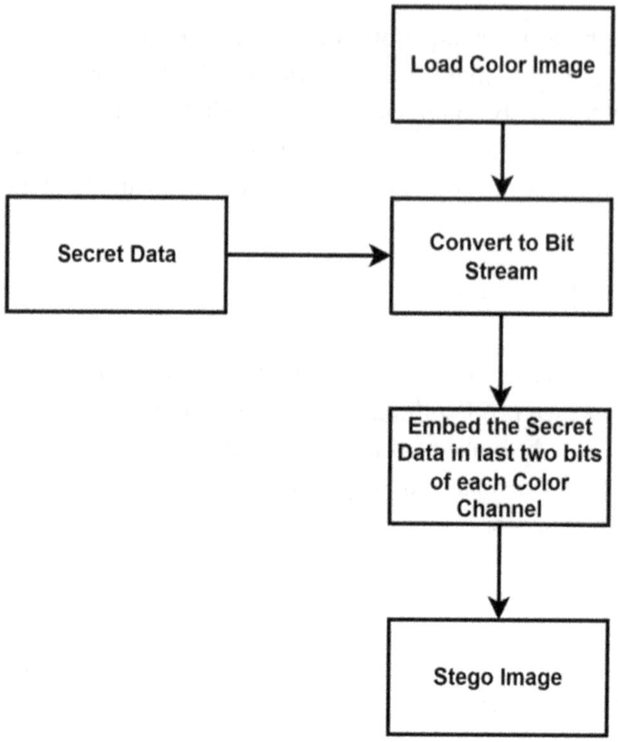

4.5 Extraction Process

It is process of extracting the original message at the receiver side. The stego-image, which holds the hidden message, is obtained first in the extraction technique. Next, a sequential scan of the image is performed, pixel by pixel. Since the two least significant bits were previously used to incorporate the secret information, they are retrieved for each pixel and placed in an array. After gathering all the necessary bits, the array is divided into 8-bit segments, each of which represents a single binary letter. After that, the original hidden message from the stego-image is gradually reconstructed using these 8-bit groups, which are transformed into their respective characters. This technique ensures that the hidden data can be reliably recovered without compromising the image's visual impact and the steps are shown in Figure 5.

Figure 5. Block Diagram of LSB Extraction

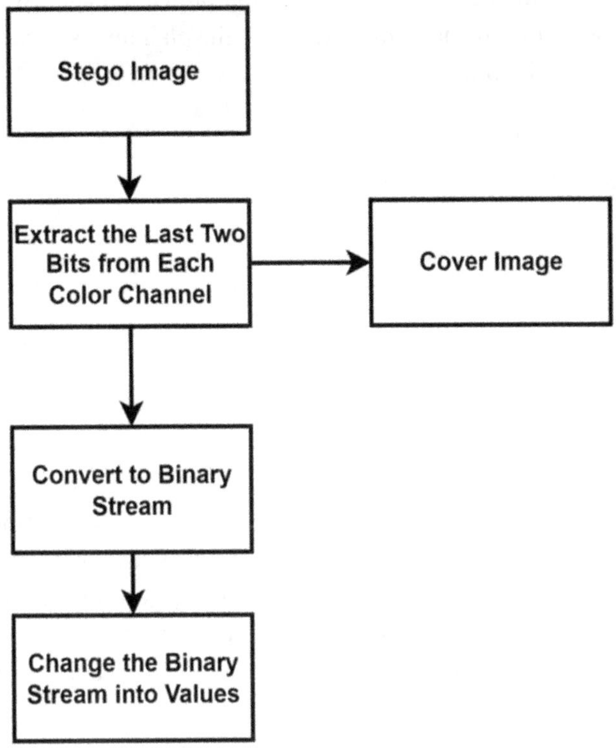

4.6 ElGamal Decryption

Decryption is the reverse process of encryption at the receiver side. It is applied to the encrypted message after extracting from the stego-image. The Diffie-Hellman based exchange algorithm is used to share the secret key between the sender and the receiver. Using that key the message is decrypted and the steps are given in Algorithm 2 (Given in Appendix A).

4.7 ANS Unscrambling

The final step of decryption is accurately reconstructing the original plain text by unscrambling the deciphered alphanumeric symbols (ANS). This phase restores the right symbol sequence while maintaining message integrity by acting as the opposite of the special scrambling process used during encryption. By adding an extra transformation layer and making it much harder for adversaries to decipher the information without knowing the scrambling function, ANS unscrambling helps to improve security. In addition to strengthening protection against statistical and differential assaults, our method guarantees that the plaintext is accurately restored in its original semantic form.

5. RESULTS & DISCUSSION

5.1 Performance Metrics

The performance of the proposed work is compared in terms of entropy, NPCR, peak signal-to-noise ratio and Mean square error.

5.1.1. Entropy

It is the measure of randomness. It determines the amount of information contained in the image. The adaption level of intensity that each pixel of an image can accept. The stronger performance of the encryption algorithm can be determined by higher values of entropy shown in Table 2 and Figure 6, which compares the entropy values of original image i.e cover image and stego image. The formula used to calculate the entropy is given in equation 1.

Entropy=-

$$\sum_{i=1}^{m} pi \log2 pi \qquad (1)$$

Where pi is the normalized histogram values of an image.

Table 2. Comparison of Entropy Values

Images	Original Image Entropy	Stego Entropy
Fox_128.jpeg	6.332	6.332
Apple_128.jpeg	6.552	6.569
Panda_128.jpeg	5.005	5.007
Star_256.jpeg	3.929	3.940
Woman_256.jpeg	7.757	7.757
Einstein_256.jpeg	6.228	6.228
Bird_512.jpeg	2.857	2.862

continued on following page

Table 2. Continued

Images	Original Image Entropy	Stego Entropy
Burger_512.jpeg	7.320	7.320
Capsicum_512.jpg	7.718	7.718

Figure 6. Graphical Representation of Entropy Values

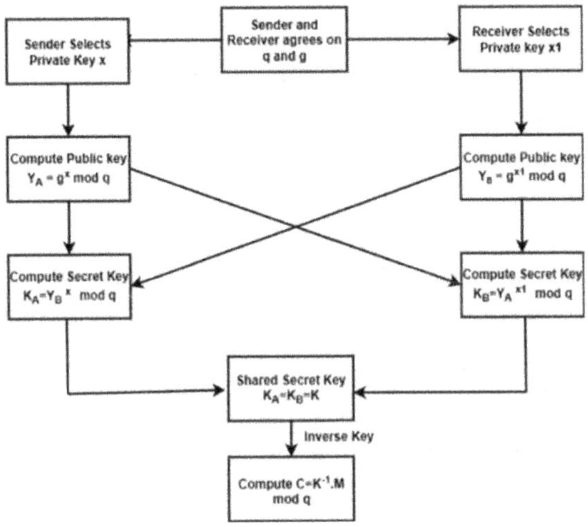

The results from the table1 and Figure 6 demonstrates that thc entropy between cover and stego images is nearly identically preserved by the steganographic process. It is difficult to identify hidden data using cntropy-based analysis since this suggests that the hidden data embedding does not substantially change statistical features.

PSNR Value:

Peak signal -to-noise Ratio (PSNR) is the ratio between the maximum intensity of images and the mean squared error of the images. It determines the quality of an image and calculated using equation 2.

PSNR=

$$10 \log_{10}\left(\frac{MAX^2}{MSE}\right) \quad (2)$$

Here, MAX-maximum intensity of pixels, MSE-Mean Squared Error.

MSE Value:

Mean Squared Error (MSE) is the squared difference between average of Stego image values and the cover image values.

MSE=

$$\frac{1}{m \times n} \sum_{i=0}^{m-1} \sum_{j=0}^{n-1} [I(i,j) - K(i,j)]^2 \tag{3}$$

Here, m, n denotes the row and column of image pixels; I, K denotes the cover and stego image values.

NPCR Value:

Number of Pixel Change Rate (NPCR) is the number of pixels got changed from cover image to stego-image.

NPCR= $\frac{\sum_{i=1}^{M} \sum_{j=1}^{N} D(i,j)}{M \times N} \times 100$

where D(i,j) is an indicator function that equals 1 if the pixel values differ at position (i,j) and 0 otherwise. The values for NPCR, PSNR and MSE are tabulated in Table 3 and Figure [8-9].

Table 3. Comparison of NPCR, PSNR and MSE Values

Images	NPCR	PSNR	MSE
Fox_128.jpeg	**0.011**	**67.548**	**0.011**
Apple_128.jpeg	**0.0111**	**67.65**	**0.0111**
Panda_128.jpeg	**0.011**	**67.579**	**0.011**
Star_256.jpeg	0.002	73.600	0.002
Woman_256.jpeg	0.002	73.42	0.002
Einstein_256.jpeg	0.002	73.373	0.002
Bird_512.jpeg	7.09×e-04	79.621	7.09×e-04
Burger_512.jpeg	7.565×e-04	79.3922	7.565×e-04
Capsicum_512.jpg	7.057×e-04	79.622	7.057×e-04

Figure 7. Graphical representation of PSNR values

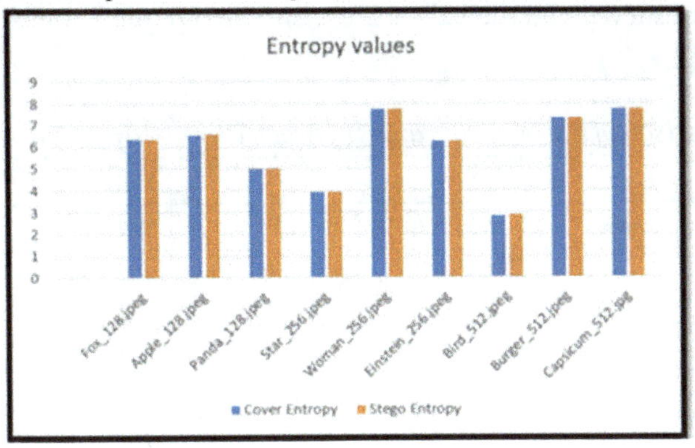

Figure 8. Graphical representation of NPCR and MSE values

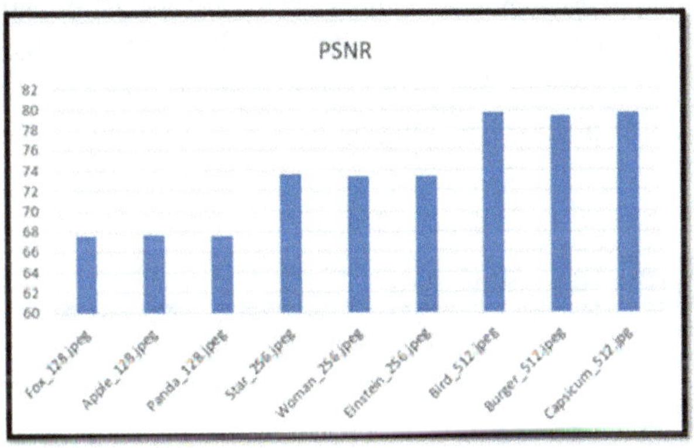

NPCR, PSNR, and MSE measures are used to evaluate performance, and the results show how effective the proposed steganographic method is. As can be seen in Table 2 and Figure [7-8], all test images have PSNR values between 67 and 79 dB, which is much higher than the generally used cutoff of 40 dB. This indicates good imperceptibility and preservation of visual quality. Pixel-wise differences between cover and stego pictures are insignificant, as confirmed by the corresponding MSE values, which range from 0.011 to 7.56×10−4. The NPCR values show that only a small percentage of pixels were altered during data embedding, staying extremely close to zero and ranging from 0.011 for smaller images to around 10^{-4} for larger images. All of these findings support the notion that the system is appropriate for real-world covert communication applications since it provides high security and invisibility, maintains statistical features, and introduces very little distortion. The proposed algorithm is also compared against with the existing techniques present in the Literature survey and the values are mentioned in the Table 4.

Table 4: Comparison of PSNR, MSE values between Proposed and Existing Techniques

	PSNR	**MSE**
S-P Box with Steganography	36.2 -37.9	38.2
DNA Cryptography and Steganography	44.92-55.15	0.41-2.29
SPT	42-92-51.15	1.27-3.18
DNA based Steganography	43.18-53.64	1.93-2.90
ANS+EEG+LSB	67.5-79.6	0.01-7.09×e-04

The table indicates that the proposed system has a smallest distortion between the images shows that the concealed information is not detectable by the human eye.

The security of the proposed algorithm is also analysed using statistical tests like histogram analysis. The histogram representation between the original image and the stegoimage for an Apple_128.jpeg is shown in the following Figure 9. In this the x-axis consists of pixel values ranging from 0 to 255 and the y-axis represents the intensities.

Figure 9. **Histogram Representation**

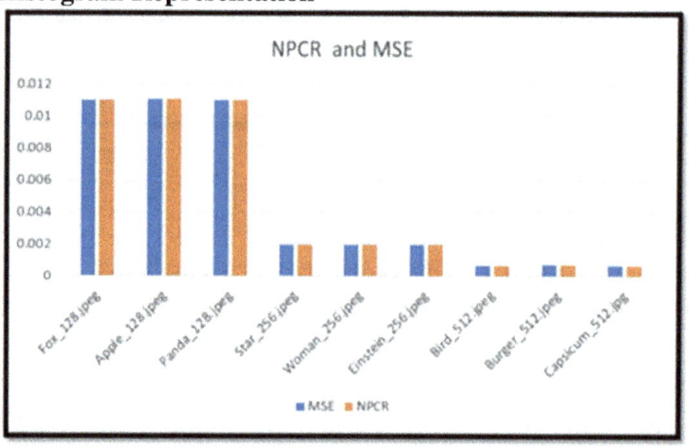

The histogram of the original and stego images shows that the pixel intensities are distributed identically across the range. The statistical features of the stego image are compatible with those of the original image, making it difficult for the intruder to observe the concealed data. There are no new peaks in the histograms, indicating that the smaller modifications occurred during the embedding process, which maintains the characteristics of the images like brightness, mean and variance.

The Enhanced ElGamal algorithm uses modular arithmetic, which guarantees nonlinear patterns in ciphertext and satisfies the avalanche effect with a value of 50.99%. This indicates that the minor modifications in the input generate random patterns in the ciphertext.

Inferences

The proposed work ensures three-level security by combining techniques from cryptography and steganography. Diffusion is offered at the character level using Alphanumeric scrambling which guarantees that the message is statistically obscured. The encryption algorithm generates the nonlinear patterns of the ciphertext and protects against attacks. The metrics like PSNR, entropy, MSE and NPCR values preserves the randomness in pixel positions ensures secure transmission, maintains quality with minimum distortion and protects against the attacks.

CONCLUSION

A robust cryptosystem is proposed to strengthen the security of the medical data by combining cryptography and steganography. The methods used are ANS scrambling, Enhanced Elgamal Encryption and 2-bit LSB embedding in an image. The message is scrambled using ANS scrambling and then encrypted using EEG encryption. Then it is concealed in an image. The performance of the proposed algorithm is measured using Peak signal to noise ratio, Mean square error and Number of pixel change rate. The results that the system offers high security, maintains image quality, guarantees that modifications are statistically invisible and makes it suitable for medical data transmission. In the future, the work can be extended to combine blockchain and machine learning based methods for secure transmission of medical images.

REFERENCES

Alifah Roslan, N., Izura Udzir, N., Mahmod, R., & Gutub, A. (2022). Systematic literature review and analysis for Arabic text steganography method practically. *Egyptian Informatics Journal*, *23*(4), 177–191. DOI: 10.1016/j.eij.2022.10.003

Aparna, H., & Madhumitha, J. (2023). Combined image encryption and steganography technique for enhanced security using multiple chaotic maps ☆. *Computers & Electrical Engineering*, *110*(February), 108824. DOI: 10.1016/j.compeleceng.2023.108824

Arya, A., & Soni, S. (2022). A Literature Review on Various Recent Steganography Techniques A Literature Review on Various Recent Steganography Techniques. September.

Basu, S., Karuppiah, M., Nasipuri, M., & Kumar, A. (2019). Bio-inspired cryptosystem with DNA cryptography and neural networks. *Journal of Systems Architecture*, *94*(February), 24–31. DOI: 10.1016/j.sysarc.2019.02.005

Brunet, T. D. P. (2016). Aims and methods of biosteganography. *Journal of Biotechnology*, *226*, 56–64. DOI: 10.1016/j.jbiotec.2016.03.044

Gupta, T., Selwal, A., & Sharma, A. K. (2025). A survey on image cryptography mechanisms : Hitherto, and future directions. *Computer Science Review*, *58*(January), 100783. DOI: 10.1016/j.cosrev.2025.100783

Li, N., Qin, J., Xiang, X., & Tan, Y. (2024). Journal of Information Security and Applications Robust coverless video steganography based on pose estimation and object tracking. *Journal of Information Security and Applications*, *87*(November), 103912. DOI: 10.1016/j.jisa.2024.103912

Liu, Y., Liu, S., Wang, Y., Zhao, H., & Liu, S. (2019). Neurocomputing Video steganography : A review. *Neurocomputing*, *335*, 238–250. DOI: 10.1016/j.neucom.2018.09.091

Marwan, S., Shawish, A., & Nagaty, K. (2016). BioSystems DNA-based cryptographic methods for data hiding in DNA media. *Bio Systems*, *150*, 110–118. DOI: 10.1016/j.biosystems.2016.08.013

Masdari, M., Band, S. S., Qasem, S. N., Sayed, B. T., & Pai, H. T. (2024). ECG signals-based security and steganography approaches in WBANs: A comprehensive survey and taxonomy. Sustainable Computing: Informatics and Systems, 41(April 2023), 100937. https://doi.org/DOI: 10.1016/j.suscom.2023.100937

Mojisola, F. O., Misra, S., Febisola, C. F., Abayomi-Alli, O., & Sengul, G. (2022). An improved random bit-stuffing technique with a modified RSA algorithm for resisting attacks in information security (RBMRSA). *Egyptian Informatics Journal*, *23*(2), 291–301.

Nahar, M., Kamal, A. H. M., & Hossain, G. (2023). Journal of Network and Computer Applications Protecting health data in the cloud through steganography : A table-driven, blind method using neural networks and bit-shuffling algorithm . *Journal of Network and Computer Applications*, *217*(May), 103689. DOI: 10.1016/j.jnca.2023.103689

Namasudra, S. (2022). A secure cryptosystem using DNA cryptography and DNA steganography for the cloud-based IoT infrastructure. Computers and Electrical Engineering, 104(PA), 108426. https://doi.org/DOI: 10.1016/j.compeleceng.2022.108426

Osamor, V. C., & Edosomwan, I. B. (2021). Employing scrambled alpha-numeric randomization and RSA algorithm to ensure enhanced encryption in electronic medical records. *Informatics in Medicine Unlocked*, •••, 25.

Pandey, H. M. (2020). Secure medical data transmission using a fusion of bit mask oriented genetic algorithm, encryption and steganography. *Future Generation Computer Systems*, *111*, 213–225. DOI: 10.1016/j.future.2020.04.034

Patil, K. S., Mandal, I., & Rangaswamy, C. (2022). Hybrid and Adaptive Cryptographic-based secure authentication approach in IoT based applications using hybrid encryption. *Pervasive and Mobile Computing*, *82*, 101552. DOI: 10.1016/j.pmcj.2022.101552

Patwari, B., Nandi, U., Dey, S., Dhar, S., Ghosal, S. K., & Si, T. (2025). Blockchain-Integrated Image Steganography using xDoG Edge Detection for Authentication. *Cyber Security and Applications*, *3*(March), 100091. DOI: 10.1016/j.csa.2025.100091

Shah, D., Shah, T., Naseer, Y., Jamal, S. S., & Hussain, S. (2022). Cryptographically strong S-P boxes and their application in steganography. *Journal of Information Security and Applications*, *67*(April), 103174. DOI: 10.1016/j.jisa.2022.103174

Sun, S. (2016). A novel edge based image steganography with 2 k correction and Huffman encoding. *Information Processing Letters*, *116*(2), 93–99. DOI: 10.1016/j.ipl.2015.09.016

APPENDIX A

Algorithm 1

Enhanced Elgamal Encryption

Input: Prime number, primitive root

Output: Ciphertext

Step 1: Two parties, sender A and receiver B agree upon a prime number q and a primitive root g. (g<q)

Step 2: Sender A chooses one random number x (private key) x<q and calculates public key YA=gx mod q

Step 3: B chooses one random number x1 (private key) and calculates public key YB=gx1 mod q

Step 4: Both parties share their public keys, mutually and calculate a common shared secret key KA=Y_A^x mod q & KB=Y_B^x1 mod q, whereas KA=KB=K.

Step 5: Using this key, compute cipher text C=K.M mod q where M<q

Algorithm 2

Diffie-Hellman based Enhanced Elgamal Decryption

Input: Ciphertext

Output: Plaintext

Step 1: Two parties, sender A and receiver B agree upon a prime number q and a primitive root g. (g<q)

Step 2: Sender A chooses one random number x (private key) x<q and calculates public key YA=gx mod q

Step 3: B chooses one random number x1 (private key) and calculates public key YB=gx1 mod q

Step 4: Both parties share their public keys, mutually and calculate a common shared secret key KA=Y_A^x mod q & KB=Y_B^x1 mod q, whereas KA=KB=K.

Step 5: Compute the inverse Key.

Step 6: Recover the plain text using P=K-1 .C mod q

Chapter 17
Artificial Intelligence-Based System for Detection and Treatment Planning of Kidney Disease Using CT Imaging

Aparna Shriniwas Yemul
https://orcid.org/0009-0009-3728-088X
Walchand Institute of Technology, Solapur, India

Vijay Anant Athavale
https://orcid.org/0000-0002-6812-5198
Walchand Institute of Technology, Solapur, India

Rashmi Kamlakar Dixit
https://orcid.org/0000-0003-2754-2304
Walchand Institute of Technology, Solapur, India

Shubham Suresh Vyavahare
https://orcid.org/0009-0009-4451-6635
Walchand Institute of Technology, Solapur, India

L. M. R. J. Lobo
https://orcid.org/0000-0002-8572-2082
Walchand Institute of Technology, Solapur, India

Janhavi Rajendra Kale
https://orcid.org/0009-0009-0441-6509
Walchand Institute of Technology, Solapur, India

ABSTRACT

When damaged kidneys are unable to filter blood effectively, waste and fluid buildup result. This is known as renal disease. It can be acute or chronic and is frequently associated with excessive blood pressure and diabetes. Because CT scans are more accurate than ultrasound, they are crucial for detecting anomalies such tumors,

DOI: 10.4018/979-8-3373-5641-9.ch017

stones, cysts, and structural alterations. In order to create a strong diagnostic framework, this research will use deep learning and image processing techniques to identify key signs and a generative AI model to recommend treatments.

1. INTRODUCTION

Although kidney tumors, stones, and cysts can occur anywhere in the world, India has particular difficulties and high rates of occurrence. Renal cysts can lead to infections and renal damage, even though they are often asymptomatic. Renal stones are a prevalent issue that can lead to chronic renal damage and severe discomfort (Gharahbagh et al., 2024). A major public health concern in India is chronic kidney disease (CKD). The term chronic kidney disease, or chronic kidney failure, refers to a progressive decrease of renal function. The most common causes of kidney failure include cysts, stones, and tumors. Chronic renal illness may not show any signs in its early stages.

However, kidney disease can occur and go unnoticed until it's too late. Kidney tumors are a significant worldwide problem with varying risk factors and survival rates. As humans age, fluid-filled sacs called cysts may form in the kidneys. They are usually little (Nadeem et al., 2023). Some people have many cysts, whereas others only have one. Cysts may develop in one kidney or both kidneys. Simple cysts make up the majority of them. They're not malignant. They don't make the kidneys bigger or change how they work. People over 50 are more likely to have simple kidney cysts. Men are more likely than women to have them (Chen et al., 2019).

A renal tumor, also known as a kidney tumor (KT), is an abnormal development of cells within the kidney. Kidney tumors are usually found by chance when imaging for other conditions (Dong et al., 2022). Early detection and treatment are essential for successful outcomes. Urine contains substances that cause kidney stones, which are hard, pebble-like pieces of material that form in the kidneys. Some kidney stones can be very painful and require medical intervention, however most kidney stones naturally move via the urine canal (Nithya et al., 2019).

Early detection of kidney illness is crucial for preventing major issues like renal failure since it allows for timely action to halt or even stop its progression. Since many individuals with kidney disease do not show clear symptoms in the early stages, regular testing and awareness of risk factors are crucial, especially for those with diabetes, high blood pressure, or a family history of renal disease (Lobo, L. M. R. J et al., 2023).In medical imaging, Convolutional Neural Networks (CNNs) and U-Net are useful tools for detecting kidney disease, perhaps resulting in an early diagnosis. When used in conjunction with CNN designs, U Nets are particularly good in analysing medical photos to identify subtle signs of kidney impairment (Caroli et al., 2021). By facilitating the early diagnosis of conditions including chronic kidney disease (CKD) and other kidney-related issues, this may enhance patient outcomes.

Generative AI is revolutionizing renal care with its potential for early detection, treatment plans, and improved patient outcomes. AI algorithms can evaluate large-scale statistics to predict how a disease would progress, enhance dialysis regimens, and boost kidney transplant success rates. Despite challenges including data privacy and ethical concerns, the use of AI to nephrology holds great promise for the future of renal care (Pan et al., 2023).

We used a Kaggle dataset that is openly accessible for this investigation. A wide range of CT Scan images depicting different diseases, including tumors, stones, cysts, and normal kidneys, are included in the dataset.

The originality of this work is its integrated framework, which sets it apart from other studies that have separately used CNNs, U-Nets for renal disease identification. To guarantee pixel-level accuracy and trustworthy disease classification across a variety of renal diseases (cyst, stone, tumor, and normal), the suggested method integrates segmentation using U-Net and classification using CNN in a dual-path pipeline. By including a generative AI-based treatment recommendation module with a real-time conversational interface that enables users to inquire about symptoms, management alternatives, and preventive measures, the model goes beyond simple diagnosis. The method differs from previous studies that mostly concentrate on diagnostic accuracy since it combines detection, categorization, and therapy advice into a single system.

The main unique feature of this study is the integration of automated disease detection with practical treatment planning and intelligent, context-aware clinical support, even though dataset augmentation and balanced handling of multi-class CT images further enhance performance and robustness. The system provides an interactive platform for trainee doctors to study various types of kidney disorders using AI-generated insights.

Using machine learning methods like logistic regression, SVM, KNN, and decision tree classifiers, Charleonnan et al. (2016) created a model for predicting kidney disease which is shown in Figure 1. According to their findings, the SVM classifier was the most accurate, demonstrating how well it predicts kidney illness. Although contemporary research continues to focus on deep learning models for even greater accuracy and automated feature extraction, this work shows the potential of machine learning for medical diagnosis.

Figure 1. Prediction Model

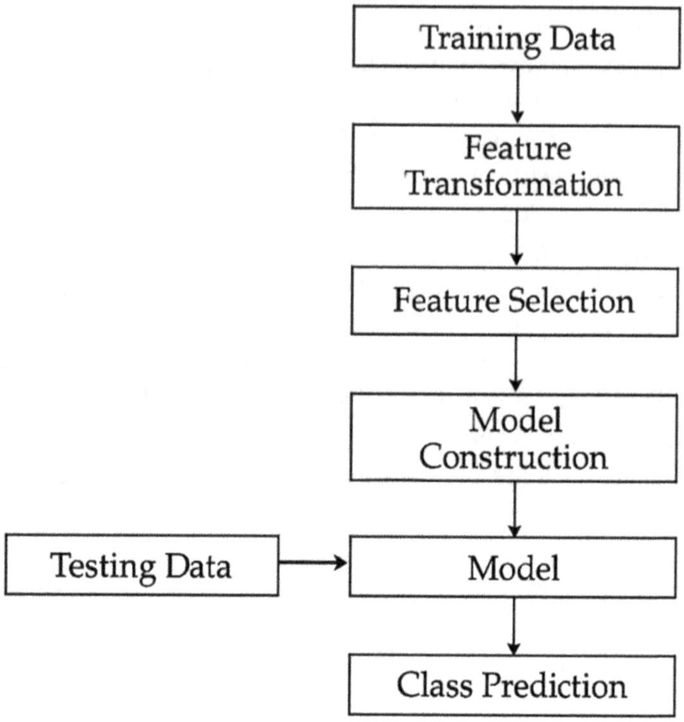

2. RELATED WORK

The following section presents the literature review conducted for our system

For the multi-class classification of kidney CT images, Sharma et al. (2025) presented a hybrid CNN model that paired a custom convolutional network with ResNet101. A dataset of CT images depicting tumor, cyst, stone, and normal conditions was used to train their model. The model's remarkable test accuracy demonstrated the advantages of combining optimized hyperparameter tuning with deep residual learning. The study demonstrates how sophisticated CNN architectures can reliably differentiate between different kidney diseases, enhancing early diagnosis.

In order to classify kidney X-ray images as either healthy or pathological, Aksakalli et al. (2021) created a deep learning-based framework, proving that artificial intelligence (AI) can be used for diagnostic purposes even when data is scarce. A thorough preprocessing pipeline comprising six steps resampling, evaluation, scaling, resizing, gray-level value extraction, and the creation of a CSV-format dataset appropriate for model input—was a component of their methodology. Given the small dataset of only 221 renal X-ray images used for both training and evaluation, these preprocessing techniques were essential in standardizing and improving the quality of the input data. The model produced encouraging results despite the small sample size, highlighting the potential of deep learning in conjunction with well-optimized preprocessing.

A morphological cascade CNN model based on multiple intersection over union (IOU) thresholds was proposed by Hui Zhang et al. (2019) for the diagnosis of kidney lesions. To efficiently detect minor injuries, their method included two morphological convolution layers, four IOU threshold cascade RCNNs, and customized feature pyramid networks (FPNs) in a quicker RCNN architecture. This study showed that the detection accuracy of subtle lesions in medical imaging can be improved by combining deep learning architectures with morphological operations.

A Heterogeneous Modified Artificial Neural Network (HMANN) was proposed by Ma et al. (2020) for the detection of chronic renal failure and the multi-classification of kidney stones. To improve diagnostic accuracy, their model incorporated crucial phases like preprocessing, feature extraction, segmentation, and classification. The system was able to handle a variety of intricate data patterns that are frequently seen in medical imaging thanks to its heterogeneous architecture. High performance in classifying a variety of kidney-related conditions was attained by HMANN through the efficient isolation of pertinent kidney structures and the analysis of their features. The study demonstrated the model's potential in handling challenging imaging tasks and emphasized the value of deep learning in nephrology. A promising development in automated diagnosis, HMANN facilitates the precise and effective detection of renal disorders in clinical settings.

A YOLOv8-based model was presented by S. D. Pande et al. (2024) to improve the detection accuracy of kidney cysts, stones, and tumors. Their method demonstrated the efficiency of YOLOv8 in quickly and precisely identifying diverse renal problems, and it offered a new and flexible platform for the clinical identification of different kidney illnesses. This study emphasizes how sophisticated object identification algorithms can increase the accuracy of renal disease diagnosis.

Using deep learning techniques, Yildirim et al. (2021) created an automated detection and localization system for kidney stone diagnosis. They used a four-stage XResNet-50 model, which is a ResNet architecture variation that was trained using 1,799 CT scans. The model successfully distinguished between pictures with and without kidney stones by acting as a binary classifier. In detecting kidney stones, their method showed excellent accuracy and dependability, demonstrating the power of deep convolutional neural networks in managing challenging medical imaging tasks. The study demonstrated the potential for automated, effective, and precise kidney stone detection in clinical settings by incorporating this architecture into diagnostic workflows. This would cut down on diagnostic delays and provide radiologists with reliable, real-time analysis.

Convolutional Neural Networks (CNNs) are a dependable and efficient method for classifying medical images, according to P. T. Akkasaligar et al. (2024), who also highlighted the accuracy and adaptability of CNNs in clinical diagnostics. In contrast to manual feature engineering, which is frequently laborious and subjective, their study demonstrated how CNNs can automatically learn and extract significant features from raw image data. Improved diagnostic performance resulted from the model's ability to recognize complex patterns linked to a range of medical conditions by utilizing deep layers of convolutional operations. The study showed that CNNs improve disease classification accuracy while also streamlining the process of medical image analysis.

In order to autonomously segment kidneys and cystic renal lesions on non-contrast computed tomography (CT) scans, Aronson et al. (2024) created a convolutional neural network (CNN) model. A dataset of 150 hand annotated images was used to train the model, allowing it to pick up intricate clinical and anatomical details. Strong overlap between the automated and manual segmentations was indicated by the renal segmentation's high Dice similarity coefficient of 0.934. A useful tool for automating large-scale picture annotation tasks, the model also showed remarkable accuracy in volumetric measurement of kidney structures. This study demonstrates how deep learning may be used to improve consistency and decrease manual workload in renal imaging analysis, especially in clinical and research workflows that call for accurate measurements of organs and lesions.

Özbay et al. (2024) developed a masked auto encoder (MAE) model incorporating self-supervised learning (SSL) and self-distillation (SD) techniques for kidney tumor detection using transfer learning. Their approach achieved a high classification accuracy of 98.04% on the kidney dataset, demonstrating that SSL-based deep learning models can effectively extract tumor features even with limited data. This study highlights the potential of such models to assist radiologists in clinical diagnosis and reduce diagnostic errors.

For kidney tumor segmentation, Gianmarco Santini et al. (2019) presented the Ensembling Multistage Deep Learning Approach (EMS-DLA). Their approach improved overall segmentation accuracy by combining prediction results from several phases using an ensembling technique to reflect variances across different models. In kidney tumor segmentation tasks, this work showed that multistage ensembling can successfully increase the robustness and accuracy of deep learning models. Using an ensemble Multiple Support Vector Machine (MSVM) classification model, Sudharson et al. (2019) presented an automated method for detecting kidney-related problems. They started by removing the need for manual feature engineering by automatically extracting deep features from renal ultrasound (US) images using pre-trained Convolutional Neural Networks (CNNs). Important structural and textural details pertaining to kidney abnormalities were captured by these extracted features. The features were then fed into an ensemble MSVM model, which enhanced classification accuracy and robustness by combining the predictive capabilities of several SVM classifiers. The model showed promise in combining deep learning and conventional machine learning techniques for accurate and automated kidney disease diagnosis when tested on a dataset of 2,085 ultrasound images.

A Deep Neural Network (DNN) model was presented by Susan Sheehan et al. (2019) with the goal of identifying and categorizing new histologic abnormalities in kidney tissue. In order to detect subtle and complex structural abnormalities that might be challenging to identify through manual examination, the model was created to process and analyze high-resolution histopathology images. The DNN was trained on a wide range of kidney histology samples, and the system showed excellent accuracy in a number of classification tasks, such as identifying glomerular changes, fibrosis, and inflammation. The study demonstrated how DNNs can handle complex visual data with ease and effectiveness, which could improve the accuracy and productivity of histopathological analysis.

Kaushik et al. (2024) utilized two deep learning architectures, VGG16 and DenseNet201, to classify renal CT scans for kidney disease diagnosis. Their study evaluated the performance of these convolutional neural network models in accurately identifying kidney diseases from CT images. The results demonstrated the effectiveness of both architectures, highlighting the potential of deep learning models in improving diagnostic accuracy for renal disorders.

A CNN-based kidney segmentation model that improves ultrasound images using a modified Contrast Limited Adaptive Histogram Equalization (CLAHE) technique was proposed by Buriboev et al (2024). For kidney structures, this technique successfully increased segmentation accuracy and edge clarity. In low-contrast imaging settings, their solution showed the promise of deep learning in conjunction with preprocessing techniques.

A thorough examination of kidney stone diagnosis utilizing image processing techniques on CT scans were carried out by Santhosh S. et al. (2023). Their research showed that because ultrasonography may overlook smaller stones, CT scans are the most reliable method for identifying kidney stones. This study highlights the value of CT imaging in conjunction with cutting-edge image processing techniques for accurate and consistent kidney stone detection in clinical settings.

A machine learning-based framework was created by Gill et al. (2023) to automatically identify and categorize various forms of kidney disease, with an emphasis on tumor identification. By using labeled datasets that included a variety of kidney tumor images and clinical information, their method enabled supervised learning algorithms to identify and distinguish between different pathological patterns. Accurately classifying renal cell carcinoma (RCC), angiomyolipoma (AML), oncocytoma, and a variety of other benign and malignant kidney tumors was the main goal of the study. The system demonstrated the efficacy of machine learning in assisting with clinical assessment by achieving dependable diagnostic performance through the use of well-annotated data for model training.

Using a specially created convolutional neural network (CNN) architecture, M.M. Ali et al. (2023) presented a deep learning method for categorizing different kidney diseases and normal renal conditions. Their proprietary CNN was designed especially for kidney image analysis, which enables it to more successfully capture disease-specific features than conventional pre-trained models. The study focused a lot of attention on improving the model's performance through the methodical adjustment and validation of important hyperparameters like activation functions, batch size, learning rate, and the number of convolutional layers. Significant gains in classification robustness and accuracy across various kidney disease categories were the result of this optimization process. Their study emphasizes how important it is to use personalized deep learning models and meticulous hyperparameter adjustment to achieve high diagnostic accuracy when detecting renal disease.

By using a variety of classification algorithms on medical datasets, Gada (2022) created an intelligent, automated, and flexible disease prediction system. Building a trustworthy predictive model that can provide extremely accurate results for a range of medical conditions, including kidney-related disorders, was the goal of their research. The authors thoroughly tested a number of supervised machine learning algorithms, including Random Forest, Decision Trees, Support Vector Machines (SVM), and Logistic Regression. They assessed each model's performance using accuracy, precision, recall, and F1-score. They developed a strong and effective prediction framework by concentrating on algorithms that continuously produced the best results for particular disease datasets.

The Region of Interest (ROI) approach enhances model performance by using adversarial examples to fine-tune the weight values, making the model more robust and accurate. A Convolutional Neural Network (CNN) is then used for classification, benefiting from the refined focus on important image regions. K. Arun Kumar et al. (2023) compared this proposed method with existing techniques, particularly in the object counting stage, and reported improved accuracy, showing the effectiveness of combining ROI and adversarial training with CNN.

The Guided Bilateral Filter (GBF) is a novel image processing technique that Ravi et al. (2024) proposed to improve feature detection in computed tomography (CT) images, with a focus on kidney stone identification and classification. Image preprocessing, feature enhancement using GBF, key feature extraction, and classification were the four main stages of their methodology. Edge-preserving smoothing, made possible by the Guided Bilateral Filter, successfully decreased noise while maintaining important structural details of the kidney and stone regions. A Support Vector Machine (SVM), which helped to reduce computational complexity while maintaining high diagnostic accuracy, was then used to process the refined feature set in order to ensure effective and accurate classification. The system's performance and dependability were enhanced by this hybrid approach, showcasing its potential as a strong and lightweight.

Recent developments in radiomics and artificial intelligence (AI) have greatly improved the ability to diagnose and prognosticate renal disease, especially with ultrasound imaging. Comprehensive reviews by Liang et al. (2023) and Xu et al. (2024) focused on the use of AI techniques, particularly deep learning models, for tasks like automatic kidney segmentation, kidney volume estimation, renal function prediction, and kidney pathology detection. These studies demonstrated how AI algorithms improve diagnostic speed, decrease inter-observer variability, and facilitate more consistent interpretations. In order to increase model robustness and clinical applicability, they also emphasized the necessity of standardized imaging protocols and high-quality annotated datasets. Their results highlight how AI-based ultrasound tools have the potential to revolutionize contemporary radiological and nephrology workflows.

Alzu'bi D et al. (2022) presented a detection model for identifying kidney tumors in CT scans using two-dimensional convolutional neural networks (2D-CNN). Their final classification model, CNN-4, consisted of four layers and demonstrated effective performance in classifying and detecting kidney tumors. This study highlights the potential of lightweight 2D-CNN architectures in accurately identifying renal tumors, contributing to improved diagnostic support in medical imaging.

In order to segment kidney tumors on non-contrast CT scans, Hatsutani et al. (2023) presented the Protuberance Detection Network, a specialized deep learning framework. Their method, in contrast to traditional models, focuses on locating protruded tumor regions, which are frequently difficult to differentiate because of their hazy borders and resemblance to the surrounding kidney tissue. The model outperformed the popular 3D U-Net architecture, achieving a Dice score of 0.615 and a sensitivity of 0.721 when tested on the publicly available KiTS19 dataset. The Protuberance Detection Network showed promise in improving automated kidney cancer detection in clinical imaging by addressing the complex morphology of renal tumors and improving segmentation accuracy in challenging cases.

Pujitha et al. (2023) proposed a comprehensive disease diagnosis system by first applying data preprocessing to clean and normalize the dataset, followed by feature selection to identify the most relevant attributes influencing the diagnosis. They implemented and tested several machine learning algorithms, including Logistic Regression, Extreme Gradient Boosting (XGBoost), Random Forest, Support Vector

Machine (SVM), Decision Tree, and Naive Bayes. Each model was trained on the processed data, and their performance was evaluated based on accuracy and predictive capability. By comparing these models, the study aimed to determine which algorithm provided the most reliable and accurate disease forecasts, supporting better clinical decision-making. The Learning Model for Kidney Cancer Detection (LMKCD), a cutting-edge learning framework created by S. Niranjana et al. (2024), is intended to detect kidney cancer intelligently from medical imaging data. To increase detection accuracy and dependability, the LMKCD model integrated customized learning strategies and enhanced feature extraction methods. The model was cross-validated against a standard Convolutional Neural Network (CNN), a commonly used deep learning benchmark in medical image analysis, in order to assess its efficacy. According to comparative results, LMKCD performed competitively—and occasionally better—in terms of accuracy, sensitivity, and robustness. This study emphasized the potential of LMKCD as a more flexible and effective substitute for traditional CNNs, highlighting its suitability in clinical diagnostic workflows for the early and accurate detection of kidney cancer.

V.S. Shri et al. (2023) introduced the RCNN model to categorize the tumor region in the renal X-ray image. They compared the Deep Learning Methods of the Mask RCNN Model with those of other models. The evaluated model was compared to other models using metrics from the Tuned Hyperparameter CNN Model and the Mask R-CNN Model. It gave the best accuracy in the fifth epoch of the Mask RCNN algorithm.

Balamanikandan et al. (2024) introduced two deep learning models based on machine learning techniques: Convolutional Neural Network and Mobile Net. Their study evaluated and compared the accuracy of these models for medical image analysis, demonstrating their effectiveness in classifying kidney-related conditions. The findings highlighted the potential of both CNN and Mobile Net architectures for reliable and efficient kidney disease detection.

The efficacy of various classification methods in medical data processing was assessed by Gupta et al (2020), who concentrated on decision trees, logistic regression, and random forest algorithms. The study evaluated these models on a variety of performance metrics, such as accuracy, precision, recall, and F1-score, using publicly accessible datasets from the UCI Machine Learning Repository. Gupta's study emphasized the distinct advantages and disadvantages of each approach, such as the interpretability of decision trees, the effectiveness of logistic regression for linear problems, and the resilience of random forests when dealing with intricate, non-linear relationships. The results gave useful information about how well each algorithm performed on particular classification tasks and offered suggestions for choosing the best models for predictive diagnostics and healthcare analytics.

In order to predict Chronic Kidney Disease (CKD), Polat et al. (2017) combined Support Vector Machine (SVM) with wrapper and filter-based feature selection methods. Their research highlighted how crucial it is to choose the most pertinent features in order to increase the accuracy and resilience of the model. The wrapper method employed a best-first search strategy, which selects feature subsets that produce the best performance after training the model. The filter method, on the other hand, used a greedy stepwise search strategy that ranks features according to statistical metrics. Combining the two methods allowed them to successfully decrease dataset redundancy, improve classification performance, and show how effective SVM is in medical diagnosis, especially when it comes to early CKD prediction using clinical attributes.

According to Mara et al. (2019), who applied the filter feature selection approach on attributes, hemoglobin, albumin, and specific gravity are feature characteristics in the CKD dataset. They trained and validated the dataset using 10-fold cross-validation after feature selection. Ogunleye et al. (2020) proposed the extreme gradient boosting (XGBoost) method for CKD classification. The 25-attribute dataset that was taken from the UCI repository was used by them. The reduced model, which used around half of the original full features, outperformed and had a greater accuracy than models based on individual feature selection strategies.

An ensemble-based model improved using explainable AI (XAI) techniques was presented by Jawad et al. (2024) for the early prediction of chronic kidney disease (CKD) utilizing structured clinical data. Three potent machine learning algorithms—XGBoost, Random Forest, and Decision Trees—were combined in the suggested method to maximize predicted accuracy by utilizing their combined advantages. Notably, the model not only performed well in classification but also offered interpretability using feature attribution techniques, enabling physicians to determine which factors had the biggest impact on the predictions. In medical situations, where adoption of AI technologies depends on user confidence, this transparency is vital. The study promoted models that are not only accurate but also interpretable and in line with clinical decision-making procedures, highlighting the significance of explainability in healthcare-focused AI.

The U-Net architecture, introduced by Ronneberger et al. (2015), features an encoder-decoder structure with skip connections that has proven highly effective for biomedical image segmentation tasks, including kidney and lesion segmentation. The encoder compresses the input image into abstract features, while the decoder reconstructs the segmented output. Skip connections link corresponding layers of the encoder and decoder, preserving spatial details lost during down sampling and improving segmentation accuracy. This design allows U-Net to perform well even with limited training data, making it a popular choice in medical imaging applications, particularly for delineating complex anatomical structures like kidneys.

Kappelhof et al. (2021) utilized the U-Net architecture for automatic segmentation of renal tumors and cysts. Their study achieved a high dice similarity coefficient of over 0.95, demonstrating the effectiveness of U-Net in accurately segmenting kidney abnormalities. This research highlights the strong performance of deep learning-based segmentation models in supporting precise and automated analysis of renal imaging. More than half of renal cell carcinomas (RCCs) are unintentionally discovered using noninvasive imaging methods, according to Tsili et al. (2021), underscoring the crucial role multimodality imaging plays in the management of renal masses. The study covered the diagnostic and prognostic utility of multiparametric MRI (mpMRI), CT, contrast-enhanced ultrasonography (CEUS), and conventional ultrasound in detecting and describing kidney masses.

Generative AI techniques such as Generative Adversarial Networks (GANs) have been applied to augment tiny annotated datasets in medical imaging to enhance model resilience and generalisation Bogacsovics et al. (2022) used GAN-based augmentation to improve the diagnosis accuracy of kidney disease.

Using 24 predictive clinical features extracted from patient data, Salekin et al. (2016) created a machine learning-based method to identify Chronic Kidney Disease (CKD). By carefully choosing the most pertinent and instructive characteristics that greatly aid in CKD prediction, their study aimed to increase model accuracy. In order to do this, they used feature selection techniques that improved model performance and reduced noise by ranking features according to their individual predictive strength. Classifiers like support vector machines and decision trees were then trained using the improved feature set. Their findings supported the early detection and treatment of CKD by demonstrating that good feature selection not only lowers computational complexity but also significantly improves diagnostic precision.

Suganthi et al. (2022) utilized a dataset from the UCI repository containing 24 clinical parameters, such as sugar levels and age, to develop a system for predicting Chronic Kidney Disease (CKD). The study employed the AdaBoosting ensemble method alongside the K-Fold Cross Validation technique to ensure robust model evaluation and reduce the risk of overfitting. A variety of machine learning algorithms, including K-Nearest Neighbors (KNN), Decision Trees (DT), Random Forest (RF), Naive Bayes (NB), and Logistic Regression (LR), were applied, along with their ensemble versions, to classify the data and improve prediction accuracy. The comparative analysis aimed to identify the most effective approach for CKD prediction based on performance metrics.

K.S et al. (2024) contributed to the advancement of automatic object recognition in ultrasonic images by developing an application aimed at assisting medical professionals in identifying stone regions within ultrasound scans. The system employed a semi-automated approach, allowing practitioners to manually select regions of interest where potential kidney stones were suspected. Once the region was selected, various feature extraction algorithms were applied to analyze texture, shape, and intensity characteristics, aiding in accurate detection and classification of stones. This method combined human expertise with computational efficiency, enhancing diagnostic precision and reducing the workload in clinical settings.

In order to identify urinary tract stones on non-contrast CT scans, Parakh et al. (2019) created a cascading deep learning system using Inception-v3 CNNs. Urinary tract slices were localized in the first network, whereas the presence of stones was classified in the second. Their model proved to be robust and generalizable, exhibiting strong diagnostic performance across a variety of CT protocols. The study demonstrated how well two-stage CNNs work for automated kidney stone detection in terms of both localization and classification.

In order to detect kidney stones in CT images, Elton et al. (2018) proposed a system that combines a 13-layer CNN classifier with 3D U-Net for kidney segmentation. To improve performance, denoising and densitometry were used in the preprocessing stages. Their model demonstrated the advantages of integrating segmentation and classification networks in a pipeline for precise stone detection by achieving high sensitivity and precision.

3. METHODOLOGY

The system is divided into two models Model no 1. Region-Based Prediction Model and Model no 2. Content Generation Model.

The application of the method for kidney disease diagnosis is demonstrated in Figure 2. Region-Based Prediction Model, which focuses on using CT scan images to segment and classify kidney anomalies such cysts, stones, tumors, and normal instances. The system starts with a dataset of CT scan images that are employed in two concurrent operations. The first method involves feeding a U-Net model with CT scan image and mask image. Following analysis of these inputs, kidney regions of interest, such as possible tumors, stones, or cysts, are highlighted by segmented regions produced by U-Net, a convolutional neural network architecture designed for medical image segmentation.

In the second option, the original CT scan images are sent through a CNN (Convolutional Neural Network), which acts as a prediction model. Classification is the job of this model. The results are separated into four categories: cyst, tumor, stone, and normal. The method is a helpful tool for aiding in the diagnosis of renal disease since its segmentation and classification routes work together to ensure correct detection of kidney abnormalities.

Figure 2. Region-Based Prediction Model

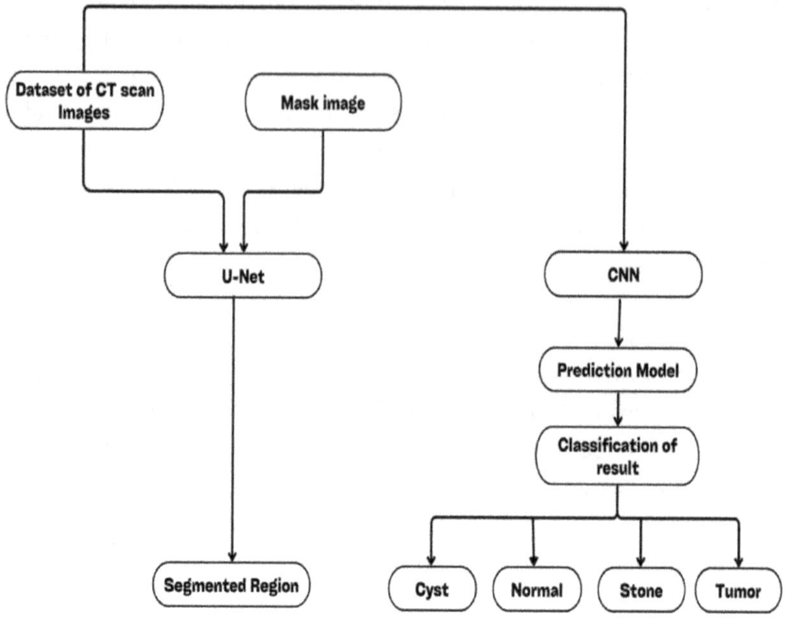

The Content Generation Model, a generative AI model for next-word prediction, is depicted in Figure 3. The input text is the first thing that is transformed into a numerical form via input embedding, in which each word is represented as a dense vector that captures its position and meaning. In order to better understand the context, attention transformers analyse the relationships between each word in the sequence using self-attention mechanisms after processing these embedding.

The final output is subjected to a softmax layer, which transforms the model's raw output scores into a probability distribution across the entire vocabulary. As a result, word probabilities are produced, and the model selects the word that has the best chance of being the next predicted word. The model can provide content that is logical and pertinent to the context thanks to this organized workflow.

The system also includes a real-time chat interface where users can ask questions about kidney disease, such as symptoms, causes, diagnosis, treatments, and prevention. Designed to provide intelligent, context-aware responses, it serves as a valuable tool for trainee doctors, enhancing interaction and simplifying medical information.

Figure 3. Content Generation Model

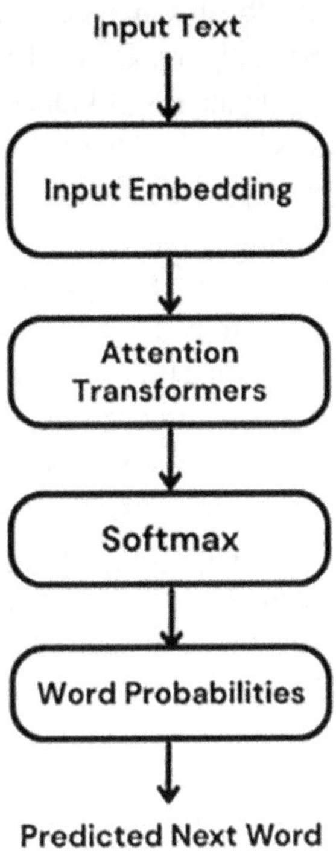

3.1. Algorithm

The projected model, which makes use of big data sets and a deep learning algorithm to build its output, is for the estimation of kidney disease and provides the type of disease in its output.

3.1.1. Segmentation

The U-Net architecture is a potent tool in the diagnosis and tracking of kidney disease since it is very good at separating kidney structures and anomalies from CT scan pictures. Imaging can identify structural abnormalities, such as cysts, tumors, stones, or changed kidney shapes, which are common signs of renal disease. Because of its encoder-decoder architecture, which captures both the fine-grained features, and the global context required to identify and characterize kidney tissues and anomalies, U-Net is especially well-suited for this purpose.

To create ground truth masks for this application, a dataset of CT scans with kidneys and related anomalies manually annotated is first prepared. The U-Net model can learn the spatial and structural patterns of kidney areas. The network receives each CT scan and Mask images as input, and the result is a segmented image where each pixel is identified as belonging to the kidney, a diseased area (such a tumor, cyst, or stone), or the background.

In detection tasks like identifying cyst, stone, normal, and tumor in medical images, deep learning models are commonly trained to predict the bounding boxes or regions of interest (ROIs) surrounding the kidney ailment that has been detected. The accuracy of the predicted regions can be evaluated using the IoU measure by contrasting them with the ground truth annotations. A higher IoU indicates more overlap between the actual and projected disease regions. IoU is commonly used to assess the segmentation masks accuracy by linking the separation masks to the ground truth masks. The IoU metric helps to estimate the quality of the segmentation output by evaluating the degree of overlap between the expected and actual segmentations. The relationship between the expected and actual segmentation masks. IoU is computed as follows:

IoU = union of forecast and ground truth masks / connection of predicted and ground truth masks (1).

In order to determine the intersection and union of two masks, the masks must first be converted into binary arrays. The background pixels are assigned a value of 0, the item of interest pixels are assigned a value of 1, and so on.

Metrics like Intersection over Union (IoU), which are used to evaluate performance during training, assist guarantee that the model correctly delineates kidney borders and identifies anomalous structures. Given the variation in kidney size, shape, and orientation among patients, data augmentation is essential for enhancing robustness and generalization. The U-Net model can help physicians locate illness areas, design treatments, and monitor the course of a disease over time by automatically segmenting kidneys from fresh CT scans once it has been taught.

3.1.2. Classification

By building a classification or detection model that can recognize these categories based on spatial and intensity information inside the scans, Convolutional Neural

Networks (CNNs) is used to identify cysts, stones, tumors, and normal kidney from CT scan pictures

Unlike traditional algorithms that require manual feature engineering, CNNs process input images through multiple layers, starting with convolutional layers that apply filters to identify features such as edges, textures, and shapes within CT scans. This is followed by activation functions like ReLU, which introduce non-linearity, and pooling layers that reduce the spatial dimensions of feature maps, making the model more efficient and robust to variations in input images. The final fully connected layers integrate these learned features to classify images into categories, such as normal kidney, kidney stone, or cyst. In renal disease diagnosis, CNNs analyze CT images to detect abnormalities with high accuracy, enabling rapid and automated screening for clinicians.

Measures like accuracy, precision, recall, and F1-measure are used to assess the CNN's performance after it has been trained using a loss function categorical cross-entropy. Techniques like transfer learning and data augmentation (such as flipping, rotation, and contrast modification) are used to improve the model's capacity for generalization. In actual use, radiologists can quickly check for anomalies by using CNN to categorize each input CT picture into one of the four disease categories.

When segmentation is necessary and the objective is only to categorize or identify the existence of a condition, this approach is especially helpful. CNN-based classification provides a quicker and more computationally effective method for automated illness diagnosis from CT images, even though it is less comprehensive than pixel-level segmentation using U-Net.

4. EXPERIMENTAL SETUP

4.1. Software Requirements

- **VS Code (Development):** VS Code is lightweight yet powerful for development, especially when working with machine learning and deep learning libraries like TensorFlow.
- **TensorFlow:** TensorFlow is primarily used for deep learning and machine learning problems, such as classification, perception, understanding, discovery, prediction, and creation.
- **Python 3.10:** It brings performance improvements and new syntax features like pattern matching, which can help with cleaner and more efficient code.

4.2. Hardware Requirements

- **Processor i3/i5:** Processor i3/i5 is used for best performance. The i3/i5 is a powerful machine suitable for developing machine learning models.
- **RAM 16GB and above:** With 16 GB of RAM, there would be enough memory to run a few lightweight programs simultaneously. It allows opening multiple browser tabs and handling various operations efficiently.
- **GPU 8GB VRAM Graphics Card with CUDA Support:** An 8GB VRAM GPU with CUDA support will allow for efficient parallel computing, making deep learning tasks like training classification models much faster. With your analytical approach, you might find it helpful to optimize batch sizes and leverage mixed precision training to further enhance performance.

5. RESULTS AND DISCUSSIONS

5.1 Experimental Equations and Calculations:

To coordinate with the system's utilities, the system is created in Python utilizing generic code. The data set required is downloaded from Kaggle.

The accuracy is a ratio based on predicted output and actual output for system, which is labeled as follows:

$$A = \frac{Nc}{Nt} \qquad (2)$$

Where A is Accuracy, Nc is Number of correctly identified data points and Nt is Total number of data points

For e.g. If there are 98 classified data points properly classified and 100 data points consider for the experimentation:

Accuracy = 98 / 100 = 0.98 or 98%

The F1-measure is particularly useful in image processing tasks, as it provides a balance between precision and recall. In object detection, for example, a high precision score is important to avoid false positives.

The traditional F1-measure is designed as follows:

$$\text{F1} - \text{Measure} = 2 \times \frac{\text{Precision} \times \text{Recall}}{\text{Precision} + \text{Recall}} \qquad (3)$$

It can first define the accurate positives (TP), wrong positives (FP), and wrong negatives (FN) as follows in order to simplify the equation:

$$\text{Precision} = \frac{\text{TP}}{\text{TP} + \text{FP}} \tag{4}$$

$$\text{Recall} = \frac{\text{TP}}{\text{TP} + \text{FN}}. \tag{5}$$

Calculated Precision is as follows:

Precision = Accurate Positives / (Accurate Positives + Wrong Positives)... (a)

Precision = 1778 / (1778 + 17).

Precision = 0.990529

It can calculate the Recall as follows:

Recall=Accurate Positives / (Accurate Positives + Wrong Negatives) ... (b)

Recall = 1778 / (1778 + 16)

Recall = 0.991081.

Finally, it can analyze the F1-Measure as follows:

F1-Measure = (2 × Precision× Recall) / (Precision + Recall)... (c)

F1-Measure = (2 × 0.990529× 0.991081) / (0.990529+ 0.991081)

F1-Measure = (2 × 0.981694) / 1.98161

F1-Measure = 1.963388 / 1.98161

F1-Measure = 0.90805.

A thorough assessment of the classification model's performance by class is shown in Table 1. The Normal, Cyst, Stone, and Tumor classifications have different results. To evaluate the model's ability to identify each class, three important performance measures are taken into account: precision, recall, and F1-measure.

The effectiveness of a multi-class classification model intended to differentiate between four medical conditions tumor, stone, cyst, and normal is evaluated in this study. The model's performance was assessed using key performance metrics such as accuracy, recall, precision, and F1-measure. According to the overall accuracy of 98%, predictions were produced in each area.

For cyst classification, the precision, recall, and F1- measure of 0.9905, 0.9911, and 0.9908, respectively, show excellent consistency and a very low number of false positives or false negatives.

The greatest precision of 0.9942 for normal situations indicates that the model is quite good at identifying cases that are genuinely normal. While the F1-measure is still high at 0.9909, the recall is slightly lower at 0.9877. Despite its power, stone detection's precision (0.9658) is marginally lower than that of other classes, which might be a sign of a higher false-positive rate. However, the high recall (0.9878) results in a decent F1-measure of 0.9767 to compensate for this. With 0.9833 precision and 0.9842 recall, the tumor classification remains balanced, yielding a reliable detection F1-measure of 0.9838.

Several steps were taken to prevent overfitting and guarantee the reliability of the results, even though the system obtained high accuracy 98%. Using a variety of data augmentation techniques, such as flipping, rotation, contrast modification, and scaling, the dataset was balanced among four classifications (cyst, stone, tumor, and normal). These techniques lessened model bias toward the majority class and broadened the variety of training data. The CNN model was initialized with pre-trained weights using transfer learning, which increased feature extraction effectiveness and decreased the possibility of overfitting on a small dataset. To guarantee that assessment metrics were obtained from CT scan images, the dataset was divided into subsets for training (70%), validation (20%), and testing (10%). Additionally, class-specific metrics and confusion matrices were used to track performance in addition to overall accuracy, confirming that predictions were consistent across all categories.

Table 1. Class-Specific Evaluation Metrics (Source: author)

Kidney Disease	Precision	Recall	F1-measure
Cyst	0.990529	0.991081	0.990805
Normal	0.994186	0.987678	0.990921
Stone	0.965774	0.987823	0.976674
Tumor	0.983302	0.984215	0.983759

The Performance Evaluation Metrics of Kidney Disease chart for a model that is used to identify and classify renal disease based on tumor, stone, cyst, and normal is displayed in Figure 4.

Figure 4. Performance Metrics of Kidney disease

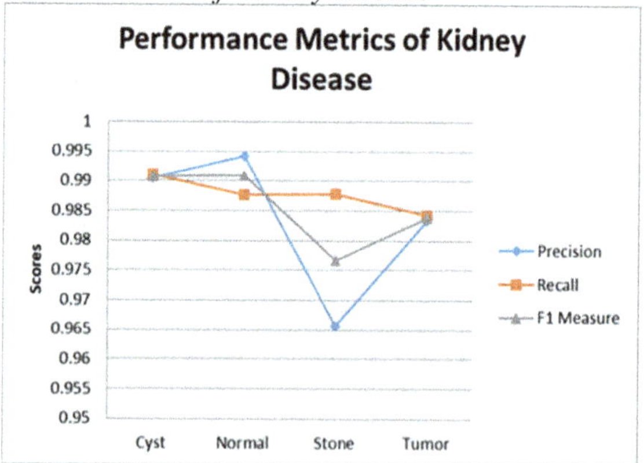

The confusion matrix in Figure 5, shows the high performance of the kidney disease classification model across four classes: Normal, Cyst, Stone, and Tumor.

Most predictions are correct, with values mainly along the diagonal, indicating minimal misclassifications.

Figure 5. Confusion matrix for kidney disease

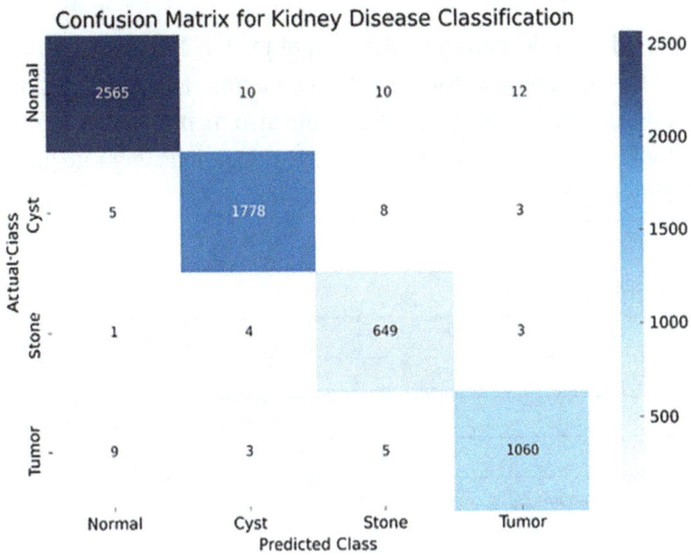

Table 2 presents the input data format, processing methods, features extracted, and accuracy of our system.

Table 2. Results for accuracy of System.

Model of Machine Learning Using CNN Algorithm			
Format of Input Data	**Processing Technique**	**Feature's extraction**	**Accuracy**
Scanned Images of Kidney Disease	Normalization and augmentation	Normal, Cyst, Stone, Tumor, Shape	98%

Table 3 compares the outcomes obtained by earlier authors with the anticipated increases in accuracy.

Specifically, comparisons are drawn with CNN-based classifiers Tsili et al., YOLO-based detection models Pande et al., these studies report accuracies ranging from 90–95% depending on task complexity, dataset size, and imaging modality. By incorporating such references into Table 3, the performance of the system can be contextualized within the current state of the art, demonstrating its accuracy.

Table 3. Comparisons of existing systems with Standard literature

Model of Machine Learning Using CNN Algorithm		
Name of model	**Accuracy achieved by other authors**	**Accuracy achieved**
CNN	95%	98%

Table 4 provides the Simulation variables of the CNN model used in this study. It outlines the dataset division for training, validation, and testing, along with the maximum number of training cycles. The table also mentions the number of filters in the convolutional layer, and specifies the optimizer, learning rate, and minibatch size used during training.

Table 4. Simulation variables

Specifications	Amounts
CNN Variables	
Dataset division	70% training, 20% validation, 10% testing
Max epochs	2000
Number of filters in convolution 2d layer	16
Solver name	Adam learning rate 3×10^{-4}
Minibatch size	8

The Table 5, Dataset details provides information about the dataset used in the study. It includes the total number of images and specifies that the dataset is divided into four classes, namely cyst, normal, stone, and tumor. It also mentions the image size used for model training and gives the distribution of image counts for each class.

The study uses a comprehensive dataset of 6125 CT scans, collected from Kaggle. Each scan was annotated by expert radiologists for kidney structure and disease labels.

In the preprocessing stage, all kidney images were normalized to a standard intensity range to ensure consistent brightness and contrast across samples. The images were then resampled to a uniform voxel size and cropped to focus specifically on the kidney region, eliminating irrelevant background information. To improve the model's ability to generalize and prevent overfitting, various data augmentation techniques were applied, including rotation, flipping, scaling, elastic deformation, and contrast adjustment. These transformations helped simulate diverse imaging conditions and anatomical variations. Furthermore, to address the issue of class imbalance where certain kidney disease categories were underrepresented over-sampling of minority classes and weighted loss functions were implemented during training. This approach minimized bias toward majority classes and improved the model's overall classification performance across all categories.

Table 5. Dataset details

Dataset	
Total image count	6125
Number of classes	4 (Cyst, Normal, Stone, Tumor)
Size of the image	512 × 512
Cyst image count	1794
Normal image count	2597
Stone image count	657
Tumor image count	1077

Table 6, describes the CNN summary used in this study. It includes an input layer for image data, followed by a convolutional layer with specified filter size and stride. An activation function is applied after convolution. The model also contains a fully connected layer to process the extracted features, followed by a softmax activation function for classification. Finally, it uses categorical cross-entropy as the loss function for training.

Table 6. CNN Summary

Layer	Details
Input Layer	512 ×512 ×3
Convolutional	2D CNN 3×3×3 with stride 1
Activation Function	Adam
Fully connected layer	128 ×4
Activation Function	Softmax
Loss	Categorial cross entrophy

Figure 6. CT scan image and segmented image of different kidney disease (i) Normal, (ii) Cyst, (iii) Stone, (iv) Tumor.

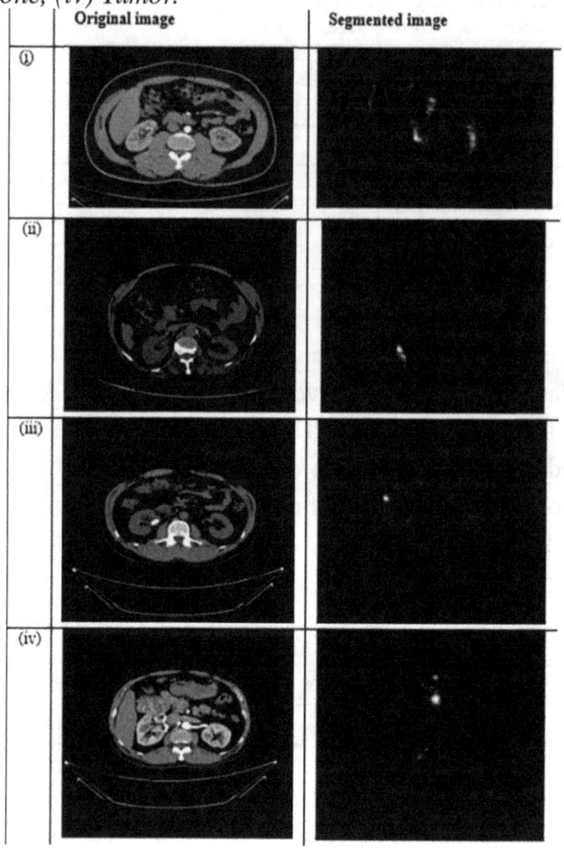

Figure 6, shows CT scan images with their segmented outputs for different kidney conditions: normal, cyst, stone, and tumor. The normal image shows no abnormalities. The cyst image highlights a fluid-filled area. The stone image identifies a bright calcified region, and the tumor image marks an irregular mass. These segmentations demonstrate the model's ability to accurately detect and differentiate each kidney disease.

5.2 Screenshots of Result

Figure 7. Selecting the image from folder

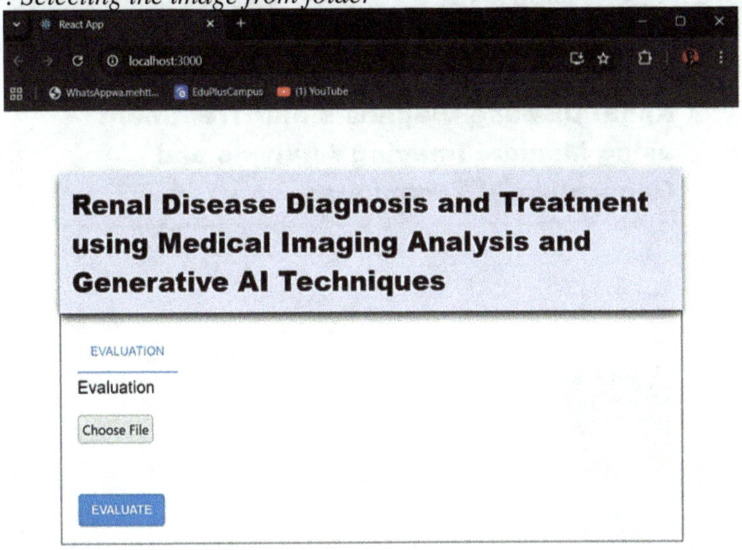

In Figure 7, shows the purpose of the system, there is an evaluation module, where users can upload medical imaging files (CT scans) for analysis. The interface includes a file input button labeled Choose File, allowing users to browse and select an image file from their local system. After file selection, users can initiate the evaluation process by clicking on the EVALUATE button, which will process the input through the integrated AI model to diagnose renal diseases such as cysts, stones, or tumors.

Figure 8. After selection of input image

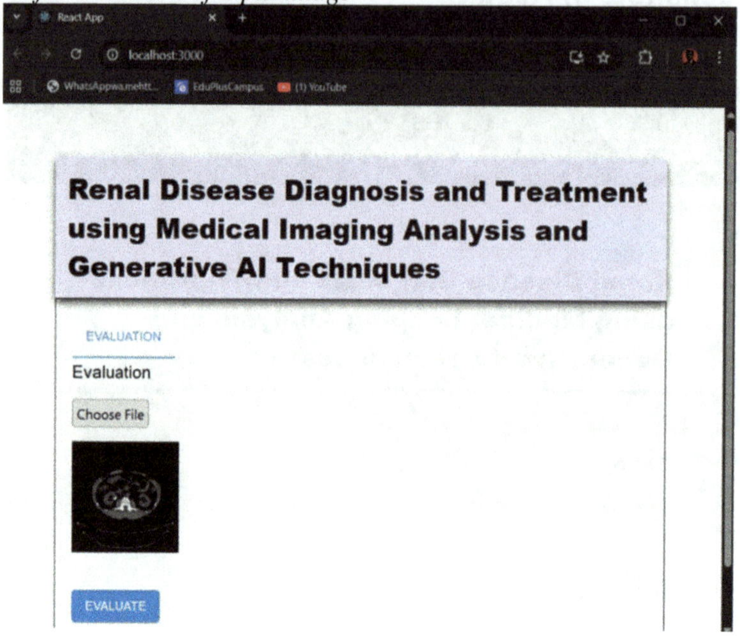

Figure 8, shows the functionality of the developed expert system where the user has selected an input image, and the selected image is displayed on the interface for confirmation.

Figure 9. Kidney disease classification and segmented image

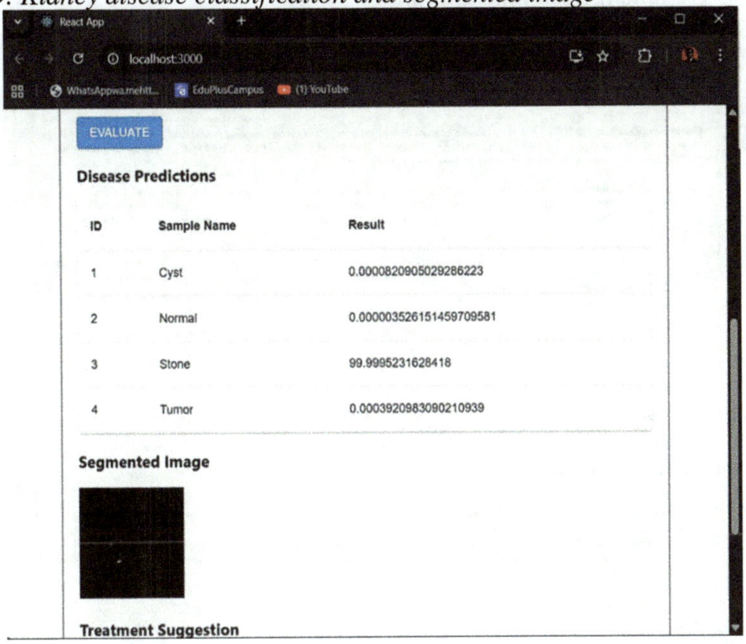

Above Figure 9, shows the predictions table, there is a Segmented Image section, which displays the processed output image after segmentation by the AI model. This image highlights the region of interest (ROI) within the kidney, such as the detected stone in this case

Figure 10. Treatment Recommendations

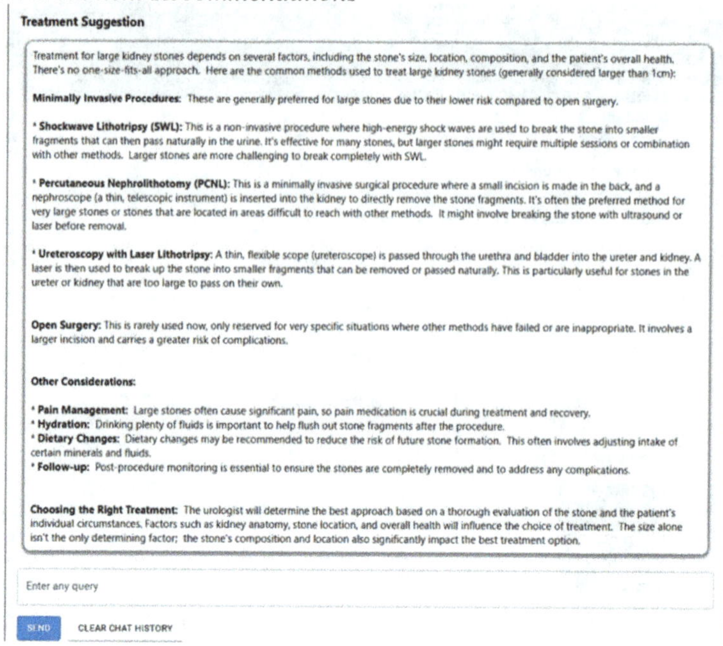

Figure 10. displays the treatment recommendations output for kidney stone.

6. CONCLUSION AND FUTURE SCOPE

6.1 Conclusion

This system utilizes advanced and efficient feature extraction techniques applied to CT scan images to accurately identify various renal diseases. By leveraging deep learning algorithms and image processing methods, it effectively captures intricate patterns and features within the CT images that are indicative of specific kidney conditions. This high level of precision allows the model to categorize multiple kidney disease such as cysts, stones, and tumor.

Furthermore, beyond mere classification, the model is designed to treatment recommendations based on the identified condition. This means that once the disease is detected, the system suggests treatment options tailored to the patient's needs, enhancing clinical decision-making. Such recommendations can include medical management strategies, follow-up imaging, or surgical interventions, depending on the type of the detected disease.

Ultimately, this integrated system offers a comprehensive solution for kidney disease management by combining diagnostic capabilities with actionable therapeutic guidance. The system also includes a chat interface enabling real-time communication. It aids trainee doctors in their workflow by enabling early detection and timely, appropriate treatment, reducing potential complications and promoting better overall renal health care.

6.2 Future Scope

This system can be enhanced in a number of ways in the future. To validate the model's practicality, clinical validation using actual hospital data and physician input will be crucial. By integrating imaging data with lab findings and patient history, the system may be connected to electronic health records (EHRs) to offer more individualized diagnostic and treatment recommendations. Incorporating explainable AI techniques will raise the system's transparency by providing the rationale behind a prediction or recommendation, potentially boosting patient and physician trust. By taking these actions, the system will transition from a research model to actual clinical application.

Although the system shows good results, it has some limitations. The dataset was taken from Kaggle and may not cover all patient types. There are ethical concerns with using AI to recommend treatments, including patient privacy, and the possibility of physicians becoming overly reliant on the system. To make the model more applicable in practice, we intend to test it on a wider range of datasets in subsequent research, incorporate ethical checks, and increase computational efficiency.

AI DISCLOSURE

This book chapter, "*Artificial Intelligence-Based System for Detection and Treatment Planning of Kidney Disease using CT Imaging*" was primarily authored by [Aparna Yemul, Rashmi Dixit, Dr. L.M.R.J. Lobo, Dr. Vijay Anant Athavale, Mr. Shubham Vyavahare, Janhavi Kale.] with intellectual contributions, analysis, and writing done by the authors. Artificial Intelligence (AI)-based tools, including but not limited to ChatGPT and other text-processing software, were used to assist in specific aspects of the writing process. Portions of this paper were developed with the assistance of artificial intelligence tools. Canva was used for creating diagrams, and Grammarly was utilized for language refinement and summarization support. However, the conceptualization, analysis, interpretation of results, and conclusions presented in this paper are solely the work of the authors. The AI tools were used only to support the writing and presentation process, and all final content has been thoroughly reviewed and approved by the authors.

ACKNOWLEDGMENT

The authors acknowledge the Department of Information Technology, Walchand Institute of Technology, Solapur, India for provision of support and resources for, the project. Special appreciation to L.M.R.J. Lobo by assisting with quality guidance and feedbacks throughout the research. The research made use of the CT scan images available from Kaggle, to train and test the models. The authors also used open-source tool like TensorFlow to train the models and evaluate the system. The authors thank their peers and co-researchers for their valuable suggestions and technical support for the different component of this work.

REFERENCES

Akkasaligar, P. T., Pattar, S., Uppin, A., Kori, K., & Kulakarni, A. (2024). Kidney tumor detection using computed tomography scan images through CNN. In *Proceedings of the 2024 International Conference on Distributed Computing and Optimization Techniques (ICDCOT)* (pp. 1–6). IEEE. DOI: 10.1109/ICDCOT61034.2024.10516254

Aksakalli, I., Kaçdioğlu, S., & Hanay, Y. S. (2021). Kidney X-ray Images Classification using Machine Learning and Deep Learning Methods. *Balkan Journal of Electrical and Computer Engineering*, *9*(2), 144–151. DOI: 10.17694/bajece.878116

Ali, M. M., Agrawal, J., Mishra, T., & Raj, M. (2023). An automated deep learning approach for kidney disease detection. In *Proceedings of the 2023 International Conference on Integrated Intelligence and Communication Systems (ICIICS)* (pp. 1–6). IEEE._DOI: 10.1109/ICIICS59993.2023.10421534

Alzu'bi, D., Abdullah, M., Hmeidi, I., AlAzab, R., Gharaibeh, M., El-Heis, M., Almotairi, K. H., Forestiero, A., Hussein, A. M., & Abualigah, L. (2022). Kidney tumor detection and classification based on deep learning approaches: A new dataset in CT scans. *Journal of Healthcare Engineering*, *2022*, 3861161. Advance online publication. DOI: 10.1155/2022/3861161 PMID: 37323471

Aronson, L., Massaa, R. N., Gardezi, S. J. S., & Wentland, A. L. (2024). Automatic segmentation of the kidneys and cystic renal lesions on non-contrast CT using a convolutional neural network. /arXiv.2405.08282DOI: 10.48550

Arunkumar, K., Eshwar, S., Mohammed Saleem, D., & Vamsikrishna, C. (2023). Implementation of kidney stone detection using CNN. In 2023 5th International Conference on Smart Systems and Inventive Technology (ICSSIT) (pp. 1320–1324). IEEE. DOI: 10.1109/ICSSIT55814.2023.10061142

Balamanikandan, A., Saravanakumar, M., Gunasekaran, S., Anjum, V., Gurusamy, P., & Ashokkumar, N. (2024). Deep learning in the detection of chronic kidney disease. In *Proceedings of the 2024 4th International Conference on Intelligent Technologies (CONIT)* (pp. 1–6). IEEE. DOI: 10.1109/CONIT61985.2024.10627434

Bogacsovics, G., Toth, J., Hajdu, A., & Harangi, B. (2022). Enhancing CNNs through the use of hand-crafted features in automated fundus image classification. *Biomedical Signal Processing and Control, 76*, 103685. DOI: 10.1016/j.bspc.2022.103685

Buriboev, A., Bobakulov, A., Yusupova, Z., Fayzullaev, A., Nematov, D., & Rakhmonov, A. (2024). Kidney segmentation in ultrasound images based on CNN using modified CLAHE. *Sensors (Basel), 24*(23), 7703. DOI: 10.3390/s24237703 PMID: 39686240

Caroli, A., Remuzzi, A., & Lerman, L. O. (2021). Basic principles and new advances in kidney imaging. *Kidney International, 100*(5), 1001–1011. DOI: 10.1016/j.kint.2021.04.032 PMID: 33984338

Charleonnan, A., Fufaung, T., Niyomwong, T., Chokchueypattanakit, W., Suwannawach, S., & Ninchawee, N. (2016). Predictive analytics for chronic kidney disease using machine learning techniques. In *Proceedings of the 2016 Management and Innovation Technology International Conference (MITicon)* (pp. MIT-80–MIT-83). IEEE. DOI: 10.1109/MITICON.2016.8025242

Chen, T. K., Knicely, D. H., & Grams, M. E. (2019). Chronic kidney disease diagnosis and management: A review. *Journal of the American Medical Association, 322*(13), 1294–1304. DOI: 10.1001/jama.2019.14745 PMID: 31573641

Dong, Y., Liu, Q., Du, B., & Zhang, L. (2022). Weighted feature fusion of convolutional neural network and graph attention network for hyperspectral image classification. IEEE Transactions on Image Processing, PP, 1–1. DOI: 10.1109/TIP.2022.3144017

Elton, D. M., Zhang, Y., & Wong, S. T. C. (2018). A deep learning system for automated kidney stone detection and volumetric segmentation on non-contrast CT scans. *Medical Physics*. Advance online publication. DOI: 10.1002/mp.13490 PMID: 35156216

Gada, D. (2022). Disease Prediction System using Machine Learning. 2022 6th International Conference on Computing, Communication, Control and Automation (ICCUBEA, 1–5. DOI: 10.1109/ICCUBEA54992.2022.10011002

Gharahbagh, A. A., Hajihashemi, V., Machado, J. J. M., & Tavares, J. M. R. S. (2024). Feature Extraction Based on Local Histogram with Unequal Bins and a Recurrent Neural Network for the Diagnosis of Kidney Diseases from CT Images. *Bioengineering (Basel, Switzerland), 11*(3), 220. DOI: 10.3390/bioengineering11030220 PMID: 38534494

Gill, K. S., Anand, V., Chauhan, R., Singh, P., & Gupta, R. (2023). Detection of kidney disease in X-ray images using machine learning on MobileNetV3 CNN model. In *Proceedings of the 2023 2nd International Conference on Futuristic Technologies (INCOFT)* (pp. 1–4). IEEE. DOI: 10.1109/INCOFT60753.2023.10425269

Gupta, R., Koli, N., Mahor, N., & Tejashri, N. (2020). Performance analysis of Machine Learning classifier for predicting chronic kidney Disease. *2020 International Conference for Emerging Technology (INCET)*, 1–4. DOI: 10.1109/INCET49848.2020.9154147

Hatsutani, T., Ichinose, A., Nakamura, K., & Kitamura, Y. (2023). Segmentation of kidney tumors on non-contrast CT images using Protuberance Detection Network. /arXiv.2312.04796DOI: 10.1007/978-3-031-43990-2_2

Jawad, M., Zahoor, M., Iqbal, T., Khan, I., & Alouffi, B. (2024). An ensemble learning-based explainable AI framework for early diagnosis of chronic kidney disease. https://arxiv.org/abs/2406.06728

K. S., R., L., A. C. P., V., & G. V. (2024). Enhancing kidney stone recognition in ultrasound imaging using hybrid feature extraction techniques. In Proceedings of the 2024 Second International Conference on Intelligent Cyber Physical Systems and Internet of Things (ICoICI) (pp. 1–5). IEEE. DOI: 10.1109/ICoICI62503.2024.10696452

Kappelhof, N., Ramos, L., Kappelhof, M., Van Os, H., Chalos, V., Van Kranendonk, K., Kruyt, N., Roos, Y., Van Zwam, W., Van Der Schaaf, I., Van Walderveen, M., Wermer, M., Van Oostenbrugge, R., Lingsma, H., Dippel, D., Majoie, C., & Marquering, H. (2021). Evolutionary algorithms and decision trees for predicting poor outcome after endovascular treatment for acute ischemic stroke. *Computers in Biology and Medicine, 133*, 104414. DOI: 10.1016/j.compbiomed.2021.104414 PMID: 33962154

Kaushik, P., & Sharma, P. (2024). Advanced kidney CT scan diagnosis: A comparative study of VGG16 and DenseNet201 deep learning models. In *Proceedings of the 2024 International Conference on Cybernation and Computation (CYBERCOM)* (pp. 350–355). IEEE. DOI: 10.1109/CYBERCOM63683.2024.10803203

Liang, X., Du, M., & Chen, Z. (2023). Artificial intelligence-aided ultrasound in renal diseases: A systematic review. *Quantitative Imaging in Medicine and Surgery, 13*(6), 3988–4001. DOI: 10.21037/qims-22-1428 PMID: 37284081

Lobo, L. M. R. J., & Markandeya, D. L. (2023). Expert system for medical diagnosis and consultancy using prediction algorithms of machine learning. In Algorithms for intelligent systems (pp. 381–391).DOI: 10.1007/978-981-99-1435-7_33

Ma, F., Sun, T., Liu, L., & Jing, H. (2020). Detection and diagnosis of chronic kidney disease using deep learning-based heterogeneous modified artificial neural network. *Future Generation Computer Systems, 111*, 17–26. DOI: 10.1016/j.future.2020.04.036

. Nadeem, M., Tan, G., Altaf, M., Mumtaz, M. K., Fatima, A., & Noshi. (2023). Evaluation and classification of kidney stone detection using deep learning techniques. In 2023 6th International Conference on Software Engineering and Computer Science (CSECS) (pp. 1–6). IEEE. DOI: 10.1109/CSECS60003.2023.10428612

Niranjana, S., Titus, A., Venkat, S., Arulanantham, D., & Begum, A. S. (2024). Experimental Evaluation in Identification of Kidney Cancer using Modified Learning Scheme. *2022 International Conference on Advances in Computing, Communication and Applied Informatics (ACCAI)*, 1–6. DOI: 10.1109/ACCAI61061.2024.10601727

Nithya, A., Appathurai, A., Venkatadri, N., Ramji, D. R., & Anna Palagan, C. (2019). Kidney disease detection and segmentation using artificial neural network and multi-kernel k-means clustering for ultrasound images. *Measurement, 149*, 106952. DOI: 10.1016/j.measurement.2019.106952

Ogunleye, A., & Wang, Q. G. (2020). XGBoost model for chronic kidney disease diagnosis. *IEEE/ACM Transactions on Computational Biology and Bioinformatics, 17*(6), 2131–2140. DOI: 10.1109/TCBB.2019.2911071 PMID: 30998478

Özbay, E., Altunbey Özbay, F., & Soleimanian Gharehchopogh, F. (2024). Kidney tumor classification on CT images using self-supervised learning. *Computers in Biology and Medicine, 176*, 108554. DOI: 10.1016/j.compbiomed.2024.108554 PMID: 38744013

Pande, S. D., & Agarwal, R. (2024). Multi-class kidney abnormalities detecting novel system through computed tomography. *IEEE Access : Practical Innovations, Open Solutions, 12*, 21147–21155. DOI: 10.1109/ACCESS.2024.3351181

Parakh, A., Lee, H., & Singh, P.. (2019). Urinary stone detection on CT images using deep convolutional neural networks: Evaluation of model performance and generalization. *Radiology. Artificial Intelligence, 1*(6), e190018. DOI: 10.1148/ryai.2019180066 PMID: 33937795

Polat, H., Mehr, H. D., & Cetin, A. (2017). Diagnosis of chronic kidney disease based on support vector machine by feature selection methods. *Journal of Medical Systems, 41*(4), 55. Advance online publication. DOI: 10.1007/s10916-017-0703-x PMID: 28243816

Pujitha, K., Soni, N. B., Eram, L. F., Sai, P. N., Divija, S., & Supriya, R. S. (2023). Chronic kidney disease detection using machine learning approach. In *Proceedings of the 2023 2nd International Conference on Vision Towards Emerging Trends in Communication and Networking Technologies (ViTECoN)* (pp. 1–5). IEEE. DOI: 10.1109/ViTECoN58111.2023.10157496

. R, M., S, P., Ravi, V., Stephan, T., Mazroa, A. A., Singh, P., Diwakar, M., & Gupta, I. (2024). Automatic Kidney Stone Detection System using Guided Bilateral Feature Detector for CT Images. The Open Public Health Journal, 17(1). DOI: 10.2174/01 18749445334602240820074311

Ronneberger, O., Fischer, P., & Brox, T. (2015). U-NET: Convolutional Networks for Biomedical Image Segmentation. In Lecture notes in computer science (pp. 234–241). DOI: 10.1007/978-3-319-24574-4_28

Salekin, A., & Stankovic, J. (2016). Detection of chronic kidney disease and selecting important predictive attributes. In *Proceedings of the 2016 IEEE International Conference on Healthcare Informatics (ICHI)* (pp. 262–270). IEEE. DOI: 10.1109/ICHI.2016.36

Santhosh, S., A. S. M., A. D. S., P. G. S., & V. P. T. (2023). Deep learning based kidney stone detection using CT scan images. In Proceedings of the 2023 First International Conference on Advances in Electrical, Electronics and Computational Intelligence (ICAEECI) (pp. 1–7). IEEE. DOI: 10.1109/ICAEECI58247.2023.10370804

Santini, G., Moreau, N., & Rubeaux, M. (2019). Kidney tumor segmentation using an ensembling multi-stage deep learning: A contribution to the KiTS19 challenge. arXiv. /arXiv.1909.00735DOI: 10.24926/548719.023

Sharma, A., Sinha, A., & Ahmed, S. (2025). Automated kidney disease classification using deep hybrid CNN architecture on CT images, arXiv:2502.04367. https://arxiv.org/abs/2502.04367

Sheehan, S., Mawe, S., Cianciolo, R. E., Korstanje, R., & Mahoney, J. M. (2019). Detection and classification of novel renal histologic phenotypes using deep neural networks. *American Journal of Pathology, 189*(9), 1786–1796. DOI: 10.1016/j.ajpath.2019.05.019 PMID: 31220455

Sri, V. S., & Lakshmi, G. R. J. (2023). Detection analysis of abnormality in kidney using deep learning techniques and its optimization. In *Proceedings of the 2023 Second International Conference on Electrical, Electronics, Information and Communication Technologies (ICEEICT)* (pp. 1–6). IEEE. DOI: 10.1109/ICEEICT56924.2023.10157637

Sudharson, S., & Kokil, P. (2019). Abnormality detection in the renal ultrasound images using ensemble MSVM model. In *Proceedings of the 2019 International Conference on Wireless Communications Signal Processing and Networking (WiSPNET)* (pp. 378–382). IEEE. DOI: 10.1109/WiSPNET45539.2019.9032737

Suganthi, N. M., VM, J., Rama, P., & Chandralekha, E. (2022). Chronic Kidney Disease Detection using AdaBoosting Ensemble Method and K-Fold Cross Validation. *2022 International Conference on Automation, Computing and Renewable Systems (ICACRS)*, 979–983. DOI: 10.1109/ICACRS55517.2022.10029047

Tsili, A. C., Andriotis, E., Gkeli, M. G., Krokidis, M., Stasinopoulou, M., Varkarakis, I. M., & Moulopoulos, L.-A. (2021). The role of imaging in the management of renal masses. *European Journal of Radiology*, *141*, 109777. DOI: 10.1016/j.ejrad.2021.109777 PMID: 34020173

Yildirim, K., Bozdag, P. G., Talo, M., Yildirim, O., Karabatak, M., & Acharya, U. R. (2021). Deep learning model for automated kidney stone detection using coronal CT images. *Computers in Biology and Medicine*, *135*, 104569. Advance online publication. DOI: 10.1016/j.compbiomed.2021.104569 PMID: 34157470

Zhang, H., Chen, Y., Song, Y., Xiong, Z., Yang, Y., & Wu, Q. M. J. (2019). Automatic kidney lesion detection for CT images using morphological cascade convolutional neural networks. *IEEE Access : Practical Innovations, Open Solutions*, *7*, 83001–83011. DOI: 10.1109/ACCESS.2019.2924207

Compilation of References

Abadi, M., Chu, A., Goodfellow, I., McMahan, H. B., Mironov, I., Talwar, K., & Zhang, L. (2016). Deep learning with differential privacy. *Proceedings of the 2016 ACM SIGSAC Conference on Computer and Communications Security*, 308–318. https://doi.org/DOI: 10.1145/2976749.2978318

Abbasi-Sureshjani, S., Dashtbozorg, B., ter Haar Romeny, B. M., & Fleuret, F. (2018). Exploratory Study on Direct Prediction of Diabetes Using Deep Residual Networks. *Lecture Notes in Computational Vision and Biomechanics*, *27*, 797–802. DOI: 10.1007/978-3-319-68195-5_86

Abbas, Q., Fondon, I., Sarmiento, A., Jiménez, S., & Alemany, P. (2017a). Automatic recognition of severity level for diagnosis of diabetic retinopathy using deep visual features. *Medical & Biological Engineering & Computing*, *55*(11), 1959–1974. DOI: 10.1007/s11517-017-1638-6 PMID: 28353133

Abousaber, I., Abdallah, H. F., & El-Ghaish, H. (2025). Robust predictive framework for diabetes classification using optimized machine learning on imbalanced datasets. *Frontiers in Artificial Intelligence*, *7*, 1499530. DOI: 10.3389/frai.2024.1499530 PMID: 39839971

Adepoju, V. A., Adejumo, O. A., Adepoju, O. E., Adeniyi, M. O., Etuk, V., Nzekwe, I., Inegbeboh, J. O., Adelekan, A., & Oladimeji, O. (2022). Do private health providers adhere to National Tuberculosis Guideline while assigning treatment outcome? Findings from a lower middle-income country. *Frontiers in Public Health*, *10*, 924132. DOI: 10.3389/fpubh.2022.924132 PMID: 36211674

Adrion, J. R., Cole, C. B., Dukler, N., Galloway, J. G., Gladstein, A. L., Gower, G., Kyriazis, C. C., Ragsdale, A. P., Tsambos, G., Baumdicker, F., Carlson, J., Cartwright, R. A., Durvasula, A., Gronau, I., Kim, B. Y., McKenzie, P., Messer, P. W., Noskova, E., Del Vecchyo, D. O., & Kern, A. D. (2020). A community-maintained standard library of population genetic models. *eLife*, *9*, e54967. Advance online publication. DOI: 10.7554/eLife.54967 PMID: 32573438

Ağraz, M., Eğrioğlu, E., Baş, E., Chen, M. Y., Göksülük, D., & Burak, M. F. (2025). Diabetes Development Prediction Using a Hybrid Model Combining Dendritic Artificial Neuron Model and Logistic Regression. *Endocrinology Research & Practice, 29*(2).

Ağraz, M., Eğrioğlu, E., Baş, E., Chen, M. Y., Göksülük, D., & Burak, M. F. (2025). Diabetes Development Prediction Using a Hybrid Model Combining Dendritic Artificial Neuron Model and Logistic Regression. *Endocrinology Research and Practice*, *29*(2), 84–93. DOI: 10.5152/erp.2025.24585

Ahmed, H. S. (2024). Uncover this tech term: Generative adversarial networks. *Korean Journal of Radiology*, *25*(5), 493. DOI: 10.3348/kjr.2023.1306 PMID: 38627875

Ahmed, S. R. A., Barazanchi, I. A., Mhana, A., & Abdulshaheed, H. R. (2019). Lung cancer classification using data mining and supervised learning algorithms on multi-dimensional data set. [PEN]. *Periodicals of Engineering and Natural Sciences*, *7*(2), 438. DOI: 10.21533/pen.v7i2.483

Akhtar, S., Aftab, S., Ali, O., Ahmad, M., Khan, M. A., Abbas, S., & Ghazal, T. M. (2025). A deep learning based model for diabetic retinopathy grading. *Scientific Reports*, *15*(1), 1–20. DOI: 10.1038/s41598-025-87171-9 PMID: 39885230

Akintunde, T. Y., Musa, T. H., Musa, H. H., Musa, I. H., Chen, S., Ibrahim, E., Tassang, A. E., & Helmy, M. S. E. D. M. (2021). Bibliometric analysis of global scientific literature on effects of COVID-19 pandemic on mental health. *Asian Journal of Psychiatry*, *63*, 102753. DOI: 10.1016/j.ajp.2021.102753 PMID: 34280888

Akiya, I., Ishihara, T., & Yamamoto, K. (2024). Comparison of Synthetic Data Generation Techniques for Control Group Survival Data in Oncology Clinical Trials: Simulation Study. *JMIR Medical Informatics*, *12*, e55118. DOI: 10.2196/55118 PMID: 38889082

Akkasaligar, P. T., Pattar, S., Uppin, A., Kori, K., & Kulakarni, A. (2024). Kidney tumor detection using computed tomography scan images through CNN. In *Proceedings of the 2024 International Conference on Distributed Computing and Optimization Techniques (ICDCOT)* (pp. 1–6). IEEE. DOI: 10.1109/ICDCOT61034.2024.10516254

Akpinar, M. H., Sengur, A., Salvi, M., Seoni, S., Faust, O., Mir, H., Molinari, F., & Acharya, U. R. (2024). Synthetic data generation via generative adversarial networks in healthcare: A systematic review of image- and signal-based studies. *IEEE Open Journal of Engineering in Medicine and Biology*, *6*, 183–192. DOI: 10.1109/OJEMB.2024.3508472 PMID: 39698120

Aksakalli, I., Kaçdioğlu, S., & Hanay, Y. S. (2021). Kidney X-ray Images Classification using Machine Learning and Deep Learning Methods. *Balkan Journal of Electrical and Computer Engineering*, *9*(2), 144–151. DOI: 10.17694/bajece.878116

Al Mamari, H. I. B., Al Washahi, N. A. A., Al Busaidi, M. H. K., & Hajamohideen, F. (2023). Deep neural network based composting processing technology: A solution for municipality and fertilizer companies. *IET Conference Proceedings,* 2022(26), 422–430. DOI: 10.1049/icp.2023.0642

Alberts, C. J., Boyd, A., Bruisten, S. M., Heijman, T., Hogewoning, A., Rooijen, M. V., Siedenburg, E., & Sonder, G. J. B. (2019). Hepatitis A incidence, seroprevalence, and vaccination decision among MSM in Amsterdam, the Netherlands. *Vaccine*, *37*(21), 2849–2856. DOI: 10.1016/j.vaccine.2019.03.048 PMID: 30992222

Aldausari, N., Sowmya, A., Marcus, N., & Mohammadi, G. (2023). Video Generative Adversarial Networks: A Review. *ACM Computing Surveys*, *55*(2), 1–25. DOI: 10.1145/3487891

Alifah Roslan, N., Izura Udzir, N., Mahmod, R., & Gutub, A. (2022). Systematic literature review and analysis for Arabic text steganography method practically. *Egyptian Informatics Journal*, *23*(4), 177–191. DOI: 10.1016/j.eij.2022.10.003

Ali, M. M., Agrawal, J., Mishra, T., & Raj, M. (2023). An automated deep learning approach for kidney disease detection. In *Proceedings of the 2023 International Conference on Integrated Intelligence and Communication Systems (ICIICS)* (pp. 1–6). IEEE. DOI: 10.1109/ICIICS59993.2023.10421534

AlJaberi, O. A., Hussain, M., & Drake, P. R. (2020). A framework for measuring sustainability in healthcare systems. *International Journal of Healthcare Management*, *13*(4), 276–285. Advance online publication. DOI: 10.1080/20479700.2017.1404710

Al-Maniri, A. A., Al-Rawas, O. A., Al-Ajmi, F., De Costa, A., Eriksson, B., & Diwan, V. K. (2008). Tuberculosis suspicion and knowledge among private and public general practitioners: Questionnaire Based Study in Oman. *BMC Public Health*, *8*(1), 1–7. DOI: 10.1186/1471-2458-8-177 PMID: 18501022

Al-Nouti, A. F., & Yaseen, Z. M. (2025). Integration of a hybrid machine learning model with a differential evolution algorithm for underground pipeline corrosion prediction. *Engineering Applications of Artificial Intelligence*, *158*, 111511. Advance online publication. DOI: 10.1016/j.engappai.2025.111511

Alruwaili, R. F., Alsadaan, N., Alruwaili, A. N., & Alrumayh, A. G. (2023). Unveiling the symbiosis of Environmental Sustainability and Infection Control in Health Care settings: A systematic review. *Sustainability (Basel)*, *15*(22), 15728. DOI: 10.3390/su152215728

Altuhaifa, F. A., Win, K. T., & Su, G. (2023). Predicting lung cancer survival based on clinical data using machine learning: A review. *Computers in Biology and Medicine*, *165*, 107338. Advance online publication. DOI: 10.1016/j.compbiomed.2023.107338 PMID: 37625260

Al-Worafi, Y. M. (2023). Tuberculosis Management in Developing Countries. In *Handbook of Medical and Health Sciences in Developing Countries: Education, Practice, and Research* (pp. 1–40). Springer International Publishing., DOI: 10.1007/978-3-030-74786-2_52-1

Alyoubi, W. L., Shalash, W. M., & Abulkhair, M. F. (2020a). Diabetic retinopathy detection through deep learning techniques: A review. *Informatics in Medicine Unlocked*, *20*, 100377. DOI: 10.1016/j.imu.2020.100377

Alzu'bi, D., Abdullah, M., Hmeidi, I., AlAzab, R., Gharaibeh, M., El-Heis, M., Almotairi, K. H., Forestiero, A., Hussein, A. M., & Abualigah, L. (2022). Kidney tumor detection and classification based on deep learning approaches: A new dataset in CT scans. *Journal of Healthcare Engineering*, *2022*, 3861161. Advance online publication. DOI: 10.1155/2022/3861161 PMID: 37323471

Ananthakrishnan, R., Richardson, M. A., van den Hof, S., Rangaswamy, R., Thiagesan, R., Auguesteen, S., & Kamp, N. (2019). Successfully engaging private providers to improve diagnosis, notification, and treatment of TB and drug-resistant TB: The EQUIP public-private model in Chennai, India. *Global Health, Science and Practice*, *7*(1), 41–53. DOI: 10.9745/GHSP-D-18-00318 PMID: 30926737

Anderson, S. (2012). Public, private, neither, both? Publicness theory and the analysis of healthcare organisations. *Social Science & Medicine*, *74*(3), 313–322. DOI: 10.1016/j.socscimed.2011.07.021 PMID: 21893377

Aparna, H., & Madhumitha, J. (2023). Combined image encryption and steganography technique for enhanced security using multiple chaotic maps ☆. *Computers & Electrical Engineering*, *110*(February), 108824. DOI: 10.1016/j.compeleceng.2023.108824

Apellaniz, P. A., Galende, B. A., Jim, A., Parras, J., & Zazo, S. (2025). Advancing Cancer Research with Synthetic Data Generation in Low-Data Scenarios. *IEEE Journal of Biomedical and Health Informatics*, 1–15. DOI: 10.1109/JBHI.2025.3595371 PMID: 40758491

Ardabili, S., Mosavi, A., Ghamisi, P., Ferdinand, F., Varkonyi-Koczy, A., Reuter, U., Rabczuk, T., & Atkinson, P. (2020). COVID-19 Outbreak Prediction with Machine Learning. *Algorithms*, *13*(10), 249. DOI: 10.3390/a13100249

Ardila, D., Kiraly, A. P., Bharadwaj, S., Choi, B., Reicher, J. J., Peng, L., & Corrado, G. S. (2019). End-to-end lung cancer screening with three-dimensional deep learning on low-dose chest computed tomography. *Nature Medicine*, *25*(6), 954–961. https://pubmed.ncbi.nlm.nih.gov/31110349/. DOI: 10.1038/s41591-019-0447-x PMID: 31110349

Arora, L., Singh, S. K., Kumar, S., Gupta, H., Alhalabi, W., Arya, V., Bansal, S., Chui, K. T., & Gupta, B. B. (2024). Ensemble deep learning and EfficientNet for accurate diagnosis of diabetic retinopathy. *Scientific Reports*, *14*(1), 1–16. DOI: 10.1038/s41598-024-81132-4 PMID: 39695310

Arpaci, I., Huang, S., Al-Emran, M., Al-Kabi, M. N., & Peng, M. (2021). Predicting the COVID-19 infection with fourteen clinical features using machine learning classification algorithms. *Multimedia Tools and Applications*, *80*(8), 11943–11957. DOI: 10.1007/s11042-020-10340-7 PMID: 33437173

Arslan, A. K., Yagin, F. H., Algarni, A., Karaaslan, E., Al-Hashem, F., & Ardigò, L. P. (2024). Enhancing type 2 diabetes mellitus prediction by integrating metabolomics and tree-based boosting approaches. *Frontiers in Endocrinology*, *15*, 1444282. DOI: 10.3389/fendo.2024.1444282 PMID: 39588339

Arunkumar, K., Eshwar, S., Mohammed Saleem, D., & Vamsikrishna, C. (2023). Implementation of kidney stone detection using CNN. In 2023 5th International Conference on Smart Systems and Inventive Technology (ICSSIT) (pp. 1320–1324). IEEE. DOI: 10.1109/ICSSIT55814.2023.10061142

Arya, A., & Soni, S. (2022). A Literature Review on Various Recent Steganography Techniques A Literature Review on Various Recent Steganography Techniques. September.

Ashrafi, N., Schmitt, V., Spang, R. P., Möller, S., & Voigt-Antons, J. N. (2023, June). Protect and extend-using GANs for synthetic data generation of time-series medical records. In *2023 15th International Conference on Quality of Multimedia Experience (QoMEX)* (pp. 171-176). IEEE. DOI: 10.1109/QoMEX58391.2023.10178496

Assaf, D., Gutman, Y., Neuman, Y., Segal, G., Amit, S., Gefen-Halevi, S., Shilo, N., Epstein, A., Mor-Cohen, R., Biber, A., Rahav, G., Levy, I., & Tirosh, A. (2020). Utilization of machine-learning models to accurately predict the risk for critical COVID-19. *Internal and Emergency Medicine*, *15*(8), 1435–1443. DOI: 10.1007/s11739-020-02475-0 PMID: 32812204

Athieniti, E., & Spyrou, G. M. (2023). A guide to multi-omics data collection and integration for translational medicine. In *Computational and Structural Biotechnology Journal* (Vol. 21). DOI: 10.1016/j.csbj.2022.11.050

Attaran, M. (2022). Blockchain technology in healthcare: Challenges and opportunities. *International Journal of Healthcare Management*, *15*(1), 70–83. DOI: 10.1080/20479700.2020.1843887

Atta-ur-Rahman, , Sultan, K., Naseer, I., Majeed, R., Musleh, D., Abdul Salam Gollapalli, M., Chabani, S., Ibrahim, N., Yamin Siddiqui, S., & Adnan Khan, M.Atta-ur-Rahman. (2021). Supervised Machine Learning-Based Prediction of COVID-19. *Computers, Materials & Continua*, *69*(1), 21–34. DOI: 10.32604/cmc.2021.013453

Auffray, C., Balling, R., Barroso, I., Bencze, L., Benson, M., Bergeron, J., Bernal-Delgado, E., Blomberg, N., Bock, C., Conesa, A., Del Signore, S., Delogne, C., Devilee, P., Di Meglio, A., Eijkemans, M., Flicek, P., Graf, N., Grimm, V., Guchelaar, H.-J., & Zanetti, G. (2016). Making sense of big data in health research: Towards an EU action plan. *Genome Medicine*, *8*(1), 1–10. DOI: 10.1186/s13073-016-0323-y PMID: 26750923

Aviv-Reuven, S., & Rosenfeld, A. (2021). Publication patterns' changes due to the COVID-19 pandemic: A longitudinal and short-term scientometric analysis. *Scientometrics*, *126*(8), 6761–6784. DOI: 10.1007/s11192-021-04059-x PMID: 34188333

Ayilara, O. F., Platt, R. W., Dahl, M., Coulombe, J., Ginestet, P. G., Chateau, D., & Lix, L. M. (2023). Generating synthetic data from administrative health records for drug safety and effectiveness studies. *International Journal of Population Data Science*, *8*(1). Advance online publication. DOI: 10.23889/ijpds.v8i1.2176 PMID: 38414538

Azizi, Z., Zheng, C., Mosquera, L., Pilote, L., & El Emam, K. (2021). Can synthetic data be a proxy for real clinical trial data? A validation study. *BMJ Open*, *11*(4), e043497. Advance online publication. DOI: 10.1136/bmjopen-2020-043497 PMID: 33863713

Babar, F. F., Jamil, F., Alsboui, T., Babar, F. F., Ahmad, S., & Alkanhel, R. I. (2024, May). Federated active learning with transfer learning: Empowering edge int Gaoelligence for enhanced lung cancer diagnosis. In *Proceedings of the 20th International Wireless Communications and Mobile Computing Conference (IWCMC)* (pp. 1333–1338). IEEE. https://doi.org/DOI: 10.1109/IWCMC61514.2024.10592390

Baião, A. R., Cai, Z., Poulos, R. C., Robinson, P. J., Reddel, R. R., Zhong, Q., Vinga, S., & Gonçalves, E. (2025). A technical review of multi-omics data integration methods: From classical statistical to deep generative approaches. *Briefings in Bioinformatics*, *26*(4), bbaf355. Advance online publication. DOI: 10.1093/bib/bbaf355 PMID: 40748323

Balamanikandan, A., Saravanakumar, M., Gunasekaran, S., Anjum, V., Gurusamy, P., & Ashokkumar, N. (2024). Deep learning in the detection of chronic kidney disease. In *Proceedings of the 2024 4th International Conference on Intelligent Technologies (CONIT)* (pp. 1–6). IEEE. DOI: 10.1109/CONIT61985.2024.10627434

Bappi, M. I., Juthy, J. A., & Kim, K. (2025). Deep learning-based diabetic retinopathy recognition and grading: Challenges, gaps, and an improved approach — A survey. *ICT Express*, *11*(August), 993–1013. Advance online publication. DOI: 10.1016/j.icte.2025.08.001

Barr, A. A., Quan, J., Guo, E., & Sezgin, E. (2025). Large language models generating synthetic clinical datasets: A feasibility and comparative analysis with real-world perioperative data. *Frontiers in Artificial Intelligence*, *8*, 1533508. Advance online publication. DOI: 10.3389/frai.2025.1533508 PMID: 39974356

Barriga, E. S., Murray, V., Agurto, C., Pattichis, M., Bauman, W., Zamora, G., & Soliz, P. (2010). Automatic system for diabetic retinopathy screening based on AM-FM, partial least squares, and support vector machines. *2010 7th IEEE International Symposium on Biomedical Imaging: From Nano to Macro, ISBI 2010 - Proceedings*, 1349–1352. DOI: 10.1109/ISBI.2010.5490247

Basri, M. A. (2024). *Evaluating the Usefulness of Synthetic Data in Healthcare: Applications in Predictive Modeling and Privacy Protection.*

Bassani, T., Cina, A., Galbusera, F., Cazzato, A., Pellegrino, M. E., Albano, D., & Sconfienza, L. M. (2025). Feasibility of generating sagittal radiographs from coronal views using GAN-based deep learning framework in adolescent idiopathic scoliosis. *European Radiology Experimental*, *9*(1), 11. DOI: 10.1186/s41747-025-00553-6 PMID: 39881022

Basu, S., Karuppiah, M., Nasipuri, M., & Kumar, A. (2019). Bio-inspired cryptosystem with DNA cryptography and neural networks. *Journal of Systems Architecture*, *94*(February), 24–31. DOI: 10.1016/j.sysarc.2019.02.005

Beaulieu-Jones, B. K., Wu, Z. S., Williams, C., Lee, R., Bhavnani, S. P., Byrd, J. B., & Greene, C. S. (2019). Privacy-preserving generative deep neural networks support clinical data sharing. *Circulation: Cardiovascular Quality and Outcomes*, *12*(7), e005122. Advance online publication. DOI: 10.1161/CIRCOUTCOMES.118.005122 PMID: 31284738

Beaumont, J. (2021). *Synthetic data for the privacy-conscious Luddite*. Towards Data Science.

Behera, M. K. (2020). Prediction of different stages in Diabetic retinopathy from retinal fundus images using radial basis function based SVM. *Indian Journal of Science and Technology*, *13*(20), 2030–2040. DOI: 10.17485/IJST/v13i20.322

Belsti, Y., Moran, L., Du, L., Mousa, A., De Silva, K., Enticott, J., & Teede, H. (2023). Comparison of machine learning and conventional logistic regression-based prediction models for gestational diabetes in an ethnically diverse population: The Monash GDM machine learning model. *International Journal of Medical Informatics*, *179*, 105228. Advance online publication. DOI: 10.1016/j.ijmedinf.2023.105228 PMID: 37774429

Bengesi, S., El-Sayed, H., Sarker, M. K., Houkpati, Y., Irungu, J., & Oladunni, T. (2024). *Advancements in Generative AI: A Comprehensive Review of GANs, GPT, Autoencoders, Diffusion Model, and Transformers*. IEEE., DOI: 10.1109/ACCESS.2024.3397775

Bhanot, K., Qi, M., Erickson, J. S., Guyon, I., & Bennett, K. P. (2021). The Problem of Fairness in Synthetic Healthcare Data. *Entropy (Basel, Switzerland)*, *23*(9), 1165. DOI: 10.3390/e23091165 PMID: 34573790

Bhat, S. S., Selvam, V., & Ansari, G. A. (2023). Predicting Life Style of Early Diabetes Mellitus Using Machine Learning.

Bhatt, J., & Bathija, P. (2018). Ensuring access to quality health care in vulnerable communities. *Academic Medicine*, *93*(9), 1271–1275. DOI: 10.1097/ACM.0000000000002254 PMID: 29697433

Bhavana, S., Akula, A., Rao, V. N., & Swetha, C. (2025). Advanced AI Approaches in Education. In *Supporting Personalized Learning and Students' Skill Development With AI* (pp. 1–16). IGI Global Scientific Publishing. DOI: 10.4018/979-8-3693-8965-2.ch001

Bhuyan, S. S., Sateesh, V., Mukul, N., Galvankar, A., Mahmood, A., Nauman, M., Rai, A., Bordoloi, K., Basu, U., & Samuel, J. (2025). Generative artificial intelligence Use in healthcare: Opportunities for clinical excellence and administrative efficiency. *Journal of Medical Systems*, *49*(1), 10. DOI: 10.1007/s10916-024-02136-1 PMID: 39820845

Bibikova, M., & Fan, J. (2023). Liquid biopsy for early detection of lung cancer. *Chinese Medical Journal Pulmonary and Critical Care Medicine*, *1*(4), 200–206. DOI: 10.1016/j.pccm.2023.08.005 PMID: 39171286

Bietsch, D., Stahlbock, R., & Voß, S. (2023). Synthetic Data as a Proxy for Real-World Electronic Health Records in the Patient Length of Stay Prediction. *Sustainability (Basel)*, *15*(18), 13690. Advance online publication. DOI: 10.3390/su151813690

Birajdar, P. S., & Lobo, L. M. R. J. (2023). Advancing cancer research: Intelligent prediction and analysis system based on deep learning. [JETIR]. *Journal of Emerging Technologies and Innovative Research*, *10*(8). https://www.jetir.org/indexx?v=10&i=8&j=August%202023

Biswal, S., Singh, D., & Pentyala, S.. (2021). SynthEHR: A Transformer-based approach for generating synthetic electronic health records. *2021 IEEE International Conference on Bioinformatics and Biomedicine (BIBM)*, 2686-2693.

Biswas, A., Md Abdullah Al, N., Imran, A., Sejuty, A. T., Fairooz, F., Puppala, S., & Talukder, S. (2023). Generative Adversarial Networks for Data Augmentation. In *Data Driven Approaches on Medical Imaging*. DOI: 10.1007/978-3-031-47772-0_8

Bogacsovics, G., Toth, J., Hajdu, A., & Harangi, B. (2022). Enhancing CNNs through the use of hand-crafted features in automated fundus image classification. *Biomedical Signal Processing and Control*, *76*, 103685. DOI: 10.1016/j.bspc.2022.103685

Bogale, B., Scambler, S., Mohd Khairuddin, A. N., & Gallagher, J. E. (2024). Health system strengthening in fragile and conflict-affected states: A review of systematic reviews. *PLoS One*, *19*(6), e0305234. DOI: 10.1371/journal.pone.0305234 PMID: 38875266

Brown, T., Mann, B., Ryder, N., Subbiah, M., Kaplan, J. D., Dhariwal, P., Neelakantan, A., Shyam, P., Sastry, G., Askell, A., Agarwal, S., Herbert-Voss, A., Krueger, G., Henighan, T., Child, R., Ramesh, A., Ziegler, D., Wu, J., Winter, C., . . . Amodei, D. (2020). Language Models are Few-Shot Learners. *Advances in Neural Information Processing Systems*, *33*, 1877–1901. https://proceedings.neurips.cc/paper/2020/hash/1457c0d6bfcb4967418bfb8ac142f64a-Abstract.html

Brunet, T. D. P. (2016). Aims and methods of biosteganography. *Journal of Biotechnology, 226*, 56–64. DOI: 10.1016/j.jbiotec.2016.03.044

Buriboev, A., Bobakulov, A., Yusupova, Z., Fayzullaev, A., Nematov, D., & Rakhmonov, A. (2024). Kidney segmentation in ultrasound images based on CNN using modified CLAHE. *Sensors (Basel), 24*(23), 7703. DOI: 10.3390/s24237703 PMID: 39686240

Cao, H., Tan, C., Gao, Z., Xu, Y., Chen, G., Heng, P. A., & Li, S. Z. (2024). A Survey on Generative Diffusion Models. *IEEE Transactions on Knowledge and Data Engineering, 36*(7), 2814–2830. Advance online publication. DOI: 10.1109/TKDE.2024.3361474

Cao, X. (2020). COVID-19: Immunopathology and its implications for therapy. *Nature Reviews. Immunology, 20*(5), 269–270. DOI: 10.1038/s41577-020-0308-3 PMID: 32273594

Cao, Y., Mao, J., Yu, H., Zhang, Q., Wang, H., Zhang, Q., Guo, L., & Gao, F. (2020). A novel hybrid active contour model for intracranial tuberculosis MRI segmentation applications. *IEEE Access : Practical Innovations, Open Solutions, 8*, 149569–149585. DOI: 10.1109/ACCESS.2020.3016746

CARE. T. I. (2023). THE STATE OF TB. https://cisp.cachefly.net/assets/articles/attachments/90339_2023-state-of-tb-report-.pdf

Caroli, A., Remuzzi, A., & Lerman, L. O. (2021). Basic principles and new advances in kidney imaging. *Kidney International, 100*(5), 1001–1011. DOI: 10.1016/j.kint.2021.04.032 PMID: 33984338

Cascella, M., Scarpati, G., Bignami, E. G., Cuomo, A., Vittori, A., Di Gennaro, P., Crispo, A., & Coluccia, S. (2023). Utilizing an artificial intelligence framework (conditional generative adversarial network) to enhance telemedicine strategies for cancer pain management. *Journal of Anesthesia, Analgesia and Critical Care, 3*(1), 19. Advance online publication. DOI: 10.1186/s44158-023-00104-8 PMID: 37386680

Cavinato, T., Rubinacci, S., Malaspinas, A. S., & Delaneau, O. (2024). A resampling-based approach to share reference panels. *Nature Computational Science, 4*(5), 360–366. DOI: 10.1038/s43588-024-00630-7 PMID: 38745108

Chakaya, J., Khan, M., Ntoumi, F., Aklillu, E., Fatima, R., Mwaba, P., Kapata, N., Mfinanga, S., Hasnain, S. E., Katot, P. D.M.C., Bulabula, A. N. H, Sam-Agudu, N. A, Nachega, J. B., Tiberi, S., McHugh, T. D., Abubakar, I., & Zumla, A. (2021).

Chandra, S., Prakash, P. K. S., Samanta, S., & Chilukuri, S. (2024a). ClinicalGAN: Powering patient monitoring in clinical trials with patient digital twins. *Scientific Reports*, *14*(1), 12236. DOI: 10.1038/s41598-024-62567-1 PMID: 38806536

Chang, K., Shlezinger, N., & Eldar, Y. C. (2020). Federated learning for privacy-preserving medical data generation. *arXiv preprint arXiv:2009.07062*.

Chang, L., Yan, Y., & Wang, L. (2020). Coronavirus Disease 2019: Coronaviruses and Blood Safety. *Transfusion Medicine Reviews*, *34*(2), 75–80. DOI: 10.1016/j.tmrv.2020.02.003 PMID: 32107119

Chan, T. F., & Vese, L. A. (2001). Active contours without edges. *IEEE Transactions on Image Processing*, *10*(2), 266–277. DOI: 10.1109/83.902291 PMID: 18249617

Charleonnan, A., Fufaung, T., Niyomwong, T., Chokchueypattanakit, W., Suwannawach, S., & Ninchawee, N. (2016). Predictive analytics for chronic kidney disease using machine learning techniques. In *Proceedings of the 2016 Management and Innovation Technology International Conference (MITicon)* (pp. MIT-80–MIT-83). IEEE. DOI: 10.1109/MITICON.2016.8025242

Chaves, L., & Marques, G. (2021). Data mining techniques for early diagnosis of diabetes: A comparative study. *Applied Sciences (Basel, Switzerland)*, *11*(5), 2218. DOI: 10.3390/app11052218

Chenchu, S., Kandem, V., Dattaram, T., & Rao, T. V. N. (2025). The convergence of artificial intelligence and graphical user interface. In *Supply Chain Transformation Through Generative AI and Machine Learning* (pp. 69–102). IGI Global Scientific Publishing. DOI: 10.4018/979-8-3693-4433-0.ch004

Chen, I., Johansson, F. D., & Sontag, D. (2023). Why is my model unfair? A systematic review of sources of unfairness in machine learning for healthcare. *Nature Medicine*, *29*(6), 1344–1354.

Chen, T. K., Knicely, D. H., & Grams, M. E. (2019). Chronic kidney disease diagnosis and management: A review. *Journal of the American Medical Association*, *322*(13), 1294–1304. DOI: 10.1001/jama.2019.14745 PMID: 31573641

Chijioke-Akaniro, O., Ubochioma, E., Omoniyi, A., Omosebi, O., Olarewaju, O., Etolue, M., Asuke, S., Aniwada, E., Ndubisi, A. U., Ombeka, V., Agbajes, A., Lawanson, A., & Anyaike, C. (2022). Strategic engagement of private facilities to increase public-private mix (PPM) contribution to Nigeria tuberculosis case notification. *Journal of Tuberculosis Research*, *10*(3), 99–110. DOI: 10.4236/jtr.2022.103008

Chilala, S. B., Silumbwe, A., Zulu, J. M., Tetui, M., Bulawayo, M., Chewe, M., & Hangoma, P. (2024). Individual, community and health systems factors influencing time to notification of tuberculosis: Situating software and hardware bottlenecks in local health systems. *BMC Health Services Research, 24*(1), 1–11. DOI: 10.1186/s12913-024-11697-3 PMID: 39415167

Chitale, R., Shah, B., Bhalgat, S., Pandey, A., & Jakhete, S. A. (2023, August). Utilization of CNN and ensemble methods to support medical practitioners in categorizing lung cancer: A research paper. In *Proceedings of the 7th International Conference on Computing, Communication, Control and Automation (ICCUBEA)* (pp. 1–5). IEEE. https://doi.org/DOI: 10.1109/ICCUBEA58933.2023.10392016

Choi, E., Biswal, S., Malin, B., Duke, J., Stewart, W. F., & Sun, J. (2017).[98] Generating multi-label discrete patient records using generative adversarial networks. *Machine Learning for Healthcare Conference*, 286–305. PMLR.

Choi, E., Biswal, S., Malin, B., Duke, J., Stewart, W. F., & Sun, J. (2017, November 6). Generating Multi-label Discrete Patient Records using Generative Adversarial Networks. *Proceedings of the 2nd Machine Learning for Healthcare Conference.* https://proceedings.mlr.press/v68/choi17a.html

Cole, B., Nilsen, D. M., Will, L., Etkind, S. C., Burgos, M., & Chorba, T. (2020). Essential components of a public health tuberculosis prevention, control, and elimination program: Recommendations of the Advisory Council for the Elimination of Tuberculosis and the National Tuberculosis Controllers Association. *MMWR. Recommendations and Reports, 69*(7), 1–27. Advance online publication. DOI: 10.15585/mmwr.rr6907a1 PMID: 32730235

Confusion Matrix - Clearly Explained | Towards Data Science. (n.d.). Retrieved August 5, 2025, from https://towardsdatascience.com/confusion-matrix-clearly-explained-fee63614dc7/

Convolutional Neural Network (CNN) | TensorFlow Core. (n.d.). Retrieved August 5, 2025, from https://www.tensorflow.org/tutorials/images/cnn

Convolutional Neural Network with Implementation in Python. (n.d.). Retrieved August 5, 2025, from https://www.analyticsvidhya.com/blog/2021/08/beginners-guide-to-convolutional-neural-network-with-implementation-in-python/

Costaner, L., Informatika, T., Ilmu Komputer, F., & Lancang Kuning -Riau, U. (2024). Feature Extraction Analysis for Diabetic Retinopathy Detection Using Machine Learning Techniques. *SISTEMASI, 13*(5), 2268–2276. DOI: 10.32520/stmsi.v13i5.4600

Costa, P., Galdran, A., Smailagic, A., & Campilho, A. (2018). A Weakly-Supervised Framework for Interpretable Diabetic Retinopathy Detection on Retinal Images. *IEEE Access : Practical Innovations, Open Solutions*, *6*, 18747–18758. DOI: 10.1109/ACCESS.2018.2816003

Cyril, S., Smith, B. J., Possamai-Inesedy, A., & Renzaho, A. M. (2015). Exploring the role of community engagement in improving the health of disadvantaged populations: A systematic review. *Global Health Action*, *8*(1), 29842. DOI: 10.3402/gha.v8.29842 PMID: 26689460

Dahmen, J., & Cook, D. (2019a). SynSys: A Synthetic Data Generation System for Healthcare Applications. *Sensors (Basel)*, *19*(5), 1181. DOI: 10.3390/s19051181 PMID: 30857130

Dankar, F. K., & Ibrahim, M. (2021). Fake It Till You Make It: Guidelines for Effective Synthetic Data Generation. *Applied Sciences 2021, Vol. 11, Page 2158*, *11*(5), 2158. DOI: 10.3390/app11052158

Das, D., Biswas, S. K., & Bandyopadhyay, S. (2022). A critical review on diagnosis of diabetic retinopathy using machine learning and deep learning. In *Multimedia Tools and Applications* (Vol. 81, Issue 18). Multimedia Tools and Applications. DOI: 10.1007/s11042-022-12642-4

Das, S., Kharbanda, K., M, S., Raman, R., & D, E. D. (2021). Deep learning architecture based on segmented fundus image features for classification of diabetic retinopathy. *Biomedical Signal Processing and Control*, *68*, 102600. DOI: 10.1016/j.bspc.2021.102600

de Vries, G., van Hest, R. A., & Richardus, J. H. (2007). Impact of mobile radiographic screening on tuberculosis among drug users and homeless persons. *American Journal of Respiratory and Critical Care Medicine*, *176*(2), 201–207. DOI: 10.1164/rccm.200612-1877OC PMID: 17413123

Demissie Gizaw, G., Aderaw Alemu, Z., & Kibret, K. T. (2015). Assessment of knowledge and practice of health workers towards tuberculosis infection control and associated factors in public health facilities of Addis Ababa, Ethiopia: A cross-sectional study. *Archives of Public Health = Archives Belges de Santé Publique*, *73*(1), 1–9. DOI: 10.1186/s13690-015-0062-3 PMID: 25821581

Devaraj, J., Madurai Elavarasan, R., Pugazhendhi, R., Shafiullah, G. M., Ganesan, S., Jeysree, A. K., Khan, I. A., & Hossain, E. (2021). Forecasting of COVID-19 cases using deep learning models: Is it reliable and practically significant? *Results in Physics*, *21*, 103817. DOI: 10.1016/j.rinp.2021.103817 PMID: 33462560

Devi, D. (2024). Towards real-time earthquake forecasting in Chile: Integrating intelligent technologies and machine learning. *Computers & Electrical Engineering*, *117*, 109285. DOI: 10.1016/j.compeleceng.2024.109285

Dhaliwal, L. K. (2020). Health equity and sustainable development goals: role and the complexity. *Good health and well-being*, 316-324. DOI: 10.1007/978-3-319-95681-7_66

Diabetic Retinopathy Columbus | Diabetes Norfolk | Eye Physicians P.C. (n.d.). Retrieved August 5, 2025, from https://www.eyephysicianspc.com/ocular-disease-treatments-columbus/diabetic-retinopathy/

Dong, Y., Liu, Q., Du, B., & Zhang, L. (2022). Weighted feature fusion of convolutional neural network and graph attention network for hyperspectral image classification. IEEE Transactions on Image Processing, PP, 1–1. DOI: 10.1109/TIP.2022.3144017

Draghi, B., Wang, Z., Myles, P., & Tucker, A. (2024). Identifying and handling data bias within primary healthcare data using synthetic data generators. *Heliyon*, *10*(2), e24178. DOI: 10.1016/j.heliyon.2024.e24164 PMID: 38288010

Dutta, S., Manideep, B. C. S., Basha, S. M., Caytiles, R. D., & Iyengar, N. C. S. N. (2018). Classification of diabetic retinopathy images by using deep learning models. *International Journal of Grid and Distributed Computing*, *11*(1), 89–106. DOI: 10.14257/ijgdc.2018.11.1.09

Dwork, C. (2008). Differential privacy: A survey of results. In *International Conference on Theory and Applications of Models of Computation* (pp. 1-19). Springer, Berlin, Heidelberg.

Elaraby, M. E., Ewees, A. A., & Anter, A. M. (2024). A robust IoT-based cloud model for COVID-19 prediction using advanced machine learning technique. *Biomedical Signal Processing and Control*, *87*, 105542. DOI: 10.1016/j.bspc.2023.105542

Elton, D. M., Zhang, Y., & Wong, S. T. C. (2018). A deep learning system for automated kidney stone detection and volumetric segmentation on non-contrast CT scans. *Medical Physics*. Advance online publication. DOI: 10.1002/mp.13490 PMID: 35156216

Elvatun, S., Knoors, D., Brant, S., Jonasson, C., & Nygård, J. F. (2025). Synthetic data as external control arms in scarce single-arm clinical trials. *PLOS Digital Health*, *4*(1), e0000581. DOI: 10.1371/journal.pdig.0000581 PMID: 39847598

Erdaş, Ç. B., & Sümer, E. (2024). CNN-Based Neurodegenerative Disease Classification Using QR-Represented Gait Data. *Brain and Behavior*, *14*(10), e70100.

Esteban, C., Hyland, S. L., & Rätsch, G. (2017). Real-valued (medical) time series generation with recurrent conditional GANs. *arXiv preprint arXiv:1706.02633.*

Esteva, A., Robicquet, A., Ramsundar, B., Kuleshov, V., DePristo, M., Chou, K., Cui, C., Corrado, G., Thrun, S., & Dean, J. (2019). A guide to deep learning in healthcare. *Nature Medicine*, *25*(1), 24–29. DOI: 10.1038/s41591-018-0316-z PMID: 30617335

Fan, R., Liu, Y., & Zhang, R. (2021). Multi-scale feature fusion with adaptive weighting for diabetic retinopathy severity classification. *Electronics (Basel)*, *10*(12), 1369. Advance online publication. DOI: 10.3390/electronics10121369

Farnoodian, M. E., Moridani, M. K., & Mokhber, H. (2023). Detection and prediction of diabetes using effective biomarkers. *Computer Methods in Biomechanics and Biomedical Engineering. Imaging & Visualization*, •••, 1–13.

Fayyaz, A. M., Sharif, M. I., Azam, S., Karim, A., & El-Den, J. (2023). Analysis of Diabetic Retinopathy (DR) Based on the Deep Learning. *Information (Basel)*, *14*(1), 30. Advance online publication. DOI: 10.3390/info14010030

Field, M., Vinod, S., Delaney, G. P., Aherne, N., Bailey, M., Carolan, M., Dekker, A., Greenham, S., Hau, E., Lehmann, J., Ludbrook, J., Miller, A., Rezo, A., Selvaraj, J., Sykes, J., Thwaites, D., & Holloway, L. (2024). Federated learning survival model and potential radiotherapy decision support impact assessment for non–small cell lung cancer using real-world data. *Clinical Oncology*, *36*(7), e197–e208. DOI: 10.1016/j.clon.2024.03.008 PMID: 38631978

Figueira, A., & Vaz, B. (2022). Survey on Synthetic Data Generation, Evaluation Methods and GANs. *Mathematics 2022, Vol. 10, Page 2733, 10*(15), 2733. DOI: 10.3390/math10152733

Foomani, F. H., Anisuzzaman, D. M., Niezgoda, J., Niezgoda, J., Guns, W., Gopalakrishnan, S., & Yu, Z. (2022). Synthesizing time-series wound prognosis factors from electronic medical records using generative adversarial networks. *Journal of Biomedical Informatics*, *125*, 103972. DOI: 10.1016/j.jbi.2021.103972 PMID: 34920125

Foraker, R., Morrow, J. D., Johnson, J. A., Wilcox, A. B., Forster, A. J., & Payne, P. R. O. (2025). Understanding synthetic data: Artificial datasets for real-world evidence. *BMJ Evidence-Based Medicine*, bmjebm-2024-113617. DOI: 10.1136/bmjebm-2024-113617

Francesca, T. (2019). *Comparing privacy laws: GDPR v. CCPA*. https://futurium.ec.europa.eu/en/european-ai-alliance/open-library/comparing-privacy-laws-gdpr-v-ccpa

Frederick, A., Das, M., Mehta, K., Kumar, G., & Satyanarayana, S. (2021). Pharmacy based surveillance for identifying missing tuberculosis cases: A mixed methods study from South India. *The Indian Journal of Tuberculosis*, *68*(1), 51–58. DOI: 10.1016/j.ijtb.2020.09.017 PMID: 33641851

Gada, D. (2022). Disease Prediction System using Machine Learning. 2022 6th International Conference on Computing, Communication, Control and Automation (ICCUBEA, 1–5. DOI: 10.1109/ICCUBEA54992.2022.10011002

Galal, A., Moustafa, A., & Salama, M. (2024), Transforming Neurodegenerative Disorder Care with Machine Learning: Strategies and Applications. Available at *SSRN*: https://ssrn.com/abstract=5114443 or http://dx.doi.org/DOI: 10.2139/ssrn.5114443

Gao, C., Wu, L., Wu, W., Huang, Y., Wang, X., Sun, Z., Xu, M., & Gao, C. (2025). Deep learning in pulmonary nodule detection and segmentation: A systematic review. *European Radiology*, *35*(1), 255–266. DOI: 10.1007/s00330-024-10907-0 PMID: 38985185

Garg, P. P., Jayashree, J., & Vijayashree, J. (2025). Revolutionizing healthcare: The transformative role of artificial intelligence. In *Responsible and Explainable Artificial Intelligence in Healthcare* (pp. 1–23). Elsevier. DOI: 10.1016/B978-0-443-24788-0.00001-7

Gautam, A., & Shanker, R. (2025). Diabetic retinopathy detection from fundus images: A wide survey from grading to segmentation of lesions. *Computers in Biology and Medicine*, *196*(July), 110715. Advance online publication. DOI: 10.1016/j.compbiomed.2025.110715 PMID: 40683101

Gebru, T., Morgenstern, J., Vecchione, B., Vaughan, J. W., Wallach, H., Daumé, H.III, & Crawford, K. (2021). Datasheets for datasets. *Communications of the ACM*, *64*(12), 86–92. DOI: 10.1145/3458723

Gharahbagh, A. A., Hajihashemi, V., Machado, J. J. M., & Tavares, J. M. R. S. (2024). Feature Extraction Based on Local Histogram with Unequal Bins and a Recurrent Neural Network for the Diagnosis of Kidney Diseases from CT Images. *Bioengineering (Basel, Switzerland)*, *11*(3), 220. DOI: 10.3390/bioengineering11030220 PMID: 38534494

Gill, K. S., Anand, V., Chauhan, R., Singh, P., & Gupta, R. (2023). Detection of kidney disease in X-ray images using machine learning on MobileNetV3 CNN model. In *Proceedings of the 2023 2nd International Conference on Futuristic Technologies (INCOFT)* (pp. 1–4). IEEE. DOI: 10.1109/INCOFT60753.2023.10425269

Giuffrè, M., & Shung, D. L. (2023a). Harnessing the power of synthetic data in healthcare: Innovation, application, and privacy. *NPJ Digital Medicine*, *6*(1), 186. Advance online publication. DOI: 10.1038/s41746-023-00927-3 PMID: 37813960

Glaziou, P., Floyd, K., & Raviglione, M. C. (2018). Global epidemiology of tuberculosis. In *Seminars in respiratory and critical care medicine* (Vol. 39, No. 03, pp. 271-285). Thieme Medical Publishers. DOI: 10.1055/s-0038-1651492

Global Tuberculosis Report 2020–Reflections on the Global TB burden, treatment and prevention efforts. *International journal of infectious diseases, 113*, S7-S12. DOI: 10.1016/j.ijid.2021.02.107

Goel, S., Gupta, S., Panwar, A., Kumar, S., Verma, M., Bourouis, S., & Ullah, M. A. (2021). Deep Learning Approach for Stages of Severity Classification in Diabetic Retinopathy Using Color Fundus Retinal Images. *Mathematical Problems in Engineering*, *2021*, 1–8. Advance online publication. DOI: 10.1155/2021/7627566

Goncalves, A., Ray, P., Soper, B., Stevens, J., Coyle, L., & Sales, A. P. (2020). Generation and evaluation of synthetic patient data. *BMC Medical Research Methodology*, *20*(1), 108. Advance online publication. DOI: 10.1186/s12874-020-00977-1 PMID: 32381039

Gong, J., Wang, T., Wang, Z., Chu, X., Hu, T., Li, M., Peng, W., Feng, F., Tong, T., & Gu, Y. (2024). Enhancing brain metastasis prediction in non-small cell lung cancer: A deep learning-based segmentation and CT radiomics-based ensemble learning model. *Cancer Imaging; the Official Publication of the International Cancer Imaging Society*, *24*(1), 1. Advance online publication. DOI: 10.1186/s40644-023-00623-1 PMID: 38167564

Gong, W., Pu, Y., Ning, T., Zhu, Y., Mu, G., & Li, J. (2025). Deep learning for enhanced prediction of diabetic retinopathy: A comparative study on the diabetes complications data set. *Frontiers in Medicine*, *12*(June), 1591832. Advance online publication. DOI: 10.3389/fmed.2025.1591832 PMID: 40589972

Gonzales, A., Guruswamy, G., & Smith, S. R. (2023). Synthetic data in health care: A narrative review. *PLOS Digital Health*, *2*(1), e0000082. DOI: 10.1371/journal.pdig.0000082 PMID: 36812604

Goodfellow, I. J., Pouget-Abadie, J., Mirza, M., Xu, B., Warde-Farley, D., Ozair, S., Courville, A., & Bengio, Y. (2014). Generative Adversarial Nets. *Advances in Neural Information Processing Systems, 27*. https://www.github.com/goodfeli/adversarial

Goodfellow, I., Pouget-Abadie, J., Mirza, M., Xu, B., Warde-Farley, D., Ozair, S., Courville, A., & Bengio, Y. (2014). Generative adversarial nets. In *Advances in Neural Information Processing Systems* (Vol. 27, pp. 2672-2680).

Goodfellow, I., Bengio, Y., & Courville, A. (2016). *Deep learning*. The MIT Press.

Goodfellow, I., Pouget-Abadie, J., Mirza, M., Xu, B., Warde-Farley, D., Ozair, S., Courville, A., & Bengio, Y. (2014). Generative adversarial nets. *Advances in Neural Information Processing Systems*, •••, 27.

Govindarajan, P., Abhishek, M., Niharika, K., & Tesfahun, A. (2024). Lungcanary-Pioneering Early Lung Cancer Detection using Machine Learning Algorithms. *8th IEEE International Conference on Computational System and Information Technology for Sustainable Solutions, CSITSS 2024*. DOI: 10.1109/CSITSS64042.2024.10816854

Govindarajan, P., Shreya, N. S., Tesfahun, A., & Amrithavarshini Bhargava, S. (2024). Computing Approach to Detect the Factors and their Impact in Prevalence of Thyroid. *Proceedings of the 18th INDIAcom; 2024 11th International Conference on Computing for Sustainable Global Development, INDIACom 2024*, 1493–1500. DOI: 10.23919/INDIACom61295.2024.10498625

Groß, B., & Wunder, G. (2023). Differentially private synthetic data generation via lipschitz-regularised variational autoencoders. *2023 IEEE Smart World Congress (SWC)*, 1–8.

Guan, H., Yap, P. T., Bozoki, A., & Liu, M. (2024). Federated learning for medical image analysis: A survey. In *Pattern Recognition* (Vol. 151). DOI: 10.1016/j.patcog.2024.110424

Gupta, P., Kumar, D., Malviya, M., & Choudhury, T. (2021). Cancer chatbot: An NLP-based conversational system for cancer diagnosis and support. *IEEE Access : Practical Innovations, Open Solutions*, *9*, 145857–145869.

Gupta, R., Koli, N., Mahor, N., & Tejashri, N. (2020). Performance analysis of Machine Learning classifier for predicting chronic kidney Disease. *2020 International Conference for Emerging Technology (INCET)*, 1–4. DOI: 10.1109/INCET49848.2020.9154147

Gupta, S., Granich, R., Lepere, P., Hersh, B., Gouws, E., & Samb, B. (2014). Review of policy and status of implementation of collaborative HIV-TB activities in 23 high-burden countries. *The International Journal of Tuberculosis and Lung Disease : the Official Journal of the International Union against Tuberculosis and Lung Disease*, *18*(10), 1149–1158. DOI: 10.5588/ijtld.13.0889 PMID: 25216827

Gupta, T., Selwal, A., & Sharma, A. K. (2025). A survey on image cryptography mechanisms : Hitherto, and future directions. *Computer Science Review, 58*(January), 100783. DOI: 10.1016/j.cosrev.2025.100783

Halpern, G. A., Nemet, M., Gowda, D. M., Kilickaya, O., & Lal, A. (2024). Advances and utility of digital twins in critical care and acute care medicine: A narrative review. *Journal of Yeungnam Medical Science*. Advance online publication. DOI: 10.12701/jyms.2024.01053 PMID: 39587767

Hamidian, S., Sahiner, B., Petrick, N., & Pezeshk, A. (2017). 3D convolutional neural network for automatic detection of lung nodules in chest CT. *Proceedings of SPIE - the International Society for Optical Engineering, 10134*, 1013409. Advance online publication. DOI: 10.1117/12.2255795 PMID: 28845077

Hanahan, D. (2022). Hallmarks of cancer: New dimensions. *Cancer Discovery, 12*(1), 31–46. DOI: 10.1158/2159-8290.CD-21-1059 PMID: 35022204

Hanna, M. G., Pantanowitz, L., Dash, R., Harrison, J. H., Deebajah, M., Pantanowitz, J., & Rashidi, H. H. (2025a). Future of Artificial Intelligence—Machine Learning Trends in Pathology and Medicine. *Modern Pathology, 38*(4), 100705. DOI: 10.1016/j.modpat.2025.100705 PMID: 39761872

Haque, M., Islam, T., Rahman, N. A. A., McKimm, J., Abdullah, A., & Dhingra, S. (2020). Strengthening primary health-care services to help prevent and control long-term (chronic) non-communicable diseases in low-and middle-income countries. *Risk Management and Healthcare Policy, 13*, 409–426. DOI: 10.2147/RMHP.S239074 PMID: 32547272

Hasan, S. S., Fury, M. S., Woo, J. J., Kunze, K. N., & Ramkumar, P. N. (2025). Ethical application of generative artificial intelligence in medicine. *Arthroscopy, 41*(4), 874–885. DOI: 10.1016/j.arthro.2024.12.011 PMID: 39689842

Hassan, M. M., Mollick, S., & Yasmin, F. (2022). An unsupervised cluster-based feature grouping model for early diabetes detection. *Healthcare Analytics, 2*, 100112. DOI: 10.1016/j.health.2022.100112

Hatsutani, T., Ichinose, A., Nakamura, K., & Kitamura, Y. (2023). Segmentation of kidney tumors on non-contrast CT images using Protuberance Detection Network. /arXiv.2312.04796DOI: 10.1007/978-3-031-43990-2_2

Heckel, R., Jacob, M., Chaudhari, A., Perlman, O., & Shimron, E. (2024). Deep learning for accelerated and robust MRI reconstruction: A review. Magnetic Resonance Materials in Physics. *Biology and Medicine (Aligarh), 37*(3), 335–368. DOI: 10.1007/s10334-024-01173-8 PMID: 39042206

He, K., Zhang, X., Ren, S., & Sun, J. (2016). Deep residual learning for image recognition. In *Proceedings of the IEEE Conferencepr Conference on Computer Vision and Pattern Recognition (CVPR)* (pp. 770–778). IEEE. https://doi.org/DOI: 10.1109/CVPR.2016.90

Hernandez, M., & Hernandez, M. (2022). Incorporation of Synthetic Data Generation Techniques within a Controlled Data Processing Workflow in the Health and Wellbeing Domain. *Electronics (Basel)*, *11*(5), 812–812. DOI: 10.3390/electronics11050812

Ho, J., Jain, A., & Abbeel, P. (2020). Denoising diffusion probabilistic models. *Advances in Neural Information Processing Systems, 2020-December.*

Hogeweg, L., Sánchez, C. I., Maduskar, P., Philipsen, R., Story, A., Dawson, R., Theron, G., Dheda, K., Peters-Bax, L., & van Ginneken, B. (2015). Automatic detection of tuberculosis in chest radiographs using a combination of textural, focal, and shape abnormality analysis. *IEEE Transactions on Medical Imaging*, *34*(12), 2429–2442. DOI: 10.1109/TMI.2015.2405761 PMID: 25706581

Ho, J., Jain, A., & Abbeel, P. (2020). Denoising diffusion probabilistic models. *Advances in Neural Information Processing Systems*, *33*, 6840–6851.

Houssein, E. H., & Sayed, A. (2023). A modified weighted mean of vectors optimizer for chronic kidney disease classification. *Computers in Biology and Medicine*, *155*, 106691. DOI: 10.1016/j.compbiomed.2023.106691 PMID: 36805229

Houston, A., & Cosma, G. (2023). A genetically-optimised artificial life algorithm for complexity-based synthetic dataset generation. *Information Sciences*, *619*, 540–561. Advance online publication. DOI: 10.1016/j.ins.2022.11.015

Huang, G., Li, R., Bai, Q., & Alty, J. (2023, July 22). Multimodal learning of clinically accessible tests to aid diagnosis of neurodegenerative disorders: A scoping review. *Health Information Science and Systems*, *11*(1), 32. DOI: 10.1007/s13755-023-00231-0 PMID: 37489153

Hu, C., Yun, K. H., Su, Z., & Xi, C. (2022). Effective crisis management during adversity: Organizing resilience capabilities of firms and sustainable performance during COVID-19. *Sustainability (Basel)*, *14*(20), 13664. DOI: 10.3390/su142013664

Husainy, A. S., Mangave, S. S., Patil, C. C., & Mane, S. D. (2024). Harmonizing Responsibilities: Challenges and Opportunities in the Integration of Climate Change and Sustainable Development Goals (SDGs). *The Asian Review of Civil Engineering*, *13*(1), 30–43. DOI: 10.70112/tarce-2024.13.1.4232

Hyun, J., Yongho Lee, Lee, Y., Ha Min Son, Son, H. M., Seo Hu Lee, Lee, S. H., Vinh Pham, Pham, V., Park, J. U., Ji Ung Park, Park, J. U., Tai-Myoung Chung, Chung, T. M., & Chung, T.-M. (2021). *Synthetic Data Generation System for AI-Based Diabetic Foot Diagnosis. 2*(5), 1–9. DOI: 10.1007/s42979-021-00667-9

Hyun, S. H., Ahn, M. S., Koh, Y. W., & Lee, S. J. (2019). A machine-learning approach using PET-based radiomics to predict the histological subtypes of lung cancer. *Clinical Nuclear Medicine, 44*(12), 956–960. DOI: 10.1097/RLU.0000000000002810 PMID: 31689276

Ibeneme, S., Karamagi, H., Muneene, D., Goswami, K., Chisaka, N., & Okeibunor, J. (2022). Strengthening health systems using innovative digital health technologies in Africa. *Frontiers in Digital Health, 4*, 854339. DOI: 10.3389/fdgth.2022.854339 PMID: 35434700

Ibrahim, M., Al Khalil, Y., Amirrajab, S., Sun, C., Breeuwer, M., Pluim, J., & Dumontier, M. (2025). Generative AI for synthetic data across multiple medical modalities: A systematic review of recent developments and challenges. *Computers in Biology and Medicine, 189*, 109834. DOI: 10.1016/j.compbiomed.2025.109834 PMID: 40023073

Image Classification using CNN : Python Implementation - Analytics Vidhya. (n.d.). Retrieved August 5, 2025, from https://www.analyticsvidhya.com/blog/2021/06/image-classification-using-convolutional-neural-network-with-python/

Imam Basha, S. K., & Jana, S. (2025). Review: Machine learning-based lung diseases classification by using chest X-ray image. In *Proceedings of the 2025 International Conference on Visual Analytics and Data Visualization (ICVADV)* (pp. 1241–1245). IEEE. https://doi.org/DOI: 10.1109/ICVADV63329.2025.10961453

Ince, V., Bader-El-Den, M., & Sari, O. F. (2024, August). Enhanced dataset synthesis using CTGAN for metagenomic dataset. In *2024 IEEE 12th International Conference on Intelligent Systems (IS)* (pp. 1-6). IEEE. DOI: 10.1109/IS61756.2024.10705275

Jabir, M., & Choolayil, A. C. (2024). *Social Work with Populations Vulnerable to Neglected Tropical Diseases: Evidence and Insights from India*. Springer Nature., DOI: 10.1007/978-3-031-68997-0

Jadon, A., & Kumar, S. (2023, July 25). Leveraging Generative AI Models for Synthetic Data Generation in Healthcare: Balancing Research and Privacy. *2023 International Conference on Smart Applications, Communications and Networking (SmartNets).* 2023 International Conference on Smart Applications, Communications and Networking (SmartNets), Istanbul, Turkiye. DOI: 10.1109/SmartNets58706.2023.10215825

Jaeger, S., Karargyris, A., Candemir, S., Folio, L., Siegelman, J., Callaghan, F., Xue, Z., Palaniappan, K., Singh, R. K., Antani, S., Thoma, G., Wang, Y.-X., Lu, P.-X., & McDonald, C. J. (2014). Automatic tuberculosis screening using chest radiographs. *IEEE Transactions on Medical Imaging*, *33*(2), 233–245. DOI: 10.1109/TMI.2013.2284099 PMID: 24108713

James, S., Harbron, C., Branson, J., & Sundler, M. (2021). Synthetic data use: Exploring use cases to optimise data utility. *Discover Artificial Intelligence*, *1*(1), 15. Advance online publication. DOI: 10.1007/s44163-021-00016-y

Javanparast, S., Windle, A., Freeman, T., & Baum, F. (2018). Community health worker programs to improve healthcare access and equity: Are they only relevant to low-and middle-income countries? *International Journal of Health Policy and Management*, *7*(10), 943–954. DOI: 10.15171/ijhpm.2018.53 PMID: 30316247

Jawad, M., Zahoor, M., Iqbal, T., Khan, I., & Alouffi, B. (2024). An ensemble learning-based explainable AI framework for early diagnosis of chronic kidney disease. https://arxiv.org/abs/2406.06728

Jindal, V., Kukreja, V., Singh, D. P., Vats, S., & Mehta, S. (2023, October). Pushing diagnostic frontiers: Federated learning CNN for diverse lung disease. In *Proceedings of the 2023 4th IEEE Global Conference for Advancement in Technology (GCAT)* (pp. 1–6). IEEE. https://doi.org/DOI: 10.1109/GCAT59970.2023.10353284

Jumper, J., Evans, R., Pritzel, A., Green, T., Figurnov, M., Ronneberger, O., Tunyasuvunakool, K., Bates, R., Žídek, A., Potapenko, A., Bridgland, A., Meyer, C., Kohl, S. A. A., Ballard, A. J., Cowie, A., Romera-Paredes, B., Nikolov, S., Jain, R., Adler, J., & Hassabis, D. (2021). Highly accurate protein structure prediction with AlphaFold. *Nature*, *596*(7873), 583–589. Advance online publication. DOI: 10.1038/s41586-021-03819-2 PMID: 34265844

Ju, W., Xiang, D., Zhang, B., Wang, L., Kopriva, I., & Chen, X. (2015). Random walk and graph cut for co-segmentation of lung tumor on PET-CT images. *IEEE Transactions on Image Processing*, *24*(12), 5854–5867. DOI: 10.1109/TIP.2015.2488902 PMID: 26462198

K. S., R., L., A. C. P., V., & G. V. (2024). Enhancing kidney stone recognition in ultrasound imaging using hybrid feature extraction techniques. In Proceedings of the 2024 Second International Conference on Intelligent Cyber Physical Systems and Internet of Things (ICoICI) (pp. 1–5). IEEE. DOI: 10.1109/ICoICI62503.2024.10696452

Kalagotla, S. K., Gangashetty, S. V., & Giridhar, K. (2021). A novel stacking technique for prediction of diabetes. *Computers in Biology and Medicine*, *135*, 104554. DOI: 10.1016/j.compbiomed.2021.104554 PMID: 34139440

Kaliappan, J., Saravana Kumar, I. J., Sundaravelan, S., Anesh, T., Rithik, R. R., Singh, Y., Vera-Garcia, D. V., Himeur, Y., Mansoor, W., Atalla, S., & Srinivasan, K. (2024). Analyzing classification and feature selection strategies for diabetes prediction across diverse diabetes datasets. *Frontiers in Artificial Intelligence*, *7*, 1421751. DOI: 10.3389/frai.2024.1421751 PMID: 39233892

Kamath, S., Poojary, M., Shetty, H., Umesh, K., Kar, S., Lakshmi Ramesh, V., Hajare, G., Thomas, A., Brand, H., Jahangir, S., & Kamath, R. (2024). "Private Hospitals Generally Offer Better Treatment and Facilities": Out-of-Pocket Expenditure on Healthcare and the Preference for Private Healthcare Providers in South India. *International Journal of Environmental Research and Public Health, 21*(10), 1287. DOI: 10.3390/ijerph21101287 PMID: 39457260

Kanungo, Y. S., Srinivasan, B., & Choudhary, S. (2017). Detecting diabetic retinopathy using deep learning. *RTEICT 2017 - 2nd IEEE International Conference on Recent Trends in Electronics, Information and Communication Technology, Proceedings, 2018-January*, 801–804. DOI: 10.1109/RTEICT.2017.8256708

Kappelhof, N., Ramos, L., Kappelhof, M., Van Os, H., Chalos, V., Van Kranendonk, K., Kruyt, N., Roos, Y., Van Zwam, W., Van Der Schaaf, I., Van Walderveen, M., Wermer, M., Van Oostenbrugge, R., Lingsma, H., Dippel, D., Majoie, C., & Marquering, H. (2021). Evolutionary algorithms and decision trees for predicting poor outcome after endovascular treatment for acute ischemic stroke. *Computers in Biology and Medicine, 133*, 104414. DOI: 10.1016/j.compbiomed.2021.104414 PMID: 33962154

Kaushik, P., & Sharma, P. (2024). Advanced kidney CT scan diagnosis: A comparative study of VGG16 and DenseNet201 deep learning models. In *Proceedings of the 2024 International Conference on Cybernation and Computation (CYBERCOM)* (pp. 350–355). IEEE. DOI: 10.1109/CYBERCOM63683.2024.10803203

Keerthi, B., Powmika, K. K., Narendra, P., & Karthik, N. (n.d.). Diabetic Retinopathy Detection Using Deep Learning. *2024 International Conference on Signal Processing, Computation, Electronics, Power and Telecommunication, IConSCEPT 2024 - Proceedings, 10*(04), 154–159. DOI: 10.1109/IConSCEPT61884.2024.10627921

Kenneweg, P., Dandinasivara, R., Luo, X., Hammer, B., & Schönhuth, A. (2024). Generating Synthetic Genotypes using Diffusion Models. *ArXiv Preprint ArXiv:2412.03278.*

Khanday, A. M. U. D., Rabani, S. T., Khan, Q. R., Rouf, N., & Mohi Ud Din, M. (2020). Machine learning based approaches for detecting COVID-19 using clinical text data. *International Journal of Information Technology : an Official Journal of Bharati Vidyapeeth's Institute of Computer Applications and Management*, *12*(3), 731–739. DOI: 10.1007/s41870-020-00495-9 PMID: 32838125

Khan, M. S., Mehboob, N., Rahman-Shepherd, A., Naureen, F., Rashid, A., Buzdar, N., & Ishaq, M. (2019). What can motivate Lady Health Workers in Pakistan to engage more actively in tuberculosis case-finding? *BMC Public Health*, *19*(1), 1–9. DOI: 10.1186/s12889-019-7326-8 PMID: 31345194

Khan, S. A. R., Zhang, Y., Kumar, A., Zavadskas, E., & Streimikiene, D. (2020). Measuring the impact of renewable energy, public health expenditure, logistics, and environmental performance on sustainable economic growth. *Sustainable Development (Bradford)*, *28*(4), 833–843. DOI: 10.1002/sd.2034

Khan, S., Siddiqui, F., & Ahad, M. A. (2025). Integrating CNN-based feature fusion and spatial attention for tuberculosis detection with Bayesian optimized XGBoost. *International Journal of Data Science and Analytics*, *20*(6), 5415–5434. DOI: 10.1007/s41060-025-00778-z

Khan, Z., Khan, F. G., Khan, A., Rehman, Z. U., Shah, S., Qummar, S., Ali, F., & Pack, S. (2021). Diabetic Retinopathy Detection Using VGG-NIN a Deep Learning Architecture. *IEEE Access : Practical Innovations, Open Solutions*, *9*, 61408–61416. DOI: 10.1109/ACCESS.2021.3074422

Khurshid, M. R., Manzoor, S., Sadiq, T., Hussain, L., Khan, M. S., & Dutta, A. K. (2025). Unveiling diabetes onset: Optimized XGBoost with Bayesian optimization for enhanced prediction. *PLoS One*, *20*(1), e0310218. DOI: 10.1371/journal.pone.0310218 PMID: 39854291

Kibria, H. B., Nahiduzzaman, M., Goni, M. O. F., Ahsan, M., & Haider, J. (2022). An ensemble approach for the prediction of diabetes mellitus using a soft voting classifier with an explainable AI. *Sensors (Basel)*, *22*(19), 7268. DOI: 10.3390/s22197268 PMID: 36236367

Kim, T. H., Krichen, M., Ojo, S., Alamro, M. A., & Sampedro, G. A. (2024). TSSG-CNN: A tuberculosis semantic segmentation-guided model for detecting and diagnosis using the adaptive convolutional neural network. *Diagnostics (Basel)*, *14*(11), 1174. Advance online publication. DOI: 10.3390/diagnostics14111174 PMID: 38893700

Kingma, D. P., & Welling, M. (2013). Auto-encoding variational bayes. *arXiv preprint arXiv:1312.6114*.

Kingma, D. P., & Welling, M. (2014). Auto-encoding variational bayes. *2nd International Conference on Learning Representations, ICLR 2014 - Conference Track Proceedings*. DOI: 10.61603/ceas.v2i1.33

Kiran, A., & Kumar, S. S. (2023). A Comparative Analysis of GAN and VAE based Synthetic Data Generators for High Dimensional, Imbalanced Tabular data. *2023 2nd International Conference for Innovation in Technology, INOCON 2023*. DOI: 10.1109/INOCON57975.2023.10101315

Kiran, A., Rubini, P., & Kumar, S. S. (2025). Comprehensive Review of Privacy, Utility, and Fairness Offered by Synthetic Data. *IEEE Access : Practical Innovations, Open Solutions*, *13*, 15795–15811. DOI: 10.1109/ACCESS.2025.3532128

Knevel, R., & Liao, K. P. (2023). From real-world electronic health record data to real-world results using artificial intelligence. *Annals of the Rheumatic Diseases*, *82*(3), 306–311. DOI: 10.1136/ard-2022-222626 PMID: 36150748

Koetzier, L. R., Wu, J., Mastrodicasa, D., Lutz, A., Chung, M., Koszek, W. A., Pratap, J., Chaudhari, A. S., Rajpurkar, P., Lungren, M. P., & Willemink, M. J. (2024). Generating Synthetic Data for Medical Imaging. *Radiology*, *312*(3), e232471. DOI: 10.1148/radiol.232471 PMID: 39254456

Kotelnikov, A., Barannikov, S., Kiani, A., & Burnaev, E. (2023). TabDDPM: Modelling Tabular Data with Diffusion Models. *International Conference on Learning Representations*.

Kreis, K., Gao, R., & Vahdat, A. (2022, June). Denoising diffusion-based generative modeling: Foundations and applications. In *Proceedings of the IEEE/CVF Conference on Computer Vision and Pattern Recognition (CVPR)* (Tutorial).

Kumar, C. U. O., Singh, I., & Suguna, M. (2024). Optimizing Patient Recruitment for Clinical Trials: A Hybrid Classification Model and Game-Theoretic Approach for Strategic Interaction. *IEEE Access : Practical Innovations, Open Solutions*, *12*, 10254–10280. DOI: 10.1109/ACCESS.2024.3351688

Kumar, R.. (2018). Lung cancer classification using deep learning. *Procedia Computer Science*, *132*, 1228–1236. DOI: 10.1016/j.procs.2018.05.118

Kundu, D., Chopra, K., Khanna, A., Babbar, N., & Padmini, T. J. (2016). Accelerating TB notification from the private health sector in Delhi, India. *indian journal of tuberculosis, 63*(1), 8-12. DOI: 10.1016/j.ijtb.2016.02.002

Kuriakose, S. M., Joseph, J. A. R., & Kollinal, R. (2024). The Rise of Digital Twins in Healthcare: A Mapping of the Research Landscape. *Cureus*. Advance online publication. DOI: 10.7759/cureus.65358 PMID: 39184791

Kwan, A., Daniels, B., Saria, V., Satyanarayana, S., Subbaraman, R., McDowell, A., Bergkvist, S., Das, R. K., Das, V., Das, J., & Pai, M. (2018). Variations in the quality of tuberculosis care in urban India: A cross-sectional, standardized patient study in two cities. *PLoS Medicine*, *15*(9), e1002653. DOI: 10.1371/journal.pmed.1002653 PMID: 30252849

Lal, S. S. (2010). The role of private health sector engagement in TB control in India. *The Hospital*, *2006*(07), 11.

Lam, C., Yi, D., Guo, M., & Lindsey, T. (n.d.). *Automated Detection of Diabetic Retinopathy using Deep Learning*.

Lee, G., Kweon, S., Bae, S., & Choi, E. (2024). Overview of the EHRSQL 2024 Shared Task on Reliable Text-to-SQL Modeling on Electronic Health Records. In Naumann, T., Ben Abacha, A., Bethard, S., Roberts, K., & Bitterman, D. (Eds), *Proceedings of the 6th Clinical Natural Language Processing Workshop* (pp. 644–654). Association for Computational Linguistics. DOI: 10.18653/v1/2024.clinicalnlp-1.62

Lee, G., Lee, H. Y., Park, H., Schiebler, M. L., van Beek, E. J. R., Ohno, Y., Seo, J. B., & Leung, A. (2017). Radiomics and its emerging role in lung cancer research, imaging biomarkers and clinical management: State of the art. *European Journal of Radiology*, *86*, 297–307. DOI: 10.1016/j.ejrad.2016.09.005 PMID: 27638103

Leeming, M. G., Ang, C. S., Nie, S., Varshney, S., & Williamson, N. A. (2023). Simulation of mass spectrometry-based proteomics data with Synthedia. *Bioinformatics Advances*, *3*(1), vbac096. Advance online publication. DOI: 10.1093/bioadv/vbac096 PMID: 36698761

Lee, T. K., Kim, S. Y., Choi, H. J., Choe, E. K., & Sohn, K. A. (2025). Vision transformer based interpretable metabolic syndrome classification using retinal Images. *NPJ Digital Medicine*, *8*(1), 205. Advance online publication. DOI: 10.1038/s41746-025-01588-0 PMID: 40216912

Lee, Y. G., Kwak, M.-S., Kim, J. E., Kim, M. S., No, D. U., & Chai, H. Y. (2025). Synthetic data production for biomedical research. *Osong Public Health and Research Perspectives*, *16*(2), 94–99. DOI: 10.24171/j.phrp.2024.0335 PMID: 40262847

Lei, X., Liu, Q., Escobar, E., Philogene, J., Zhu, H., Wang, Y., & Tang, S. (2015). Public–private mix for tuberculosis care and control: A systematic review. *International Journal of Infectious Diseases*, *34*, 20–32. DOI: 10.1016/j.ijid.2015.02.015 PMID: 25722284

Levin, A., & Kaddar, M. (2011). Role of the private sector in the provision of immunization services in low-and middle-income countries. *Health Policy and Planning*, *26*(suppl_1), i4–i12. DOI: 10.1093/heapol/czr037 PMID: 21729916

Li, H., Yu, L., & He, W. (2019). The Impact of GDPR on Global Technology Development. In *Journal of Global Information Technology Management* (Vol. 22, Issue 1). DOI: 10.1080/1097198X.2019.1569186

Liang, X., Du, M., & Chen, Z. (2023). Artificial intelligence-aided ultrasound in renal diseases: A systematic review. *Quantitative Imaging in Medicine and Surgery*, *13*(6), 3988–4001. DOI: 10.21037/qims-22-1428 PMID: 37284081

Liang, Z., Liu, W., & Yao, R. (2016). Contrast enhancement by nonlinear diffusion filtering. *IEEE Transactions on Image Processing*, *25*(2), 673–686. DOI: 10.1109/TIP.2015.2507405 PMID: 26685234

Li, C., Kao, C.-Y., Gore, J. C., & Ding, Z. (2008). Minimization of region-scalable fitting energy for image segmentation. *IEEE Transactions on Image Processing*, *17*(10), 1940–1949. DOI: 10.1109/TIP.2008.2002304 PMID: 18784040

Li, F., Liu, Z., Chen, H., Jiang, M., Zhang, X., & Wu, Z. (2019). Automatic detection of diabetic retinopathy in retinal fundus photographs based on deep learning algorithm. *Translational Vision Science & Technology*, *8*(6), 4. Advance online publication. DOI: 10.1167/tvst.8.6.4 PMID: 31737428

Lile, R., Ocnean, M., Balan, I. M., & KIBA, D. (2023). Challenges for Zero Hunger (SDG 2): Links with Other SDGs. *Transitioning to Zero Hunger. Chapter, MDPI*, 9-66. DOI: 10.3390/books978-3-03897-863-3

Li, N., Qin, J., Xiang, X., & Tan, Y. (2024). Journal of Information Security and Applications Robust coverless video steganography based on pose estimation and object tracking. *Journal of Information Security and Applications*, *87*(November), 103912. DOI: 10.1016/j.jisa.2024.103912

Little, C., Elliot, M., & Allmendinger, R. (2023). Federated learning for generating synthetic data: A scoping review. *International Journal of Population Data Science*, *8*(1), 2158. DOI: 10.23889/ijpds.v8i1.2158 PMID: 38414544

Liu, Z., Gao, A., Sheng, H., & Wang, X. (2025). Identification of diabetic retinopathy lesions in fundus images by integrating CNN and vision mamba models. *PLoS ONE, 20*(1 January), 1–19. DOI: 10.1371/journal.pone.0318264

Liu, H., Zhang, Y., Wang, X., Chen, J., & Li, Q. (2022). Deep learning-based detection of lung cancer in chest X-rays. *Biomedical Signal Processing and Control*, *76*, 103977. DOI: 10.1016/j.bspc.2022.103977

Liu, J., Peng, B., & Yin, Z. (2023, January). A Hybrid Machine Learning Method for Diabetes Detection based on Unsupervised Clustering. In *Proceedings of the 2023 7th International Conference on Machine Learning and Soft Computing* (pp. 144-149). DOI: 10.1145/3583788.3583809

Liu, P., Yang, X., Jin, B., & Zhou, Q. (2021). Diabetic retinal grading using attention-based bilinear convolutional neural network and complement cross entropy. *Entropy (Basel, Switzerland), 23*(7), 816. Advance online publication. DOI: 10.3390/e23070816 PMID: 34206941

Liu, R., Wang, S., Tian, F., & Yi, L. (2025). SIR-3DCNN: A framework of multivariate time series classification for lung cancer detection. *IEEE Transactions on Instrumentation and Measurement, 74*, 1–13. Advance online publication. DOI: 10.1109/TIM.2025.3563000

Liu, Y., Acharya, U. R., & Tan, J. H. (2025). Preserving privacy in healthcare: A systematic review of deep learning approaches for synthetic data generation. *Computer Methods and Programs in Biomedicine, 260*, 108571. DOI: 10.1016/j.cmpb.2024.108571 PMID: 39742693

Liu, Y., Liu, S., Wang, Y., Zhao, H., & Liu, S. (2019). Neurocomputing Video steganography : A review. *Neurocomputing, 335*, 238–250. DOI: 10.1016/j.neucom.2018.09.091

Liu, Z. G., Ji, T. Y., Chen, J. W., Zhang, L. J., Zhang, L. L., & Wu, Q. H. (2024). Conditional-TimeGAN for realistic and high-quality appliance trajectories generation and data augmentation in nonintrusive load monitoring. *IEEE Transactions on Instrumentation and Measurement, 73*, 1–15. DOI: 10.1109/TIM.2024.3381263

Li, W., Peng, Y., & Peng, K. (2024). Diabetes prediction model based on GA-XGBoost and stacking ensemble algorithm. *PLoS One, 19*(9), e0311222. DOI: 10.1371/journal.pone.0311222 PMID: 39348356

Li, X., Hu, J., & Zhang, L.. (2021). Applications of Artificial Intelligence in Ophthalmology: Current and Future Directions. *. *The Lancet. Digital Health, 3*(10), e682–e694. DOI: 10.1016/S2589-7500(21)00107-6 PMID: 34479825

Li, Y., Rao, S., Solares, J. R. A., & Ramakrishnan, N. (2020). Gena-bert: A new method for generating electronic health records. *2020 IEEE International Conference on Healthcare Informatics (ICHI)*, 1-10.

Li, Y., Wu, X., Yang, P., Jiang, G., & Luo, Y. (2022). Machine learning for lung cancer diagnosis, treatment, and prognosis. *Genomics, Proteomics & Bioinformatics, 20*(5), 850–866. DOI: 10.1016/j.gpb.2022.11.003 PMID: 36462630

Lobo, L. M. R. J., & Markandeya, D. L. (2023). Expert system for medical diagnosis and consultancy using prediction algorithms of machine learning. In Algorithms for intelligent systems (pp. 381–391). https://doi.org/DOI: 10.1007/978-981-99-1435-7_33

Loni, M., Poursalim, F., Asadi, M., & Gharehbaghi, A. (2025). A review on generative AI models for synthetic medical text, time series, and longitudinal data. *npj. Digital Medicine*, *8*(1), 281. DOI: 10.1038/s41746-024-01373-1 PMID: 40374917

Lopez, R., Regier, J., Cole, M. B., Jordan, M. I., & Yosef, N. (2018). Deep generative modeling for single-cell transcriptomics. *Nature Methods*, *15*(12), 1053–1058. Advance online publication. DOI: 10.1038/s41592-018-0229-2 PMID: 30504886

Lu, Y., Chen, L., Zhang, Y., Shen, M., Wang, H., Wang, X., van Rechem, C., Fu, T., & Wei, W. (2025a). *Machine Learning for Synthetic Data Generation: A Review* (No. arXiv:2302.04062). arXiv. https://doi.org//arXiv.2302.04062DOI: 10.48550

Lugner, M., Rawshani, A., Helleryd, E., & Eliasson, B. (2024). Identifying top ten predictors of type 2 diabetes through machine learning analysis of UK Biobank data. *Scientific Reports*, *14*(1), 2102. DOI: 10.1038/s41598-024-52023-5 PMID: 38267466

Lu, L., & Huang, T. (2022). Effects of early nursing monitoring on pregnancy outcomes of pregnant women with gestational diabetes mellitus under the Internet of Things. *Computational and Mathematical Methods in Medicine*, *2022*(1), 8535714. DOI: 10.1155/2022/8535714 PMID: 35693264

Luo, J., Yang, L., Liu, Y., Hu, C., Wang, G., Yang, Y., Yang, T.-L., & Zhou, X. (2025). Review of diffusion models and its applications in biomedical informatics. *BMC Medical Informatics and Decision Making 2025 25:1*, *25*(1), 1–21. DOI: 10.1186/s12911-025-03210-5

Luo, T., Gast, T. J., Vermeer, T. J., & Burns, S. A. (2017b). Retinal Vascular Branching in Healthy and Diabetic Subjects. *Investigative Ophthalmology & Visual Science*, *58*(5), 2685. DOI: 10.1167/iovs.17-21653 PMID: 28525557

Lutkevich, B. (2019). What is HIPAA (Health Insurance Portability and Accountability Act)? In *WhatIs.com.*

Mackay, P. (2025). *Compiling Complex Medical Reports using a Generic LLM: Exploring Hybrid Prompt Engineering Strategies for Language Improvement and Hallucination Mitigation* [Thesis, University of Lincoln]. DOI: 10.24385/lincoln.29596808.v1

Maduskar, P., Philipsen, R. H. H. M., Melendez, J., Scholten, E. T., Chanda-Kapata, P., Ayles, H., & van Ginneken, B. (2013). Detection of tuberculosis using digital chest radiography: Automated reading vs. interpretation by clinical officers. *The International Journal of Tuberculosis and Lung Disease : the Official Journal of the International Union against Tuberculosis and Lung Disease*, *17*(12), 1613–1620. DOI: 10.5588/ijtld.13.0325 PMID: 24200278

Ma, F., Sun, T., Liu, L., & Jing, H. (2020). Detection and diagnosis of chronic kidney disease using deep learning-based heterogeneous modified artificial neural network. *Future Generation Computer Systems*, *111*, 17–26. DOI: 10.1016/j.future.2020.04.036

Mainga, T. M. (2023). *Critical assessment of the intersection between mental health and Tuberculosis (TB) during TB treatment and beyond in a Sub-Saharan context with a focus on Zambia* (Doctoral dissertation, London School of Hygiene & Tropical Medicine). DOI: 10.17037/pubs.04670902

Marchesi, R., Micheletti, N., I-Hsien Kuo, N., Barbieri, S., Jurman, G., & Osmani, V. (2025a). Generative AI mitigates representation bias and improves model fairness through synthetic health data. *PLoS Computational Biology*, *21*(5), e1013080. DOI: 10.1371/journal.pcbi.1013080 PMID: 40388536

Marino, S., Cassidy, R., Nanni, J., Wang, Y., Liu, Y., Tang, M., Yuan, Y., Chen, T., Sinha, A., Pandian, B., Dinov, I. D., & Burns, M. L. (2025). Medical data sharing and synthetic clinical data generation – maximizing biomedical resource utilization and minimizing participant re-identification risks. *NPJ Digital Medicine*, *8*(1), 526. DOI: 10.1038/s41746-025-01935-1 PMID: 40818998

Marouf, M., Machart, P., Bansal, V., Kilian, C., Magruder, D. S., Krebs, C. F., & Bonn, S. (2020). Realistic in silico generation and augmentation of single-cell RNA-seq data using generative adversarial networks. *Nature Communications*, *11*(1), 166. Advance online publication. DOI: 10.1038/s41467-019-14018-z PMID: 31919373

Marwan, S., Shawish, A., & Nagaty, K. (2016). BioSystems DNA-based cryptographic methods for data hiding in DNA media. *Bio Systems*, *150*, 110–118. DOI: 10.1016/j.biosystems.2016.08.013

Masdari, M., Band, S. S., Qasem, S. N., Sayed, B. T., & Pai, H. T. (2024). ECG signals-based security and steganography approaches in WBANs: A comprehensive survey and taxonomy. Sustainable Computing: Informatics and Systems, 41(April 2023), 100937. https://doi.org/DOI: 10.1016/j.suscom.2023.100937

Mateen, M., Wen, J., Hassan, M., Nasrullah, N., Sun, S., & Hayat, S. (2020). Automatic Detection of Diabetic Retinopathy: A Review on Datasets, Methods and Evaluation Metrics. *IEEE Access : Practical Innovations, Open Solutions*, *8*, 48784–48811. DOI: 10.1109/ACCESS.2020.2980055

Mekala, V. K., Vadlamudi, G., Firdaus, A., Vemuru, N., Aramandla, K., & Rajeswara Rao, D. (2021). Early Detection of Diabetic Retinopathy. *International Journal for Research in Applied Science and Engineering Technology*, *9*(IX), 429–435. Advance online publication. DOI: 10.22214/ijraset.2021.37918

Mendes, J. M., Barbar, A., & Refaie, M. (2025). Synthetic data generation: A privacy-preserving approach to accelerate rare disease research. *Frontiers in Digital Health*, *7*, 1563991. DOI: 10.3389/fdgth.2025.1563991 PMID: 40171526

Miletic, M., & Sariyar, M. (2024). Large language models for synthetic tabular health data: A benchmark study. In Ugon, A., Karlsson, D., Klein, G. H., & Moen, A. (Eds.), *Digital Health and Informatics Innovations for Sustainable Health Care Systems* (pp. 963–967). IOS Press., DOI: 10.3233/SHTI240571

Miletic, M., & Sariyar, M. (2025). Synthetic data generation methods for longitudinal and time series health data. In *Global Healthcare Transformation in the Era of Artificial Intelligence and Informatics* (pp. 367–371). IOS Press. DOI: 10.3233/SHTI250740

Mishra, A., Pandey, M., & Singh, L. (2024). Segmentation and Classification of Diabetic Retinopathy using Ensemble Deep Neural Network. *Procedia Computer Science, 233*(2023), 226–234. DOI: 10.1016/j.procs.2024.03.212

Mishra, S., & Venkatesh, M. (2024). Rare disease clinical trials in the European Union: Navigating regulatory and clinical challenges. *Orphanet Journal of Rare Diseases*, *19*(1), 285. DOI: 10.1186/s13023-024-03146-5 PMID: 39085891

Mohanty, C., Mahapatra, S., Acharya, B., Kokkoras, F., Gerogiannis, V. C., Karamitsos, I., & Kanavos, A. (2023). Using Deep Learning Architectures for Detection and Classification of Diabetic Retinopathy. *Sensors (Basel)*, *23*(12), 1–18. DOI: 10.3390/s23125726 PMID: 37420891

Mohanty, P. K., Francis, S. A. J., Barik, R. K., Roy, D. S., & Saikia, M. J. (2024). Leveraging Shapley additive explanations for feature selection in ensemble models for diabetes prediction. *Bioengineering (Basel, Switzerland)*, *11*(12), 1215. DOI: 10.3390/bioengineering11121215 PMID: 39768033

Mohd Aman, A. H., Hassan, W. H., Sameen, S., Attarbashi, Z. S., Alizadeh, M., & Latiff, L. A. (2021). IoMT amid COVID-19 pandemic: Application, architecture, technology, and security. *Journal of Network and Computer Applications*, *174*, 102886. DOI: 10.1016/j.jnca.2020.102886 PMID: 34173428

Mojisola, F. O., Misra, S., Febisola, C. F., Abayomi-Alli, O., & Sengul, G. (2022). An improved random bit-stuffing technique with a modified RSA algorithm for resisting attacks in information security (RBMRSA). *Egyptian Informatics Journal*, *23*(2), 291–301.

Moon, K. R., van Dijk, D., Wang, Z., Gigante, S., Burkhardt, D. B., Chen, W. S., Yim, K., van den Elzen, A., Hirn, M. J., Coifman, R. R., Ivanova, N. B., Wolf, G., & Krishnaswamy, S. (2019). Visualizing structure and transitions in high-dimensional biological data. *Nature Biotechnology*, *37*(12), 1482–1492. Advance online publication. DOI: 10.1038/s41587-019-0336-3 PMID: 31796933

Mortimer, F., Isherwood, J., Wilkinson, A., & Vaux, E. (2018). Sustainability in quality improvement: Redefining value. *Future Healthcare Journal*, *5*(2), 88–93. DOI: 10.7861/futurehosp.5-2-88 PMID: 31098540

Moulaei, K., Shanbehzadeh, M., Mohammadi-Taghiabad, Z., & Kazemi-Arpanahi, H. (2022). Comparing machine learning algorithms for predicting COVID-19 mortality. *BMC Medical Informatics and Decision Making*, *22*(1), 2. DOI: 10.1186/s12911-021-01742-0 PMID: 34983496

Mukherjee, S., Huang, X., & Bhagalia, R. R. (2017). Lung nodule segmentation using deep learned prior based graph cut. In *2017 IEEE 14th International Symposium on Biomedical Imaging (ISBI 2017)* (pp. 1205–1208). IEEE. https://doi.org/DOI: 10.1109/ISBI.2017.7950733

Muna, A., Amjad, A., Abdulhafeez, J., & Ishaque, M. (2025). AI-powered cancer analysis: A secure and innovative approach to early diagnosis and prognosis. In *Proceedings of the 2025 2nd International Conference on Advanced Innovations in Smart Cities (ICAISC)* (pp. 1–8). IEEE. https://doi.org/DOI: 10.1109/ICAISC64594.2025.10959580

Munadi, K., Muchtar, K., Maulina, N., & Pradhan, B. (2020). Image enhancement for tuberculosis detection using deep learning. *IEEE Access : Practical Innovations, Open Solutions*, *8*, 217897–217907. DOI: 10.1109/ACCESS.2020.3041867

Muñoz-Mata, B. G., Dorantes-Méndez, G., & Piña-Ramírez, O. (2024). Classification of Parkinson's disease severity using gait stance signals in a spatiotemporal deep learning classifier. *Medical & Biological Engineering & Computing*, *62*(11), 3493–3506.

Murtaza, H., Ahmed, M., Khan, N. F., Murtaza, G., Zafar, S., & Bano, A. (2023). Synthetic data generation: State of the art in health care domain. In *Computer Science Review* (Vol. 48). DOI: 10.1016/j.cosrev.2023.100546

Nahar, M., Kamal, A. H. M., & Hossain, G. (2023). Journal of Network and Computer Applications Protecting health data in the cloud through steganography : A table-driven, blind method using neural networks and bit-shuffling algorithm . *Journal of Network and Computer Applications, 217*(May), 103689. DOI: 10.1016/j.jnca.2023.103689

Nahiduzzaman, M., Robiul Islam, M., Omaer Faruq Goni, M., Shamim Anower, M., Ahsan, M., Haider, J., & Kowalski, M. (2023). Diabetic retinopathy identification using parallel convolutional neural network based feature extractor and ELM classifier. *Expert Systems with Applications, 217*(December 2022), 119557. DOI: 10.1016/j.eswa.2023.119557

Namasudra, S. (2022). A secure cryptosystem using DNA cryptography and DNA steganography for the cloud-based IoT infrastructure. Computers and Electrical Engineering, 104(PA), 108426. https://doi.org/DOI: 10.1016/j.compeleceng.2022.108426

Nandini, K., & Rahimunnisa, K. (2025). Intelligent maternal-fetal healthcare monitoring and abnormality detection using deep belief networks optimized by a bacterial foraging algorithm. *Biomedical Signal Processing and Control, 110*, 108175. DOI: 10.1016/j.bspc.2025.108175

NarainPonraj. D., Christy, E., A, G., S, G., & Sharu, M. (2018). Analysis of LBP and LOOP based textural feature extraction for the classification of CT lung images. In 2018 4th International Conference on Devices, Circuits and Systems (ICDCS). IEEE. https://doi.org/DOI: 10.1109/ICDCSyst.2018.8605138

Nayak, J., Bhat, P. S., Acharya, U. R., Lim, C. M., & Kagathi, M. (2008). Automated identification of diabetic retinopathy stages using digital fundus images. *Journal of Medical Systems, 32*(2), 107–115. DOI: 10.1007/s10916-007-9113-9 PMID: 18461814

Nazera, F., Tanvir, K., & Kabir, Md. S., Hasan, Md. S., Hena, K. T., & Gomes, D. (2025). Hybrid Vision Transformer Naive Bayes Model for Mosquito Species Recognition with Virus Colony Search Optimization. *2025 International Conference on Quantum Photonics, Artificial Intelligence, and Networking (QPAIN)*, 1–6. DOI: 10.1109/QPAIN66474.2025.11171832

Needham, D. M., Bowman, D., Foster, S. D., & Godfrey-Faussett, P. (2004). Patient care seeking barriers and tuberculosis programme reform: A qualitative study. *Health Policy (Amsterdam)*, *67*(1), 93–106. DOI: 10.1016/S0168-8510(03)00065-4 PMID: 14726009

Neely, B. A., Dorfer, V., Martens, L., Bludau, I., Bouwmeester, R., Degroeve, S., Deutsch, E. W., Gessulat, S., Käll, L., Palczynski, P., Payne, S. H., Rehfeldt, T. G., Schmidt, T., Schwämmle, V., Uszkoreit, J., Vizcaíno, J. A., Wilhelm, M., & Palmblad, M. (2023). Toward an Integrated Machine Learning Model of a Proteomics Experiment. In *Journal of Proteome Research* (Vol. 22, Issue 3). DOI: 10.1021/acs.jproteome.2c00711

Negandhi, H., Tiwari, R., Sharma, A., Nair, R., Zodpey, S., Reddy Allam, R., & Oruganti, G. (2017). Rapid assessment of facilitators and barriers related to the acceptance, challenges and community perception of daily regimen for treating tuberculosis in India. *Global Health Action*, *10*(1), 1290315. DOI: 10.1080/16549716.2017.1290315 PMID: 28485693

Nguyen, H. T., Butler, M., Roychoudhry, A., Shannon, A. G., Flack, J., & Mitchell, P. (1996). Classification of diabetic retinopathy using neural networks. *Annual International Conference of the IEEE Engineering in Medicine and Biology - Proceedings, 4*, 1548–1549. DOI: 10.1109/IEMBS.1996.647546

Nikolentzos, G., Vazirgiannis, M., Xypolopoulos, C., Sarrah, H., & Chatzianastasis, M. (2023). Synthetic electronic health records generated with variational graph autoencoders. *npj. Digital Medicine*, *6*(1), 83. DOI: 10.1038/s41746-023-00822-x PMID: 37120594

Niranjana, S., Titus, A., Venkat, S., Arulanantham, D., & Begum, A. S. (2024). Experimental Evaluation in Identification of Kidney Cancer using Modified Learning Scheme. *2022 International Conference on Advances in Computing, Communication and Applied Informatics (ACCAI)*, 1–6. DOI: 10.1109/ACCAI61061.2024.10601727

Nithya, A., Appathurai, A., Venkatadri, N., Ramji, D. R., & Anna Palagan, C. (2019). Kidney disease detection and segmentation using artificial neural network and multi-kernel k-means clustering for ultrasound images. *Measurement*, *149*, 106952. DOI: 10.1016/j.measurement.2019.106952

NN in Deep Learning: Algorithm and Machine Learning Uses. (n.d.). Retrieved August 5, 2025, from https://www.simplilearn.com/tutorials/deep-learning-tutorial/convolutional-neural-network

Noise filtering in Digital Image Processing | by Anisha Swain | Medium. (n.d.). Retrieved August 5, 2025, from https://medium.com/@anishaswain/noise-filtering-in-digital-image-processing-d12b5266847c

Norval, M., Wang, Z., & Sun, Y. (2019). Pulmonary tuberculosis detection using deep learning convolutional neural networks. In *Proceedings of the 3rd International Conference on Video and Image Processing (ICVIP 2019)* (pp. 47–51). ACM. https://doi.org/DOI: 10.1145/3376067.3376068

Obermeyer, Z., Abbott-Klafter, J., & Murray, C. J. (2008). Has the DOTS strategy improved case finding or treatment success? An empirical assessment. *PLoS One*, *3*(3), e1721. DOI: 10.1371/journal.pone.0001721 PMID: 18320042

Obermeyer, Z., Powers, B., Vogeli, C., & Mullainathan, S. (2019). Dissecting racial bias in an algorithm used to manage the health of populations. *Science*, *366*(6464), 447–453. DOI: 10.1126/science.aax2342 PMID: 31649194

Ogunleye, A., & Wang, Q. G. (2020). XGBoost model for chronic kidney disease diagnosis. *IEEE/ACM Transactions on Computational Biology and Bioinformatics*, *17*(6), 2131–2140. DOI: 10.1109/TCBB.2019.2911071 PMID: 30998478

Olabanjo, O., Wusu, A., Olabanjo, O., Asokere, M., Afisi, O., & Akinnuwesi, B. (2025). A novel deep learning model for early diabetes risk prediction using attention-enhanced deep belief networks with highly imbalanced data. *International Journal of Information Technology : an Official Journal of Bharati Vidyapeeth's Institute of Computer Applications and Management*, *17*(4), 1–23. DOI: 10.1007/s41870-025-02459-3

Olorunfemi, B. O., Ogunde, A. O., Almogren, A., Adeniyi, A. E., Ajagbe, S. A., Bharany, S., Altameem, A., Rehman, A. U., Mehmood, A., & Hamam, H. (2025). Efficient diagnosis of diabetes mellitus using an improved ensemble method. *Scientific Reports*, *15*(1), 3235. DOI: 10.1038/s41598-025-87767-1 PMID: 39863685

Omer, H. K. (2024). Diabetic retinopathy detection using Bilayered Neural Network classification model with resubstitution validation. *MethodsX*, *12*(April), 102705. DOI: 10.1016/j.mex.2024.102705 PMID: 38633420

Oprisanu, B., Ganev, G., & De Cristofaro, E. (2022). On Utility and Privacy in Synthetic Genomic Data. *29th Annual Network and Distributed System Security Symposium, NDSS 2022*. DOI: 10.14722/ndss.2022.24092

Orujov, F., Maskeliūnas, R., Damaševičius, R., & Wei, W. (2020). Fuzzy based image edge detection algorithm for blood vessel detection in retinal images. *Applied Soft Computing*, *94*, 106452. DOI: 10.1016/j.asoc.2020.106452

Osamor, V. C., & Edosomwan, I. B. (2021). Employing scrambled alpha-numeric randomization and RSA algorithm to ensure enhanced encryption in electronic medical records. *Informatics in Medicine Unlocked*, •••, 25.

Özbay, E., Altunbey Özbay, F., & Soleimanian Gharehchopogh, F. (2024). Kidney tumor classification on CT images using self-supervised learning. *Computers in Biology and Medicine*, *176*, 108554. DOI: 10.1016/j.compbiomed.2024.108554 PMID: 38744013

Pande, S. D., & Agarwal, R. (2024). Multi-class kidney abnormalities detecting novel system through computed tomography. *IEEE Access : Practical Innovations, Open Solutions*, *12*, 21147–21155. DOI: 10.1109/ACCESS.2024.3351181

Pandey, H. M. (2020). Secure medical data transmission using a fusion of bit mask oriented genetic algorithm, encryption and steganography. *Future Generation Computer Systems*, *111*, 213–225. DOI: 10.1016/j.future.2020.04.034

Papadopoulos, D., & Karalis, V. D. (2023). Variational Autoencoders for Data Augmentation in Clinical Studies. *Applied Sciences (Basel, Switzerland)*, *13*(15), 8793. Advance online publication. DOI: 10.3390/app13158793

Papri, N. J., Ahmed, A., & Chowdhury, A. (2025). IoT and cloud-based non-invasive diabetes detection system from photoplethysmogram. *Discover Internet of Things*, *5*(1), 57. DOI: 10.1007/s43926-025-00158-w

Paproki, A., Salvado, O., & Fookes, C. (2024). Synthetic data for deep learning in computer vision & medical imaging: A means to reduce data bias. *ACM Computing Surveys*, *56*(11), 1–37. DOI: 10.1145/3663759

Parakh, A., Lee, H., & Singh, P.. (2019). Urinary stone detection on CT images using deep convolutional neural networks: Evaluation of model performance and generalization. *Radiology. Artificial Intelligence*, *1*(6), e190018. DOI: 10.1148/ryai.2019180066 PMID: 33937795

Pardeshi, G., Wang, W., Kim, J., Blossom, J., Kim, R., & Subramanian, S. V. (2021). TB notification rates across parliamentary constituencies in India: A step towards data-driven political engagement. *Tropical Medicine & International Health*, *26*(7), 730–742. DOI: 10.1111/tmi.13574 PMID: 33715264

Parkhi, D., Periyathambi, N., Ghebremichael-Weldeselassie, Y., Patel, V., Sukumar, N., Siddharthan, R., & Saravanan, P. (2023). Prediction of postpartum prediabetes by machine learning methods in women with gestational diabetes mellitus. *iScience*, *26*(10), 107846. Advance online publication. DOI: 10.1016/j.isci.2023.107846 PMID: 37767000

Pasculli, G., Virgolin, M., Myles, P., Vidovszky, A., Fisher, C., Biasin, E., Mourby, M., Pappalardo, F., D'Amico, S., Torchia, M., Chebykin, A., Carbone, V., Emili, L., & Roeshammar, D. (2025). Synthetic Data in Healthcare and Drug Development: Definitions, Regulatory Frameworks, Issues. *CPT: Pharmacometrics & Systems Pharmacology, 14*(5), 840–852. DOI: 10.1002/psp4.70021 PMID: 40193292

Patil, K. S., Mandal, I., & Rangaswamy, C. (2022). Hybrid and Adaptive Cryptographic-based secure authentication approach in IoT based applications using hybrid encryption. *Pervasive and Mobile Computing, 82*, 101552. DOI: 10.1016/j.pmcj.2022.101552

Patwari, B., Nandi, U., Dey, S., Dhar, S., Ghosal, S. K., & Si, T. (2025). Blockchain-Integrated Image Steganography using xDoG Edge Detection for Authentication. *Cyber Security and Applications, 3*(March), 100091. DOI: 10.1016/j.csa.2025.100091

Pezoulas, V. C., Zaridis, D. I., Mylona, E., Androutsos, C., Apostolidis, K., Tachos, N. S., & Fotiadis, D. I. (2024). Synthetic data generation methods in healthcare: A review on open-source tools and methods. *Computational and Structural Biotechnology Journal, 23*, 2892–2910. DOI: 10.1016/j.csbj.2024.07.005 PMID: 39108677

Phridviraj, M. S. B., Bhukya, R., Madugula, S., Manjula, A., Vodithala, S., & Waseem, M. S. (2023). A bi-directional Long Short-Term Memory-based Diabetic Retinopathy detection model using retinal fundus images. *Healthcare Analytics, 3*(January), 100174. DOI: 10.1016/j.health.2023.100174

Piccazzo, R., Paparo, F., & Garlaschi, G. (2014). Diagnostic accuracy of chest radiography for the diagnosis of tuberculosis (TB) and its role in the detection of latent TB infection: A systematic review. *The Journal of Rheumatology. Supplement, 91*(0), 32–40. DOI: 10.3899/jrheum.140100 PMID: 24788998

Pinaya, W. H., Scarpiniti, M., Kikas, P., Tudosiu, P. D., Dighum, W., & Cardoso, M. J. (2022). Brain imaging generation with latent diffusion models. *arXiv preprint arXiv:2209.07162*. DOI: 10.1007/978-3-031-18576-2_12

Polat, H., Mehr, H. D., & Cetin, A. (2017). Diagnosis of chronic kidney disease based on support vector machine by feature selection methods. *Journal of Medical Systems, 41*(4), 55. Advance online publication. DOI: 10.1007/s10916-017-0703-x PMID: 28243816

Poucin, F., Kraus, A., & Simon, M. (2021). Boosting Instance Segmentation with Synthetic Data: A study to overcome the limits of real world data sets. *Proceedings of the IEEE International Conference on Computer Vision, 2021-October*. DOI: 10.1109/ICCVW54120.2021.00110

Prakash, K. B. (2020). Analysis, Prediction and Evaluation of COVID-19 Datasets using Machine Learning Algorithms. *International Journal of Emerging Trends in Engineering Research*, *8*(5), 2199–2204. DOI: 10.30534/ijeter/2020/117852020

Prasanna Das, H., Tran, R., Singh, J., Yue, X., Tison, G., Sangiovanni-Vincentelli, A., & Spanos, C. J. (2022). Conditional Synthetic Data Generation for Robust Machine Learning Applications with Limited Pandemic Data. *Proceedings of the AAAI Conference on Artificial Intelligence*, *36*(11), 11792–11800. DOI: 10.1609/aaai.v36i11.21435

Prathibha, S., & Siddappaji, . (2024). Advancing diabetic retinopathy diagnosis with fundus imaging: A comprehensive survey of computer-aided detection, grading and classification methods. *Global Transitions*, *6*, 93–112. DOI: 10.1016/j.glt.2024.04.001

Prema, N. S., & Pushpalatha, M. P. (2019). An ensemble model for the prediction of gestational diabetes mellitus (GDM). *Indian Journal of Public Health Research & Development*, *10*(8), 1234–1239. DOI: 10.5958/0976-5506.2019.02399.4

Price, W. N., & Cohen, I. G. (2019). Privacy in the age of medical big data. In *Nature Medicine* (Vol. 25, Issue 1). DOI: 10.1038/s41591-018-0272-7

Priya, R., & Aruna, P. (2012). SVM and Neural Network based Diagnosis of Diabetic Retinopathy. *International Journal of Computer Applications*, *41*(1), •••. DOI: 10.5120/5503-7503

Pujitha, K., Soni, N. B., Eram, L. F., Sai, P. N., Divija, S., & Supriya, R. S. (2023). Chronic kidney disease detection using machine learning approach. In *Proceedings of the 2023 2nd International Conference on Vision Towards Emerging Trends in Communication and Networking Technologies (ViTECoN)* (pp. 1–5). IEEE. DOI: 10.1109/ViTECoN58111.2023.10157496

Punnose, J., Malhotra, R. K., Sukhija, K., Mathew, A., Sharma, A., & Choudhary, N. (2020). Glycated hemoglobin in the first trimester: A predictor of gestational diabetes mellitus in pregnant Asian Indian women. *Diabetes Research and Clinical Practice*, *159*, 107953. Advance online publication. DOI: 10.1016/j.diabres.2019.107953 PMID: 31794807

Puri, C., Sharma, M., & Reddy, K. T. V. (2025). Lung cancer detection: A comparative approach using regressor methods. In *Proceedings of the 2025 4th International Conference on Sentiment Analysis and Deep Learning (ICSADL)* (pp. 722–726). IEEE. https://doi.org/DOI: 10.1109/ICSADL65848.2025.10933212

Pustozerov, E. A., Chernykh, V. Y., Popova, P. V., Vasyukova, E. A., Tkachuk, A. S., & Yuldashev, Z. M. (2020). Health monitoring system for patients with gestational diabetes mellitus based on nutrition diaries and fitness bracelets. *Biomedical Engineering*, *53*(5), 305–308. DOI: 10.1007/s10527-020-09931-3

Qiao, L., Zhu, Y., & Zhou, H. (2020). Diabetic Retinopathy Detection Using Prognosis of Microaneurysm and Early Diagnosis System for Non-Proliferative Diabetic Retinopathy Based on Deep Learning Algorithms. *IEEE Access : Practical Innovations, Open Solutions*, *8*, 104292–104302. DOI: 10.1109/ACCESS.2020.2993937

Quellec, G., Charrière, K., Boudi, Y., Cochener, B., & Lamard, M. (2017). Deep image mining for diabetic retinopathy screening. *Medical Image Analysis*, *39*, 178–193. DOI: 10.1016/j.media.2017.04.012 PMID: 28511066

Radhika, P. R., Nair, R., & Gangadharan, V. (2019). A comparative study of lung cancer detection using machine learning algorithms. In *2019 Fifth International Conference on Electrical Energy Systems (ICEES)* (pp. 1–4). IEEE. https://doi.org/ DOI: 10.1109/ICECCT.2019.8869001

Rajabi, M., Ebrahimi, P., & Aryankhesal, A. (2021). Collaboration between the government and nongovernmental organizations in providing health-care services: A systematic review of challenges. *Journal of Education and Health Promotion*, *10*(1), 242. DOI: 10.4103/jehp.jehp_1312_20 PMID: 34395679

Raja, J., Rajeswari, J., & Jayashri, S. (2023). A secured QR pattern based e-health care CAD system for CXR image analyzes. *Optik (Stuttgart)*, *273*, 170344. Advance online publication. DOI: 10.1016/j.ijleo.2022.170344

Rajendra, P., & Latifi, S. (2021). Prediction of diabetes using logistic regression and ensemble techniques. *Computer Methods and Programs in Biomedicine Update*, *1*, 100032. DOI: 10.1016/j.cmpbup.2021.100032

Rajotte, J. F., Bergen, R., Buckeridge, D. L., El Emam, K., Ng, R., & Strome, E. (2022). Synthetic data as an enabler for machine learning applications in medicine. In *iScience* (Vol. 25, Issue 11). DOI: 10.1016/j.isci.2022.105331

Rakesh, P. S., & Shannawaz, M. (2024). Ensuring universal access to quality care for persons with presumed tuberculosis reaching the private sector: Lessons from Kerala. *International Journal for Equity in Health*, *23*(1), 101. DOI: 10.1186/s12939-024-02151-1 PMID: 38760667

Rakesh, P. S., Shannawaz, M., Mathew, M. E., & Sachdeva, K. S. (2024). Facilitators and barriers for private health sector engagement for tb care in india: A systematic review and meta-synthesis of qualitative research. *Global Health, Science and Practice*, *12*(4). Advance online publication. DOI: 0.9745/GHSP-D-24-00034 PMID: 39019586

Ramachandranpillai, R., Sikder, M. F., Bergström, D., & Heintz, F. (2024). Bt-GAN: Generating Fair Synthetic Healthdata via Bias-transforming Generative Adversarial Networks. *Journal of Artificial Intelligence Research*, *79*, 1313–1341. DOI: 10.1613/jair.1.15317

Raman, G., Ashraf, B., Demir, Y. K., Kershaw, C. D., Cheruku, S., Atis, M., Atis, A., Atar, M., Chen, W., Ibrahim, I., Bat, T., & Mete, M. (2023). Machine learning prediction for COVID-19 disease severity at hospital admission. *BMC Medical Informatics and Decision Making*, *23*(1), 46. DOI: 10.1186/s12911-023-02132-4 PMID: 36882829

Ramasamy, L. K., Padinjappurathu, S. G., Kadry, S., & Damaševičius, R. (2021). Detection of Diabetic Retinopathy Using a Fusion of Textural and Ridgelet Features of Retinal Images and Sequential Minimal Optimization Classifier. *PeerJ. Computer Science*, *7*, 1–21. DOI: 10.7717/peerj-cs.456 PMID: 34013026

Rani, S., Kumar, R., Panda, B. S., Kumar, R., Muften, N. F., Abass, M. A., & Lozanović, J. (2025). Machine Learning-Powered Smart Healthcare Systems in the Era of Big Data: Applications, Diagnostic Insights, Challenges, and Ethical Implications. *Diagnostics (Basel)*, *15*(15), 1914. DOI: 10.3390/diagnostics15151914 PMID: 40804880

Rao, H., Zeng, M., Zhao, X., & Miao, C. (2025). A survey of artificial intelligence in gait-based neurodegenerative disease diagnosis, Neurocomputing, Volume 626,, 129533, ISSN 0925-2312, DOI: 10.1016/j.neucom.2025.129533

Rao, R., Liu, J., Verkuil, R., Meier, J., Canny, J. F., Abbeel, P., Sercu, T., & Rives, A. (2021). MSA Transformer. *BioRxiv*, 2021.02.12.430858. DOI: 10.1101/2021.02.12.430858

Rashid, Z., Ahmed, H., Nadeem, N., Zafar, S. B., & Yousaf, M. Z. (2025). The paradigm of digital health: AI applications and transformative trends. *Neural Computing & Applications*, *37*(17), 1–32. DOI: 10.1007/s00521-025-11081-0

Raviglione, M., & Sulis, G. (2016). Tuberculosis 2015: Burden, challenges and strategy for control and elimination. *Infectious Disease Reports*, *8*(2), 6570. DOI: 10.4081/idr.2016.6570 PMID: 27403269

Ravindran, D., Pillai, R. H., Srinivasa, D., & Somashekaraiah, S. (2024). Service Quality Evaluation of Healthcare Sustainability: Patient Satisfaction, Service Delivery, and Clinical Outcomes. In *Business Resilience and Digital Technology in the Post-Pandemic Era: A Global Case* (pp. 57-76). Cham: Springer Nature Switzerland. DOI: 10.1007/978-3-031-48075-1_6

Regulation—2016/679—EN - gdpr—EUR-Lex. (n.d.). Retrieved 6 September 2025, from https://eur-lex.europa.eu/eli/reg/2016/679/oj/eng

Rigla, M., Martínez-Sarriegui, I., García-Sáez, G., Pons, B., & Hernando, M. E. (2018). Gestational diabetes management using smart mobile telemedicine. *Journal of Diabetes Science and Technology*, *12*(2), 260–264. DOI: 10.1177/1932296817704442 PMID: 28420257

Rikta, S. T., Uddin, K. M. M., Biswas, N., Mostafiz, R., Sharmin, F., & Dey, S. K. (2023). XML-GBM lung: An explainable machine learning-based application for the diagnosis of lung cancer. *Journal of Pathology Informatics*, *14*, 100307. Advance online publication. DOI: 10.1016/j.jpi.2023.100307 PMID: 37025326

Ritoré, Á., Jiménez, C. M., González, J. L., Rejón-Parrilla, J. C., Hervás, P., Toro, E., Parra-Calderón, C. L., Celi, L. A., Túnez, I., & Armengol De La Hoz, M. Á. (2024). The role of Open Access Data in democratizing healthcare AI: A pathway to research enhancement, patient well-being and treatment equity in Andalusia, Spain. *PLOS Digital Health*, *3*(9), e0000599. DOI: 10.1371/journal.pdig.0000599 PMID: 39283912

Rodríguez, R., Svensson, G., & Ferro, C. (2021). Assessing the future direction of sustainable development in public hospitals: Time-horizon, path and action. *Health Policy (Amsterdam)*, *125*(4), 526–534. DOI: 10.1016/j.healthpol.2020.10.012 PMID: 33309182

Rodtook, A., & Makhanov, S. S. (2013). Multi-feature gradient vector flow snakes for adaptive segmentation of the ultrasound images of breast cancer. *Journal of Visual Communication and Image Representation*, *24*(8), 1414–1430. DOI: 10.1016/j.jvcir.2013.09.009

Rom, Y., Aviv, R., Cohen, G. Y., Friedman, Y. E., Ianchulev, T., & Dvey-Aharon, Z. (2024). Diabetes detection from non-diabetic retinopathy fundus images using deep learning methodology. *Heliyon*, *10*(16), e36592. DOI: 10.1016/j.heliyon.2024.e36592 PMID: 39258195

Ronneberger, O., Fischer, P., & Brox, T. (2015). U-NET: Convolutional Networks for Biomedical Image Segmentation. In Lecture notes in computer science (pp. 234–241). DOI: 10.1007/978-3-319-24574-4_28

Rosenthal, S., Adler-Milstein, J., & Patel, V. (2024). Public Health Data Exchange Through Health Information Exchange Organizations: National Survey Study. *JMIR Public Health and Surveillance*, *10*, e64969. DOI: 10.2196/64969 PMID: 39588746

Roychowdhury, S., Koozekanani, D. D., & Parhi, K. K. (2014). DREAM: Diabetic Retinopathy Analysis Using Machine Learning. *IEEE Journal of Biomedical and Health Informatics*, *18*(5), 1717–1728. DOI: 10.1109/JBHI.2013.2294635 PMID: 25192577

Rujas, M., Martín Gómez Del Moral Herranz, R., Fico, G., & Merino-Barbancho, B. (2025a). Synthetic data generation in healthcare: A scoping review of reviews on domains, motivations, and future applications. *International Journal of Medical Informatics*, *195*, 105763. DOI: 10.1016/j.ijmedinf.2024.105763 PMID: 39719743

Said, A., Yahyaoui, A., & Abdellatif, T. (2024). HIPAA and GDPR Compliance in IoT Healthcare Systems. *Communications in Computer and Information Science, 2071 CCIS*, 198–209. DOI: 10.1007/978-3-031-55729-3_16

Saini, K., Dewal, M. L., & Rohit, M. (2012). A fast region-based active contour model for boundary detection of echocardiographic images. *Journal of Digital Imaging*, *25*(2), 271–278. DOI: 10.1007/s10278-011-9408-8 PMID: 21779946

Sairam, M. V. S., & Egala, R. (2024). A review on medical image analysis using deep learning. *Engineering Proceedings*, *66*(1), 7. DOI: 10.3390/engproc2024066007

Salekin, A., & Stankovic, J. (2016). Detection of chronic kidney disease and selecting important predictive attributes. In *Proceedings of the 2016 IEEE International Conference on Healthcare Informatics (ICHI)* (pp. 262–270). IEEE. DOI: 10.1109/ICHI.2016.36

Sandler, M., Howard, A., Zhu, M., Zhmoginov, A., & Chen, L.-C. (2018). MobileNetV2: Inverted residuals and linear bottlenecks. In *Proceedings of the IEEE/CVF Conference on Computer Vision and Pattern Recognition (CVPR)* (pp. 4510–4520). IEEE. https://doi.org/DOI: 10.1109/CVPR.2018.00474

Sangeetha, J., & Govindarajan, P. (2023). Prediction of agricultural waste compost maturity using fast regions with convolutional neural network(R-CNN). *Materials Today: Proceedings*. Advance online publication. DOI: 10.1016/j.matpr.2023.01.112

Santangelo, G., Nicora, G., Bellazzi, R., & Dagliati, A. (2025a). How good is your synthetic data? SynthRO, a dashboard to evaluate and benchmark synthetic tabular data. *BMC Medical Informatics and Decision Making*, *25*(1), 89. DOI: 10.1186/s12911-024-02731-9 PMID: 39966793

Santhakumar, R., Tandur, M., Rajkumar, E. R., Geetha, K. S., Haritz, G., & Rajamani, K. T. (2017). Machine learning algorithm for retinal image analysis. *IEEE Region 10 Annual International Conference, Proceedings/TENCON*, 1236–1240. DOI: 10.1109/TENCON.2016.7848208

Santhosh, S., A. S. M., A. D. S., P. G. S., & V. P. T. (2023). Deep learning based kidney stone detection using CT scan images. In Proceedings of the 2023 First International Conference on Advances in Electrical, Electronics and Computational Intelligence (ICAEECI) (pp. 1–7). IEEE. DOI: 10.1109/ICAEECI58247.2023.10370804

Santiago-Mozos, R., Pérez-Cruz, F., Madden, M. G., & Artés-Rodríguez, A. (2013). An automated screening system for tuberculosis. *IEEE Journal of Biomedical and Health Informatics*, *18*(3), 855–862. DOI: 10.1109/JBHI.2013.2282874 PMID: 24132025

Santini, G., Moreau, N., & Rubeaux, M. (2019). Kidney tumor segmentation using an ensembling multi-stage deep learning: A contribution to the KiTS19 challenge. arXiv. /arXiv.1909.00735DOI: 10.24926/548719.023

Santoso, A. S., & Nelloh, L. A. M. (2017). *Hasil Peer Reviewer Juril Elsevier2-LN*. https://doi.org/DOI: 10.1016/J.PROCS

Sarkis, J. (2020). Supply chain sustainability: Learning from the COVID-19 pandemic. *International Journal of Operations & Production Management*, *41*(1), 63–73. DOI: 10.1108/IJOPM-08-2020-0568

Saxena, D., & Cao, J. (2021). Generative Adversarial Networks (GANs). In *ACM Computing Surveys* (Vol. 54, Issue 3). DOI: 10.1145/3446374

Seeram, E., & Kanade, V. (2024). Ethical and Regulatory Considerations. In E. Seeram & V. Kanade, *Artificial Intelligence in Medical Imaging Technology* (pp. 151–167). Springer Nature Switzerland. DOI: 10.1007/978-3-031-64049-0_9

Setiawan, F., & Lin, C. W. (2021). Identification of neurodegenerative diseases based on vertical ground reaction force classification using time–frequency spectrogram and deep learning neural network features. *Brain Sciences*, *11*(7), 902.

Shah, D., Shah, T., Naseer, Y., Jamal, S. S., & Hussain, S. (2022). Cryptographically strong S-P boxes and their application in steganography. *Journal of Information Security and Applications*, *67*(April), 103174. DOI: 10.1016/j.jisa.2022.103174

Shakola, F., Palejev, D., & Ivanov, I. (2022). A Framework for Comparison and Assessment of Synthetic RNA-Seq Data. *Genes*, *13*(12), 2362. Advance online publication. DOI: 10.3390/genes13122362 PMID: 36553629

Shao, H., Liu, X., Zong, D., & Song, Q. (2024). Optimization of diabetes prediction methods based on combinatorial balancing algorithm. *Nutrition & Diabetes*, *14*(1), 63. DOI: 10.1038/s41387-024-00324-z PMID: 39143066

Sharma, A., Sinha, A., & Ahmed, S. (2025). Automated kidney disease classification using deep hybrid CNN architecture on CT images, arXiv:2502.04367. https://arxiv.org/abs/2502.04367

Sheehan, S., Mawe, S., Cianciolo, R. E., Korstanje, R., & Mahoney, J. M. (2019). Detection and classification of novel renal histologic phenotypes using deep neural networks. *American Journal of Pathology*, *189*(9), 1786–1796. DOI: 10.1016/j.ajpath.2019.05.019 PMID: 31220455

Shen, Y., Yu, J., Zhou, J., & Hu, G. (2025). Twenty-five years of evolution and hurdles in electronic health records and interoperability in medical research: Comprehensive review. *Journal of Medical Internet Research*, *27*, e59024. DOI: 10.2196/59024 PMID: 39787599

Shinde, S. G., & Lobo, L. M. R. J. (2019). A secured prediction system for human diseases using a genetic algorithm approach to data mining. *International Journal of Emerging Technologies and Innovative Research*, *6*(1), 266–274. https://www.jetir.org/papers/JETIRW006059.pdf

Shivappriya, S. N., Alagumeenaakshi, M., & Sasikala, S. (2024). Deep Learning-Based Diabetic Retinopathy Severity Classification and Progression Time Estimation. *IFAC-PapersOnLine*, *58*(3), 78–83. DOI: 10.1016/j.ifacol.2024.07.129

Shi, Y., & Sun, J. (2024). Integrated bagging-RF learning model for diabetes diagnosis in middle-aged and elderly population. *PeerJ. Computer Science*, *10*, e2436. DOI: 10.7717/peerj-cs.2436 PMID: 39650520

Shoeibi, A., Khodatars, M., Jafari, M., Ghassemi, N., Sadeghi, D., Moridian, P., Khadem, A., Alizadehsani, R., Hussain, S., Zare, A., Sani, Z. A., Khozeimeh, F., Nahavandi, S., Acharya, U. R., & Gorriz, J. M. (2024). Automated detection and forecasting of COVID-19 using deep learning techniques: A review. *Neurocomputing*, *577*, 127317. DOI: 10.1016/j.neucom.2024.127317

Shokri, R., Stronati, M., Song, C., & Shmatikov, V. (2017). Membership inference attacks against machine learning models. *2017 IEEE Symposium on Security and Privacy (SP)*, 3–18. DOI: 10.1109/SP.2017.41

Showkatian, E., Salehi, M., Ghaffari, H., Reiazi, R., & Sadighi, N. (2022). Deep learning-based automatic detection of tuberculosis disease in chest X-ray images. *Polish Journal of Radiology / Polish Medical Society of Radiology*, *87*(1), 118–124. DOI: 10.5114/pjr.2022.113435 PMID: 35280947

Silva Filho, T. M., Pimentel, B. A., Souza, R. M. C. R., & Oliveira, A. L. I. (2015). Hybrid methods for fuzzy clustering based on fuzzy c-means and improved particle swarm optimization. *Expert Systems with Applications*, *42*(17–18), 6315–6328. DOI: 10.1016/j.eswa.2015.04.032

Singh, G. (2025). Wearable IoT (w-IoT) artificial intelligence (AI) solution for sustainable smart healthcare. *International Journal of Information Management Data Insights*, *5*(1), 100291. DOI: 10.1016/j.jjimei.2024.100291

SMART Health IT. (2017). *SMART on FHIR sandbox*. https://docs.smarthealthit.org/

Soares, J. V. B., Leandro, J. J. G., Cesar, R. M., Jelinek, H. F., & Cree, M. J. (2006). Retinal vessel segmentation using the 2-D Gabor wavelet and supervised classification. *IEEE Transactions on Medical Imaging*, *25*(9), 1214–1222. DOI: 10.1109/TMI.2006.879967 PMID: 16967806

Sohl-Dickstein, J., Weiss, E., Maheswaranathan, N., & Ganguli, S. (2015). Deep unsupervised learning using nonequilibrium thermodynamics. *International Conference on Machine Learning*, 2256–2265. PMLR.

Sonal, D., Pattanaik, S., Nayak, K., Vyas, R. R., Sharma, T., & Kohli, A. (2025). An approach for detecting and classification of lung cancer using deep learning and machine learning. In *Proceedings of the 2025 IEEE 14th International Conference on Communication Systems and Network Technologies (CSNT)* (pp. 53–58). IEEE. https://doi.org/DOI: 10.1109/CSNT64827.2025.10968546

Soomro, T. A., Afifi, A. J., Zheng, L., Soomro, S., Gao, J., Hellwich, O., & Paul, M. (2019). Deep Learning Models for Retinal Blood Vessels Segmentation: A Review. In *IEEE Access* (Vol. 7, pp. 71696–71717). Institute of Electrical and Electronics Engineers Inc. DOI: 10.1109/ACCESS.2019.2920616

Srinivasan, S. (2025). Patient-Centric Care in Tuberculosis Management: Addressing Challenges and Improving Health Outcomes. In *Convergence of Population Health Management, Pharmacogenomics, and Patient-Centered Care* (pp. 265-282). IGI Global. DOI: 10.4018/979-8-3693-3260-3.ch012

Srinivasan, S., & Praba Lama (2025). Patient-Centered Care for TB Patients: An Effective Approach to Corporate Social Responsibility. In Corporate Social Responsibility in Health and Social Care (pp. 183-218). IGI Global. DOI: 10.4018/979-8-3693-5991-4.ch008

Srinivasan, S., & Vallipriya, R. (2025). Bias: Understanding and Addressing Disparities in Patient Care Across Multiple Demographics. In *Cases on Physician Cultural Responsibility, Ethics, and Biases* (pp. 21-38). IGI Global Scientific Publishing. DOI: 10.4018/979-8-3693-3683-0.ch002

Srinivasan, S., & Vallipriya, R. (2025). Intercultural Communication: An Effective Strategy for the Patient Physician Relationship. In *Cases on Physician Cultural Responsibility, Ethics, and Biases* (pp. 171-192). IGI Global Scientific Publishing. DOI: 10.4018/979-8-3693-3683-0.ch008

Srinivasan, S., Vallipriya, R., & Singh, A. K. (2025). Integrated Public-Private Partnerships to Combat Tuberculosis for Improving Economic Development. In *Public Private Partnership Dynamics for Economic Development* (pp. 323–356). IGI Global Scientific Publishing., DOI: 10.4018/979-8-3693-9153-2.ch015

Sri, V. S., & Lakshmi, G. R. J. (2023). Detection analysis of abnormality in kidney using deep learning techniques and its optimization. In *Proceedings of the 2023 Second International Conference on Electrical, Electronics, Information and Communication Technologies (ICEEICT)* (pp. 1–6). IEEE. DOI: 10.1109/ICEEICT56924.2023.10157637

Srivastava, R., Duan, L., Wong, D. W. K., Liu, J., & Wong, T. Y. (2017). Detecting retinal microaneurysms and hemorrhages with robustness to the presence of blood vessels. *Computer Methods and Programs in Biomedicine*, *138*, 83–91. DOI: 10.1016/j.cmpb.2016.10.017 PMID: 27886718

Srivastava, R., Wong, D. W. K., Duan, L., Liu, J., & Wong, T. Y. (2015). Red lesion detection in retinal fundus images using Frangi-based filters. *Proceedings of the Annual International Conference of the IEEE Engineering in Medicine and Biology Society, EMBS, 2015-November*, 5663–5666. DOI: 10.1109/EMBC.2015.7319677

Stallworthy, G., Dias, H. M., & Pai, M. (2020). Quality of tuberculosis care in the private health sector. *Journal of Clinical Tuberculosis and Other Mycobacterial Diseases*, *20*, 100171. DOI: 10.1016/j.jctube.2020.100171 PMID: 32642560

Stop, T. B. Initiative. (2001). *Global DOTS expansion plan: progress in TB control in high-burden countries, 2001 one year after the Amsterdam Ministerial Conference* (No. WHO/CDS/STB/2001.11). World Health Organization. https://iris.who.int/bitstream/handle/10665/66800/WHO_CDS_STB_2001.11.pdf

Story, A., Murad, S., Roberts, W., Verheyen, M., & Hayward, A. C. (2007). Tuberculosis in London: The importance of homelessness, problem drug use and prison. *Thorax*, *62*(8), 667–671. DOI: 10.1136/thx.2006.065409 PMID: 17289861

Sudharson, S., & Kokil, P. (2019). Abnormality detection in the renal ultrasound images using ensemble MSVM model. In *Proceedings of the 2019 International Conference on Wireless Communications Signal Processing and Networking (WiSPNET)* (pp. 378–382). IEEE. DOI: 10.1109/WiSPNET45539.2019.9032737

Suganthi, N. M., VM, J., Rama, P., & Chandralekha, E. (2022). Chronic Kidney Disease Detection using AdaBoosting Ensemble Method and K-Fold Cross Validation. *2022 International Conference on Automation, Computing and Renewable Systems (ICACRS)*, 979–983. DOI: 10.1109/ICACRS55517.2022.10029047

Sun, W., Huang, X., Tseng, T.-L. B., & Qian, W. (2017). Automatic lung nodule graph cuts segmentation with deep learning false positive detection. In *Medical Imaging 2017: Computer-Aided Diagnosis* (Article 101343E). SPIE. https://doi.org/DOI: 10.1117/12.2251302

Sun, S. (2016). A novel edge based image steganography with 2 k correction and Huffman encoding. *Information Processing Letters*, *116*(2), 93–99. DOI: 10.1016/j.ipl.2015.09.016

Suseela, R. P., & Shannawaz, M. (2023). Engaging the Private Health Service Delivery Sector for TB Care in India—Miles to Go! *Tropical Medicine and Infectious Disease*, *8*(5), 265. DOI: 10.3390/tropicalmed8050265 PMID: 37235313

Sushith, M., Sathiya, A., Kalaipoonguzhali, V., & Sathya, V. (2025). A hybrid deep learning framework for early detection of diabetic retinopathy using retinal fundus images. *Scientific Reports*, *15*(1), 1–31. DOI: 10.1038/s41598-025-99309-w PMID: 40307328

Susser, D., Schiff, D. S., Gerke, S., Cabrera, L. Y., Cohen, I. G., Doerr, M., Harrod, J., Kostick-Quenet, K., McNealy, J., Meyer, M. N., Price, W. N.II, & Wagner, J. K. (2024). Synthetic Health Data: Real Ethical Promise and Peril. *The Hastings Center Report*, *54*(5), 8–13. DOI: 10.1002/hast.4911 PMID: 39487776

Taha, A., Flury, D. V., Enodien, B., Taha-Mehlitz, S., & Schmid, R. A. (2022). The development of machine learning in lung surgery: A narrative review. *Frontiers in Surgery*, *9*, 914903. DOI: 10.3389/fsurg.2022.914903 PMID: 36171812

Taifa, I. A., Setu, D. M., Islam, T., Dey, S. K., & Rahman, T. (2024). A hybrid approach with customized machine learning classifiers and multiple feature extractors for enhancing diabetic retinopathy detection. *Healthcare Analytics*, *5*(March), 100346. DOI: 10.1016/j.health.2024.100346

Teli, A. (2025). Uncover this tech term: Variational autoencoders. *Korean Journal of Radiology*, *26*(6), 616. DOI: 10.3348/kjr.2025.0073 PMID: 40341889

Templin, T., Perez, M. W., Sylvia, S., Leek, J., & Sinnott-Armstrong, N. (2024). Addressing 6 challenges in generative AI for digital health: A scoping review. *PLOS Digital Health*, *3*(5), e0000503. DOI: 10.1371/journal.pdig.0000503 PMID: 38781686

Teo, Z. L., Tham, Y. C., Yu, M., Chee, M. L., Rim, T. H., Cheung, N., Bikbov, M. M., Wang, Y. X., Tang, Y., Lu, Y., Wong, I. Y., Ting, D. S. W., Tan, G. S. W., Jonas, J. B., Sabanayagam, C., Wong, T. Y., & Cheng, C. Y. (2021). Global Prevalence of Diabetic Retinopathy and Projection of Burden through 2045: Systematic Review and Meta-analysis. *Ophthalmology*, *128*(11), 1580–1591. DOI: 10.1016/j.ophtha.2021.04.027 PMID: 33940045

Thambawita, V., Salehi, P., Sheshkal, S. A., Hicks, S. A., Hammer, H. L., Parasa, S., de Lange, T., Halvorsen, P., & Riegler, M. A. (2022). SinGAN-Seg: Synthetic training data generation for medical image segmentation. *PLoS ONE, 17*(5 May). DOI: 10.1371/journal.pone.0267976

Thanki, R. (2023). A deep neural network and machine learning approach for retinal fundus image classification. *Healthcare Analytics, 3*(December 2022), 100140. DOI: 10.1016/j.health.2023.100140

Tian, M., Chen, B., Guo, A., Jiang, S., & Zhang, A. R. (2024a). Reliable generation of privacy-preserving synthetic electronic health record time series via diffusion models. *Journal of the American Medical Informatics Association : JAMIA*, *31*(11), 2529–2539. DOI: 10.1093/jamia/ocae229 PMID: 39222376

Tisha, S. N., & Ani, S. A. (2024). Predictive Insights: Empowering early detection of lung cancer using machine learning excellence. 2017 IEEE Region 10 Symposium (TENSYMP), 1–6. https://doi.org/DOI: 10.1109/TENSYMP61132.2024.10752136

Tjoa, E., & Guan, C. (2021). A survey on explainable artificial intelligence (XAI): Toward medical XAI. *IEEE Transactions on Neural Networks and Learning Systems*, *32*(11), 4793–4813. DOI: 10.1109/TNNLS.2020.3027314 PMID: 33079674

Tong, L., Shi, W., Isgut, M., Zhong, Y., Lais, P., Gloster, L., Sun, J., Swain, A., Giuste, F., & Wang, M. D. (2023). Integrating multi-omics data with EHR for precision medicine using advanced artificial intelligence. *IEEE Reviews in Biomedical Engineering*, *17*, 80–97. DOI: 10.1109/RBME.2023.3324264 PMID: 37824325

Topol, E. J. (2019). High-performance medicine: The convergence of human and artificial intelligence. *Nature Medicine*, *25*(1), 44–56. DOI: 10.1038/s41591-018-0300-7 PMID: 30617339

Tran, B. X., Ha, G. H., Nguyen, L. H., Vu, G. T., Hoang, M. T., Le, H. T., Latkin, C. A., Ho, C. S. H., & Ho, R. C. M. (2020). Studies of Novel Coronavirus Disease 19 (COVID-19) Pandemic: A Global Analysis of Literature. *International Journal of Environmental Research and Public Health*, *17*(11), 4095. DOI: 10.3390/ijerph17114095 PMID: 32521776

Trent, R. J. (2012). Public Health, Communicable Diseases and Global Health. *Molecular Medicine (Cambridge, Mass.)*, *169*, 169–201. Advance online publication. DOI: 10.1016/B978-0-12-381451-7.00006-2

Trowman, R., Migliore, A., & Ollendorf, D. A. (2024). Designing collaborations involving health technology assessment: Discussions and recommendations from the 2024 health technology assessment international global policy forum. *International Journal of Technology Assessment in Health Care*, *40*(1), e41. DOI: 10.1017/S0266462324000436 PMID: 39494818

Tsili, A. C., Andriotis, E., Gkeli, M. G., Krokidis, M., Stasinopoulou, M., Varkarakis, I. M., & Moulopoulos, L.-A. (2021). The role of imaging in the management of renal masses. *European Journal of Radiology*, *141*, 109777. DOI: 10.1016/j.ejrad.2021.109777 PMID: 34020173

Tumuhimbise, W., & Musiimenta, A. (2021). A review of mobile health interventions for public private mix in tuberculosis care. *Internet Interventions : the Application of Information Technology in Mental and Behavioural Health*, *25*, 100417. DOI: 10.1016/j.invent.2021.100417 PMID: 34401376

Ul Abideen, Z., Ghafoor, M., Munir, K., Saqib, M., Ullah, A., Zia, T., & Tariq, A. (2020). Uncertainty assisted robust tuberculosis identification with Bayesian convolutional neural networks. *IEEE Access : Practical Innovations, Open Solutions*, *8*, 22812–22825. DOI: 10.1109/ACCESS.2020.2970023 PMID: 32391238

Ullah, A. N. Z., Huque, R., Husain, A., Akter, S., Islam, A., & Newell, J. N. (2012). Effectiveness of involving the private medical sector in the National TB Control Programme in Bangladesh: Evidence from mixed methods. *BMJ Open*, *2*(6), e001534. DOI: 10.1136/bmjopen-2012-001534 PMID: 23253871

Umer, F., & Adnan, N. (2024). Generative artificial intelligence: synthetic datasets in dentistry. In *BDJ Open* (Vol. 10, Issue 1). DOI: 10.1038/s41405-024-00198-4

Uplekar, M. (2003). Involving private health care providers in delivery of TB care: Global strategy. *Tuberculosis (Edinburgh, Scotland)*, *83*(1-3), 156–164. DOI: 10.1016/S1472-9792(02)00073-2 PMID: 12758206

Uplekar, M. (2016). Public-private mix for tuberculosis care and prevention. What progress? What prospects? *The International Journal of Tuberculosis and Lung Disease : the Official Journal of the International Union against Tuberculosis and Lung Disease*, *20*(11), 1424–1429. DOI: 10.5588/ijtld.15.0536 PMID: 27776581

Urs, M. P. R., & Babu, G. N. K. S. (2024). Performance analysis and classification of lung cancer types using machine learning. *2024 International Conference on Knowledge Engineering and Communication Systems (ICKECS)*, 1–5. https://doi.org/DOI: 10.1109/ICKECS61492.2024.10617015

Usman Akram, M., Khalid, S., Tariq, A., Khan, S. A., & Azam, F. (2014). Detection and classification of retinal lesions for grading of diabetic retinopathy. *Computers in Biology and Medicine*, *45*(1), 161–171. DOI: 10.1016/j.compbiomed.2013.11.014 PMID: 24480176

Uyanik, H., Sengur, A., Salvi, M., Tan, R. S., Tan, J. H., & Acharya, U. R. (2025). Automated Detection of Neurological and Mental Health Disorders Using EEG Signals and Artificial Intelligence: A Systematic Review. *Wiley Interdisciplinary Reviews. Data Mining and Knowledge Discovery*, *15*(1), e70002. DOI: 10.1002/widm.70002

Vaishya, R., Javaid, M., Khan, I. H., & Haleem, A. (2020). Artificial Intelligence (AI) applications for COVID-19 pandemic. *Diabetes & Metabolic Syndrome*, *14*(4), 337–339. DOI: 10.1016/j.dsx.2020.04.012 PMID: 32305024

van Breugel, B., Liu, T., Oglic, D., & van der Schaar, M. (2024). Synthetic data in biomedicine via generative artificial intelligence. *Nature Reviews Bioengineering*, *2*(12), 991–1004. DOI: 10.1038/s44222-024-00245-7

Vaswani, A., Shazeer, N., Parmar, N., Uszkoreit, J., Jones, L., Gomez, A. N., Kaiser, L., & Polosukhin, I. (2017). Attention is all you need. *Advances in Neural Information Processing Systems*, •••, 30.

Vergunst, F., Berry, H. L., Rugkåsa, J., Burns, T., Molodynski, A., & Maughan, D. L. (2020). Applying the triple bottom line of sustainability to healthcare research—A feasibility study. *International Journal for Quality in Health Care : Journal of the International Society for Quality in Health Care*, *32*(1), 48–53. DOI: 10.1093/intqhc/mzz049 PMID: 31087047

Vij, R., & Arora, S. (2023). A Systematic Review on Diabetic Retinopathy Detection Using Deep Learning Techniques. In *Archives of Computational Methods in Engineering* (Vol. 30, Issue 3). Springer Netherlands. DOI: 10.1007/s11831-022-09862-0

Vîrgolici, O., Lixandru, D., Mihai, A., tefan, D. S., Guja, C., Vîrgolici, H., & Virgolici, B. (2025). prediction of metabolic parameters of diabetic patients depending on body weight variation using machine learning techniques. *Biomedicines*, *13*(5), 1116. DOI: 10.3390/biomedicines13051116 PMID: 40426942

Virhia, J., Gilmour, M., Russell, C., Mutua, E., Nasuwa, F., Mmbaga, B. T., Mshana, S. E., Dunlea, T., Shirima, G., Seni, J., Lembo, T., & Davis, A. (2023). "If you do not take the medicine and complete the dose… It could cause you more trouble": Bringing awareness, local knowledge and experience into antimicrobial stewardship in Tanzania. *Antibiotics (Basel, Switzerland)*, *12*(2), 243. DOI: 10.3390/antibiotics12020243 PMID: 36830154

Voigt, P., & Von dem Bussche, A. (2017). The EU General Data Protection Regulation (GDPR): A Practical Guide. In *The EU General Data Protection Regulation (GDPR): a Practical Guide*. DOI: 10.1007/978-3-319-57959-7

Wagner, J. K., Cabrera, L. Y., Gerke, S., & Susser, D. (2024a). Synthetic data and ELSI-focused computational checklists—A survey of biomedical professionals' views. *PLOS Digital Health*, *3*(11), e0000666. DOI: 10.1371/journal.pdig.0000666 PMID: 39565773

Walonoski, J., Kramer, M., Nichols, J., Quina, A., Moesel, C., Hall, D., Duffett, C., Dube, K., Gallagher, T., & McLachlan, S. (2018). Synthea: An approach, method, and software mechanism for generating synthetic patients and the synthetic electronic health care record. *Journal of the American Medical Informatics Association : JAMIA*, *25*(3), 230–238. Advance online publication. DOI: 10.1093/jamia/ocx079 PMID: 29025144

Wandy, J., McBride, R., Rogers, S., Terzis, N., Weidt, S., van der Hooft, J. J. J., Bryson, K., Daly, R., & Davies, V. (2023). Simulated-to-real benchmarking of acquisition methods in untargeted metabolomics. *Frontiers in Molecular Biosciences*, *10*, 1130781. Advance online publication. DOI: 10.3389/fmolb.2023.1130781 PMID: 36959982

Wang, C., Tachimori, H., Yamaguchi, H., Sekiguchi, A., Li, Y., & Yamashita, Y. (2024). A multimodal deep learning approach for the prediction of cognitive decline and its effectiveness in clinical trials for Alzheimer's disease. *Translational Psychiatry*, *14*(1), 105. DOI: 10.1038/s41398-024-02819-w PMID: 38383536

Wang, M., Ma, C., Liu, A., Xiao, H., Ren, Y., Li, Z., Wang, Z., Xia, Q., Dou, P., Li, B., & Chen, P. (2024). A bibliometric analysis of acupuncture for Parkinson's disease non-motor symptoms from 2003 to 2023. *Complementary Therapies in Medicine*, *87*, 103111. DOI: 10.1016/j.ctim.2024.103111 PMID: 39542379

Wang, Q., Wu, B., Zhu, P., Li, P., Zuo, W., & Hu, Q. (2020). ECA-Net: Efficient channel attention for deep convolutional neural networks. In *Proceedings of the IEEE/CVF Conference on Computer Vision and Pattern Recognition (CVPR)* (pp. 11531–11539). IEEE. https://doi.org/DOI: 10.1109/CVPR42600.2020.01155

Wang, X., Li, Y., Zhang, H., Chen, J., & Liu, Q. (2020). Enhanced nodule detection in lung CT scans using deep learning. *AI*, *1*(1), 24–38. DOI: 10.3390/ai1010003

Wani, N. A., Kumar, R., & Bedi, J. (2023). DeepXplainer: An interpretable deep learning based approach for lung cancer detection using explainable artificial intelligence. *Computer Methods and Programs in Biomedicine*, *243*, 107879. Advance online publication. DOI: 10.1016/j.cmpb.2023.107879 PMID: 37897989

Way, G. P., & Greene, C. S. (2018). Extracting a biologically relevant latent space from cancer transcriptomes with variational autoencoders. *Pacific Symposium on Biocomputing*, *0*(212669), 80–91. Advance online publication. DOI: 10.1142/9789813235533_0008 PMID: 29218871

Weerasuriya, C. K. (2022). *Advancing Mathematical Models of Mycobacterium tuberculosis Transmission to Support Vaccine Introduction* (Doctoral dissertation, London School of Hygiene & Tropical Medicine). DOI: 10.17037/PUBS.04665244

Wei, R., Garcia, C., El-Sayed, A., Peterson, V., & Mahmood, A. (2020). Variations in Variational Autoencoders - A Comparative Evaluation. *IEEE Access : Practical Innovations, Open Solutions*, *8*, 153651–153670. Advance online publication. DOI: 10.1109/ACCESS.2020.3018151

Weiss, J. B., Berner, E. S., Johnson, K. B., Giuse, D. A., Murphy, B. A., & Lorenzi, N. M. (2013). Recommendations for the design, implementation and evaluation of social support in online communities, networks, and groups. *Journal of Biomedical Informatics*, *46*(6), 970–976. DOI: 10.1016/j.jbi.2013.04.004 PMID: 23583424

Wippel, C., Farroñay, S., Gilbert, H. N., Millones, A. K., Acosta, D., Torres, I., Jimenez, J., Alarcon, V. A., Lecca, L., & Yuen, C. M. (2024). Exploring the role of the private sector in tuberculosis detection and management in Lima, Peru: A mixed-methods patient pathway analysis. *The American Journal of Tropical Medicine and Hygiene, 111*(1), 168–175. DOI: 10.4269/ajtmh.23-0504 PMID: 38744270

Woo, S., Park, J., Lee, J.-Y., & Kweon, I. S. (2018). CBAM: Convolutional block attention module. In *Proceedings of the European Conference on Computer Vision (ECCV)* (pp. 3–19). Springer. https://doi.org/DOI: 10.1007/978-3-030-01234-2_1

World Health Organization. (2009). *Global tuberculosis control: a short update to the 2009 report* (No. WHO/HTM/TB/2009.426). World Health Organization. https://iris.who.int/bitstream/handle/10665/44241/9789241598866_eng.pdf

World Health Organization. (2010). *The global plan to stop TB 2011-2015: transforming the fight towards elimination of tuberculosis.* World Health Organization., DOI: 10.1098/rsif.2010.0072

World Health Organization. (2014). *Tuberculosis control* (No. SEA-TB-352). WHO Regional Office for South-East Asia. https://iris.who.int/bitstream/handle/10665/206505/B5082.pdf

World Health Organization. (2024). *WHO consolidated guidelines on tuberculosis. Module 6: tuberculosis and comorbidities.* World Health Organization.

Wu, L. (2013). Classification of diabetic retinopathy and diabetic macular edema. *World Journal of Diabetes, 4*(6), 290–296. DOI: 10.4239/wjd.v4.i6.290 PMID: 24379919

Wulczyn, E., Steiner, D. F., Moran, M., Tan, F., Flament-Auvigne, I., Brown, T., & Chen, P. H. C. (2021). Interpretable survival prediction for colorectal cancer using deep learning. *NPJ Digital Medicine, 4*(1), 1–26. DOI: 10.1038/s41746-021-00427-2 PMID: 33875798

Xiaohui, Z., & Chutatape, O. (2004). Detection and classification of bright lesions in color fundus images. *Proceedings - International Conference on Image Processing, ICIP, 1*, 139–142. DOI: 10.1109/ICIP.2004.1418709

Xiao, X., Zhang, Y., Chen, H., Ren, W., Zhang, J., & Xu, J. (2025). A differential privacy-based mechanism for preventing data leakage in large language model training. *Academic Journal of Sociology and Management, 3*(2), 33–42. DOI: 10.70393/616a736d.323732

Xie, Y., Wu, Z., Han, X., Wang, H., Wu, Y., Cui, L., & Lin, J. (2020). Computer-aided system for the detection of multicategory pulmonary tuberculosis in radiographs. *Journal of Healthcare Engineering*, *2020*, 9843260. Advance online publication. DOI: 10.1155/2020/9205082 PMID: 32908660

Xu, L., Skoularidou, M., Cuesta-Infante, A., & Veeramachaneni, K. (2019). Modeling tabular data using conditional GAN. *Advances in Neural Information Processing Systems*, •••, 32.

Xu, Q., Wang, J., & Lu, Y. P. (2016). The association of maternal body composition and dietary intake with the risk of gestational diabetes mellitus during the second trimester in a cohort of Chinese pregnant women. [Original not fully accessible; volume/issue inferred from context]. *Biomedical and Environmental Sciences*, *29*(1), 1–11. PMID: 26822508

Xu, T., & Yuan, Z. (2022). Convolution neural network with coordinate attention for the automatic detection of pulmonary tuberculosis images on chest X-rays. *IEEE Access : Practical Innovations, Open Solutions*, *10*, 86710–86717. DOI: 10.1109/ACCESS.2022.3199419

Yadav, G., Maheshwari, S., & Agarwal, A. (2014). Contrast limited adaptive histogram equalization based enhancement for real time video)); system. In *2014 International Conference on Advances in Computing, Communications and Informatics (ICACCI)* (pp. 2392–2397). IEEE. https://doi.org/DOI: 10.1109/ICACCI.2014.6968381

Yan, C., Yan, Y., Wan, Z., Zhang, Z., Omberg, L., Guinney, J., Mooney, S. D., & Malin, B. A. (2022a). A Multifaceted benchmarking of synthetic electronic health record generation models. *Nature Communications*, *13*(1), 7609. Advance online publication. DOI: 10.1038/s41467-022-35295-1 PMID: 36494374

Yan, C., Zhang, Z., Nyemba, S., & Li, Z. (2024). Generating synthetic electronic health record data using generative adversarial networks: Tutorial. *JMIR AI*, *3*, e52615. DOI: 10.2196/52615 PMID: 38875595

Yang, B., Li, T., Xie, H., Liao, Y., & Chen, Y. P. P. (2022). Classification of Diabetic Retinopathy Severity Based on GCA Attention Mechanism. *IEEE Access : Practical Innovations, Open Solutions*, *10*, 2729–2739. DOI: 10.1109/ACCESS.2021.3139129

Yang, L., Zhang, Z., Song, Y., Hong, S., Xu, R., Zhao, Y., Zhang, W., Cui, B., & Yang, M. H. (2024). Diffusion Models: A Comprehensive Survey of Methods and Applications. *ACM Computing Surveys*, *56*(4), 1–39. Advance online publication. DOI: 10.1145/3626235

Yang, X., Liu, L., & Wang, Y. (2024). A decision tree-driven IoT system for improved prenatal diagnostic accuracy. *BMC Medical Informatics and Decision Making*, *24*(1), 375. DOI: 10.1186/s12911-024-02759-x PMID: 39639288

Yasin, N. Y. (2007). Connect the" DOTS": a new era in Turkish tuberculosis control. http://193.140.201.98/handle/123456789/17477

Yassin, M. A., Kimbo, L., Wandwalo, E., Rashid, A., Dzokoto, A., Weber, U., & Stallworthy, G. (2024). Leveraging Global Fund's investments to expand innovative public-private provider engagement in TB. *IJTLD Open*, *1*(6), 250–257. DOI: 10.5588/ijtldopen.24.0162 PMID: 39021451

Yellappa, V. H. (2019). Optimising the involvement of private practitioners in tuberculosis care and control in India. DOI: 10.26481/dis.20191111vy

Yellappa, V., Lefèvre, P., Battaglioli, T., Devadasan, N., & Van der Stuyft, P. (2017). Patients pathways to tuberculosis diagnosis and treatment in a fragmented health system: A qualitative study from a south Indian district. *BMC Public Health*, *17*(1), 1–10. DOI: 10.1186/s12889-017-4627-7 PMID: 28778192

Yelmen, B., Decelle, A., Ongaro, L., Marnetto, D., Tallec, C., Montinaro, F., Furtlehner, C., Pagani, L., & Jay, F. (2021). Creating artificial human genomes using generative neural networks. *PLOS Genetics*, *17*(2), e1009303. Advance online publication. DOI: 10.1371/journal.pgen.1009303 PMID: 33539374

Yildirim, K., Bozdag, P. G., Talo, M., Yildirim, O., Karabatak, M., & Acharya, U. R. (2021). Deep learning model for automated kidney stone detection using coronal CT images. *Computers in Biology and Medicine*, *135*, 104569. Advance online publication. DOI: 10.1016/j.compbiomed.2021.104569 PMID: 34157470

Yoon, J., Jarrett, D., & van der Schaar, M. (2019). Time-series generative adversarial networks. *Advances in Neural Information Processing Systems*, •••, 32.

Yoon, J., Mizrahi, M., Ghalaty, N. F., Jarvinen, T., Ravi, A. S., Brune, P., Kong, F., Anderson, D., Lee, G., Meir, A., Bandukwala, F., Kanal, E., Arık, S., & Pfister, T. (2023). EHR-Safe: Generating high-fidelity and privacy-preserving synthetic electronic health records. *NPJ Digital Medicine*, *6*(1), 141. Advance online publication. DOI: 10.1038/s41746-023-00888-7 PMID: 37567968

Yu, H., Zhou, Z., & Wang, Q. (2020). Deep learning assisted predict of lung cancer on computed tomography images using the adaptive hierarchical heuristic mathematical model. *IEEE Access : Practical Innovations, Open Solutions*, *8*, 86400–86410. DOI: 10.1109/ACCESS.2020.2992645

Yun, C., Tang, F., Gao, Z., Wang, W., Bai, F., Miller, J. D., Liu, H., Lee, Y., & Lou, Q. (2024). Construction of risk prediction model of type 2 diabetic kidney disease based on deep learning. *Diabetes & Metabolism Journal*, *48*(4), 771–779. DOI: 10.4093/dmj.2023.0033 PMID: 38685670

Zafar, A., Kim, K. S., Ali, M. U., Byun, J. H., & Kim, S. H. (2025). A lightweight multi-deep learning framework for accurate diabetic retinopathy detection and multi-level severity identification. *Frontiers in Medicine*, *12*(April), 1–11. DOI: 10.3389/fmed.2025.1551315 PMID: 40241910

Zaidi, I., Sarma, P. S., & Khayyam, K. U. (2024). Factors associated with treatment adherence among pulmonary tuberculosis patients in New Delhi. *The Indian Journal of Tuberculosis*, *71*, S52–S58. DOI: 10.1016/j.ijtb.2023.08.006 PMID: 39067956

Zamzmi, G., Subbaswamy, A., Sizikova, E., Margerrison, E., Delfino, J. G., & Badano, A. (2025a). Scorecard for synthetic medical data evaluation. *Communications Engineering*, *4*(1), 130. DOI: 10.1038/s44172-025-00450-1 PMID: 40691520

Zhang, H., Chen, Y., Song, Y., Xiong, Z., Yang, Y., & Wu, Q. M. J. (2019). Automatic kidney lesion detection for CT images using morphological cascade convolutional neural networks. *IEEE Access : Practical Innovations, Open Solutions*, *7*, 83001–83011. DOI: 10.1109/ACCESS.2019.2924207

Zhang, Q., Bai, C., Liu, Z., Yang, L. T., Yu, H., Zhao, J., & Wang, X. (2020). A GPU-based residual network for medical image classification in smart medicine. *Information Sciences*, *536*, 91–100. DOI: 10.1016/j.ins.2020.05.013

Zhang, W., Xia, Z., Cai, G., Wang, J., & Dong, X. (2025). Enhancing diabetes risk prediction through focal active learning and machine learning models. *PLoS One*, *20*(7), e0327120. DOI: 10.1371/journal.pone.0327120 PMID: 40627636

Zhang, W., Zhang, X., Zhao, J., Qiang, Y., Tian, Q., & Tang, X. (2017). A segmentation method for lung nodule image sequences based on superpixels and density-based spatial clustering of applications with noise. *PLoS One*, *12*(9), e0184290. Advance online publication. DOI: 10.1371/journal.pone.0184290 PMID: 28880916

Zhang, Y., Li, H., Chen, X., Wang, J., & Liu, Q. (2019). Hybrid PET/CT imaging for enhanced lung cancer diagnosis. *IEEE Transactions on Biomedical Engineering*, *66*(10), 2905–2913. DOI: 10.1053/j.semnuclmed.2009.03.003

Zhang, Z., Yan, C., & Malin, B. A. (2022). Membership inference attacks against synthetic health data. *Journal of Biomedical Informatics*, *125*, 103977. Advance online publication. DOI: 10.1016/j.jbi.2021.103977 PMID: 34920126

Zhou, F., Ran, X., Song, F., Wu, Q., Jia, Y., Liang, Y., Chen, S., Zhang, G., Dong, J., & Wang, Y. (2024). A stepwise prediction and interpretation of gestational diabetes mellitus: Foster the practical application of machine learning in clinical decision-making. *Heliyon, 10*(12), e32709. Advance online publication. DOI: 10.1016/j.heliyon.2024.e32709 PMID: 38975148

Zumla, A., Abubakar, I., Raviglione, M., Hoelscher, M., Ditiu, L., Mchugh, T. D., Squire, S. B., Cox, H., Ford, N., McNerney, R., Marais, B., Grobusch, M., Lawn, S. D., Migliori, G., Mwaba, P., O'Grady, J., Pletschette, M., Ramsay, A., Chakaya, J., & Atun, R. (2012). Drug-resistant tuberculosis—Current dilemmas, unanswered questions, challenges, and priority needs. *The Journal of Infectious Diseases, 205*(suppl_2), S228–S240. DOI: 10.1093/infdis/jir858 PMID: 22476720

About the Contributors

Munir Ahmad is a dedicated expert in Spatial Data Infrastructure (SDI), Geo-Information Production, Information Systems, and Information Governance, with over 25 years of experience driving innovation across the geospatial domain. Holding a PhD in Computer Science, he specializes in the production, management, analysis, visualization, and quality control of spatial data, and has led major SDI development and deployment initiatives, particularly in Pakistan. His work spans spatial database design, Web/Mobile/Desktop GIS development, and Geo Web Services architecture, complemented by significant contributions to Volunteered Geographic Information (VGI), Open Source Geoportals, and Metadata Portals. He is also at the forefront of integrating emerging technologies such as blockchain for trusted geospatial data exchange, artificial intelligence and machine learning for automated analytics, prediction, and quality assurance, and metaverse environments for immersive geospatial visualization and planning into next-generation SDI ecosystems. Beyond geospatial applications, he advances the use of AI, ML, blockchain, and metaverse technologies across sectors, including education, health, business, tourism, disaster management, environment, governance, and marketing, enabling data-driven decision-making and digital transformation. As a researcher, trainer, and mentor with more than 100 publications, he also serves as a reviewer for several reputed international journals published by Frontiers, IGI Global, Wiley, Springer, and others. He continues to expand knowledge in geo-technology, data governance, and information infrastructure while supporting R&D and guiding the next generation of geo-information professionals.

***

Vijay Anant Athavale has a rich teaching, research and administrative experience of more than 34 years of serving in Government and Private Universities and Colleges in India and abroad. He has served academic assignments in Canada, the Republic of Yemen and the Republic of Sudan. He also served as an expatriate expert for the United Nations Development Programme to Ethiopia. He has been instrumental in shaping of several Institutes of repute offering Technical and Management Education in India. He has successfully led the transformation journey of some of the institutes, which has resulted in national and international accreditations. As a thought leader and a subject-matter expert, he has presented numerous sessions at Conferences, FDPs, and Workshops as Keynote speaker, Session Chair, Organizing Committee member, TPC etc. He is a reviewer for several SCIE, Scopus, WoS indexed journals. He is also an associate editor of International Journal of Electrical and Electronic Research (IJEER) (ISSN 2347-470X) which is indexed by SCOPUS. He has contributed several chapters in books & handbooks published by IGI Global USA, Taylor and Francis Group, UK, Springer etc.

Rubidha Devi D works as an Assistant Professor in the Computer Science and Engineering Department at SASTRA Deemed University, Kumbakonam, India. She has published several research works in peer-reviewed journals. Her research area includes Deep Learning, Machine learning, and Temporal and Spatial Time-series Analysis.

Noboranjan Dey is currently serving as a Lecturer in the Computer Science department under the faculty of science and technology at American International University Bangladesh. He was granted an ICCR scholarship for his Master's degree. He pursued M.Tech in Computer Science and Engineering from National Institute of Technology Warangal, India, and a Bachelor's degree from AIUB. His current research interests include Deep Learning, Neural Networks, Computer Vision, Image Processing, Medical Imaging, and Biometrics.

Rashmi K. Dixit is an Assistant Professor in the Department of Computer Science and Engineering at Walchand Institute of Technology (WIT), Solapur. With over 22 years of teaching experience, she has made significant contributions in both academic instruction and research guidance. Dr. Dixit is a recognized Ph.D. supervisor for PAl Solapur University, Solapur and is actively involved in mentoring doctoral research in the fields of Blockchain Technology, Cloud Computing, and Data Security. Her research interests are aligned with emerging technologies and their secure implementation in distributed systems. She plays a key role in the Training and Placement (T&P) Cell of the department, contributing to student employability and industry interactions. Dr. Dixit has diligently guided students during curriculum and career planning while bridging the gap between academic learning and industry needs. Throughout her career, Dr. Dixit has taught a diverse range of core Computer Science subjects, including: Database Engineering (DBE),

Computer Organization and Architecture (COA),Distributed Systems (DMS),Design and Analysis of Algorithms (DAA),Artificial Intelligence (AI),Data Structures (DS) She remains committed to academic excellence, fostering a strong research culture among her students while providing them with the technical knowledge and practical exposure required to excel in her field.

Subha Durai is a research enthusiast, and she serves LEAD College of Management, Kerala.

Reazul Islam is a Ph.D. student in the Department of Computer Science at the University at Albany, State University of New York, where his research focuses on Internet of Things (IoT), Artificial Intelligence (AI), and Machine Learning (ML). His work explores the intersection of intelligent systems and real-world applications, aiming to design sustainable and efficient solutions for societal challenges. Before pursuing his doctoral studies, Mr. Islam served as an Assistant Professor in the Department of Computer Science at the American International University–Bangladesh (AIUB) and as a Lead Researcher at the Advanced Machine Intelligence Research Lab, specializing in AI-driven IoT systems.

Raja J serves as the Principal at Adhiparasakthi Engineering College. With a distinguished portfolio, he has authored 50+ papers in reputable journals, showcasing expertise in VLSI, Wireless Communication, and Signal Processing. His leadership role reflects his commitment to academic excellence, while his extensive publications underscore his dedication to advancing knowledge in these fields

Janhavi Rajendra Kale has completed her B.E in Computer Engineering from Pune University, India and has completed her MTech in Computer Engineering from VIT Pune, India. Her area of interest includes Artificial intelligence, Machine Learning and Theory of Computation. She is presently working as an Assistant Professor Department of Information Technology at Walchand Institute of Technology, Solapur, India. She has published her research in reputed Journals and conferences.

Babaqul Khudayqulov is a distinguished academic affiliated with the Department of Basic Medical Sciences at Termez University of Economics and Service, Termez, Uzbekistan. His educational and research pursuits focus on foundational and applied aspects of medical sciences, contributing to the advancement of healthcare education and biomedical understanding in Uzbekistan. Dr. Khudayqulov has been actively involved in teaching and mentoring students, fostering interdisciplinary learning that bridges medical theory with practical healthcare applications. His scholarly interests encompass human physiology, public health, and the integration of clinical science, reflecting a commitment to improving educational standards and community well-being through evidence-based medical education and research.

L.M.R.J. Lobo is a B.Sc in statistics and a BE in Computer Engineering from Shivaji University, Kolhapur. He has also completed his MTech in Computer and Information Technology from IIT Kharagpur, India. His area of interest include Artificial intelligence, Machine Learning, Genetic Algorithms and System software. He is presently working as a Professor and Head, Department of Information Technology at Walchand Institute of Technology, Solapur, India. He has published more than 80 Papers in reputed Journals and conferences. He also received International Luminary Award in Teaching.

Kamaladevi M received a MCA. from Government College(Autonomous) Kumbakonam in 2002 and an M.Phil. from Bharthidasan University, Trichy, Tamil Nadu, India, in the year 2007. She completed her M.Tech in Computer Science from SASTRA Deemed University, Thanjavur, Tamil Nadu, in 2010. She is currently pursuing a doctoral degree in Computer Science and Engineering from SASTRA Deemed University. With 20 years of teaching experience for UG and PG courses in Computer Science, she is presently working as an Assistant Professor in the Department of Computer Science and Engineering at SASTRA University, SRC Campus, Kumbakonam. Her research interests lie in Data Mining, Machine Learning, and Deep Learning. She has published research papers in book chapters, international conferences, Scopus, and Science Citation Indexed Journals.

Varsha Vyankatesh Manglaram is a Master of Technology graduate in Computer Science and Engineering from Walchand Institute of Technology, Solapur, Maharashtra, India. Her research interests include machine learning, big data analytics, natural language processing, cloud computing, artificial intelligence, deep learning, medical image processing, and health informatics. She has actively participated in research projects focused on deep learning and medical image analysis, particularly in healthcare applications. Her current research involves developing an AI-based system for lung cancer diagnosis and treatment recommendation using convolutional neural networks and generative AI techniques. She is proficient in Python, TensorFlow, and various image processing tools. Her primary research interests lie in AI-driven healthcare solutions and health informatics. She is based in Solapur, India.

Chiranjeevi Manike is a distinguished academician, researcher, and mentor with over 20 years of professional experience in the field of Computer Science and Engineering. He holds a Ph.D. from the prestigious Indian Institute of Technology

(IIT) Dhanbad. His academic background also includes a Master of Technology (M.Tech) in Computer Science and Engineering, as well as a Bachelor of Technology (B.Tech) in Computer Science and Engineering. Throughout his career, Dr. Manike has demonstrated a deep commitment to quality education and innovation. Over the past five years, he has focused extensively on teaching and mentoring in the areas of Data Science and Big Data Analytics. His contributions include the design of modern, industry-relevant curricula and the establishment of a state-of-the-art Big Data Lab, helping students gain hands-on experience in data-driven technologies. Dr. Manike has served in key academic leadership positions, including Head of the Department for Computer Science and Engineering (CSE), and Data Science & Computer Science (DS & CS). His expertise spans curriculum development, research supervision, and academic policy design. In addition to his academic pursuits, Dr. Manike is a passionate lifelong learner who recently completed a Master's Program in Data Science from Simplilearn, further strengthening his practical knowledge in this evolving domain. Beyond the classroom, Dr. Manike is also involved in social service. He actively contributes to a registered non-profit organization that organizes cultural and community events, reflecting his dedication to holistic societal development. He is currently engaged in research, writing, and the creation of educational content aimed at empowering individuals in the areas of health, money, and education — with the larger vision of contributing to a stronger, self-reliant India. His ambition is to become financially independent and help his family and community do the same, ultimately aspiring to become a billionaire with a purpose.

Geetha Manoharan is currently working in Telangana as an assistant professor at SR University. She is the university-level PhD program coordinator and has also been given the additional responsibility of In Charge Director of Publications and Patents under the Research Division at SR University.

S.Meganathan completed his Ph.D. in 2013 at SASTRA Deemed University. He works as an Associate Professor in the Department of Computer Science & Engineering at Srinivasa Ramanujan Centre, SASTRA Deemed University, Kumbakonam. Four research scholars are pursuing Ph.D. programme under his guidance in data mining and its applications. Their research focuses on tropical cyclone prediction, electrical consumption prediction based on climate data, patient diagnosis systems on medical data, and improved D.S.S. systems on medical database systems. There are 32 research articles published in SCOPUS-indexed journals and 8 in SCI/SCIE indexed journals. He has experience in consultancy projects in the area of Video and Image Analytics for the Mahamaham Festival 2016, held at Kumbakonam, Tamil Nadu. This project extended to various festivals conducted by the HR&CE departments and the Revenue Departments of the government of

Tamil Nadu. The student projects for B. Tech, M.Sc., and M.C.A., programmes in meteorological data have been guided for the past 20 years.

Ramya N received her B.E degree in computer science and engineering from Karpaga Vinayaga College of Engineering & Technology, Anna University, Chennai, India in 2006 and her M.E degree in computer science and engineering from Satyabhama University, Chennai, India in 2012. She is currently pursuing PhD at the department of Computer Science and Engineering, SRM University, Chennai, India and also working as an Assistant Professor in the department of Computer Science and Engineering at Sri Sai Ram Engineering College, Chennai, India. Her industry experience is about 1.5 years in Patni Computers as a software engineer. Her areas of interest are Wireless Ad-Hoc Networks, Artificial Intelligence, Security, Machine Learning and Deep Learning

Umamaheswari Purushothaman holds a B.E. in Information Technology from Periyar Maniammai College of Engineering and Technology (2003), an M.B.A. from Alagappa University, Karaikudi, Tamil Nadu (2006), and an M.Tech in Computer Science from SASTRA Deemed University, Thanjavur, Tamil Nadu (2011). She earned her Ph.D. in Computer Science and Engineering from SASTRA Deemed University. With two decades of experience, she has taught both undergraduate and postgraduate courses in Computer Science. She is currently an Assistant Professor in the Department of Computer Science and Engineering at SRC Campus, SASTRA University, Kumbakonam. Her research interests focus on Data Mining, Machine Learning, and Deep Learning. She has published numerous research papers in international conferences, SCI-indexed journals, Scopus, and book chapters.

Muzaffar Shojonov is a researcher and faculty member in the Department of Information Technology at Urgench State University, Urgench, Uzbekistan. His professional interests include information systems, software engineering, and applied IT for education and public services. He participates in collaborative projects and conferences and contributes to publications addressing practical and theoretical aspects of computing.

A. Sumathi is working as an Assistant Professor in the Department of Computer Science and Engineering, SRC, SASTRA Deemed to be University, Kumbakonam, TN, India. Received the M.Tech and Ph.D. degree in Computer Science and Engineering from SASTRA Deemed to be University, Thanjavur. Research areas include Data Mining, Machine Learning, Data Science, and Healthcare applications.

VenkataramanV. is a seasoned academician and researcher at SASTRA UNIVERSITY with over 25 years of experience in teach8ng and research. He has made significant contributions to his field, publishing 39 papers indexed in Scopus and 12 papers in prestigious SCI - indexed Journals.

M Vanitha is currently working as an Assistant Professor in the Department of Computer Science and Engineering, Srinivasa Ramanujan Centre, SASTRA Deemed University, Kumbakonam, Tamil Nadu, India. She has teaching experience for more than fifteen years. She has published several research works in peer-reviewed journals. Her research area includes Deep Learning, Machine learning and Time-series Analysis.

Srinivasan Vasan is an Assistant Professor in the Department of Humanities and Social Sciences at Graphic Era (Deemed to be University), with 14 years of teaching and field expertise. He has served in the Ministry of Health and Family Welfare, as a Guest Faculty, and as a Mobilization Training Specialist with the State Government. Recently, he contributed to a tuberculosis project funded by GFATM and USAID. He has published 60 papers, with 20 more under peer review in UGC-CARE and SCOPUS journals.

Shubham Suresh Vyavahare has completed his BCA from PAH Solapur University, India, and holds certifications in Power BI, Cloud Computing, DevOps Engineering, Automation Testing using Java & Selenium, and Generative AI Tools. His areas of interest include Artificial Intelligence, Machine Learning, and Generative AI. He is currently working as a Technical Assistant in the Department of Information Technology at Walchand Institute of Technology, Solapur, India. He has published his research in reputed journals and conferences.

Aparna Yemul holds a Master of Technology degree in Computer Science and Engineering from Walchand Institute of Technology, Solapur, Maharashtra, India. Her academic and research pursuits span across multiple domains including artificial intelligence, machine learning, blockchain technology, deep learning, natural language processing, cloud computing, medical image processing, and health informatics. She has been actively engaged in research projects focusing on the integration of deep learning methods in medical image analysis to improve healthcare outcomes. Currently, her work is centered on designing a system based on Deep Learning and Generative AI Techniques for Enhanced Diagnosis and Treatment Suggestion of Kidney Diseases. Skilled in Python, TensorFlow, and advanced image processing frameworks, she is committed to leveraging AI innovations to develop intelligent healthcare solutions that can enhance diagnostic accuracy and patient care. Aparna is based in Solapur, India.

Rajani Mahesh Yemul has completed her B.E in Computer Science & Engineering from Solapur University, India and has completed her MTech in Computer Science & Engineering from PAH Solapur University, India. Her area of interest includes Artificial intelligence, Machine Learning, Computer Networks and System Software. She is presently working as an Assistant Professor Department of Information Technology at Walchand Institute of Technology, Solapur, India. She has published her research in reputed Journals and conferences.

Index

A

B

C

H

I

K

L

M

N

O

P

R

S

T

V

X

www.ingramcontent.com/pod-product-compliance
Lightning Source LLC
LaVergne TN
LVHW081330021026
849161LV00008BA/1825
* 9 7 9 8 3 3 7 3 5 6 4 1 9 *